FROM THE EXPERTS IN ENDOCRINOLOGY

ENDO 2023
MEET THE PROFESSOR

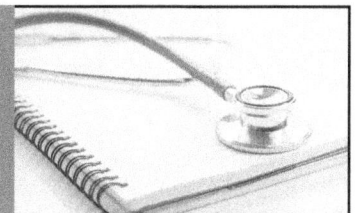

REFERENCE EDITION

ENDOCRINE
CASE MANAGEMENT

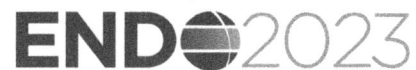

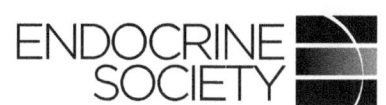

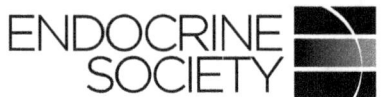

2055 L Street, NW, Suite 600
Washington, DC 20036
www.endocrine.org

Other Publications:
endocrine.org/publications

The Endocrine Society is the world's largest, oldest, and most active organization working to advance the clinical practice of endocrinology and hormone research. Founded in 1916, the Society now has more than 18,000 global members across a range of disciplines.

The Society has earned an international reputation for excellence in the quality of its peer-reviewed journals, educational resources, meetings, and programs that improve public health through the practice and science of endocrinology.

Clinical Practice Chair, ENDO 2023
Stephen M. Rosenthal, MD

ISBN: 978-1-936704-23-1
Library of Congress Control Number: 2022951736

On the Cover: © Shutterstock. Close up stethoscope on blank notepad as medical concept. (By Singha Songsak P).

ENDO 2023
CONTENTS

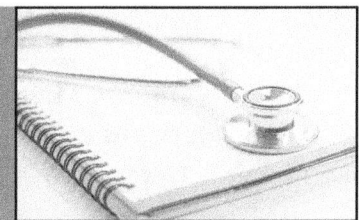

ADIPOSE TISSUE, APPETITE, OBESITY, AND LIPIDS

ADRENAL

BONE AND MINERAL METABOLISM

CARDIOVASCULAR ENDOCRINOLOGY

DIABETES MELLITUS AND GLUCOSE METABOLISM

NEUROENDOCRINOLOGY AND PITUITARY

PEDIATRIC ENDOCRINOLOGY

REPRODUCTIVE ENDOCRINOLOGY

THYROID

TUMOR BIOLOGY

MISCELLANEOUS

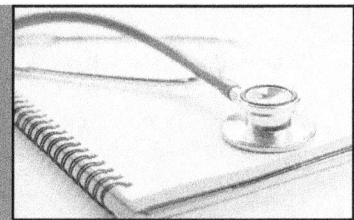
2023 Endocrine Case Management: Meet the Professor Faculty

Jaime Almandoz, MD, MBA
University of Texas Southwestern Medical Center

Bradley D. Anawalt, MD
University of Washington School of Medicine

Howard B. A. Baum, MD
Vanderbilt University Medical Center

Margaret Cristina da Silva Boguszewski, MD, PhD
Federal University of Parana

Mariëtte R. Boon, MD, PhD
Erasmus University Medical Center

Michael Buchfelder, MD, PhD
University Hospital Erlangen

Yee-Ming Chan, MD, PhD
Boston Children's Hospital and Harvard Medical School

Stephanie Crossen, MD, MPH
University of California Davis Children's Hospital

Caroline J. Davidge-Pitts, MB, BCh
Mayo Clinic Rochester

Wouter W. de Herder, MD, PhD
Erasmus MC and Erasmus MC Cancer Institute

Linda A. DiMeglio, MD, MPH
Indiana University School of Medical

Gerard M. Doherty, MD
Brigham & Women's Hospital and Harvard Medical School

Andrea Dunaif, MD
Icahn School of Medicine and Mount Sinai Health System

Richard A. Feelders, MD, PhD
Erasmus Medical Center

Gary D. Hammer, MD, PhD
University of Michigan

David J. Handelsman, AO, MBBS, PhD
University of Sydney

Alan G. Harris, MD, PhD
NYU Langone Grossman School of Medicine

Frances J. Hayes, MB BCh BAO
Massachusetts General Hospital

Megan R. Haymart, MD
University of Michigan

Ana Oliveira Hoff, MD
Faculdade de Medicina da Universidade de São Paulo (FMUSP)

Michael S. Irwig, MD
Beth Israel Deaconess Medical Center and Harvard Medical School

Niki Karavitaki, MSc, PhD
University of Birmingham

Karine Khatchadourian, MD, MSc
University of Ottawa

Michael Mannstadt, MD
Massachusetts General Hospital and Harvard Medical School

Daniel L. Metzger, MD
University of British Columbia

Susanne U. Miedlich, MD
University of Rochester Medical Center

Christiaan F. Mooij, MD, PhD
Emma Children's Hospital, Amsterdam University Medical Centers

Carla Moran, MB PhD
Beacon Hospital Dublin and St. Vincent's University Hospital

Leena Nahata, MD
The Ohio State University College of Medicine, The Abigail Wexner Research Institute, and Nationwide Children's Hospital

Matthew A. Nehs, MD
Brigham & Women's Hospital and Harvard Medical School

Connie B. Newman, MD
New York University School of Medicine

Karel Pacak, MD, PhD, DSc
Eunice Kennedy Shriver National Institute of Child Health and Human Development, National Institutes of Health

Mary Elizabeth Patti, MD
Joslin Diabetes Center

Avin Pothuloori, MD
Nebraska Methodist Physicians Clinic

Douglas S. Ross, MD
Massachusetts General Hospital and Harvard Medical School

Joshua D. Safer, MD
Mount Sinai Center for Transgender Medicine and Surgery and Icahn School of Medicine at Mount Sinai

Loren S. Schechter, MD
Rush University Medical Center

Rebecca B. Schechter, MD
Highland Park, IL

Dolores Shoback, MD
University of California, San
Francisco, and San Francisco
Veterans Affairs Medical Center

Lisa R. Tannock, MD
University of Kentucky

Stylianos Tsagarakis, MD, PhD
Evangelismos Hospital

Adina F. Turcu, MD, MS
University of Michigan

Elisabeth F. C. van
Rossum, MD, PhD
Erasmus University Medical Center

A. S. Paul van Trotsenburg,
MD, PhD
Emma Children's Hospital,
Amsterdam University
Medical Centers

Varsha Vimalananda, MD, MPH
Bedford VA Medical Center and
Boston University Chobanian and
Avedisian School of Medicine

Brielle Weinstein, MD
Rush University Medical Center

Corrine Welt, MD
University of Utah

Joy Y. Wu, MD, PhD
Stanford University
School of Medicine

Carol H. Wysham, MD
University of Washington and
MultiCare Rockwood Clinic

Jun Yang, MBBS, PhD
Hudson Institute of Medical Research

William F. Young, Jr., MD, MSc
Mayo Clinic Rochester

Kevin C. J. Yuen, MD
University of Arizona College
of Medicine and Creighton
School of Medicine

David Zangen, MD
Hadassah Medical Center

Annual Meeting Steering Committee (AMSC)

Jenny A. Visser, PhD – AMSC Chair
Erasmus MC

Stephen Rosenthal, MD –
Clinical Practice Chair
University of California,
San Francisco

Christopher McCartney, MD
– Clinical Science Chair
University of Virginia
School of Medicine

Carolyn L. Cummins, PhD
– Basic Science Chair
University of Toronto

Annual Meeting Steering Committee Clinical Peer Reviewers

Ana Paula Abreu, MD, PhD

Kimia Saleh Anaraki, MD

Irina Bancos, MD

Andrew Bauer, MD

Ernesto Bernal-Mizrachi, MD

Kristien Boelaert, MD, PhD

Massimiliano Caprio, MD, PhD

Barbara Gisella Carranza Leon, MD

Carolyn L. Cummins, PhD

Jaydira Del Rivero, MD

Adda Grimberg, MD

Ole-Petter Hamnvik,
MBBChBAO, MMSc, MRCPI

Marta Korbonits, MD, PhD

Christopher McCartney, MD

Raghavendra Mirmira, PhD, MD

Gabrielle Page-Wilson, MD

Yumie Rhee, MD, PhD

Stephen Rosenthal, MD

W. Edward Visser, MD, PhD

Bu Beng Yeap, MBBS, FRACP, PhD

Elaine Wei-Yin Yu, MD

Maria-Christina Zennaro, MD, PhD

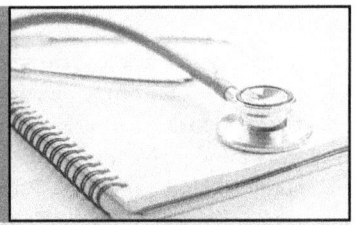

OVERVIEW

The *Endocrine Case Management: Meet the Professor* reference book is intended primarily for consultation relating to endocrinology. As a reference book, educational credits are not available. For information on educational products that include educational credit, please visit endocrine.org/store.

LEARNING OBJECTIVES

Endocrine Case Management: Meet the Professor will allow learners to assess their knowledge of all aspects of endocrinology, diabetes, and metabolism.

Completion of this educational activity enables learners to accomplish key objectives:

- Recognize clinical manifestations of endocrine and metabolic disorders and select among current options for diagnosis, management, and therapy.

- Identify risk factors for endocrine and metabolic disorders and develop strategies for prevention.

- Evaluate endocrine and metabolic manifestations of systemic disorders.

- Use existing resources pertaining to clinical guidelines and treatment recommendations for endocrine and related metabolic disorders to guide diagnosis and treatment.

TARGET AUDIENCE

Endocrine Case Management: Meet the Professor provides case-based education to clinicians interested in improving patient care.

STATEMENT OF INDEPENDENCE

The Endocrine Society has a policy of ensuring that the content and quality of this educational activity are balanced, independent, objective, and scientifically rigorous. The scientific content of this activity was developed under the supervision of the Endocrine Society's Annual Meeting Steering Committee.

DISCLOSURE POLICY

The faculty, committee members, and staff who are in position to control the content of this activity are required to disclose to the Endocrine Society and to learners any relevant financial relationship(s) of the individual or spouse/partner that have occurred within the last 12 months with any commercial interest(s) whose products or services are related to the content. Financial relationships are defined by remuneration in any amount from the commercial interest(s) in the form of grants; research support; consulting fees; salary; ownership interest (e.g., stocks, stock options, or ownership interest excluding diversified mutual funds); honoraria or other payments for participation in speakers' bureaus, advisory boards, or boards of directors; or other financial benefits. The intent of this disclosure is not to prevent planners with relevant financial relationships from planning or delivery of content, but rather to provide learners with information that allows them to make their own judgments of whether these financial relationships may have influenced the educational activity with regard to exposition or conclusion. The Endocrine Society has reviewed all disclosures and resolved or managed all identified conflicts of interest, as applicable.

The Endocrine Society has reviewed these relationships to determine which are relevant to the content of this activity and resolved any identified conflicts of interest for these individuals.

The faculty reported the following relevant financial relationship(s) during the content development process for this activity: **Jaime Almandoz, MD, MBA,** Advisory Board Member: Eli Lilly & Company, Novo Nordisk. **Margaret Cristina da Silva Boguszewski, MD, PhD,** Advisory Board Member: Novo Nordisk, Pfizer, Inc, Speaker: Novo Nordisk. **Wouter W. de Herder, MD, PhD,** Advisory Board Member: Novartis Pharmaceuticals, Ipsen, Speaker: Novartis Pharmaceuticals, Ipsen. **Linda A. DiMeglio, MD, MPH,** Advisory Board Member: Abata; Consulting Fee: Vertex, Abata; Research Investigator: Lilly USA, LLC, Mannkind Corporation, research support to my institution for a study; Medtronic Minimed, research support to my institution for a study; Dompe, Provention Bio, Zealand, research support to my institution for a study. **Andrea Dunaif, MD,** Consulting Fee: Quest Diagnostics, SLACK Incorporated, Neuocrine Biosciences, Inc, Novo Nordisk. **Gary D. Hammer, MD, PhD,** Advisory Board Member: Radionetics, Orphagen; Consulting Fee: Radionetic, Orphagen; Owner/Co-Owner: Sling therapeutics - Founder and Board member, Stock Owner: Orphagen, Sling Therapeutics. **Alan G. Harris, MD, PhD,** Royalties: Lutathera AAA/Novartis. **Ana Oliveira Hoff, MD,** Advisory Board Member: Eli Lilly & Company; Research Investigator: Eli Lilly & Company, Roche Pharmaceuticals. **Niki Karavitaki, MSc, PhD,** Grant Recipient: Pfizer, Inc; Speaker: Pfizer, Inc. **Michael Mannstadt, MD,** Advisory Board Member: Takeda, Amolyt, Calcilytix; Research Investigator: Takeda, Amolyt, Calcilytix; Other: UpToDate. **Mary Elizabeth Patti, MD,** Consulting Fee: MBX, Hanmi Pharmaceuticals, AstraZeneca; Other: Fractyl Laboratories. **Dolores Shoback, MD,** Consultant: Takeda, Ascendis, Bridge Bio. **Elisabeth F. C. van Rossum, MD, PhD,** Research Investigator: Rhythm (payment to the Erasmus MC university medical center to fund materials and human resources for a clinical trial for patients with rare genetic obesity, no commercial interest); Speaker: educational or scientific presentations (no commercial interest) for eg E-WISE (CME online), Dutch Obesity Academy, ELANN, Int Medical Press, NVE Academy, ASCEND, Public Eyes communication, SCEM; Other: Ambo Anthos (publisher). Royalties lay book "FAT, the secret organ" (minor part of the royalties are personal). **Carol H. Wysham, MD,** Investigator: Corcept, Eli Lilly, Novo Nordisk, Regeneron, Vanda.

The following faculty reported no relevant financial relationships: **Bradley D. Anawalt, MD; Howard B. A. Baum, MD; Mariëtte R. Boon, MD, PhD; Michael Buchfelder, MD, PhD; Yee-Ming Chan, MD, PhD; Stephanie Crossen, MD, MPH; Caroline J. Davidge-Pitts, MB, BCh; Gerard M. Doherty, MD; Richard Feelders, MD, PhD; David J. Handelsman, AO, MBBS, PhD; Frances J. Hayes, MB BCh BAO; Megan R. Haymart, MD; Michael S. Irwig, MD; Karine Khatchadourian, MD, MSc; Daniel L. Metzger, MD; Susanne U. Miedlich, MD; Christiaan F. Mooij, MD, PhD; Carla Moran, MB, PhD; Leena Nahata, MD; Matthew A. Nehs, MD; Connie B. Newman, MD; Karel Pacak, MD, PhD, DSc; Avin Pothuloori, MD; Douglas S. Ross, MD; Joshua Safer, MD; Loren S. Schechter, MD, FACS; Rebecca B. Schechter, MD; Lisa R. Tannock, MD; Stylianos Tsagarakis, MD, PhD; Adina F. Turcu, MD, MS; A. S. Paul van Trotsenburg, MD, PhD; Varsha Vimalananda, MD, MPH; Brielle Weinstein, MD; Corrine Welt, MD; Joy Y. Wu, MD, PhD; Jun Yang, MBBS, PhD; William F. Young, Jr., MD, MSc; Kevin C. J. Yuen, MD;** and **David Zangen, MD.**

The following AMSC peer reviewers reported relevant financial relationships: **Irina Bancos, MD,** Advisory Board: Adrenas, HRA Pharma, Corcept, Recordati; Consulting: HRA Pharma, Corcept, Sparrow Pharmaceutics, Recordati; Writer: Elsevier, Funding for Investigator Initiated Award: Recordati, NIH; Reviewer: Dynamed. **Andrew Bauer, MD,** Speaker: Hexal, AG. **Kristien Boelaert, MD, PhD,** Advisory Board: Pfizer, EISAI; Member and Awards Committee: American Thyroid Association; Member, Council Member, Clinical Committee Chair Elect: Society for Endocrinology; Member: British Thyroid Association, European Thyroid Association, European Endocrine Society, British Thyroid Association. **Massimiliano Caprio, MD, PhD,** Grant Recipient: Bayer AG; Associate Editor: Frontiers in Endocrinology. **Barbara Gisella Carranza Leon, MD,** Co-investigator: Novartis, IONIS Pharmaceutical Inc, NIH, FH Foundation, Regenxbio, Inc; Member of the Maintenance of Certification Committee: American Board of Obesity Medicine. **Carolyn L. Cummins, PhD,** Member: American Association of Pharmaceutical Scientists, Canadian Society of Pharmaceutical Sciences; Reviewer and Grantee: Canadian Institutes of Health Research. **Adda Grimberg, MD,** Advisory Board: Pfizer, Consultant: Pediatric Endocrine Society Growth Hormone Deficiency Knowledge Center, Sponsored by Sandoz; Grant Recipient: Eunice Kennedy Shriver National Institute of Child Health and Human Development; Advisory Board: Pediatric Endocrine Society, Growth Hormone Research Society; Editorial Board: Pediatric Endocrinology Reviews; Speaker: Midwest Pediatric Endocrine Society, Canadian Pediatric Endocrine Group. **Ole-Petter Hamnvik, MB BCh BAO, MMSc, MRCPI,** Education Editor: New England Journal of Medicine. **Marta Korbonits, MD, PhD,** Speaker: Pfizer, Ipsen; Associate Editor: Journal of the Endocrine Society; Scientific Advisor: ONO, NorvoNordisk, Corcept; Investigator: Crinetics. **Christopher McCartney, MD,** Grant Recipient: NIH; Reviewer: NIH. **Raghavendra Mirmira, PhD, MD,** Editor: Journal of Clinical Endocrinology and Metabolism, Advisory Board: Veralox Therapeutics; Investigator-Initiated Award: Veralox Therapeutics, HiberCell, Inc. **Gabrielle Page-Wilson, MD,** Advisory Board: Strongbridge Biopharma, Recordati Rare Diseases, Inc, Xeris BioPharma; Consultant: Xeris

BioPharma. **Yumie Rhee, MD, PhD,** Ambassador: American Society of Bone and Mineral Research; Committee: Korean Endocrine Society, Korean Society of Bone and Mineral Research. **Stephen Rosenthal, MD,** Board of Directors and Member: World Professional Association for Transgender Health. **W. Edward Visser, MD, PhD,** Royalties (Institution): Egetis Therapeutics. **Bu Beng Yeap, MBBS, FRACP, PhD,** Advisory Board: NovoNordisk, Bayer, Advisor: Lawley Pharmaceuticals; Speaker: AstraZeneca, Besins, Philippine Society for Endocrinology, Diabetes and Metabolism, View Street Medical, President: Endocrine Society of Australia; Associate Editor: Asian Journal of Andrology, Journal of Gerontology Medical Sciences; Editorial Board: Journal of Gerontology Medical Sciences, Journal of Clinical Endocrinology and Metabolism, Maturitas. **Elaine Wei-Yin Yu, MD,** Grant Recipient: Amgen; Stock Owner: Opko. **Maria-Christina Zennaro, MD, PhD,** Member: Societé Française d'Endocrinologie, Societé Française de Caridologie, European Network for the Study of Adrenal Tumors; Executive Committee: International Aldosterone Conference; President: European Section of Aldosterone Council (ESAC)-France; French network on adrenal tumors COMETE.

The following AMSC members reported no relevant financial relationships: **Ana Paula Abreu, MD, PhD; Ernesto Bernal-Mizrachi, MD; Jaydira Del Rivero, MD;** and **Kimia Saleh Anaraki, MD.**

The Endocrine Society staff associated with the development of content for this activity reported no relevant financial relationships.

DISCLAIMERS
The information presented in this activity represents the opinion of the faculty and is not necessarily the official position of the Endocrine Society.

USE OF PROFESSIONAL JUDGMENT:
The educational content in this enduring activity relates to basic principles of diagnosis and therapy and does not substitute for individual patient assessment based on the health care provider's examination of the patient and consideration of laboratory data and other factors unique to the patient. Standards in medicine change as new data become available.

DRUGS AND DOSAGES:
When prescribing medications, the physician is advised to check the product information sheet accompanying each drug to verify conditions of use and to identify any changes in drug dosage schedule or contraindications.

POLICY ON UNLABELED/OFF-LABEL USE
The Endocrine Society has determined that disclosure of unlabeled/off-label or investigational use of commercial product(s) is informative for audiences and therefore requires this information to be disclosed to the learners at the beginning of the presentation. Uses of specific therapeutic agents, devices, and other products discussed in this educational activity may not be the same as those indicated in product labeling approved by the Food and Drug Administration (FDA). The Endocrine Society requires that any discussions of such "off-label" use be based on scientific research that conforms to generally accepted standards of experimental design, data collection, and data analysis. Before recommending or prescribing any therapeutic agent or device, learners should review the complete prescribing information, including indications, contraindications, warnings, precautions, and adverse events.

ACKNOWLEDGMENT OF COMMERCIAL SUPPORT
This activity is not supported by educational grant(s) or other funds from any commercial supporter.

PUBLICATION DATE: June 2023

COMMON ABBREVIATIONS

ACTH = corticotropin

ACE inhibitor = angiotensin-converting enzyme inhibitor

ALT = alanine aminotransferase

AST = aspartate aminotransferase

BMI = body mass index

CNS = central nervous system

CT = computed tomography

DHEA = dehydroepiandrosterone

DHEA-S = dehydroepiandrosterone sulfate

DNA = deoxyribonucleic acid

DPP-4 inhibitor = dipeptidyl-peptidase 4 inhibitor

DXA = dual-energy x-ray absorptiometry

FDA = Food and Drug Administration

FGF-23 = fibroblast growth factor 23

FNA = fine-needle aspiration

FSH = follicle-stimulating hormone

GH = growth hormone

GHRH = growth hormone–releasing hormone

GLP-1 receptor agonist = glucagonlike peptide 1 receptor agonist

GnRH = gonadotropin-releasing hormone

hCG = human chorionic gonadotropin

HDL = high-density lipoprotein

HIV = human immunodeficiency virus

HMG-CoA reductase inhibitor = 3-hydroxy-3-methylglutaryl coenzyme A reductase inhibitor

IGF-1 = insulinlike growth factor 1

LDL = low-density lipoprotein

LH = luteinizing hormone

MCV = mean corpuscular volume

MIBG = *meta*-iodobenzylguanidine

MRI = magnetic resonance imaging

NPH insulin = neutral protamine Hagedorn insulin

PCSK9 inhibitor = proprotein convertase subtilisin/kexin 9 inhibitor

PET = positron emission tomography

PSA = prostate-specific antigen

PTH = parathyroid hormone

PTHrP = parathyroid hormone–related protein

SGLT-2 inhibitor = sodium-glucose cotransporter 2 inhibitor

SHBG = sex hormone–binding globulin

T_3 = triiodothyronine

T_4 = thyroxine

TPO antibodies = thyroperoxidase antibodies

TRH = thyrotropin-releasing hormone

TRAb = thyrotropin-receptor antibodies

TSH = thyrotropin

VLDL = very low-density lipoprotein

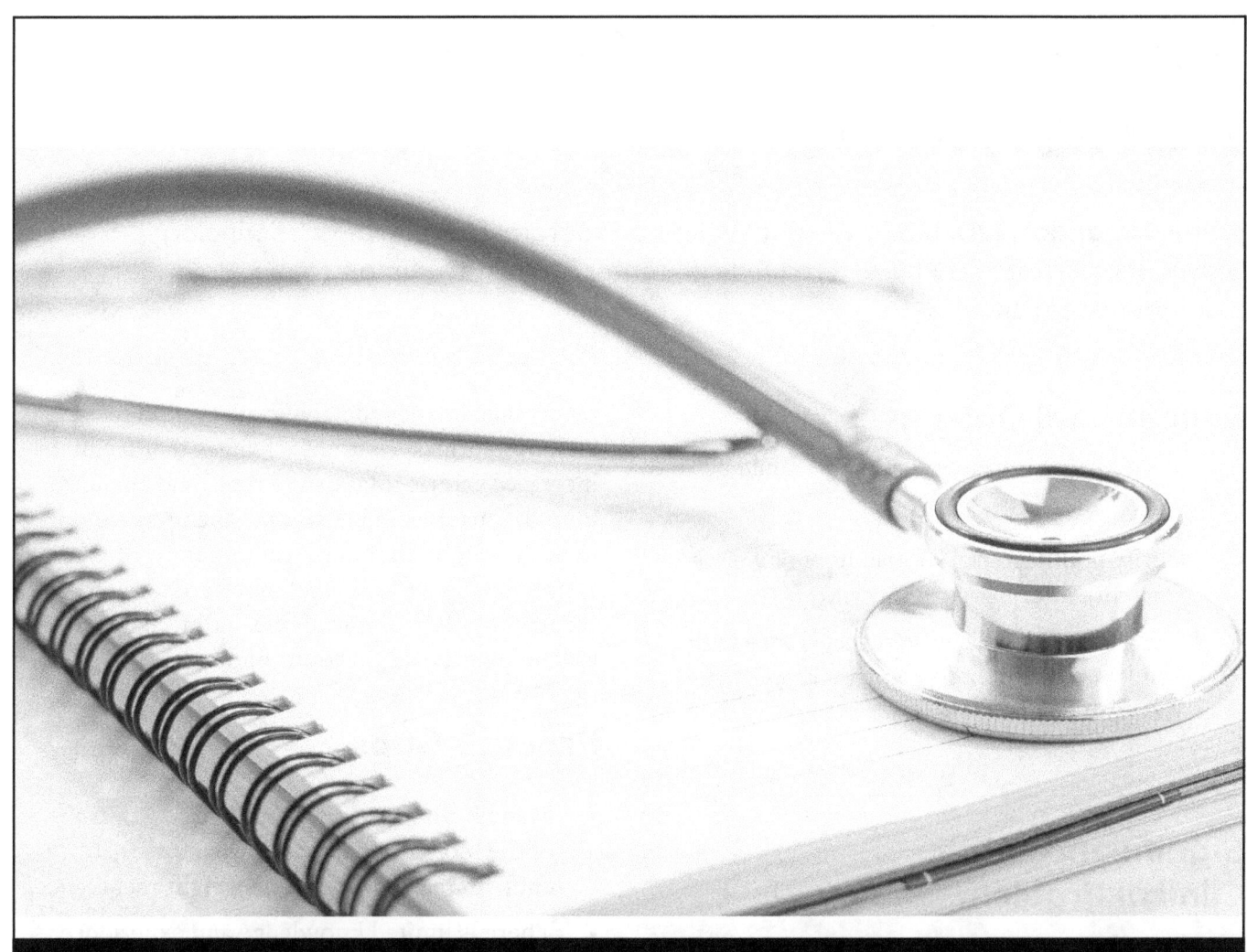

ADIPOSE TISSUE, APPETITE, OBESITY, AND LIPIDS

Weight Recurrence After Bariatric Surgery

Jaime Almandoz, MD, MBA. Weight Wellness Program; Division of Endocrinology, University of Texas Southwestern Medical Center, Dallas, TX; Email: Jaime.Almandoz@ utsouthwestern.edu

Educational Objectives

After reviewing this chapter, learners should be able to:

- Identify multifactorial contributors of weight recurrence after bariatric surgery.

- Manage postbariatric weight recurrence with considerations for endoscopic therapies and antiobesity medications.

Significance of the Clinical Problem

Obesity is the most common chronic disease in the United States, and it is a major contributor to health care expense, morbidity, and mortality. Bariatric surgery is one of the most effective tools for treating class 3 (severe) obesity and its complications, including type 2 diabetes mellitus and fatty liver disease.[1,2] Studies highlight the benefits of achieving and maintaining significant weight reduction after bariatric surgery, as disease remission frequently correlates with weight loss after bariatric surgery. Recent data suggest that those with severe obesity who undergo bariatric surgery have a lower risk of obesity-related cancers compared with the risk of those who do not undergo bariatric surgery. Greater weight loss confers greater risk reduction.[3]

Weight recurrence after bariatric surgery occurs because obesity is a chronic and multifactorial disease for which surgery is not curative. Factors associated with weight recurrence include metabolic adaptation to weight loss, postsurgical anatomic changes that facilitate increased calorie intake over time, and changes in individual health behaviors. The increase in body weight after bariatric surgery is often distressing for patients and may be associated with recurrence of cardiometabolic, biomechanical, and psychological complications of obesity.

Practice Gaps

- Many health care providers are not aware of the biologic and anatomic factors that contribute to postbariatric weight recurrence.

- There is limited knowledge and experience in using endoscopic therapies and antiobesity medications to treat weight recurrence after bariatric surgery.

Discussion

To effectively treat postbariatric weight recurrence, it is helpful to understand some of the changes in energy homeostasis and postbariatric gastrointestinal anatomy that can facilitate increases in body weight. Metabolic adaptation to weight loss is a shift in energy homeostatic systems that promotes weight recurrence by increasing energy intake and decreasing energy expenditure by 300 to 400 kcal/day less than predicted, which is due to a decrease in physical activity energy expenditure and an increase in skeletal muscle work efficiency (*figure 1*).[4] Metabolic adaptation to weight loss appears to be proportional to the

Figure 1. Changes from baseline in energy balance and homeostatic systems during maintenance of reduced body weight.

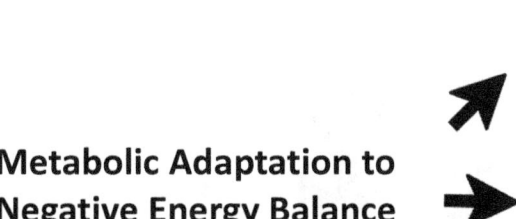

Neurohormonal Regulation
Decreased Leptin
Decreased TSH, T4, T3
Autonomic nervous system
- Decreased sympathetic tone
- Increased parasympathetic tone

Energy Intake
Decreased satiety
Greater responsiveness to food
Decreased perception of portions consumed
Decreased restraint in response to food

Energy Expenditure
Decreased EE at rest and activity
300-400 kcal/day less than predicted
Mainly due to:
- Lower physical activity EE
- Higher skeletal muscle work efficiency
    - Increased MHCI/II
    - Decreased SERCA

MCH, myosin heavy chain; PNS, parasympathetic nervous system; SERCA, sarcoplasmic endoplasmic reticulum Ca++-dependent ATPase; SNS, sympathetic nervous system. Adapted from Aronne LJ et al. Obesity, 2021; 29(S1): S9-S24. © The Obesity Society.

magnitude of reduction in circulating leptin levels, which correlates with the magnitude of adipose tissue loss.

Beyond metabolic adaptations that promote positive energy balance and weight recurrence, anatomic changes after surgery can also facilitate changes in energy intake, which include dilatations in gastric sleeves, gastric-bypass pouches, and gastrointestinal anastomoses. Over the last few decades, advances in endoscopic therapies have demonstrated effectiveness for treating weight recurrence in place of bariatric surgery revisions. These include revisional-endoscopic sleeve gastroplasty[5] and reductions in both gastric-bypass pouches and gastro-jejunal anastomoses, which are comparable to operative revisions for weight reduction.[6]

Although lifestyle modification is foundational for optimizing health and body weight, several antiobesity medications have been approved by the US FDA for treating obesity (*figure 2*). In addition, antiobesity medications have proven to be effective tools for treating weight recurrence and insufficient weight loss after bariatric surgery. Combinations of antiobesity medications may be necessary to treat weight recurrence effectively, and studies have shown that patients treated with antiobesity medication regimens containing GLP-1 receptor agonists achieve greater weight loss.[7,8] Unfortunately, less that 2% of people who are eligible for antiobesity medications in the United States receive treatment and most receive older, less effective antiobesity medications because of challenges with insurance coverage and affordability for more effective, newer medications.[9,10]

Many patients with postbariatric weight recurrence feel frustrated and embarrassed by their weight gain. They are often given the same generalized lifestyle recommendations that were ineffective prior to bariatric surgery. Insufficient understanding of the biological mechanisms that

Figure 2. Total body weight loss percentage with FDA-approved antiobesity medications.

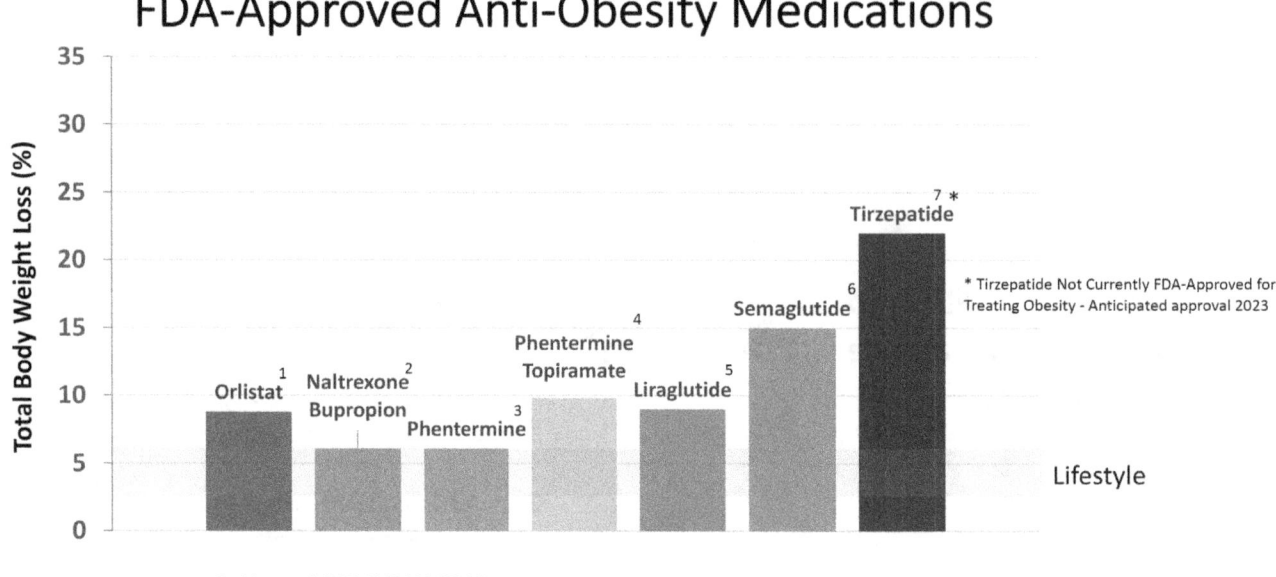

Davidson et al. JAMA 1999;281:235-242

1. Davidson et al. JAMA. 1999;281(3):235-242.

2. Greenway et al. Lancet. 2010;376(9741):595-605.

3. Yanovski et al. JAMA. 2014;311(1):74-86.

4. Gadde et al. Lancet. 2011;377(9774):1341-1352.

5. Pi-Sunyer et al. N Engl J Med. 2015;373(1):11-22.

6. Wilding et al. N Engl J Med. 2021;384:989-1002.

7. Jastreboff et al. N Engl J Med. 2022;387(3):205-216.
   (Color—web and EPUB only)

promote postbariatric weight recurrence and limited knowledge regarding advanced endoscopic therapies and antiobesity medications may limit clinicians and patients from pursuing treatment. More research is needed to determine the timing and sequence of therapies to treat postbariatric weight recurrence. Given that obesity is a chronic and complex disease that is often not addressed by lifestyle modification alone. People with severe obesity may require a combination of bariatric procedures and antiobesity medications to achieve and maintain clinically significant reductions in body weight, in addition to treating postbariatric weight recurrence.

Clinical Case Vignettes

Case 1

A 55-year-old man underwent Roux-en-Y gastric bypass 8 years ago at a weight of 331 lb (150 kg) (BMI = 44.8 kg/m²). He has a history of hypertension and type 2 diabetes that have been in remission since surgery. One year after surgery, his weight was 216 lb (98 kg) (BMI = 29.3 kg/m²), which increased gradually to 273 lb (124 kg) (BMI = 37 kg/m²) over the past 7 years.

The patient's primary care provider recommended an intermittent fasting dietary pattern and a walking program, which resulted in a transient weight reduction of 6.6 lb (3 kg). He is frustrated that his weight did not decrease more.

Which of the following neurohormonal change is associated with metabolic adaptation to weight loss and postbariatric weight recurrence?

A. Increased sympathetic nervous system tone

B. Increased free T_4 levels

C. Decreased leptin levels

D. Increased leptin levels

E. Increased TSH

Answer: C) Decreased leptin levels

Metabolic adaptation is the decrease in energy expenditure below predicted following weight loss. After bariatric surgery, metabolic adaptation has been found to be proportional to the degree of energy imbalance and the decrease in circulating leptin levels (Answer C).[11] Additional changes within the body's systems of energy homeostasis that promote weight recurrence after weight loss include decreased sympathetic nervous system tone, increased parasympathetic nervous system tone, decreased TSH, decreased T_4 levels, and decreased T_3 levels.[4]

Increases in body weight may be associated with recurrence in cardiometabolic, biomechanical, and psychological obesity-related complications. Beyond this, many patients who experience postbariatric weight regain are made to feel that it is their fault, which can lead to avoidance of health professionals who can help to address their weight and health concerns.

The incorporation of concepts such as metabolic adaptation can help determine more appropriate calorie intake goals for patients after bariatric surgery. Commonly used predictive equations for resting metabolic rate and calorie needs are derived from people who are not in a weight-reduced state and may overestimate calorie needs after bariatric surgery.

The understanding that obesity is a chronic and complex disease and that postbariatric weight recurrence is the result of factors that include metabolic adaptation and anatomic changes within the gastrointestinal tract can inform discussions between health care professionals and patients and help avoid blaming patients for weight regain.

Case 1 (continued)

The patient decides to follow-up with the bariatric surgeon who performed his surgery. He would like to avoid further operations, and a referral to consider advanced endoscopic therapies is placed.

Which of the following endoscopic therapies can be used to treat weight recurrence after gastric bypass?

A. Ethanol ablation of ghrelin-producing oxyntic glands
B. Revisional endoscopic sleeve gastroplasty
C. Duodenal mucosal resurfacing with hydrothermal ablation
D. Suturing of the gastro-jejunal anastomosis to decrease diameter
E. Magnetic enteral bypass with self-assembling magnets

Answer: D) Suturing of the gastro-jejunal anastomosis

Increased gastro-jejunal stoma diameter is a predictor of weight recurrence after Roux-en-Y gastric bypass.[12] Several endoscopic interventions have shown promise for treating postbariatric weight gain. For patients with a history of Roux-en-Y gastric bypass, endoscopic gastro-jejunal revision (Answer D) leads to comparable weight loss vs surgical revision at 1, 3, and 5 years.[6]

For patients with a history of sleeve gastrectomy, which is currently the most commonly performed bariatric surgery, revisional endoscopic sleeve gastroplasty (Answer B) results in 16% weight loss at 12 months.

Ethanol ablation of ghrelin-producing cells (Answer A) is not practical given the diffuse distribution of these cells throughout the gastric fundus and duodenum, which would also be difficult to access trans-orally after Roux-en-Y gastric bypass.

Similarly, hydrothermal duodenal mucosal resurfacing (Answer C) would be difficult to perform after Roux-en-Y gastric bypass and has not been evaluated for postbariatric weight management.

Magnetic enteral bypass (Answer E) has been evaluated as a primary metabolic procedure and as an adjunct to sleeve gastrectomy. Self-assembling magnets have not been evaluated in patients with a history of Roux-en-Y gastric bypass who already have a surgical intestinal bypass.

For patients with a history of bariatric surgery, beyond metabolic adaptation, anatomic factors such as dilatation of the gastric sleeve dilatation and gastro-jejunal anastomosis can be associated with weight recurrence. Recent advances in endoscopic therapies have provided effective treatment options for postbariatric weight recurrence without resorting to surgical revision. Endoscopic revisions can be considered in addition to lifestyle modification and pharmacotherapies for treating and stabilizing postbariatric weight gain.

Case 1 (continued)

The patient's annual postbariatric micronutrient screening and laboratory testing does not show any evidence of nutritional deficiencies. However, his hemoglobin A_{1c} value is elevated at 6.2% (44 mmol/mol), and his blood pressure is 145/90 mm Hg. He had not seen his endocrinologist since the Roux-en-Y gastric bypass, and he is advised to go back to discuss treatments.

Based on his history, which of the following FDA-approved antiobesity medications would be the best treatment option for weight reduction?

A. Phentermine

B. Metformin

C. Naltrexone/bupropion

D. Liraglutide

E. Semaglutide

Answer: E) Semaglutide

Multiple medications are approved by the FDA for treating obesity (*figure 2*), but there is a lack of prospective, randomized data for patients with persistent obesity or weight recurrence after bariatric surgery. Studies suggest that combination antiobesity medications therapies and those containing GLP-1 receptor agonists result in greater weight reduction for patients with postbariatric weight recurrence.[7] Data

from the STEP-8 trial, comparing liraglutide, 3 mg daily, with semaglutide, 2.4 weekly, show that semaglutide (Answer E) leads to greater weight loss compared with liraglutide (Answer D) in a nonbariatric population.[13] Recent data from Murvelashvili et al suggest that antiobesity medication regimens with semaglutide, 1 mg weekly (lower than the 2.4-mg weekly dose approved for treating obesity), lead to greater weight reduction than those containing liraglutide, 3 mg daily, for treating postbariatric weight recurrence.[14] In addition to incretin-based therapies, older data suggest that combinations of medications used both on- and off-label for weight loss can be effective for postbariatric weight reduction (eg, topiramate, phentermine, and metformin).[8]

Beyond weight gain, this patient has experienced recurrence of both hypertension and hyperglycemia. GLP-1 receptor agonists are a logical choice because of their effectiveness for reducing both weight and blood glucose. The elevated blood pressure makes phentermine (Answer A) and naltrexone/bupropion (Answer C) less attractive as first-line therapies for weight management.

Although metformin (Answer B) can be used to treat hyperglycemia and may have a modest effect on lowering body weight, it is not FDA-approved for weight management.

The optimal time to start antiobesity medication in the context of bariatric surgery is unknown. For example, should antiobesity medication be started prior to surgery, empirically after surgery, when weight loss slows, when weight plateaus, or after weight recurrence occurs. Regardless, published data suggest that antiobesity medications are effective for treating postbariatric weight recurrence and insufficient weight reduction.

Obesity is a complex, chronic disease, and therapies, which include lifestyle modifications, antiobesity medications, and bariatric surgery, should be used in combination to help patients achieve and maintain a healthier body weight, cardiometabolic health outcomes, and quality of life. Bariatric care should be coordinated among the primary care provider, bariatric surgeon, and obesity medicine specialist to ensure that patients have the information and tools to be successful. In addition to lifestyle modification, providers should discuss a variety of treatment options for excess body weight after bariatric surgery that can include revisional procedures and antiobesity medications.

Key Learning Points

- Bariatric surgery is one of the most effective treatments for class 3 or severe obesity; but postbariatric weight recurrence is common because obesity is a chronic and complex disease. Weight reduction after bariatric surgery confers many improvements in health that are proportional to weight loss. Metabolic adaptation to weight loss is also proportional to weight reduction and is due to changes in energy homeostasis that promote weight recurrence. Lifestyle modification is foundational for optimizing health and body weight but is often insufficient in isolation to treat significant weight recurrence.

- Postbariatric anatomic dilatations in gastric sleeves, gastric-bypass pouches, and gastrointestinal anastomoses commonly occur over time and increase the capacity to ingest excess calories. Several endoscopic therapies have been developed to treat postbariatric weight regain, which lead to similar reductions in body weight when compared with surgical revision.

- Advances in antiobesity medications, especially incretin-based therapies, have demonstrated greater effectiveness for treating postbariatric weight recurrence than older classes of antiobesity medications. Further research is needed to determine the timing and sequence of obesity therapies with bariatric surgery to optimize postbariatric weight reduction, promote weight maintenance, and treat weight recurrence.

References

1. Barthold D, Brouwer E, Barton LJ, et al. Minimum threshold of bariatric surgical weight loss for initial diabetes remission. *Diabetes Care.* 2022;45(1):92-99. PMID: 34518376

2. Lassailly G, Caiazzo R, Ntandja-Wandji L-C, et al. Bariatric surgery provides long-term resolution of nonalcoholic steatohepatitis and regression of fibrosis. *Gastroenterology.* 2020;159(4):1290-1301.e5. PMID: 32553765

3. Aminian A, Wilson R, Al-Kurd A, et al. Association of bariatric surgery with cancer risk and mortality in adults with obesity. *JAMA.* 2022;327(24):2423-2433. PMID: 35657620

4. Aronne LJ, Hall KD, Jakicic JM, et al. Describing the weight-reduced state: physiology, behavior, and interventions. *Obesity (Silver Spring).* 2021;29(Suppl 1):S9-S24. PMID: 33759395

5. Maselli DB, Alqahtani AR, Abu Dayyeh BK, et al. Revisional endoscopic sleeve gastroplasty of laparoscopic sleeve gastrectomy: an international, multicenter study. *Gastrointest Endosc.* 2021;93(1):122-130. PMID: 32473252

6. Dolan RD, Jirapinyo P, Thompson CC. Endoscopic versus surgical gastrojejunal revision for weight regain in Roux-en-Y gastric bypass patients: 5-year safety and efficacy comparison. *Gastrointest Endosc.* 2021;94(5):945-950. PMID: 34126065

7. Gazda CL, Clark JD, Lingvay I, Almandoz JP. Pharmacotherapies for post-bariatric weight regain: real-world comparative outcomes. *Obesity (Silver Spring).* 2021;29(5):829-836. PMID: 33818009

8. Stanford FC, Alfaris N, Gomez G, et al. The utility of weight loss medications after bariatric surgery for weight regain or inadequate weight loss: a multi-center study. Surg Obes Relat Dis. 2017;13(3):491-500. PMID: 27986587

9. Xia Y, Kelton CM, Guo JJ, Bian B, Heaton PC. Treatment of obesity: pharmacotherapy trends in the United States from 1999 to 2010. *Obesity (Silver Spring).* 2015;23(8):1721-1728. PMID: 26193062

10. Saxon DR, Iwamoto SJ, Mettenbrink CJ, et al. Antiobesity medication use in 2.2 million adults across eight large health care organizations: 2009-2015. *Obesity (Silver Spring).* 2019;27(12):1975-1981. PMID: 31603630

11. Knuth ND, Johannsen DL, Tamboli RA, et al. Metabolic adaptation following massive weight loss is related to the degree of energy imbalance and changes in circulating leptin. *Obesity (Silver Spring).* 2014;22(12):2563-2569. PMID: 25236175

12. Dayyeh ABK, Lautz DB, Thompson CC. Gastrojejunal stoma diameter predicts weight regain after Roux-en-Y gastric bypass. *Clin Gastroenterol Hepatol.* 2011;9(3):228-233. PMID: 21092760

13. Rubino DM, Greenway FL, Khalid U, et al; STEP 8 Investigators. Effect of weekly subcutaneous semaglutide vs daily liraglutide on body weight in adults with overweight or obesity without diabetes: the STEP 8 Randomized Clinical Trial. *JAMA.* 2022;327(2):138-150. PMID: 35015037

14. Murvelashvili N, Xie L, Schellinger JN, et al. Effectiveness of semaglutide versus liraglutide for treating post-metabolic and bariatric surgery weight recurrence. *Obesity (Silver Spring).* 2023 [Online ahead of print]. PMID: 36998152

Evaluation and Management of Nonalcoholic Fatty Liver Disease in Adults

Avin Pothuloori, MD. Department of Endocrinology, Diabetes, and Metabolism, Creighton University School of Medicine, CHI Medical Center, Omaha, NE; Email: Apothuloorimd@gmail.com

Educational Objectives

After reviewing this chapter, learners should be able to:

- Identify the patient population that should be evaluated for nonalcoholic fatty liver disease (NAFLD).

- Explain the available screening tools and diagnostic tests for NAFLD apart from liver biopsy.

- Describe current evidence-based management options for patients with NAFLD.

Significance of the Clinical Problem

NAFLD is a global public health problem and the most common cause of chronic liver disease, affecting 25% of the global population. Nonalcoholic steatohepatitis (NASH) is a more aggressive form of NAFLD, which can progress to advanced liver fibrosis, cirrhosis, or liver cancer.[1] Type 2 diabetes mellitus is a significant driver of disease progression. Age older than 50 years, insulin resistance, and features of metabolic syndrome all increase the chances of developing NASH with a more severe fibrosis stage. Interventions that promote weight loss in obesity, type 2 diabetes, prediabetes, and insulin resistance are first-line treatments.

In this Meet the Professor chapter, we will focus on identifying patients who should be screened for NAFLD. We will also explain the recommended methods to risk stratify. We will review the methods for further evaluation and intervention based on risk of progression to advanced fibrosis or cirrhosis.

The prevalence of NAFLD is expected to increase. Without early detection and intervention, a disproportionate increase in advanced disease is expected. NASH is the second most common cause of hepatocellular carcinoma in those on the waiting list for liver transplant in the United States after hepatitis C.[2] The growth is increasing at alarming rates in Asia, the Middle East, and North African regions, the countries with the highest prevalence.[3]

Practice Gaps

- Plasma aminotransferase levels are normal in many individuals with NAFLD, resulting in lack of further risk stratification if monitoring of liver enzymes alone is used.

- Liver ultrasonography has an accuracy of greater than 80% in detecting moderate to severe steatosis.[4] Detection of mild steatosis is lower with a sensitivity of 60.9% to 65%.[4]

Discussion

Definitions

- **Hepatic Steatosis**—Defined as intrahepatic fat of at least 5% of liver weight[5]

- **Nonalcoholic Fatty Liver Disease**—The definition is based on the presence of hepatic steatosis >5% of hepatocytes in the absence of significant ongoing or recent alcohol consumption and other known causes of liver disease

- **Significant alcohol consumption**—More than 21 standard drinks per week for men and more than 14 standard drinks per week for women; 1 drink = 14 g of pure alcohol

- **NASH**—Diagnosed by liver biopsy; defined by the presence of greater than or equal to 5% hepatic steatosis and hepatocyte injury (also known as hepatocyte ballooning), with or without evidence of liver fibrosis

Pathophysiology of NAFLD

Hepatic steatosis occurs when fatty acids accumulate in liver cells due to increased intrahepatic deposition of triglycerides, which can be explained by 4 different mechanisms[6]:

1. Increased inflow of fatty acids from the peripheral circulation

2. Increased hepatic synthesis of fatty acids

3. Reduced intrahepatic and peripheral fatty acid oxidation

4. Reduced release of triglycerides in the circulation through VLDL

Insulin resistance is an important factor for the development of NASH. Insulin resistance facilitates lipolysis, increasing the flow of free fatty acids to the liver and hepatic lipogenesis. Hepatic adipose tissue releases adipokines and inflammatory cytokines, such as IL-6 and TNF-α1, with a decrease in the anti-inflammatory adiponectin. The down-regulation of adiponectin paired with up-regulation of inflammatory cytokines is a progressive process that can lead to hepatocyte damage, apoptosis, and fibrosis.[7]

Diagnosis

The optimal noninvasive strategy to diagnose NAFLD is not yet known. Few guidelines exist in the diagnosis and management of NAFLD internationally. Although the gold standard for diagnosis of NAFLD is liver biopsy, the procedure can be painful and is associated with bleeding and infection. Therefore, noninvasive modalities have increasingly been used to screen patients for NAFLD. The diagnosis section of this chapter will focus on some of the options available for screening patients for NAFLD.

The most important first step is to identify those who are at high risk of NAFLD.

High-risk groups are defined as those who have an increased prevalence of hepatic steatosis.

Who Is At High Risk for NAFLD?

- Patients with obesity (BMI >30 kg/m²). The prevalence of obesity among patients with NASH and NAFLD is 81% and 51%, respectively.[7]

- Patients with prediabetes or type 2 diabetes. According to recent studies, the prevalence of NAFLD in patients with type 2 diabetes is 60% to 70%.[8]

- Patients with features of metabolic syndrome and/or insulin resistance.

- Patients with imaging studies that show evidence of hepatic steatosis.

- Patients with persistently elevated plasma aminotransferase levels over 6 months (American Association of Clinical Endocrinology [AACE] guidelines).

Not all patients with NASH/NAFLD have elevated liver enzymes. In those with elevated liver enzymes, it is important to assess for secondary causes of liver disease. These conditions include—but are not limited to—hemochromatosis, hepatitis

C, lipodystrophy, or HELLP syndrome (hemolysis, elevated liver enzymes, and low platelets).

Imaging Modalities to Screen for NAFLD

- **Ultrasonography**—According to the European Association for the Study of the Liver (EASL), ultrasonography is the preferred first-line diagnostic procedure for imaging of NAFLD, as it is widely available and is low cost. The accuracy of liver ultrasonography for the detection of moderate and severe steatosis was greater than 80% in a meta-analysis when compared with detection by liver histology (AACE guidelines). However, ultrasonography has been shown to be less sensitive for mild to moderate steatosis.

- **Controlled Attenuation Parameter**—An imaging technique used to diagnose steatosis but has limited ability to discriminate histologic grades.

- **Elastography—Vibration-Controlled Transient Elastography**

  - Vibration-controlled transient elastography (VCTE) measures shear wave velocity at a depth of 25 to 65 mm and is converted to a liver stiffness measurement (LSM) by using Hook's Law.[9] A shear wave is expressed by Young's modulus in kilopascals (kPA). A limitation to VCTE use is decreased sensitivity in those with higher BMI.

  - LSM <8.0 kPA—considered low risk for clinically significant fibrosis. Recommended to repeat surveillance in 2 to 3 years.

  - LSM >12.0 kPA—risk of advanced fibrosis is high.

  - LSM = 8.0-12.0 kPA—indeterminate risk.

- Referral to hepatologist is recommended for indeterminate- and high-risk groups.

- **MRI**—92% to 100% sensitivity and 92% to 92% specificity for evaluation of hepatic steatosis

compared ultrasonography but is considerably more expensive (EASL guidelines). MRI with elastography is a better method for the identification of the degrees of fibrosis in patients with NAFLD.

Scoring Methods to Estimate Steatosis or Fibrosis

Fibrosis-4 Index

According to the AACE clinical practice guidelines, the fibrosis-4 index (FIB-4) is the preferred calculation to assess for clinically significant fibrosis.

The formula is as follows:

- FIB-4 = age (years) × AST (U/L) / [platelets (× 10^9/L) × ALT (U/L)]

- FIB-4 score <1.45—negative predictive value of 90% for advanced fibrosis

- FIB-4 score >3.25—97% specificity and positive predictive value of 65% for advanced fibrosis

- Indeterminate values warrant further diagnostic testing for LSM

An algorithm adopted from the AACE guidelines for NAFLD (*figure*), may be used to determine the next steps after calculation of the FIB-4 score.[10]

Application of FIB-4 Index According to the 2022 AACE Guidelines

- **Low-risk group**—According to the 2022 AACE guidelines, patients in the low-risk group may be managed in the primary care setting with a focus on obesity management and cardiovascular disease prevention.

- **Indeterminate-risk group**—Patients should undergo either LSM by transient elastography or an enhanced liver fibrosis (ELF) blood test, which is further explained below. If a patient is found to be at high risk or is at indeterminant risk after 2 noninvasive tests, referral should be placed to a hepatologist.

- **High-risk group**—Referral to a liver specialist with a multidisciplinary team is recommended

Figure. Cirrhosis prevention in NAFLD.

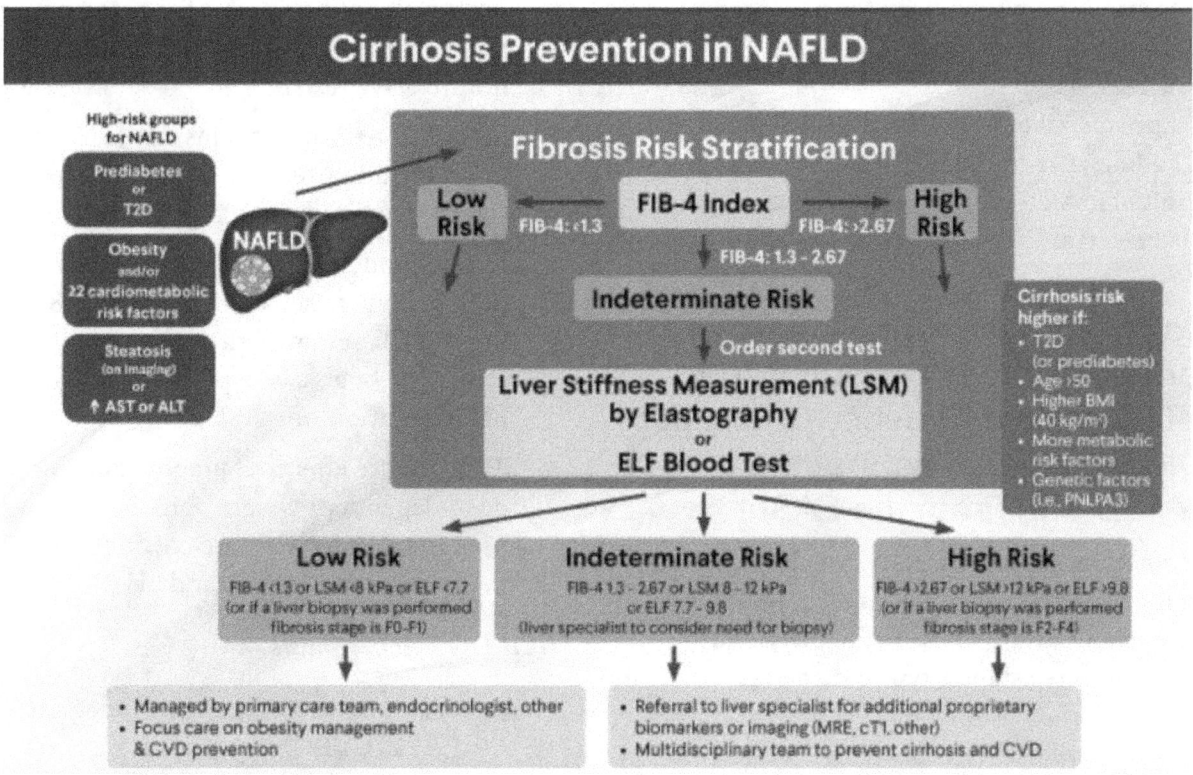

to mitigate the risk of cardiovascular disease and progression to cirrhosis.

According to the AACE clinical practice guidelines, persons with an indeterminate risk on FIB-4 calculation should undergo further evaluation with LSM or the ELF blood test.

- **ELF blood test**—Measures 3 direct markers of liver fibrosis:

  ○ **Hyaluronic acid**—a glycosaminoglycan that is produced by hepatic stellate cells

  ○ **Type III procollagen peptide (PIIINP)**—a marker of early fibrogenesis and inflammation

  ○ **Tissue inhibitor of matrix metalloproteinase 1 (TMP-1)**—circulating inhibitor of matrix metalloproteinase enzymes that can enhance fibrogenesis

Risk cutoffs are used with the ELF test to assess the likelihood of progression to cirrhosis within 3.9 years:

> **Lower risk:** <9.80
> **Medium risk:** 9.80-11.29
> **High risk:** >11.29

In a clinical setting, the use of ELF score and the FIB-4 index can be used to rule out advanced fibrosis[11] and may help providers identify patients with NAFLD who are not likely to develop adverse outcomes. Those in the lower risk group may be followed by their primary care providers to manage their cardiometabolic risks. Those in the medium- to high-risk group should be considered for additional evaluation by a hepatologist. However, guidelines on management based on the ELF score do not exist thus far.

In a study by Younossi et al, the utility of the ELF score was tested as a noninvasive approach in ruling in or ruling out advanced fibrosis in comparison to liver biopsy. The ELF score was associated with high specificity for advanced fibrosis, reaching close to 100% when an ELF cutoff of 11.3 was used.[11]

In a prospective longitudinal cohort study of 3012 adults, use of the FIB-4 index and ELF test resulted in 88% reduction in unnecessary specialist referrals.[12]

Therapy/Management Recommendations (Adopted from the 2022 Clinical Practice Guidelines for Diagnosis and Management of NAFLD and From the EASL)

Management of patients with NAFLD should focus on the treatment of associated cardiometabolic risks. These include visceral obesity, insulin resistance, type 2 diabetes, hypertension, and dyslipidemia.

In adults with NAFLD or NASH, weight loss of at least 5% is associated with greater liver histologic benefit. Clinicians should therefore recommend participation in a structured weight-loss program. Exercise 3 times a week for 12 weeks (30 to 60 minutes each session) showed decrease in hepatic steatosis.[13]

Dietary modifications recommended in persons with NAFLD/NASH include reduction in micronutrients, with emphasis placed on reduction of starches, sugars, saturated fat, and transfat.

Treatment/Interventions in Patients With Type 2 Diabetes and Biopsy-Proven NASH

Presently, there are no US FDA-approved drugs for the treatment of NASH. Some available treatment options are discussed here.

Pioglitazone

- According to the AACE guidelines and the EASL, pioglitazone is recommended for persons with type 2 diabetes and biopsy-proven NASH. Additionally, clinicians should consider treating type 2 diabetes with pioglitazone when there is an increased probability of having NASH based on elevated plasma aminotransferase levels and results of noninvasive tests.

- Pioglitazone improves insulin resistance by targeting adipose tissue and improves lipid storage/redistribution and glucose use.

- In one randomized controlled trial with pioglitazone dosed at 45 mg daily, 58% of individuals achieved the primary outcome of reduction of at least 2 points in NASH and 51% had resolution of NASH.[14]

- The adverse effects of pioglitazone include dose-dependent weight gain, heart failure if used in persons with preexisting heart disease, increased fracture risk, and bladder cancer.

GLP-1 Receptor Agonists

- According to the AACE guidelines and the EASL, GLP-1 receptor agonists are recommended for persons with type 2 diabetes and biopsy-proven NASH. Additionally, clinicians must consider GLP-1 receptor agonists in the treatment of type 2 diabetes and in those with increased risk of NASH based on elevated aminotransferase levels and results of noninvasive tests.

- Multiples studies suggest that GLP-1 receptor agonists reduce plasma aminotransferase levels and reduce liver fat content on imaging in individuals with type 2 diabetes and NAFLD.[15-17]

- According to the 2022 AACE guidelines, when used for weight management in patients with type 2 diabetes and BMI greater than or equal to 27 kg/m^2, studies suggest greatest benefit for NAFLD/NASH with semaglutide, 2.4 mg weekly, or liraglutide, 3 mg daily.

SGLT-2 Inhibitors

- SGLT-2 inhibitors have been shown to decrease liver fat, but the effect on steatohepatitis is unknown.[10]

Vitamin E

- Vitamin E has been shown to ameliorate steatohepatitis, but not fibrosis, in individuals without type 2 diabetes and with biopsy-proven NASH in a 2-year randomized controlled trial.[18]

- Conclusions of studies of vitamin E in patients with NAFLD/NASH and type 2 diabetes have been mixed. Therefore, vitamin E is not a recommended medication intervention based on current evidence for use in patients with type 2 diabetes and NAFLD/NASH.

Medications Not Shown to Improve NAFLD/NASH in Persons With Type 2 Diabetes

According to the 2022 AACE guidelines and the EASL, due to lack of evidence of efficacy, metformin, acarbose, DPP-4 inhibitors, and insulin are not recommended for the treatment of steatohepatitis (no benefit on necrosis or inflammation). However, these may be continued as needed for the treatment of hyperglycemia in those with type 2 diabetes and NAFLD or NASH.

Bariatric Surgery

- Bariatric surgery performed at well-established centers should be considered in individuals who meet criteria with clinically significant fibrosis in the setting of type 2 diabetes and obesity.

- In a prospective study evaluating the impact of bariatric surgery, 85% had resolution of NASH at 1 year, 90.5% at 5 years, and 70% had regression of fibrosis.[19]

- Caution should be exercised in recommending bariatric surgery to patients with cirrhosis and advanced fibrosis due to a higher risk of bleeding and higher mortality.

Clinical Case Vignettes

Case 1

A 42-year-old man with obesity and hypertension is referred to endocrinology for management of type 2 diabetes mellitus. His hemoglobin A_{1c} value is 7.5% (169 mmol/mol). He is currently managed with metformin, 1000 mg orally twice daily, and empagliflozin, 25 mg once daily. His BMI is 31.2 kg/m². His blood pressure is 148/88 mm Hg. Hemoglobin and hematocrit are normal. His glomerular filtration rate is 75 mL/min per 1.73 m².

Additional laboratory test results:

Platelet count = 200 × 10³/µL (SI: 200 × 10⁹/L)
Total cholesterol = 193 mg/dL (SI: 5.00 mmol/L)
Triglycerides = 141.6 mg/dL (SI: 1.60 mmol/L)
HDL cholesterol = 19.3 mg/dL (SI: 0.50 mmol/L)
LDL cholesterol = 89 mg/dL (SI: 2.31 mmol/L)
AST = 55 U/L (SI: 0.92 µkat/L)
ALT = 100 U/L (SI: 1.67 µkat/L)

Concerned about the elevated liver enzymes, which of the following should be done as the best next step?

A. Perform liver ultrasonography

B. Calculate a FIB-4 score

C. Evaluate for secondary causes of liver disease

D. Refer to a hepatologist

E. Start a GLP-1 receptor agonist

Answer: C) Evaluate for secondary causes of liver disease

The diagnosis of NAFLD involves ruling out other conditions associated with elevated liver enzymes (Answer C). Initial evaluation should include investigations to rule out other causes of hepatic steatosis and liver disease.

Secondary causes of liver disease:

1. Excessive alcohol consumption

2. Hepatitis C (genotype 3)

3. Hepatitis B—HBsAg, HBsAb, HBcAb

4. Lipodystrophy—no specific lab study exists to diagnose lipodystrophy.

5. Abetalipoproteinemia—fasting lipid panel and apolipoprotein B measurement

6. Reye syndrome

7. Pregnancy associated—HELLP syndrome

8. Hemochromatosis—iron panel

9. Autoimmune hepatitis—antinuclear antibodies, antismooth muscle antibodies, ALT, AST

10. Review of medications associated with liver disease

Case 2

Which of the following patients should be evaluated further for NAFLD?

A. 19-year-old woman with a BMI of 34 kg/m^2 and insulin resistance

B. 32-year-old man with prediabetes, BMI of 27 kg/m^2, and hypertension

C. 62-year-old woman with type 2 diabetes and elevated liver enzymes for 7 months

D. 28-year-old man with type 1 diabetes, BMI of 18 kg/m^2, hemoglobin A$_{1c}$ of 6.4%, normal liver enzymes

E. All of the above

F. A, B, and C only

Answer: F) A, B, and C only

Persons with prediabetes, type 2 diabetes, BMI greater than or equal to 30 kg/m^2, persistently elevated aminotransferase levels (6 months or more), and those with imaging studies that reveal hepatic steatosis should be further assessed for NAFLD/NASH. Thus, the patients described in

Answers A, B, and C should be evaluated further for NAFLD.

In a 2020 *Journal of Clinical Endocrinology and Metabolism* article, "Prevalence of non-alcoholic fatty liver disease in patients with type 1 diabetes mellitus: a systematic review and meta-analysis," the prevalence of NAFLD/NASH in persons with type 1 diabetes is reported to be low (less than or equal to 10% with MRI-based methods).

Case 3

A 51-year-old man with type 2 diabetes presents for follow-up in endocrine clinic. His treatment regimen is metformin, 500 mg daily, and pioglitazone, 30 mg daily. He has difficulty losing weight. His BMI is 34 kg/m^2. His liver enzymes are elevated (AST, 96 U/L; ALT, 155 U/L). His FIB-4 score is 2.1, which is considered indeterminate. Elastography documents an LSM of 10 kPA.

Which of the following is the best next step in management?

A. Start semaglutide and titrate the dosage up to 2.4 mg once weekly

B. Increase the pioglitazone dosage to 45 mg once daily

C. Advise the patient to stop drinking alcohol and repeat studies for NAFLD 3 months after alcohol cessation

D. Refer to a liver specialist

Answer: D) Refer to a liver specialist

Although all the above answers would be considered appropriate, the most important next step is to establish a multidisciplinary team involving a liver specialist (Answer D). Risk assessment with additional tests, including liver biopsy, may be warranted.

REFERENCES

1. Younossi ZM, Koenig AB, Abdelatif D, Fazel Y, Henry L, Wymer M. Global epidemiology of nonalcoholic fatty liver disease-meta-analytic assessment of prevalence, incidence, and outcomes. *Hepatology*. 2016;64(1):73-84. PMID: 26707365

2. Younossi ZM, Stepanova M, Ong JP, et al; Global Nonalcoholic Steatohepatitis Council. Nonalcoholic steatohepatitis is the fastest growing cause of hepatocellular carcinoma in liver transplant candidates. *Clin Gastroenterol Hepatol*. 2019;17(4):748-755. PMID: 29908364

3. Golabi P, Paik JM, AlQahtani S, Younossi Y, Tuncer G, Younossi ZM. Burden of non-alcoholic fatty liver disease in Asia, the Middle East and North Africa: data from global burden of disease 2009-2019. *J Hepatol.* 2021;75(4):795-809. PMID: 34081959

4. Hernaez R, Lazo M, Bonekamp S, et al. Diagnostic accuracy and reliability of ultrasonography for the detection of fatty liver: a meta-analysis. *J Hepatol.* 2011;54(3);1082-1090. PMID: 21618575

5. Nassir F, Rector RS, Hammoud G, Ibdah JA. Pathogenesis and prevention of hepatic steatosis. *J Hepatol.* 2015;11(3):167-175. PMID: 27099587

6. Divella R, Mazzocca, Daniele A, Sabba C, Paradiso A. Obesity, nonalcoholic fatty liver disease and adipocytokines network in promotion of cancer. *Int J Biol Sc.* 2019;15(3):610-616. PMID: 30745847

7. Godoy-Matos AF, Silva W, Valerio CM. NAFLD as a continuum: from obesity to metabolic syndrome and diabetes. *Diabetol Metab Syndr.* 2020;12:60. PMID: 32684985

8. Lomonaco R, Leiva EG, Bril F, et al. Advanced liver fibrosis is common in patients with type 2 diabetes followed in the outpatient setting: the need for systematic screening. *Diabetes Care.* 2021;44(2):399-406. PMID: 33355256

9. Tapper et.al. FibroScan (vibration-controlled transient elastography): where does it stand in the United States practice. *Clin Gastroenterol Hepatol.* 2015;13(1):27-36. PMID: 24909907

10. Cusi K, Isaacs S, Barb D, et al. American Association of Clinical Endocrinology clinical practice guideline for the diagnosis and management of nonalcoholic ratty liver disease in primary care and endocrinology clinical settings: co-sponsored by the American Association for the Study of Liver Diseases (AASLD). *Endocr Pract.* 20233;28(5)528-562. PMID: 35569886

11. Younossi ZM, Felix S, Jeffers T. Performance of the enhanced liver fibrosis test to estimate advanced fibrosis among patients with nonalcoholic fatty liver disease. *JAMA Netw Open.* 2021;4(9):e2123923. PMID: 34529067

12. Srivastava A, Gailer R, Tanwar S, et.al. Prospective evaluation of a primary care referral pathway for patients with non-alcoholic fatty liver disease. *J Hepatol.* 2019;71(2):371-378. PMID: 30965069

13. Keating SE, Hackett DA, Parker HM, et.al. Effect of aerobic exercise training dose on liver fat and visceral adiposity. *J Hepatol.* 2015;63(1):174-182. PMID: 25863524

14. Cusi K, Orsak B, Bril F, et al. Long term pioglitazone treatment for patients with non-alcoholic steatohepatitis and prediabetes or type 2 diabetes mellitus: a randomized trial. *Ann Intern Med.* 2016;165(5):305-315. PMID: 27322798

15. Stefan N, Haring HU, Cusi K. Non-alcoholic fatty liver disease: causes, diagnosis, cardiometabolic consequences, and treatment strategies. *Lancet Diabetes Endocrinol.* 2019;7(4):313-324. PMID: 30174213

16. Cusi K. Incretin based therapies for the management of nonalcoholic fatty liver disease in patients with type 2 diabetes. *J Hepatol.* 2019;69(6):2318-2322. PMID: 31006135

17. Patel Chavez C, Cusi K, Kadiyala S. The emerging role of glucagon-like peptide-1 receptor agonists for the management of NAFLD. *J Clin Endocrinol Metab.* 2022;107(1):29-38. PMID: 34406410

18. Sanyal AJ, Chalasani N, Kowdley KV, et al; NASH CRN. Pioglitazone, vitamin E, or placebo for nonalcoholic steatohepatitis. *N Engl J Med.* 2010;362(18):1675-1685. PMID: 20427778

19. Lassailly G, Caiazzo R, Ntandja-Wandji LC, et al. Bariatric surgery provides long term resolution of nonalcoholic steatohepatitis and regression of fibrosis. *J Gastroenterol.* 2020;159(4):1290-1301.e5. PMID: 32553765

How to Diagnose Underlying Causes and Contributing Factors in Obesity

Elisabeth F. C. van Rossum, MD, PhD. Department of Internal Medicine, Division of Endocrinology and Obesity Center CGG, Erasmus University Medical Center, Rotterdam, the Netherlands; Email: e.vanrossum@erasmusmc.nl

Mariëtte R. Boon, MD, PhD. Department of Internal Medicine, Division of Endocrinology and Obesity Center CGG, Erasmus University Medical Center, Rotterdam, the Netherlands; Email: m.r.boon@erasmusmc.nl

Educational Objectives

After reviewing this chapter, learners should be able to:

- Identify underlying causes of obesity.

- Identify and optimize factors that can impair the effects of obesity treatments such as lifestyle intervention, pharmacotherapy, or bariatric surgery.

- Recommend appropriate treatment strategies to address the underlying causes of obesity.

Significance of the Clinical Problem

Obesity is a chronic relapsing disease, and its prevalence is increasing at an alarming rate. Before starting treatment to reduce weight, adequate diagnostic assessments should be performed to identify all (potential) underlying causes and contributing factors, and these should be optimized when possible. After the diagnostic phase, a more effective individualized treatment can follow. In this Meet the Professor chapter, experience- and evidence-based practical recommendations are provided (illustrated by clinical examples) to detect potential underlying causes of contributing factors to obesity. These factors can generally be divided into several categories. The more common contributing factors are linked to unhealthy lifestyle (diet, exercise, sleep, alcohol use). In addition, medications (eg, psychiatric drugs, anticonvulsant agents, [local] corticosteroids, insulin) can contribute to weight gain. Other contributing conditions are chronic stress, binge-eating disorder, and depression. Obesity also has some endocrine causes (eg, hypothyroidism, cyclic Cushing syndrome, polycystic ovary syndrome, hypogonadism, GH deficiency) or can be due to monogenic or syndromic obesity and hypothalamic obesity. The most important alarm symptoms for genetic causes are early-onset obesity, hyperphagia, and/or striking weight discrepancy among family members. In addition, in syndromic obesity, dysmorphic features, intellectual deficit, and behavioral problems are often present. Hypothalamic obesity is generally characterized by the occurrence of hyperphagia after head trauma, infection, or surgery. In addition to the above-mentioned factors, which can be addressed in individual patient care, other environmental factors (eg, urbanization, endocrine disruptors, unhealthy food environment) may also contribute to the obesity epidemic. Identifying and optimizing the underlying diseases, contributing factors, and other associated conditions of obesity in an individual patient may result in more effective and individualized treatments and have the potential to also reduce the obesity stigma.

Obesity (defined as BMI ≥30.0 kg/m²) is a chronic relapsing disease that is a growing problem worldwide. In 2016, more than 650 million adults were living with obesity, and 4.0 million deaths annually were attributable to a high BMI. It is estimated that if current trends continue, by 2030 one billion people will be living with obesity worldwide. Obesity is associated with many diseases, including type 2 diabetes mellitus, cardiovascular disease, depression, osteoarthritis, and 13 types of cancer. In addition, obesity aggravates the course of several chronic diseases, leading to increased morbidity and even mortality. Both on a societal level, as well as in clinical practice, it is widely believed that obesity is simply the consequence of overconsuming unhealthy foods and lack of exercise. This oversimplistic view contributes to the widespread stigma of obesity and generally results in suboptimal treatment of this condition.

However, on an individual level, many factors and underlying diseases are associated with weight gain and barriers to weight loss. When facing a patient with obesity, it is thus important that clinicians not merely focus on treating the associated comorbidities and/or simply recommend weight loss but perform a proper diagnostic obesity workup. In this respect, it is curious that in other endocrine-related diseases, such as hypertension, endocrinologists are more alert to consider a variety of secondary causes. The importance of the diagnostic workup is evidenced by the fact that specific underlying causes can hamper the effect of common antiobesity treatments, such as lifestyle intervention, pharmacotherapy, or bariatric surgery.[1] The aim of this Meet the Professor session is to help clinicians deepen the diagnostic phase of evaluating obesity with a comprehensive overview of possible contributors to weight gain for individual patients.

Practice Gaps

- Although current nonpharmacological antiobesity treatments are quite effective in some patients, efficacy can be significantly hampered by the presence of underlying causes of obesity. These conditions should be properly diagnosed and, if possible, addressed to increase treatment efficacy.

- While it is crucial to perform a proper diagnostic phase in the obesity workup, most clinicians have not been formally trained to do this. Furthermore, clinicians often lack the time required to adequately workup patients with obesity.

Discussion

General Concepts

Obesity results from a chronic imbalance between energy intake and energy expenditure. Although it is generally thought that this imbalance is merely caused by a mismatch between dietary intake (eg, high caloric intake, unhealthy diet) and little exercise, this view is far too simplistic. Several other factors that influence basal metabolic rate, appetite regulation, etc, influence this balance. Understanding the effects of these factors aids in the diagnosis of underlying causes of obesity, paving the way for effective treatment. Factors influencing body-weight regulation can generally be divided into common causes (lifestyle, mental disorders, and medication) and more rare causes (endocrine diseases, hypothalamic causes, and monogenic or syndromic causes) (table).[2]

Common Causes of Obesity

Lifestyle-Related Factors

Globally, increased energy consumption, including consumption of ultra-processed foods is an important contributor to the current obesity pandemic.[3] However, in an individual patient, several factors may underlie this increased energy consumption due to the complex interplay that exists among social, psychological, and biological

Table. Recognizing Underlying Causes of Obesity in Adults

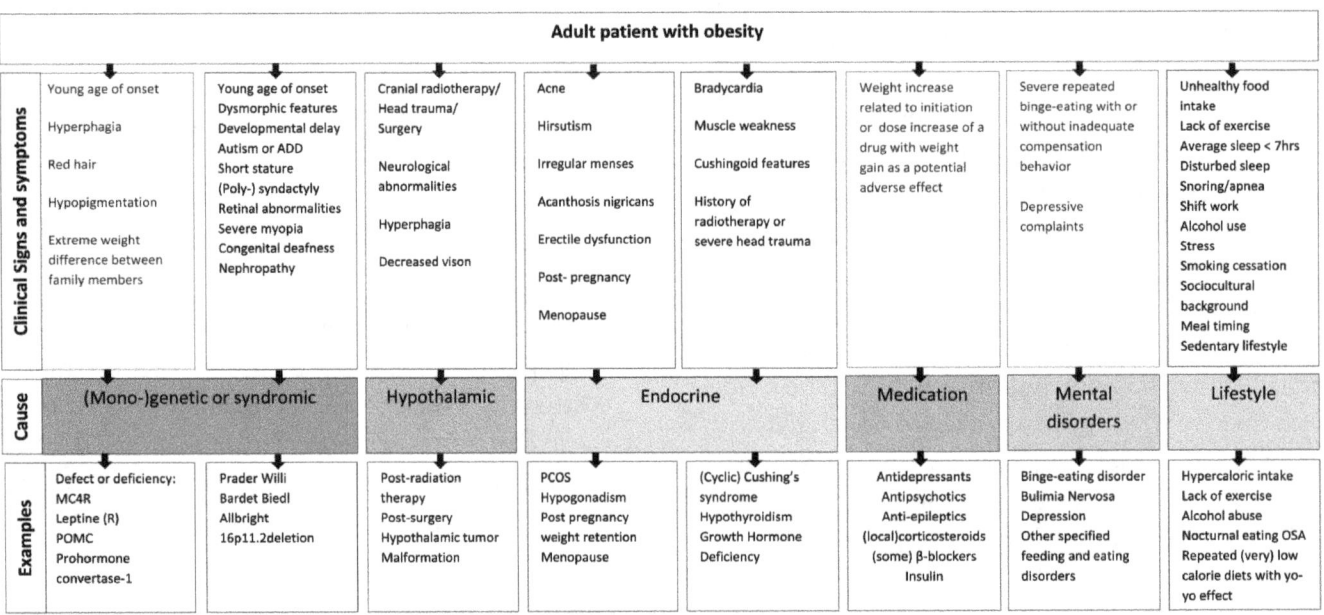

	Adult patient with obesity						
Clinical Signs and symptoms	Young age of onset Hyperphagia Red hair Hypopigmentation Extreme weight difference between family members	Young age of onset Dysmorphic features Developmental delay Autism or ADD Short stature (Poly-) syndactyly Retinal abnormalities Severe myopia Congenital deafness Nephropathy	Cranial radiotherapy/ Head trauma/ Surgery Neurological abnormalities Hyperphagia Decreased vison	Acne Hirsutism Irregular menses Acanthosis nigricans Erectile dysfunction Post- pregnancy Menopause	Bradycardia Muscle weakness Cushingoid features History of radiotherapy or severe head trauma	Weight increase related to initiation or dose increase of a drug with weight gain as a potential adverse effect	Severe repeated binge-eating with or without inadequate compensation behavior Depressive complaints	Unhealthy food intake Lack of exercise Average sleep < 7hrs Disturbed sleep Snoring/apnea Shift work Alcohol use Stress Smoking cessation Sociocultural background Meal timing Sedentary lifestyle
Cause	(Mono-)genetic or syndromic		Hypothalamic	Endocrine		Medication	Mental disorders	Lifestyle
Examples	Defect or deficiency: MC4R Leptine (R) POMC Prohormone convertase-1	Prader Willi Bardet Biedl Allbright 16p11.2deletion	Post-radiation therapy Post-surgery Hypothalamic tumor Malformation	PCOS Hypogonadism Post pregnancy weight retention Menopause	(Cyclic) Cushing's syndrome Hypothyroidism Growth Hormone Deficiency	Antidepressants Antipsychotics Anti-epileptics (local)corticosteroids (some) β-blockers Insulin	Binge-eating disorder Bulimia Nervosa Depression Other specified feeding and eating disorders	Hypercaloric intake Lack of exercise Alcohol abuse Nocturnal eating OSA Repeated (very) low calorie diets with yo-yo effect

Abbreviations: ADD, attention-deficit disorder; PCOS, polycystic ovary syndrome; MC4R, melanocortin 4 receptor; POMC, proopiomelanocortin; PPI, proton-pump inhibitors; OC, oral contraceptives; OSA, obstructive sleep apnea; OSFED, other specific feeding and eating disorders. Reprinted with permission from Van der Valk ES et al. Obes Rev, 2019; 20(6): 795-804. © The Authors. Published by John Wiley & Sons Ltd. on behalf of World Obesity Federation. (Color—web and EPUB only)

factors. Patients may overeat because they experience increased appetite. This can be an undesired consequence of having followed a very low-calorie diet without exercise or behavioral therapy, resulting in an altered balance between "hunger hormones" (eg, ghrelin) and "satiety hormones" (eg, leptin, CCK, and peptide YY). The resulting weight gain is often associated with long-term changes in these hormones, even a year after ending the initial very low-calorie diet.[4] Also, decreased quality or quantity of sleep can result in imbalance between hunger and satiety hormones and increased desire for high-caloric food, resulting in weight gain. Obstructive sleep apnea can be an underlying cause of reduced sleep quality and weight gain. However, obesity can also worsen obstructive sleep apnea. Chronic stress, resulting in increased cortisol levels, can also contribute to increased appetite, desire for high-caloric food, and increased abdominal obesity. In this respect, a strong positive correlation has been shown among hair cortisol levels, BMI, and waist circumference.[5] Stress may even counteract the effects of a healthy diet and is thus an important

factor to optimize in obesity treatment. Also, the type of food that is consumed can influence satiety. Ultra-processed food, which currently comprises more than 70% of foods in the supermarkets, may cause more caloric intake and consequently more weight gain compared with unprocessed foods.[6]

In addition to appetite, energy expenditure may be influenced by lifestyle. Sedentary lifestyle is an important contributor to decreased resting and total energy expenditure. In addition, very strict diets can not only modify hunger and satiety hormones but also reduce resting energy expenditure for a prolonged period. Energy-combusting brown adipose tissue also contributes to resting energy expenditure. Frequent exposure to cold can increase brown adipose tissue activity and resting energy expenditure with maintenance of lean mass.[7]

Mental Factors

For patients living with obesity, it is important to pay attention to mental health, as depression is more common in this population. This is a bidirectional relationship. The low-grade inflammation that occurs in obesity may contribute to the development of and/or exacerbate depression. Depression may result in binge eating and decreased physical activity, contributing to obesity. Individuals with obesity may have binge-eating disorder, which is characterized by recurrent episodes of consuming more food than normal and having feelings of lack of control. Distinguishing binge eating from hyperphagia is important, as hyperphagia is a diagnostic clue for genetic or hypothalamic obesity.

Medications That Can Induce Weight Gain
Several medications are known for their effects of inducing weight gain by increasing appetite, decreasing resting energy expenditure, or stimulating fat accumulation. The offending medications are frequently those used to treat the comorbidities of obesity (eg, antidepressants, antidiabetes agents, antihypertensive agents) and may thus further aggravate the course of obesity. We previously showed that 48% of the patients who visited our obesity clinic used potentially weight-increasing medication.[1] A brief overview of the categories of medications that can contribute to weight gain is shown in the *table*. Systemic corticosteroids are well-known for their capacity to increase weight. However, recent evidence supports the fact that even local corticosteroids may have systemic effects resulting in weight gain. This is important for clinicians to be aware of, as so many patients worldwide use corticosteroids. In a large cohort study, we recently showed that use of local corticosteroids was associated with increased BMI and waist circumference compared with these parameters in patients who did not use corticosteroids, especially in women.[8]

Rare Causes of Obesity

Endocrine Diseases
Endocrine diseases are usually associated with only modest weight gain and, therefore, are rarely an underlying cause of obesity. However, sudden weight gain should prompt the physician to screen for an underlying endocrine disease. Routine screening for hypothyroidism is advised, especially if patients also present with other symptoms such as cold intolerance, dry skin, and constipation. Routine screening for hypercortisolism in cases of sudden weight gain is not advised, except when suspicious clinical symptoms are present, such as easy bruising, proximal muscle weakness, and "fresh" purple striae. Hypogonadism in male patients (eg, low testosterone levels) may be an underlying cause of obesity. However, obesity can also result in normo- or hypogonadotropic hypogonadism that usually improves after weight loss. Testosterone supplementation is only advised in cases of overt testosterone deficiency. In that setting, testosterone has indeed been shown to improve body composition.

Hypothalamic Causes
Hypothalamic obesity is characterized by abnormal weight gain following damage of the hypothalamic region. The hypothalamus contains the control center for hunger and satiety. This signal is mediated by the consecutive action of several nuclei, including AgRP neurons and POMC neurons. Damage to the hypothalamic region caused by head trauma, surgery for entities such as craniopharyngioma, or inflammatory processes involving the hypothalamus can result in defects in hunger and/or satiety signals, typically resulting in hyperphagia and sometimes also lowering resting energy expenditure.

Monogenic or Syndromic Causes
Generally, multiple genes each contribute a small amount to the total risk of developing obesity. However, in some individuals, obesity is caused by a pathogenic variant in a single gene. Examples include melanocortin 4 receptor (MC4R) deficiency, leptin (receptor) deficiency, and POMC deficiency. Some pathogenic variants affect certain areas of the hypothalamic satiety center and are characterized by severe hyperphagia. Other clinical characteristics of monogenic obesity include early age of onset and striking weight difference compared with family members (ie, being the only family member with obesity) (*box*). Obesity can also occur as part of certain syndromes.

Syndromic obesity is defined as the presence of obesity along with additional characteristic features such as intellectual disability, dysmorphic features, and congenital abnormalities affecting specific organ systems.[9] The most well-known obesity syndromes are Prader-Willi, Bardet-Biedl, and 16p11.2 deletion syndromes. In general, important features that should spark suspicion for syndromic obesity in a person with early-onset obesity and hyperphagia are developmental delay and/or intellectual deficit, facial dysmorphism, short stature, retinitis pigmentosa, polydactyly or syndactyly, behavioral dysfunction, microcephaly or macrocephaly, autism, and congenital anomalies.[9] Our study of 1230 patients with obesity who were referred to medical centers specializing in obesity in the Netherlands showed that almost 10% had either a definitive or possible diagnosis of monogenic obesity.[10] Monogenic obesity is important to diagnose because recently targeted treatment is available for some rare types of genetic obesity, and bariatric surgery may be less effective than average in these patients.

Box. Clinical Clues for Monogenic Obesity

1. Hyperphagia
2. Early onset of obesity
3. Striking weight discrepancy with family members

Novel Tool to Aid in Diagnosing Underlying Causes of Obesity

Generally, little time is available in clinical practice to unravel the underlying causes of obesity in an individual patient and there is an unmet need to aid in this process. Therefore, we have recently developed a digital tool consisting of an extensive questionnaire coupled with an algorithm that identifies certain "red flags" that point towards underlying causes (eg, endocrine or other medical) causes or contributing factors (eg, psychological or social). These algorithms also indicate whether specific comorbidities as obstructive sleep apnea, polycystic ovary syndrome, osteoarthritis, or binge-eating disorder may be present. This tool

will soon be implemented in patient care in the Netherlands and other countries.

Clinical Case Vignettes
Case 1

A 21-year-old man is referred for obesity that has been present since early childhood. His height is 71 in (180 cm), and weight is 298 lb (135 kg) (BMI = 41.7 kg/m^2). He has an extreme appetite, has decreased satiety, and eats a large volume of food (both healthy and unhealthy). When he was a 2-year-old child, he ate from trash cans and his parents had to lock the kitchen cabinets to prevent him from continuous eating. Now, he walks 50 minutes (2.5 miles) each day to work and is engaging in sports twice weekly. His parents and his sister have a normal BMI. He is not using any medication, and his blood glucose concentration is in the prediabetes range.

Which of the following suggests a diagnosis of genetic obesity in this patient?

A. Striking weight difference with family members
B. Hyperphagia
C. Obesity since early childhood
D. Prediabetes at a relatively young age
E. A combination of 2 or more of the above-mentioned features

Answer: E) A combination of 2 or more of the above-mentioned features

Each of the above-mentioned answers—if the only symptom present—is too limited to perform genetic testing, but when a combination of these features is present in an individual (Answer E), monogenic obesity is suspected and genetic testing is recommended.

Patients with a monogenic form of obesity typically have a history of early-onset obesity in childhood and are either the only family member with obesity or have a striking weight difference when compared with their family members (Answer A). This depends on the pattern of inheritance for the given disorder (autosomal dominant, autosomal recessive, or de novo). Obesity present in all family members is more suggestive of polygenic or environmental obesity and/or social factors (eg, unhealthy food and exercise pattern).

Hyperphagia (Answer B) is an important feature of monogenic obesity and generally leads to a lot of suffering, since an all-day preoccupation with food can be very disturbing and can decrease concentration and attention for other things in life. Signs of hyperphagia include uncontrolled hunger (despite eating regularly), extreme desire to eat, preoccupation with food, tendency to eat nonfood constituents (in children), disturbed satiation and satiety, and sometimes nocturnal eating.

Obesity of early onset (Answer C) is an important clue for the presence of monogenic obesity. Monogenic (nonsyndromic) obesity generally originates from an age younger than 5 years. Syndromic obesity can also develop during childhood, but it can present during the first years of puberty as well.

Dysmorphic features commonly occur in syndromic forms of genetic obesity.[9] In monogenic obesity, however, dysmorphic features are not commonly present.

Prediabetes (Answer D) at a young adult age is an increasingly common disorder, but not a very specific sign of monogenic obesity when it is the only feature. However, since severe obesity has already been present for so long in a young adult with monogenic obesity, complications such as insulin resistance, type 2 diabetes, hypertension, and many other obesity-related comorbidities are to be expected at a relatively young age.

Case 1 (continued)

The patient is referred to an obesity-specialized university medical center for further evaluation. He has no dysmorphic features or congenital anomalies. His vision and intelligence quotient are normal, and he has no developmental delay or behavioral problems. Hyperphagia has been present from birth with no failure to thrive, feeding difficulties, or muscular hypotonia in the first year(s) of life. He has a normal IGF-1 concentration and a low-normal testosterone concentration.

Which of the following genetic obesity disorders does this patient most likely have?

A. Prader-Willi syndrome

B. Bardet-Biedl syndrome

C. *MC4R* pathogenic variant

D. 16p11.2 deletion syndrome

E. Alström syndrome

Answer: C) MC4R pathogenic variant

This patient's clinical picture is most suspicious for a monogenic nonsyndromic obesity disorder (Answer C), as he has hyperphagia, early-onset obesity, a striking weight difference compared with family members, normal intelligence quotient, no dysmorphic features, no congenital anomalies, and no developmental delay. Well-known types of monogenic obesity are due to pathogenic variants in the genes involved in the leptin-melanocortin pathway, such as *LEP*, *LEPR*, *SH2B1*, *POMC*, *PCSK1*, *MC4R*, and *MC3R*.[11] *MC4R* pathogenic variants are the most common. In contrast to monogenic nonsyndromic obesity forms, syndromic forms of genetic obesity are often associated with dysmorphic features.[9]

Prader-Willi syndrome (Answer A) is characterized by failure to thrive and feeding difficulties during infancy, obesity and hyperphagia beginning in childhood, muscular hypotonia, developmental delay, behavioral problems, GH deficiency, genital hypoplasia, short stature, and small hands and feet. A defect on chromosome 15 disrupts the normal hypothalamic functions. In most cases, Prader-Willi syndrome is caused by a de novo pathogenic variant and is not inherited.

Bardet-Biedel syndrome (Answer B), also known as Laurence-Moon-Bardet-Biedl syndrome, is characterized by retinitis pigmentosa, obesity, kidney dysfunction, polydactyly, behavioral dysfunction, and hypogonadism. The prevalence is 1 in 13,500 to 1 in 175,000.

The 16p11.2 deletion syndrome (Answer D) can be proximal or distal. Proximal 16p11.2

deletion syndrome is characterized by obesity, autism, intellectual disability, congenital anomalies, and developmental delay. Genes involved are *SH2B1* and *KCTD13*. Distal 16p11.2 deletion syndrome is characterized by obesity, developmental delay, behavioral problems, and unusual facial morphology. Both types are inherited in an autosomal dominant manner.

Alström syndrome (Answer E) is characterized by blindness, hearing impairment, childhood obesity, insulin resistance, and type 2 diabetes mellitus. This rare obesity syndrome has a prevalence of less than 1 in 1 million and is inherited in an autosomal recessive manner. The causal gene is *ALMS1*.

Case 2

A 31-year-old woman is referred to the endocrine outpatient clinic because of rapid weight gain of 35 lb (16 kg) within 2 months, abdominal obesity, and irregular menstrual cycles. She uses birth control and takes no medications.

Physical examination reveals moon facies, buffalo hump, facial acne, hirsutism, abdominal striae, bilateral ankle edema, and hypertension.

Laboratory testing documents low serum potassium levels, very low urinary cortisol excretion, and a suppressed cortisol concentration after administration of 1 mg dexamethasone. Early-morning serum cortisol and ACTH levels are low (both measured simultaneously in the early morning and midnight hours).

Which of the following is the most likely diagnosis?

A. Cushing disease due to a pituitary adenoma

B. Cushing syndrome due to ectopic ACTH production

C. Cushing syndrome due to exogenous corticosteroid use

D. Primary adrenal insufficiency

E. Central adrenal insufficiency

Answer: C) Cushing syndrome due to exogenous corticosteroid use

This is an extreme case in which Cushing syndrome occurred due to topical corticosteroid use (treatment of eczema) over a large body surface and for a long period. Often, patients may not report using locally applied medication when asked about current medications, so specifically asking about several types of corticosteroids when a patient has cushingoid symptoms can be helpful. Systemic administration of glucocorticoids is known to cause hypothalamic-pituitary-adrenal (HPA) axis suppression by reducing corticotropin (ACTH) production, which decreases cortisol secretion by the adrenal gland. The degree of HPA suppression is dependent on dose, duration, frequency, and timing of glucocorticoid administration. In addition, an individual's sensitivity to glucocorticoids (mainly genetically determined) and glucocorticoid metabolism can contribute to severe adverse effects and increased HPA suppression.[12] Accumulating evidence shows that locally administered corticosteroids can result in symptomatic HPA-axis suppression, although the risk is small. A large meta-analysis showed that the percentage of adrenal insufficiency was 7.8%, 4.2%, and 4.7% for inhalation, nasal, and topical corticosteroids, respectively, and 48.7% and 52.5% for oral and intra-articular corticosteroids, respectively.[13] In 42.7% of patients, adrenal insufficiency was present when a combination of multiple forms was used. Thus, all forms of glucocorticoid delivery have the potential to exert systemic effects and may cause Cushing syndrome.

Glucocorticoid therapies are extensively used in a wide range of medical conditions, including respiratory, allergic, inflammatory, and autoimmune diseases. They can also contribute to weight gain and/or hamper successful weight loss. It is thus important that glucocorticoids are only used for proper indications.

This patient's clinical phenotype was not caused by a pituitary adenoma (Answer A); in that case, the laboratory values would be consistent with overproduction of endogenous glucocorticoids due to endogenous ACTH overproduction (eg, high urinary cortisol, midnight ACTH and cortisol, as well as nonsuppression of cortisol after dexamethasone). The same laboratory values would be expected with Cushing syndrome due to ectopic ACTH production (Answer B).

The case is not likely to be explained by primary adrenal insufficiency (Answer D), since typical clinical symptoms and signs are not present (eg, weight loss, arthralgia, nausea, vomiting, diarrhea, dizziness, hypotension, hyperpigmentation, and salt craving). In addition, in primary adrenal insufficiency, the ACTH levels would be elevated, not low as they are in this patient.

Central adrenal insufficiency (Answer E) is also not likely, although cortisol and ACTH levels would be low in that setting too. The patient's signs and symptoms are not compatible with adrenal insufficiency but are typical for increased corticosteroid exposure.

In some hospitals, it is possible to measure exogenous corticosteroids in blood. This can also be helpful if the patient does not disclose or forgets about corticosteroid use.

Interestingly, after replacing the corticosteroid cremes with a weight-neutral medication for her eczema, the patient's weight dropped by 32 lb (14.5 kg) within a couple of months, with the same healthy lifestyle she already had.

Case 3

A 52-year-old postmenopausal woman seeks evaluation for obesity (BMI = 41.2 kg/m²). Despite optimizing her diet, she slowly keeps gaining weight. She has depression, which was treated with citalopram for the last 3 years. Her primary care provider recently switched this medication to sertraline because the depression did not improve enough with citalopram. She frequently works night shifts. She tries to exercise at least twice weekly (swimming for 1 hour) and takes daily walks with her dog. She describes her sleep quality as poor and often wakes up tired. Her partner mentions she snores and frequently seems to stop breathing. Routine bloodwork shows mildly elevated TSH (6.7 mIU/L) and a normal free T_4 concentration.

Which of the following factors is most likely to facilitate her efforts to lose weight?

A. Menopause
B. Sertraline
C. Obstructive sleep apnea
D. Subclinical hypothyroidism
E. Night shifts

Answer: B) Sertraline

The use of sertraline (Answer B) may facilitate her efforts to lose weight in the near future because its effect on weight is, on average, beneficial. In contrast, she used citalopram until recently, which is known to have weight gain as a potential adverse effect.[14] In addition, because the depression did not respond well to citalopram, depression could also be contributing to her obesity. If she loses weight after this medication switch and continues her healthy lifestyle, her depression may also improve, as obesity and depression have many shared underlying mechanisms and weight loss can also have antidepressive effects.[15]

Approximately 60% to 70% of women experience weight gain after menopause (Answer A). Although this is generally thought to be largely attributable to increase in age, some studies suggest that also hormonal factors (eg, reduction in estrogen levels and increase in FSH) independent of age contribute to the weight gain seen in some women.[16] Mechanisms include lowering lean mass, reducing resting energy expenditure, and shift in fat distribution with increased visceral fat accumulation. Menopause may increase rather than decrease fat mass.

Obstructive sleep apnea (Answer C) can aggravate obesity and does not facilitate weight loss. The precise mechanism is not clear, but it may be related to the low oxygen tension that occurs in obstructive sleep apnea, as well as dysregulation of several hormones following poor sleep quality, including hunger and satiety hormones. In the adult population, the prevalence of obstructive sleep apnea is estimated to be 25%, while it is as high as 45% in people living with obesity. Weight loss has been shown to improve obstructive sleep apnea. Obstructive sleep apnea can be diagnosed with the STOP-BANG questionnaire.

In obesity, elevated TSH and normal free T_4 levels are often mistakenly attributed to subclinical hypothyroidism (Answer D). TSH levels are often slightly increased in both children and adults with obesity and are positively correlated with BMI.[17] This is believed to be a physiological increase, possibly due to increased leptin levels that subsequently stimulate hypothalamic thyrotropin-releasing hormone release. In fact, weight loss has been shown to normalize TSH levels in patients with obesity. This patient's elevated TSH level will probably not affect her weight in a positive or negative way.

Shift workers (Answer E) have an increased risk of developing obesity and several cardiometabolic diseases, including type 2 diabetes and cardiovascular diseases. Circadian misalignment, as occurs in shift work, is associated with decreased total energy expenditure and increased caloric intake and can thus contribute to weight gain.[18] It is conceivable that it impairs her efforts and does not facilitate weight loss.

Key Learning Points

Underlying causes of obesity can be divided into common causes (lifestyle, social factors, mental disorders, medications, and common endocrine factors) and more rare causes (endocrine diseases, hypothalamic causes, and monogenic or syndromic causes)

- Clinical clues for genetic obesity include hyperphagia, early-onset obesity, and striking weight discrepancy compared with family members.

- Optimizing and/or treating underlying causes of obesity is important for successful treatment of obesity and requires personalized treatment strategies.

- Respectful and nonjudgmental discussion of obesity is important to reduce stigma of this condition.

References

1. Savas M, Wester VL, Visser JA, et al. Extensive phenotyping for potential weight-inducing factors in an outpatient population with obesity. *Obes Facts.* 2019;12(4):369-384. PMID: 31216558

2. van der Valk ES, van den Akker ELT, Savas M, et al. A comprehensive diagnostic approach to detect underlying causes of obesity in adults. *Obes Rev.* 2019;20(6):795-804. PMID: 30821060

3. Romieu I, Dossus L, Barquera S, et al. Energy balance and obesity: what are the main drivers? *Cancer Causes Control.* 2017;28(3):247-258. PMID: 28210884

4. Sumithran P, Prendergast LA, DelbridgeE, et al. Long-term persistence of hormonal adaptations to weight loss. *N Engl J Med.* 2011;365(17):1597-1604. PMID: 22029981

5. van der Valk ES, Abawi O, Mohseni M, et al. Cross-sectional relation of long-term glucocorticoids in hair with anthropometric measurements and their possible determinants: a systematic review and meta-analysis. *Obes Rev.* 2022;23(3):e13376. PMID: 34811866

6. Hall KD, Ayuketah A, Brychta R, et al. Ultra-processed diets cause excess calorie intake and weight gain: an inpatient randomized controlled trial of ad libitum food intake. *Cell Metab.* 2019;30(1):67-77. PMID: 31105044

7. Yoneshiro T, Aita S, Matsushita M, et al. Recruited brown adipose tissue as an antiobesity agent in humans. *J Clin Invest.* 2013;123(8):3404-3408. PMID: 23867622

8. Savas M, Muka T, Wester VL, et al. Associations between systemic and local corticosteroid use with metabolic syndrome and body mass index. *J Clin Endocrinol Metab.* 2017;102(10):3765-3774. PMID: 28973553

9. Kaur Y, de Souza RJ, Gibson WT, Meyre D. A systematic review of genetic syndromes with obesity. *Obes Rev.* 2017;18(6):603-634. PMID: 28346723

10. Kleinendorst L, Massink MPG, Cooiman MI, et al. Genetic obesity: next-generation sequencing results of 1230 patients with obesity. *J Med Genet.* 2018;55(9):578-586. PMID: 29970488

11. Pigeyre M, Yazdi FT, Kaur Y, Meyre D. Recent progress in genetics, epigenetics and metagenomics unveils the pathophysiology of human obesity. *Clin Sci (Lond).* 2016;130(12):943-986. PMID: 27154742

12. Wester VL, Lamberts SW, van Rossum EF. Advances in the assessment of cortisol exposure and sensitivity. *Curr Opin Endocrinol Diabetes Obes.* 2014;21(4):306-311. PMID: 24983396

13. Broersen LHA, Pereira AM, Jørgensen JOL, Dekkers OM. Adrenal insufficiency in corticosteroids sse: systematic review and meta-analysis. *J Clin Endocrinol Metab.* 2015;100(6):2171-2180. PMID: 25844620

14. Wharton S, Raiber L, Serodio KJ, Lee J, Christensen RA. Medications that cause weight gain and alternatives in Canada: a narrative review. *Diabetes Metab Syndr Obes.* 2018;11:427-438. PMID: 30174450

15. Milaneschi Y, Simmons WK, van Rossum EFC, Penninx BW. Depression and obesity: evidence of shared biological mechanisms. *Mol Psychiatry.* 2019;24(1):18-33. PMID: 29453413

16. Fenton A. Weight, shape, and body composition changes at menopause. *J Midlife Health.* 2021;12(3):187-192. PMID: 34759699

17. Biondi B. Thyroid and obesity: an intriguing relationship. *J Clin Endocrinol Metab.* 2010;95(8):3614-3617. PMID: 20685890

18. McHill AW, Wright KP Jr. Role of sleep and circadian disruption on energy expenditure and in metabolic predisposition to human obesity and metabolic disease. *Obes Rev.* 2017;18(Suppl 1):15-24. PMID: 28164449

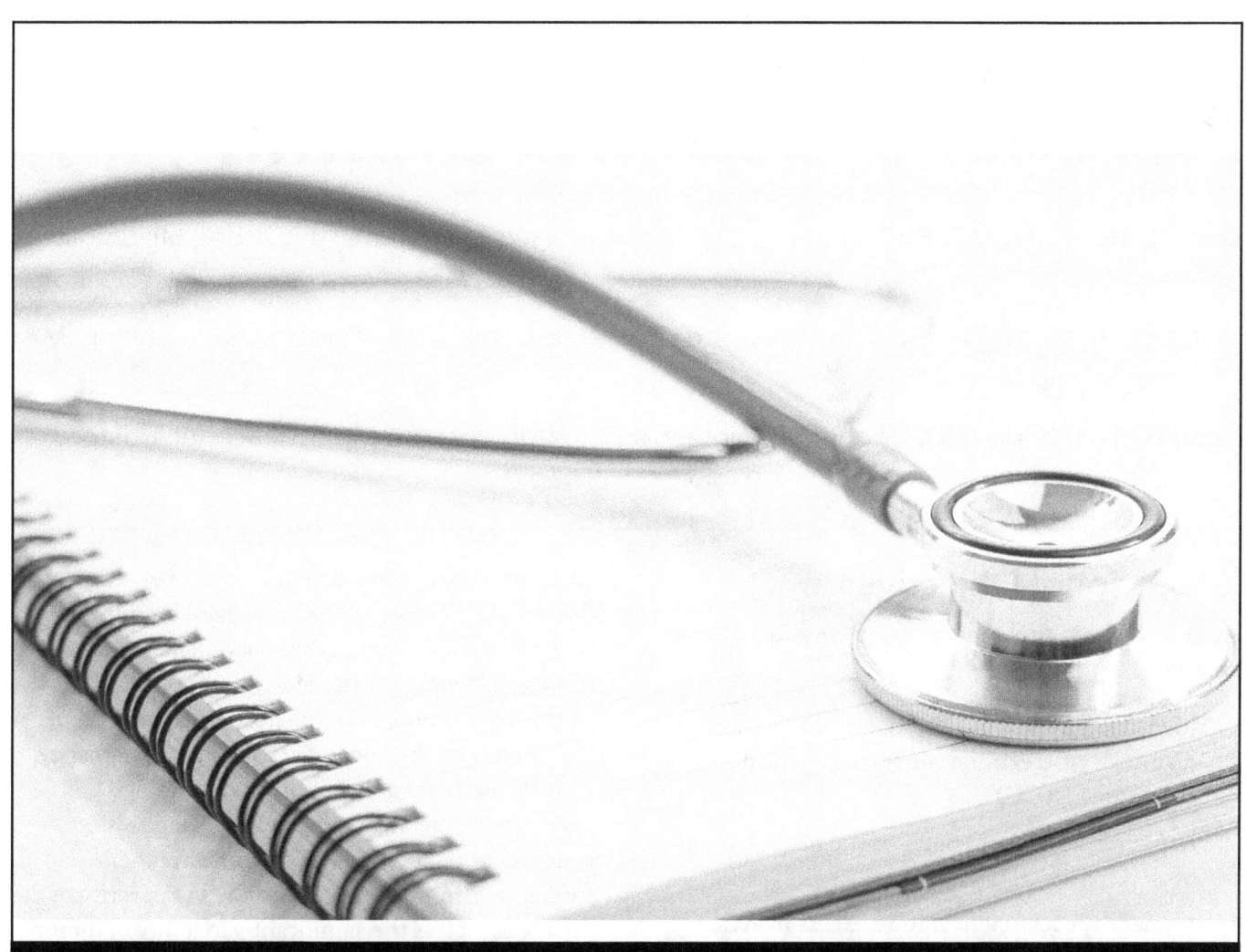

ADRENAL

Management of Adrenocortical Carcinoma

Gary D. Hammer, MD, PhD. University of Michigan Health System, Ann Arbor, MI; Email: ghammer@umich.edu

Matthew A. Nehs, MD. Brigham & Women's Hospital, Harvard Medical School, Boston, MA; Email: mnehs@bwh.harvard.edu

Gerard M. Doherty, MD. Brigham & Women's Hospital, Harvard Medical School, Boston, MA; Email: gmdoherty@bwh.harvard.edu

Educational Objectives

After reviewing this chapter, learners should be able to:

- Identify common pitfalls that lead to inaccurate diagnosis or treatment of adrenocortical carcinoma (ACC).

- Explain general principles of the management of ACC.

- Manage associated hormone excess in ACC.

- Describe the role of genetics in the biology and management of ACC.

Significance of the Clinical Problem

Adrenal tumors are very common, affecting 3% to 10% of the population, and most are small, benign nonfunctional adrenocortical adenomas (ACAs). ACC is very rare and typically lethal disease, affecting 1 to 3 per million adults per year (and 0.2 to 0.3 per million children per year), but it is difficult to treat and is associated with significant morbidity. Many affected patients present with a paucity of symptoms despite extensive metastatic disease on initial evaluation, especially if the tumor is nonfunctional. Distinguishing between a benign vs malignant mass in the adrenal is essential but not always straightforward. Most doctors have never seen a case of ACC and/or are not familiar or comfortable with the current multidisciplinary management strategies for the disease. Management requires careful attention to both the hormonal function of the tumor and the oncologic risk of the malignancy. Coordinated care between an endocrinologist, endocrine surgeon, and medical oncologist is essential, with additional support from other specialties a frequent necessity. Given the rarity of the disease as well as the significant variability in tumor behavior and patient course, we believe that ACC is best cared for in specialized centers.

The initial differential diagnosis for small adrenal tumors often includes benign and malignant lesions and tumors arising from the adrenal medulla, adrenal cortex, or metastatic lesions from other sites. When a patient presents with a large (>10 cm) adrenal mass, the differential diagnosis should also include retroperitoneal sarcoma and tumors from nearby organs (typically liver, kidney, pancreas) While the full evaluation of adrenal masses is beyond the scope of this session, the nature of these masses may become clear with biochemical testing or careful imaging review with an expert radiologist. Biopsy of potentially resectable unilateral lesions is contraindicated, as the resulting tumor spill may render resection ineffective through seeding the tract of the biopsy needle. Additionally, adrenal biopsy of ACC can produce false-negative results and is generally not diagnostically necessary.

Resection is the only potentially curative intervention to date. If the patient can have complete resection of all demonstrable tumor, that is generally advisable. Palliative resection to resolve mass effect may occasionally be helpful, but this is often rendered moot by rapid tumor progression. Moreover, new highly effective medical therapies for steroid excess make palliative resection for hormonal control a last resort. There are 2 key decisions that a clinician must make when confronted with an adrenal tumor: (1) determine the risk of malignancy of the observed lesion and (2) determine whether there is adrenal hormone excess that would support a "primary" adrenal neoplasm (benign or malignant). The answers to these questions are essential in the initial workup of any adrenal "lesion" and will guide how the endocrinologist, endocrine surgeon, surgical oncologist, and/or medical oncologist proceeds with additional diagnostic and/or therapeutic interventions.

This Meet the Professor session is designed to cover a number of important issues regarding the diagnosis and treatment of adrenocortical carcinoma by discussion of cases seen in our multidisciplinary endocrine oncology clinics.

A few of the topics to be covered are:

- Is it cancer?
- Treating the primary tumor
- Adjuvant care (to prevent recurrence) once resected
- Treating hormone excess
- Treating recurrence or nonresectable/ metastatic disease

Practice Gaps

- Lack of experience with diagnosis and treatment of ACC on presentation (diagnosis not entertained).

- Lack of referral to experienced endocrinologists or experienced endocrine surgeons for initial evaluation and treatment.
- Inappropriate therapies prior to referral to endocrinologists and endocrine surgeons.
- Challenges of mitotane therapy and proper use.
- Lack of optimal second- and third-line systemic therapies.

Discussion

There are 3 main clinical scenarios in which patients with ACC present. Forty to sixty percent of patients present with symptoms and signs of hormone excess. One-third present with nonspecific symptoms such as abdominal or flank pain, abdominal fullness, or early satiety. Lastly, 20% to 30% of ACCs are incidentally diagnosed by imaging procedures for unrelated medical concerns. All adrenal masses must be evaluated for potential hormone excess and malignancy. All adrenal masses are evaluated for cortical and medullary hormone excess using standard Endocrine Society guidelines for primary aldosteronism, Cushing syndrome, and pheochromocytoma. In addition, 11-deoxycortisol, DHEA-S, and androstenedione are measured. Biochemically or clinically apparent ACTH production is evident in up to 50% to 75% of these patients. In the setting of ACC, Cushing syndrome is the most common syndrome, and androgen excess (almost exclusively DHEA-S) is the second most common (causing rapid-onset male-pattern baldness, hirsutism, virilization, and menstrual irregularities in women). Co-secretion of 2 classes of adrenocortical hormones should raise concern for ACC, although co-secretion of cortisol and aldosterone can be seen in the setting of primary aldosteronism as well.

Radiologic Evaluation

Routine radiologic evaluation includes an unenhanced CT. Malignant masses (including ACC and metastatic deposits from other primary cancer) can be distinguished from common lipid-rich ACAs, which tend to be small (often <4 cm), homogeneous masses that measure less than 20 Hounsfield units (HU) on unenhanced CT or demonstrate loss of signal on chemical shift MR. Homogeneous adrenal tumors exhibiting greater than 20 HU can be benign, lipid-poor ACAs or nonadenomas. Such lesions can be further characterized using a dedicated adrenal protocol CT. ACAs demonstrate a greater contrast washout than adrenal nonadenomas. Most adrenal masses are benign ACAs.

While most ACCs are diagnosed late (ie, large [>4 cm]), it is important to remember that all cancers begin as 1 cell and small masses. Thus, a small, atypical-appearing mass on CT may still be malignant (although rare). In fact, we have removed a 0.8-cm ACC in a patient who was carefully followed with MRI for Li-Fraumeni syndrome. Hence, dedicated adrenal imaging is essential in the diagnosis of adrenal masses.

Biopsies are only considered when the patient has a current additional nonadrenal primary cancer *and* additional metastatic disease in the setting of a new adrenal mass. In this case, biopsy can help determine whether the adrenal mass is a metastatic lesion from the other primary or a new primary adrenal tumor that would necessitate a separate systemic approach.

The mean stages of ACC diagnosis are as follows:

- Stage 1 (<5 cm): 14%
- Stage 2 (>5 cm): 45%
- Stage 3 (local spread or regional lymphadenopathy): 27%
- Stage 4 (distant metastasis): 24% (the most common metastatic sites are lung [40%-80%], liver [40%-90%], and bone [5%-20%])

Pathologic Diagnosis

Pathologic diagnosis relies on review by an endocrine pathologist using the Weiss criteria that rely on standard histologic parameters that include invasion of tumor into capsule or adjacent vessels, necrosis, increased mitotic rates, and atypical mitotic figures. Tumors with more than 3 of these features most often behave in a malignant fashion and can be classified as ACC. Moreover, ACCs can be graded as high grade when greater than 20 mitoses per 50 high-power field (Ki67 index >10%) are present and low grade when fewer than 20 mitoses per 50 high-power field (Ki67 index <10%) are present. There is significant risk of recurrence following resected ACC. Recurrence in high-grade ACC often occurs within the first 3 to 12 months, with distant disease (liver and lungs) being more common. Low-grade ACC can present with recurrence late (2 to 3 years following resection), often with only local disease at the tumor bed or oligometastatic disease in the peritoneum or liver.

Surgical Considerations

Reasons to remove an adrenal mass include autonomous hormone excess and/or risk of malignancy. There are numerous preoperative, intraoperative, and postoperative issues to consider when selecting a surgical approach. All of these factors must be considered to achieve the best oncologic outcome and long-term functional recovery.

Resectable Lesions: Preoperative Considerations

The preoperative evaluation and preparation of the patient for surgery is highly important and includes thorough biochemical evaluation of the adrenal and hypothalamic-pituitary-adrenal axis. Electrolyte abnormalities and hypertension in Conn syndrome or Cushing syndrome should be corrected. Detailed cross-sectional imaging is obtained and studied by the surgeon in detail. We typically prefer contrast-enhanced CT to evaluate for tumor size, lymph node metastases, tumor thrombus/vascular invasion, and the patient's anthropomorphic characteristics. We occasionally use FDG-PET when attempting to distinguish benign from malignant adrenal masses that are indeterminate, although this technique does not have exceptional sensitivity or specificity for ACC. A careful consideration of the patient's cardiac, pulmonary, and nutritional status must be obtained, as these patients frequently have coexisting metabolic comorbidities.

Operative Technique

Open adrenalectomy is the preferred approach for known or suspected ACCs, including those requiring multivisceral resection. The classic anterior approach allows for full access to all organs of the peritoneal cavity and chest if necessary. The patient is positioned supine on the table. Incisions can be made in the midline or subcostal depending on preoperative factors and need for multivisceral resection. We favor large midline incisions for thin patients to preserve the rectus abdominus muscles. For rotund patients with large amounts of visceral fat, we favor a curvilinear bisubcostal incision for optimal exposure. While not often required, the thoracoabdominal approach can be useful in patients with large adrenal tumors or those involving the retrohepatic vena cava where visualization will be difficult due to body habitus or prior abdominal surgery. Although even very large right adrenal tumors can generally be removed using a subcostal incision with a midline extension and full mobilization of the liver, there are some tumors with involvement of the upper abdominal vena cava, particularly in reoperative cases, that are best performed using a thoracoabdominal approach. The patient is placed in semilateral decubitus position on a beanbag with an axillary roll beneath the axilla. The ipsilateral arm is held in place parallel over the contralateral arm with a thoracic arm holder. The pelvis remains flat. An incision is made 2 cm inferior to the ipsilateral scapula and carried from lateral to medial along the 8th or 9th intercostal space and then inferiorly along the upper midline of the abdomen to the umbilicus. The diaphragm is incised, allowing access to the chest and abdomen with excellent visualization of the retroperitoneal structures. Recovery can be delayed due to pulmonary issues or recovery of gastrointestinal function, and chronic pain from injury of the neurovascular bundle of the rib can occur.

The first operation is the best and usually only chance for long-term local control of malignancy, with the goal of a complete (R0) resection in the absence of penetration of the tumor capsule. Poor initial surgical treatment can rarely be corrected, whether by reoperation, radiotherapy, or chemotherapy. Thus, meticulous technique must be employed to avoid disrupting the tumor capsule during surgery. Complete removal of the tumor may require concomitant resection of the ipsilateral kidney, liver, spleen, pancreas, stomach, colon, or a portion of the vena cava. This decision should occur early on, rather than after handling the tumor to any great extent. Usually, the need for multivisceral resection can be predicted from preoperative CT.

Controversy surrounds the appropriateness of laparoscopic adrenalectomy for patients with ACC. ACCs can invade through the tumor capsule and are frequently microscopically present at the surface of the gland, and application of any pressure to the tumor should be avoided. Some surgeons compromise by initiating adrenalectomies laparoscopically to assess for evidence of intraperitoneal metastasis or invasion of the adrenal gland into other organs; however, this direct exploration of the tumor violates oncologic principles of resection. A recurring argument is that in "expert" hands, laparoscopic adrenalectomy may be appropriate for certain malignant adrenal tumors. However, there is no consensus definition of what constitutes adequate expertise. This does not translate to expertise for biologically aggressive, often invasive, larger adrenal cancers. Unfortunately, most ACCs are removed by low-volume and less experienced adrenal surgeons.

Surgical studies should distinguish between local/peritoneal recurrence and distant recurrence for an indication of quality of resection, as the type of operative approach most likely has less influence in the development of distant metastases compared with local/peritoneal recurrence. A retrospective study from University of Michigan reviewed 88 patients with ACC, 17 of whom underwent laparoscopic adrenalectomy. Although overall recurrence rates were similar, and despite on-average smaller tumors in the laparoscopic adrenalectomy group (7.0 cm) compared to tumor size in the open adrenalectomy group (12.3 cm), the laparoscopic adrenalectomy group had significantly earlier recurrence (9.2 months vs 19.2 months). There were more R1 or R2 resections or notation of intraoperative tumor spill (50% vs 18%) in the laparoscopic adrenalectomy group. These data suggest that although laparoscopic adrenalectomy may be technically feasible, the use of laparoscopic adrenalectomy in ACC leads to a shorter disease-free interval and a higher incidence of incomplete resections. These results were confirmed in an extended follow-up study of 110 patients undergoing open adrenalectomy and 46 undergoing laparoscopic adrenalectomy. After laparoscopic adrenalectomy, 30% had positive margins or intraoperative tumor spill compared with 16% of patients after open adrenalectomy despite larger tumors and more stage 3 tumors. Overall survival for patients with stage 2 ACC was significantly longer in those undergoing open adrenalectomy, including a subgroup of those with only R0 resections. Time to visible tumor bed recurrence or peritoneal recurrence in patients with stage 2 disease was shorter in patients who underwent laparoscopic adrenalectomy.

In summary, existing data are inconclusive and more studies are needed to better judge the equivalence of laparoscopic adrenalectomy and open adrenalectomy. In accordance with the experience gained at the authors' institutions, a conservative approach using an open technique is recommended for all adrenocortical lesions with a high preoperative probability of ACC.

Lymphadenectomy

The role of lymph node sampling or formal regional lymph node dissection in the treatment of ACC remains unknown and consensus within the field is needed. The impact of regional lymph node metastasis on overall survival provides impetus for earlier or more aggressive use of additional therapies when disease is present in the lymphatic system. In one retrospective study, performance of locoregional lymph node dissection led to improved oncologic outcome. Some of the improved outcome can be attributed to the upstaging of ACC patients with lymph node metastasis and subsequent more aggressive treatment. Similarly, more radical surgery in these patients can lead to increased clearance of disease

as opposed to a higher rate of positive margins. Nodal basins removed were not clearly reported, and lymph nodes associated with other organs during multivisceral resections were included, thereby leaving the role of prophylactic nodal dissection unknown.

Management of Invasive Tumors

Extirpation of large adrenocortical carcinomas can be extremely challenging for even the most experienced surgeon. Adequate visualization can be difficult to achieve. Partial hepatectomy may be required in some patients to achieve en bloc resection. If needed, the liver can be completely mobilized from the inferior vena cava, affording superb visualization and access to the inferior vena cava should partial resection and reconstruction be necessary, or to facilitate removal of intravascular tumor thrombus. Tumor thrombus is not a contraindication to resection and is indicated when technically feasible. In most cases, venotomy and simple closure suffices for removal of tumor; however, in certain cases, resection of a portion of the vena cava may be required. If the diameter of the vena cava is not decreased by more than 50%, resection and primary closure is adequate. For cases requiring larger segments of caval resection, autologous tissue is preferred if bowel is also resected or entered during the operation, but prosthetic material may also be used. Vascular control of the vena cava can also be achieved in the chest using a median sternotomy or by a thoracoabdominal approach. In rare circumstances, veno-venous bypass may be useful. For thrombus extending into the right atrium, cardiopulmonary bypass can facilitate complete resection. Transesophageal echocardiography should be used to help identify the level of thrombus extension if it extends into the thorax, and a cardiac anesthesiologist can be very helpful in this assessment. Should bleeding from the vena cava be encountered, it can be voluminous but is low pressure and can be controlled. Multidisciplinary consultation with vascular surgeons preoperatively can help plan for these complex resections.

Aorta and Arterial Supply

Need for resection of portions of arteries or their branches is a general but not absolute contraindication to surgery for ACC. It is uncommon but possible for the celiac axis and takeoff of the superior mesenteric artery to be partially encased with tumor. If tumor involves a short segment of the celiac axis or superior mesenteric artery, it is possible to remove this short segment prior to its branching into end arteries. The gastroduodenal artery can supply the liver in a retrograde fashion via supply from the superior mesenteric artery; however, adequacy of this alternative pathway of hepatic perfusion should be tested. The renal artery is often involved with ACC, even if the kidney parenchyma is not directly invaded. This can affect the decision to perform an en bloc nephrectomy if the vascular supply cannot be salvaged or reconstructed.

Diaphragm

En bloc resection of tumor with an accompanying portion of the diaphragm may be required to achieve negative margins. Smaller diaphragmatic defects may be closed primarily using sutures in a running locking or interrupted mattress fashion. For larger defects, various prosthetic materials may be used for closure.

Reoperative Surgery

Extent of disease and tempo of disease progression guide the decision for reoperation in the setting of recurrence. The number of organs involved by tumor at the time of the first metastasis and length of disease-free recurrence are predictors of survival. Decisions regarding resection must be individualized, and although they likely have no effect on eventual death due to disease, survival may be prolonged in some patients. Tumor grade can influence the decision for reoperation, as those with low-grade tumors generally have a slower tempo of disease progression and reoperation may be more beneficial in these patients regarding long-term survival. In contrast, those with high-grade tumors seem to benefit less, as other sites of disease often appear quickly after resection. It is not uncommon for the authors to wait several months in the setting of questionably resectable tumors or recurrences while treating with systemic therapy to assess for tumor responsiveness and/or tempo of disease progression. If progression is not rapid, surgery may proceed with greater benefit, whereas those with evidence of marked progression of disease do not undergo surgery.

Adjuvant Therapies

For reasons detailed above, adjuvant therapies are often considered, even following surgically complete R0 resections. Mitotane, an adrenolytic agent and the only US FDA–approved therapy for ACC, has been the most well-studied adjuvant treatment in this setting. Used most frequently in patients with resected high-grade ACC, a number of studies have detailed a decrease or delay in recurrence of ACC. The utility of adjuvant mitotane in low-grade ACC has recently been studied in the ADIUVO trial (NCT00777244), which suggests little benefit over placebo in the prevention of or delay in recurrence. The current ADIUVO-2 trial (NCT03723941) is underway to assess potential added benefit of combined mitotane and cisplatin-based adjuvant therapy for high-risk (high-grade) ACC. Strategies will be discussed.

Radiation therapy for local control is debated and used by a few centers in the adjuvant setting and when residual disease, spillage, or positive margins are evident following surgery. Strategies will be discussed.

Systemic Therapies

Nonresectable disease is most often treated with mitotane and/or systemic chemotherapy. The FIRM-ACT trial (**F**irst **I**nternational **R**andomized trial in locally advanced and **M**etastatic **A**drenocortical **C**arcinoma **T**reatment) was an international randomized controlled trial that compare 2 therapeutic regimens: EDP-M (etoposide, doxorubicin, cisplatin plus mitotane) vs S-M (streptozocin plus mitotane). The investigators found a significantly better response rate and progression-free survival with EDP-M than with S-M (23.2% vs 9.2 and 5.0 months vs 2.1 months, respectively). This also underscores the limitations of chemotherapy for ACC. Radiation therapy is used to treat oligometastatic disease in select cases. While small case series have shown variable benefit (4%-20% response rates) of immunotherapy in ACC, response had not correlated with mutational burden or microsatellite instability, predicted to be in part due to intratumoral cortisol production in ACC. Combination immunotherapy and glucocorticoid inhibition is currently under investigation (NCT04373265). Strategies will be discussed.

While mitotane is an adrenolytic agent, it is not used for mere hormone control in ACC. Hormone excess is treated with endocrine therapies, most often metyrapone, osilodrostat, or levoketoconazole for cortisol excess (mifepristone is challenging to implement in this population), mineralocorticoid receptor antagonists for mineralocorticoid excess, and androgen receptor antagonists for androgen excess. Strategies will be discussed.

Genetics

Genetics increasingly has a role in the diagnosis, prognosis, and management of cancer. While genetic and genomic data are more evident in thyroid cancer and neuroendocrine cancers, genetics as it pertains to ACC is emerging and will be discussed.

Although 50% to 80% of pediatric ACC cases are due to familial pathogenic variants in the *P53* gene, resulting in Li-Fraumeni syndrome, ACC is occasionally seen in Beckwith-Wiedemann syndrome due to an imprinting defect in the *IGF2* locus. Ten percent of adults with ACC have germline pathogenic variants in *P53*, while 3% have Lynch syndrome due to pathogenic variants in mismatch repair genes. Multiple endocrine neoplasia type 1, familial adenomatous polyposis, and Carney complex have also rarely been associated with ACC. All patients with ACC are therefore screened for germline pathogenic variants associated with Li-Fraumeni syndrome and Lynch syndrome. Other cancer risk syndromes are only evaluated if there is relevant and suggestive family history.

Summary

Adrenal masses are common. All masses must be evaluated for hormone excess and assessed for risk of malignancy. ACC is rare. Most ACCs are diagnosed due to hormone excess, nonspecific abdominal pain, or incidentally. Surgery is the appropriate first-line approach for resectable disease. Adjuvant therapies, most notably mitotane, are used for ACC with high risk of recurrence. Systemic therapies, most notably mitotane and EDP-M, are used as first-line therapy for nonresectable disease. Hormonal excess is controlled with standard endocrine therapies. While genetics is increasingly important in cancer care, it is only slowly emerging to develop targeted therapies for ACC.

Clinical case vignettes
Case 1

A 30-year-old man with gastroesophageal reflux presents to the emergency department with abdominal pain and is found to have an incidental adrenal mass after workup for possible appendicitis. Noncontrast CT reveals a homogeneous 7-cm left adrenal mass with an attenuation of 17 HU.

Which of the following does this lesion most likely represent?

A. ACA
B. ACC
C. Hemorrhage
D. Metastasis to the adrenal
E. Pheochromocytoma
F. None of the above

Answer: A) ACA

Case 1 (continued)

If the mass had measured 45 HU and appeared heterogeneous on noncontrast CT, which of the following diagnoses could be ruled out?

A. ACA

B. ACC

C. Hemorrhage

D. Metastasis to the adrenal

E. Pheochromocytoma

F. None of the above

Answer: F) None of the above

Recent studies have determined that an unenhanced CT tumor attenuation cutoff of 20 HU should replace that of 10 HU for diagnosis of benign ACA and exclusion of malignancy. Tumors exhibiting greater than 20 HU remain challenging to diagnose on unenhanced CT alone and can be benign or malignant processes. While not available widely, a triple test strategy of tumor diameter, imaging characteristics, and urine steroid metabolomics can improve detection of ACC, which could shorten time to surgery for patients with ACC and help to avoid unnecessary surgery in patients with benign tumors.

References

1. Irina Bancos, Taylor AE, Chortis V, et al; ENSAT EURINE-ACT Investigators. Urine steroid metabolomics for the differential diagnosis of adrenal incidentalomas in the EURINE-ACT study: a prospective test validation study. *Lancet Diabetes Endocrinol.* 2020;8(9):773-781. PMID: 32711725

2. Fassnacht M, Arlt W, Bancos I, et al. Management of adrenal incidentalomas: European Society of Endocrinology clinical practice guideline in collaboration with the European Network for the Study of Adrenal Tumors. *Eur J Endocrinol.* 2016;175(2):G1-G34. PMID: 27390021

3. Sherlock M, Scarsbrook A, Abbas A, et al. Adrenal incidentaloma. *Endocr Rev.* 2020;41(6):775-820. PMID: 32266384

4. Bancos I, Prete A. Approach to the patient with adrenal incidentaloma. *J Clin Endocrinol Metab.* 2021;106(11):3331-3353. PMID: 34260734

Case 2

A 54-year-old woman presents with a 3-year history of new hypertension (on 3 medications), diabetes mellitus treated with metformin, and a 40-lb (18.1-kg) weight gain. She has experienced spotty irregular menses for 2 years with loss of menses for the last 5 months. She notes mild hair growth on her upper lip and chin and some mild acne on her upper back.

Laboratory test results:

> Renin, undetectable
> Aldosterone = 5 ng/dL (4-21 ng/dL)
>   (SI: 138.7 pmol/L [111.0-582.5 pmol/L])
> Urinary free cortisol = 170 µg/24 h (<90 µg/24 h)
>   (SI: 469.2 nmol/d [<248.4 nmol/d])
> Baseline ACTH = <5 pg/mL (SI: <1.1 pmol/L)
>   (undetectable)
> DHEA-S = 800 µg/dL (<200 µg/dL) (SI: 21.7 µmol/L
>   [<5.4 µmol/L])
> FSH, low-normal
> Total testosterone, normal

Which of the following is this patient's most likely diagnosis?

A. ACA

B. ACC

C. Adrenal theca metaplasia

D. Congenital adrenal hyperplasia

E. Polycystic ovary syndrome

Answer: B) ACC

This is a classic case of ACTH-independent adrenocortical hormone excess. The clue that this is not congenital adrenal hyperplasia (Answer D) is the suppressed ACTH. Benign ACTH-independent Cushing syndrome due to cortisol-secreting ACA, bilateral macronodular hyperplasia, or primary pigmented nodular adrenocortical disease with suppressed ACTH would most often have suppressed DHEA-S (an ACTH-dependent hormone). ACA routinely does not secrete multiple classes of adrenocortical hormones (other than aldosterone-secreting ACA that can co-secrete low levels of cortisol). New-onset combined ACTH-independent cortisol and DHEA-S secretion is an ominous sign of what is likely to be ACC (Answer B).

Adrenal theca metaplasia (Answer C) is a rare (albeit debated) LH-dependent development of theca-like spindle cells beneath the adrenal capsule of postmenopausal females (and males). This patient has a nonelevated FSH measurement, indicating premenopausal state.

While 20% to 30% of patients with polycystic ovary syndrome (Answer E) can present with DHEA-S elevation, this case of marked DHEA-S and cortisol elevation is pathognomonic of ACTH-independent Cushing syndrome with adrenal DHEA-S elevation.

References

1. Fassnacht M, Dekkers OM, Else T, et al. European Society of Endocrinology clinical practice guidelines on the management of adrenocortical carcinoma in adults, in collaboration with the European Network for the Study of Adrenal Tumors. *Eur J Endocrinol.* 2018;179(4):G1-G46. PMID: 30299884

2. Lerario AM, Mohan DR, Hammer GD. Update on biology and genomics of adrenocortical carcinomas: rationale for emerging therapies. *Endocr Rev.* 2022;43(6):1051-1073. PMID: 35551369

3. Fidler WJ. Ovarian thecal metaplasia in adrenal glands. *Am J Clin Pathol.* 1977;67(4):318-323. PMID: 851092

4. Wassal EY, Habra MA, Vicens R, Rao P, Elsayes KM. Ovarian thecal metaplasia of the adrenal gland in association with Beckwith-Wiedemann syndrome. *World J Radiol.* 2014;6(12):919-923. PMID: 25550997

5. Mete O, Raphael S, Pirzada A, Asa SL. Is adrenal ovarian thecal metaplasia a misnomer? Report of three cases of radial scar-like spindle cell myofibroblastic nodule of the adrenal gland. *Endocr Pathol.* 2011;22(4):222-225. PMID: 21858518

6. Witchel SF, Oberfield SE, Peña AS.J Polycystic ovary syndrome: pathophysiology, presentation, and treatment with emphasis on adolescent girls. *J Endocr Soc.* 2019;3(8):1545-1573. PMID: 31384717

Case 3

A 19-year-old woman presents with apparent androgen excess and the following laboratory test results are documented:

> DHEA-S = 4000 µg/dL (<200 µg/dL)
>   (SI: 108.4 µmol/L [<5.4 µmol/L])
> Urinary free cortisol = 30 µg/24 h (<90 µg/24 h)
>   (SI: 82.8 nmol/d [<248.4 nmol/d])
> Baseline ACTH = 25 pg/mL (10-60 pg/mL)
>   (SI: 5.5 pmol/L [2.2-13.2 pmol/L])
> Cortisol following 1-mg dexamethasone-suppression
>   test = 1.2 µg/dL (SI: 33.1 nmol/L)

She has a 9.2-cm heterogeneous right adrenal mass that is abutting vs invading liver. She undergoes open adrenalectomy and partial hepatectomy that is referred to as a surgically complete resection. The pathology report notes that the mass is not invading the liver but adrenal capsular invasion is noted with microscopic extension into periadrenal fat (Ki67 index, 23%; mitotic count, 17 mitoses/50 high-power fields [high-power fields = 100x magnification]). The mass is 9.8 cm with marked necrosis, moderate nuclear atypia, and lymphovascular invasion.

An increased recurrence risk of this surgically resected lesion is predicted by which of the following observations?

A. Androgen excess

B. Female sex

C. Microscopic extension through the adrenal capsule

D. Mitotic count 17 mitoses/50 high-power fields (high-power fields = 100x magnification)

E. Young age

Answer: C) Microscopic extension through the adrenal capsule

While genetics/genomics is beginning to optimize risk stratification of recurrence following surgical resection of a variety of cancers, including ACC, clinical and pathologic assessment remains central to current prognostication. The European Network for the Study of Adrenal Tumours (ENSAT) staging system is widely used as the standard prognostic staging tool with stage 3 disease (ACC present beyond adrenal capsule), proliferation (Ki67 >10% or mitotic count >20 mitoses/50 high-power fields [Answer C]), and autonomous cortisol excess all increasing risk of recurrent disease.

References

1. Libé R, Borget I, Ronchi CL, et al; ENSAT network. Prognostic factors in stage III-IV adrenocortical carcinomas (ACC): an European Network for the Study of Adrenal Tumor (ENSAT) study. *Ann Oncol.* 2015;26(10):2119-2125. PMID: 26392430

2. Miller BS, Gauger PG, Hammer GD, Giordano TJ, Doherty GM. Proposal for modification of the ENSAT staging system for adrenocortical carcinoma using tumor grade. *Langenbecks Arch Surg.* 2010;395(7):955-961. PMID: 20694732

3. Elhassan YS, Altieri B, Berhane S, et al. S-GRAS score for prognostic classification of adrenocortical carcinoma: an international, multicenter ENSAT study. *Eur J Endocrinol.* 2021;186(1):25-36. PMID: 34709200

4. Mohan DR, Lerario AM, Else T, et al. Targeted assessment of G0S2 methylation identifies a rapidly recurrent, routinely fatal molecular subtype of adrenocortical carcinoma. *Clin Cancer Res*. 2019;25(11):3276-3288. PMID: 30770352

5. Fassnacht M, Dekkers OM, Else T, et al. European Society of Endocrinology clinical practice guidelines on the management of adrenocortical carcinoma in adults, in collaboration with the European Network for the Study of Adrenal Tumors. *Eur J Endocrinol*. 2018;179(4):G1-G46. PMID: 30299884

6. Glenn JA, Else T, Hughes DT, et al. Longitudinal patterns of recurrence in patients with adrenocortical carcinoma. *Surgery*. 2019;165(1):186-195. PMID: 30343951

7. Else T, Williams AR, Sabolch A, Jolly S, Miller BS, Hammer GD. Adjuvant therapies and patient and tumor characteristics associated with survival of adult patients with adrenocortical carcinoma. *J Clin Endocrinol Metab*. 2014;99(2):455-461. PMID: 24302750

Case 4

Case 4a

A 30-year-old woman presents with a 4-month history of new hirsutism, acne, weight gain, and amenorrhea. She has no history of menstrual irregularities or associated symptoms, and her medical history is unremarkable. Her mother and maternal aunt both had breast cancer before age 50 years, and a maternal first cousin had nonHodgkin lymphoma.

On physical examination, the patient has facial plethora and acne, male-pattern baldness, supraclavicular fat pad, proximal muscle weakness, and purple striae. Her blood pressure is 160/100 mm Hg, and pulse rate is 100 beats/min.

CT reveals a non–lipid-rich, 6-cm right adrenal mass. Adrenal biopsy reveals SF-1 positive adrenocortical tissue. She undergoes a laparoscopic resection and is referred postoperatively to the multidisciplinary endocrine/endocrine surgery clinic for management.

Case 4b

A 59-year-old man presents with severe epigastric pain associated with sweating. He reports weight loss of 61.7 lb (28 kg), diaphoresis but no fever, and new anxiety and hypertension (treated effectively with monotherapy [ACE inhibitor]) for the last 6 months. He has a history of melanoma status post excision 2 years prior and gastroesophageal reflux disease (treated with omeprazole). His family history is significant for coronary artery disease in a brother (in his 30s) and father (deceased at age 62 years).

Physical examination findings are significant for mild cachexia and blood pressure of 160/90 mm Hg with orthostasis. Bilateral masses are palpable over the left and right upper quadrants.

CT performed in the emergency department reveals bilateral adrenal masses.

Question 1 for Cases 4a and 4b

What are the indications to biopsy an adrenal mass?

A. To diagnose ACC

B. To diagnose metastasis of existing nonadrenal cancer to the adrenal

C. To rule out pheochromocytoma

Answer: B) To diagnose metastasis of existing nonadrenal cancer to the adrenal

A pheochromocytoma is first ruled out by biomedical testing. Moreover, an adrenal mass should never be biopsied until a pheochromocytoma has been ruled out biochemically (Answer C). Adrenal biopsy is not used to diagnose ACC (Answer A) but instead is best used to distinguish adrenal tissue from nonadrenal tissue. If ACC is highly suspected, resection is the diagnostic modality of choice. We recommend biopsy only when a patient has an additional known primary malignancy and biopsy would define the new adrenal mass as the known primary malignancy vs a new second malignancy (including a primary adrenal neoplasm) (Answer B).

Question 2 for Cases 4a and 4b

Which of the following is a genetic predisposition for adrenocortical neoplasia?

A. *AIRE* pathogenic variant

B. Li-Fraumeni syndrome

C. Multiple endocrine neoplasia type 2

D. *NR0B1* (formerly *DAX1*) pathogenic variant

E. *SDHB* pathogenic variant

Answer: B) Li-Fraumeni syndrome

Question 3 for Cases 4a and 4b

Which of the following is a genetic predisposition for adrenomedullary neoplasia?

A. *AIRE* pathogenic variant

B. Li-Fraumeni syndrome

C. Multiple endocrine neoplasia type 2

D. *NR0B1* (formerly *DAX1*) pathogenic variant

E. *SDHB* pathogenic variant

Answer: E) SDHB pathogenic variant

A handful of known genetic syndromes (germline and hence inherited pathogenic variants present in all cells of the body) have been associated with an increased risk of ACC. The most common of these is Li-Fraumeni syndrome due to loss-of-function of the tumor suppressor gene *TP53*. Approximately 50% to 80% of pediatric ACC cases occur in the setting of Li-Fraumeni syndrome. Recent studies have shown that up to 7.5% of adult patients with ACC harbor germline pathogenic variants in *TP53* warranting genetic screening of all patients with newly diagnosed ACC. Another cancer syndrome—Lynch syndrome (due to pathogenic variants in the *MSH* mismatch repair genes)—is present in 3.2% of adult patients with ACC. This warrants evaluation in select patients with suspicious family histories.

Approximately 40% of patients diagnosed with pheochromocytoma/paraganglioma (PPGL) carry a germline pathogenic variant in 1 of more than 20 susceptibility genes. Half of these individuals (20% of PPGL) carry a germline pathogenic variant in 1 of the succinate dehydrogenase (*SDHx*) genes (*SDHA*, *SDHB*, *SDHC*, and *SDHD*), encoding the 4 subunits of the SDH enzyme. Susceptibility genes can predispose to childhood PPGL (*VHL, RET, SDHD, EPAS1, DLST*), syndromic PPGL (*RET, VHL, EPAS1, NF1, FH*), multiple PPGL (*SDHD, TMEM127, MAX, DLST, MDH2, GOT2*), and malignant PPGL (*SDHB, FH, SLC25A11*). The discovery of a germline pathogenic variant in one of these genes changes the patient's follow-up and allows genetic screening of affected families and the presymptomatic follow-up of relatives carrying a pathogenic variant. When a pathogenic *SDHx* variant is identified in an affected patient, genetic counseling is proposed for first-degree relatives along with lifelong surveillance for all carriers.

Multiple endocrine neoplasia (MEN) type 2 is caused by pathogenic variants in the *RET* oncogene and most often presents with medullary thyroid carcinoma, pheochromocytoma, hyperparathyroidism (MEN 2A>MEN 2B), and mucosal neuromas and marfanoid habitus (MEN 2B only).

Loss-of-function of the nuclear receptor *NR0B1* (*DAX1*) gene is responsible for cytomegalic X-linked adrenal hypoplasia.

Loss-of-function of the *AIRE1* gene is responsible for polyglandular autoimmune failure type 1, also referred to as APECED (autoimmune polyendocrinopathy-candidiasis-ectodermal dystrophy). The classic triad is hypoparathyroidism, adrenal failure, and mucocutaneous candidiasis.

References

1. Yip L, Duh QY, Wachtel H, et al. American Association of Endocrine Surgeons guidelines for adrenalectomy: executive summary. *JAMA Surg.* 2022;157(10):870-877. PMID: 35976622

2. Williams AR, Hammer GD, Else T. Transcutaneous biopsy of adrenocortical carcinoma is rarely helpful in diagnosis, potentially harmful, but does not affect patient outcome. *Eur J Endocrinol.* 2014;170(6):829-835. PMID: 24836548

3. Fassnacht M, Dekkers O, Else T, et al. European Society of Endocrinology clinical practice guidelines on the management of adrenocortical carcinoma in adults, in collaboration with the European Network for the Study of Adrenal Tumors. *Eur J Endocrinol.* 2018;179(4):G1-G46. PMID: 30299884

4. Zheng S, Cherniack AD, Dewal N, et al. Comprehensive pan-genomic characterization of adrenocortical carcinoma. *Cancer Cell.* 2016;29(5):723-736. PMID: 27165744

5. Assié G, Letouzé E, Fassnacht M, et al. Integrated genomic characterization of adrenocortical carcinoma. *Nat Genet.* 2014;46(6):607-612. PMID: 24747642

6. Raymond VM, Else T, Everett JN, Long JM, Gruber SB, Hammer GD. Prevalence of germline TP53 mutations in a prospective series of unselected patients with adrenocortical carcinoma. *J Clin Endocrinol Metab.* 2013;98(1):E119-E125. PMID: 23175693

7. Raymond VM, Everett JN, Furtado LV, et al. Adrenocortical carcinoma is a lynch syndrome-associated cancer. *J Clin Oncol.* 2013;31(24):3012-3028. PMID: 23752102

8. Fishbein L, Leshchiner I, Walter V, et al. Comprehensive molecular characterization of pheochromocytoma and paraganglioma. *Cancer Cell.* 2017;31(2):181-193. PMID: 28162975

9. Amar L, Pacak K, Steichen O, et al. International consensus on initial screening and follow-up of asymptomatic SDHx mutation carriers. *Nat Rev Endocrinol.* 2021;17(7):435-444. PMID: 34021277

Additional Recommended Reading

1. Hammer GD, Lacroix A. Treatment of adrenocortical carcinoma. In Nieman LK, Pappo AS, eds. *UpToDate* (Literature review current through January 2023).

2. Lerario AM, Mohan DR, Hammer GD. Update on biology and genomics of adrenocortical carcinomas: rationale for emerging therapies. *Endocr Rev.* 2022;43(6):1051-1073. PMID: 35551369.

3. Yip L, Duh Q-Y, Wachtel H, et al. American Association of Endocrine Surgeons guidelines for adrenalectomy: executive summary. *JAMA Surg.* 2022;157(10):870-877. PMID: 35976622

4. Fassnacht M, Dekkers OM, Else T, et al. European Society of Endocrinology clinical practice guidelines on the management of adrenocortical carcinoma in adults, in collaboration with the European Network for the Study of Adrenal Tumors. *Eur J Endocrinol.* 2018;179(4):G1-G46. PMID: 30299884

5. Else T, Williams AR, Sabolch A, Jolly S, Miller BS, Hammer GD. Adjuvant therapies, patient and tumor characteristics associated with survival of adult patients with adrenocortical carcinoma. *J Clin Endocrinol Metab.* 2014;99(2):455-461. PMID: 24302750

6. Miller BS, Gauger PG, Hammer GD, Doherty GM. Resection of adrenocortical carcinoma is less complete and local recurrence occurs sooner and more often after laparoscopic adrenalectomy than after open adrenalectomy. *Surgery.* 2012;152(6):1150-1157. PMID: 23158185

7. Zheng S, Cherniack AD, Dewal N, et al; Cancer Genome Atlas Research Network. Comprehensive pan-genomic characterization of adrenocortical carcinoma. *Cancer Cell.* 2016;30(2):363. PMID: 27505681

Pearls and Myths in the Evaluation and Management of Pheochromocytoma

Karel Pacak, MD, PhD, DSc. Section on Medical Neuroendocrinology, Developmental Endocrinology, Metabolism, Genetics, and Endocrine Oncology Affinity Group, Eunice Kennedy Shriver National Institute of Child Health and Human Development, National Institutes of Health, Bethesda, MD; Email: karel@mail.nih.gov

Educational Objectives

After reviewing this chapter, learners should be able to:

- Identify and diagnose patients with either hereditary or nonhereditary pheochromocytoma based on measurements of metanephrines (plasma or urine) and 3-methoxytyramine (plasma).

- Improve ability to identify patients with pheochromocytoma based on redefined clinical signs and symptoms.

- Properly select the appropriate functional imaging modality (PET) when localizing either a hereditary or nonhereditary pheochromocytoma.

- Determine the appropriate adrenoceptor blockade needed in patients with catecholamine-producing pheochromocytomas.

Significance of the Clinical Problem

Despite improved awareness, clinical signs and symptoms of disease, increased availability of redefined diagnostic tests/criteria, and various guidelines/expert opinions in the field, the prompt and proper diagnosis of pheochromocytoma is still largely delayed. Health care professionals should provide patients with state-of-the-art clinical and biochemical evaluation. If the presence of pheochromocytoma is strongly suggested from biochemical studies, imaging studies should follow to localize the tumor and avoid unnecessary expenditures. Potency and specific action of various adrenoceptor and other receptor/channel blockers must be considered when choosing the type of blockade to block the effects of catecholamines on various organs. Errors in interpretation of biochemical test results, in the choice of the functional imaging modality, or use of improper medication can lead to a delayed diagnosis with catastrophic consequences.

Pheochromocytomas, although rare neuroendocrine tumors, present significant health risks because they produce and often release catecholamines. Consequently, patients experience cardiovascular and other complications, some of them being devastating or lethal (eg, myocardial infarction, arrhythmias, stroke, and organ ischemia). Early recognition and treatment of these tumors is paramount.[1] In this chapter, the term *pheochromocytoma* also includes its extra-adrenal counterpart, paraganglioma, unless specified in the text.

Although more than 95% of these tumors produce catecholamines, only 70% or less *release* those catecholamines into circulation. In contrast, catecholamine metabolites (metanephrines) are continuously released from tumor cells into circulation in about 95% to 99% of patients.[2] Furthermore, metanephrines are released continuously, independent from the release of catecholamines, presenting a "winning ticket" in the biochemical evaluation of these tumors. 3-Methoxytyramine, a metabolite of dopamine, adds to the biochemical diagnosis.[3] The following mnemonics may be helpful:

- Definition: *p*heochromocytoma and *p*araganglioma: *p* = production (catecholamines)
- Diagnosis: Pheochromocyto*m*a and paraganglio*m*a: *m* = metabolism (metanephrines/3-methoxytyramine)

A familiarity with catecholamine production and metabolism, age-related upper reference limits, and drug- and other health-related conditions resulting in false-positive biochemical results undoubtedly helps providers correctly and cost-effectively diagnose affected patients.[4,5] Furthermore, the myth that metanephrines, similar to catecholamines, are primarily cleared by the kidney is incorrect because only 14% to 16% of circulating metanephrines undergo renal clearance in contrast to nearly all catecholamines, which are cleared by the kidney. Therefore, proper diagnosis of pheochromocytoma in patients with impaired kidney function should be based on the measurement of plasma metanephrines with adjusted upper reference limits being 25% to 30% higher.

Early localization of these tumors is important because most patients are candidates for curative surgery. Although CT and/or MRI are essential before any surgical procedure, at present, functional imaging with PET provides a powerful tool in detecting multifocality, recurrence, or metastatic disease.[6] Functional imaging algorithms are often used to diagnose hereditary or nonhereditary pheochromocytomas, and providers should be able to order these imaging studies accordingly.

Although many medications are currently available to treat hypertension and arrhythmias, catecholamine-specific cardiovascular abnormalities require proper use of adrenoceptor blocking and other antagonizing agents (eg,

calcium-channel blockers), often in a stepwise fashion, especially in urgent or critical situations.[7,8]

Practice Gaps

- Clinical symptoms and signs related to the presence of these tumors have been newly redefined.

- Lack of comprehensive understanding of catecholamine physiology/pathophysiology and its application in the biochemical diagnosis of pheochromocytoma.

- New knowledge regarding the role of functional imaging modalities in the diagnosis of pheochromocytoma.

- Various views of adrenoceptor blockade and its use when counteracting cardiovascular and other complications of catecholamine excess (eg, the belief that blockade is only used in the preoperative setting).

Discussion

To understand pheochromocytoma or its extra-adrenal counterpart, paraganglioma, one must understand their proper definition as catecholamine-producing tumors. Further, the latest World Health Organization classification has removed the term "benign" since all of these tumors have metastatic potential and can metastasize years after a primary tumor is removed.[1] The unequivocal sites of metastases are bones and lymph nodes. Thus, the previous myth that these tumors are mainly benign is now outdated. Furthermore, tumors that are larger than 5 cm have a higher metastatic potential regardless of their genetic background.

Although clinical signs and symptoms related to the presence of these tumors are largely nonspecific, taking a careful patient history, including a detailed physical exam, is warranted since excessive catecholamine levels point toward the signs and symptoms of these tumors. Among the 3 catecholamines produced by these tumors, epinephrine and norepinephrine typically exert organ-specific effects, whereas dopamine can paradoxically cause hypotension if produced and released into the bloodstream in very high concentrations (although this is uncommon).

Catecholamines (epinephrine and norepinephrine) exert their effects via adrenoceptors if released from a tumor in sufficient amounts into the bloodstream.[7] Tumors smaller than 1 cm in largest diameter are rarely clinically apparent unless directly manipulated or in the event that release and reuptake of catecholamines from these tumors is altered (such as by antidepressants, anesthetics, psychostimulants, etc). The myth that novel antidepressants (eg, serotonin reuptake inhibitors) do not affect norepinephrine reuptake after its release from a tumor (to a much lesser extent epinephrine) is incorrect—all inhibit catecholamine reuptake. In contrast to epinephrine, norepinephrine has a strong affinity for α1-adrenoceptors followed by β1-adrenoceptors; epinephrine has a stronger affinity for β2-adrenoceptors. Metanephrines do not exert any hemodynamic or other effects. Furthermore, in contrast to norepinephrine that is released rather continuously from a tumor, epinephrine is usually released episodically. In summary, patients with norepinephrine-producing and -releasing tumors often have sustained hypertension and tachycardia with more persistent symptoms of palpitations and tremor. In contrast, patients with epinephrine-producing tumors often present with episodic hypertension and tachycardia. However, on rare occasions, epinephrine-releasing tumors can cause hypotension.[9] Therefore, the myth that all patients with elevated metanephrines should be treated first with α-adrenoceptor followed by β-adrenoceptor blockade is, albeit rarely, not entirely correct. This is because some patients with tumors secreting exclusively epinephrine (characterized by elevated metanephrine) can present with hypotension and, in such a circumstance, initial treatment with β-adrenoceptor blockade (eg, propranolol) without initial α-adrenoceptor blockade may be warranted.

It should also be noted that chronically elevated catecholamine concentrations downregulate adrenoceptors; therefore, some patients present with normal or nearly normal blood pressure and heart rate.

According to the latest reports—and dispelling yet another myth—hypertension alone is not considered a specific sign of these tumors.[10] As recently summarized, experts have identified 4 patterns suggesting the presence of a pheochromocytoma: (1) anyone who presents with paroxysmal profuse sweating, pallor, tremor, and tachycardia, especially with episodic hypertension; (2) anyone who has episodic hypertension, stroke, tachycardia, or an arrhythmia in response to anesthesia, surgery, medications, or foods known to precipitate symptoms and signs; (3) anyone with a known pathogenic variant in one of the pheochromocytoma susceptibility genes and/or a family history of pheochromocytoma; and (4) anyone with an incidentally discovered adrenal mass or mass at an extra-adrenal location that could represent a paraganglioma. Interestingly, and somewhat different from previous observations and reports, new studies have redefined clinical features that are significantly different between patients with and without these tumors, including tachycardia (>85 beats/min), lower BMI (<25 kg/m^2), pallor, sweating, palpitations, tremor, and nausea.[10] It is the author's view and the view of others that a high clinical suspicion for these tumors is also present in patients without obesity who have drug-resistant hypertension when combined with symptoms or signs related to catecholamine excess.[11] Thus, the myth that patients with isolated drug-resistant hypertension should be evaluated for pheochromocytoma is unjustified unless these patients present with additional signs and symptoms related to catecholamine excess.

In contrast to catecholamines, metanephrines and 3-methoxytyramine became pearls in the biochemical diagnosis of these tumors.[12] To properly perform biochemical evaluation, patients should rest in a recumbent position for at least 15 to 20 minutes and have drugs held that may lead to false-positive results while addressing/limiting conditions affecting sympathetic nervous system activity (positional changes, pain, anxiety). The biochemical results should be interpreted using age-specific upper reference limits (established after supine rest) while adjusting for abnormalities in renal clearance. Taken together, these measures optimize the diagnostic accuracy of biochemical evaluation. Based on the proper understanding of catecholamine physiology applied to these tumors, as well as the sympathetic nervous system, previous myths related to (1) higher frequency of false-positive results for plasma vs urinary metanephrines is incorrect; (2) the measurement of urinary dopamine or 3-methoxytyramine is no longer recommended for the diagnosis of pheochromocytoma and paraganglioma (as most is derived from the gastrointestinal tract and diet [measured as conjugated dopamine] or the renal conversion of dihydroxyphenylalanine to dopamine [measured as free dopamine]); (3) there is minimal analytic interference by drugs measuring catecholamine metabolites with the use of liquid chromatography–tandem mass spectrometry (eg, previously recommended to stop acetaminophen at least 5 days before the test is performed). The myth that a more than 3-fold increase of free metabolites above the upper reference limits suggests the presence of pheochromocytoma or paraganglioma is now replaced by a new recommendation (based on improved analytic methods) that a more than 2-fold increase of these metabolites above the upper reference limit is suspicious and warrants further investigation.[2]

According to the latest reports and discoveries, 40% of patients with pheochromocytoma have *germline* pathogenic variants. In patients without germline variants, 40% of tumors still have similar pathogenic, in this case *somatic*, variants.[13] Thus, both patients and their tumors should be tested to identify germline and somatic pathogenic variants. The myth that patients only be tested for germline variants is now outdated. Experts, including the author of this chapter, recommend performing somatic sequence variant analysis with comprehensive genetic testing in patients with these tumors.[15] Although *SDHB* pathogenic variants are considered one of the most common risk factors linked to metastatic pheochromocytoma and paraganglioma, it is not the genetic abnormality that is the most frequently associated with metastasis. This myth is outdated since 2 genetic abnormalities (pathogenic variants in *HIF2A* [*EPAS1*] and *SDHA* genes) are now considered to be very frequently related to metastatic disease.[16,17]

Due to the presence of pheochromocytoma- and paraganglioma-specific cell membrane receptors and transporters and the introduction of several novel radiopharmaceutical agents (viewed as pearls), functional imaging of these tumors has become essential and irreplaceable in diagnostic evaluation and localization. By extension, advances in functional imaging have a large role in associated systemic radiotherapies.[1] The previous myth that all of these tumors could be imaged by the same radiopharmaceutical agent is outdated. This is well-supported by discoveries that various pathogenic variants are linked to either unique or more specific expression of receptors or transporters and, by extension, which radiopharmaceutical agent provides the most accurate imaging. This has been incorporated in the newest imaging guidelines related to these tumors recommending that cluster 1A tumors (particularly *SDH* tumors) be localized by ^{68}Ga-DOTATATE PET/CT, while cluster 1B (*VHL/EPAS1*) and cluster 2 tumors be localized by ^{18}F-fluorodopa PET/CT and ^{123}I-MIBG scintigraphy.[6] Furthermore, all head and neck paragangliomas and metastatic tumors should be detected by ^{68}Ga-DOTATATE PET/CT. Recent data also suggest that ^{18}F-fluorodopa PET/CT should be used to localize apparently sporadic pheochromocytoma.[18] Two imaging pearls currently include the detection of any primary, recurrent, or metastatic pheochromocytoma associated with polycythemia using ^{18}F-fluorodopa PET/CT and the newest use of ^{64}Cu-DOTATATE PET/CT as a promising functional modality for pheochromocytomas comparable to

^{68}Ga-DOTATATE PET/CT. The longer half-life (12.7 hours) of ^{64}Cu-DOTATATE offers a longer scanning window and the ability to perform dosimetry calculations in the near future.[19]

In the past, partial adrenalectomy in patients with pheochromocytoma was recommended whenever feasible with the goal of preserving adrenocortical function. However, this approach is not recommended for patients with *SDHB*-related pheochromocytomas due to their high metastatic potential regardless of initial size. Whether the same approach applies to *SDHA*- and *HIF2A*-pheochromocytomas is currently unknown. The rule of early surgical intervention also applies for head and neck *SDHB*-related carotid body paragangliomas that should be surgically addressed when they reach the size of 1.5 cm as compared with *SDHD*-related paragangliomas that are surgically removed when they reach the size of 2 cm.[20]

Currently, there are at least 2 targeted radionuclide therapies (pearls), ^{131}I-MIBG or peptide receptor radionuclide therapy (PRRT) using ^{177}Lu- or ^{90}Y-DOTA analogues to treat metastatic or locally advanced/inoperable pheochromocytomas.[21] The use of these therapeutic approaches is guided by positivity on either ^{123}I-MIBG scintigraphy or ^{68}Ga/^{64}Cu-DOTATATE PET/CT. The myth that systemic radiotherapy with ^{123}I-MIBG should be considered for all patients is now outdated. This is particularly important for these tumors, since most metastatic pheochromocytomas (especially those related to *SDH* pathogenic variants) are not detected on ^{123}I-MIBG scintigraphy. Nevertheless, if metastatic lesions are positive on ^{123}I-MIBG scintigraphy, high-specific activity ^{131}I-MIBG can be used for systemic therapy, as this is the only radioactive treatment for these tumors approved by the US FDA.[22] Other radiotherapeutic options are low-specific activity ^{131}I-MIBG (sometimes called conventional ^{131}I-MIBG therapy, which has been used for decades) or ^{177}Lu-DOTATATE, although neither is currently approved by the US FDA for these tumors.

Starting a patient on adrenoceptor blockade is recommended in various clinical contexts. These include the moment that a catecholamine-producing pheochromocytoma is biochemically suggested and preparation before any surgical procedure, potential manipulation of a tumor, the surgical procedure itself, or the administration of certain medications (eg, antidepressants, steroids, psychostimulants). Recent reports suggest that adrenoceptor blockade is not necessary for patients with these tumors, even in preparation for surgery since anesthesiologists can easily manage catecholamine-induced variations in blood pressure and heart rate/rhythm. In the author's view, the conclusions of these reports need to be further validated. Although not every adrenoceptor blocker given to a patient before a procedure can fully counteract the effect of enormous amounts of catecholamines released during tumor manipulation, such blockade can mitigate (although not always) deleterious catecholamine effects, especially when correctly administered in a timely fashion. It is our experience and opinion that this approach upholds the Hippocratic oath "*primum non nocere*" (first, do no harm).[23] Thus, the myth related to the use of adrenoceptor blockade in patients with catecholamine-producing pheochromocytoma is currently valid and still well accepted in clinical practice.[3]

Clinical Case Vignettes
Case 1

A 45-year-old woman with metastatic and inoperable pheochromocytoma who has a germline *VHL* pathogenic variant is currently treated with doxazosin, 16 mg twice daily, and metoprolol succinate, 100 mg twice daily. She has been closely followed in clinic and now presents for her third visit within the last month with persistent sinus tachycardia (pulse rate, 110 beats/min) and hypertension (blood pressure, 150/95 mm Hg).

Which of the following is the best next step in this patient's management?

A. Add diltiazem

B. Add verapamil

C. Switch doxazosin to phenoxybenzamine

D. Switch metoprolol succinate to carvedilol

Answer: B) Add verapamil

Verapamil should be added to this patient's regimen (Answer B), as it is effective in treating both sinus tachycardia and hypertension. Moreover, the patient is on the maximum dosage of doxazosin (32 mg daily) and metoprolol succinate (200 mg daily). Providers do increase the dosages past their maximum, although this is not routinely advised. Phenoxybenzamine may treat her hypertension, but it may worsen sinus tachycardia because it can cause a decrease in blood pressure/vasodilation that can lead to reflex tachycardia. Diltiazem (Answer A) may treat sinus tachycardia, but it is not as effective as verapamil in treating hypertension (it is less potent).

Case 1 (continued)

After 3 years of effective treatment, the patient presents with persistent sinus tachycardia and hypertension. Her plasma normetanephrine concentration is now increased from 5 times the upper reference limit (last year) to 25 times the upper reference limit.

Which of the following is the best next step in this patient's management?

A. Add clonidine

B. Add metyrosine

C. Switch doxazosin to phenoxybenzamine

D. Switch metoprolol succinate to carvedilol

Answer: B) Add metyrosine

This patient has had a dramatic increase in plasma normetanephrine suggesting progression of her underlying disease. Metyrosine (Answer B) can benefit this patient, as it inhibits the synthesis of catecholamines (here, particularly norepinephrine)

and thus would be able to treat both the sinus tachycardia and hypertension that result from them.

Switching from one β-adrenoceptor blocker to another (metoprolol to carvedilol [Answer D]) may provide some benefit, especially for tachycardia, but this would likely not afford as much benefit as metyrosine.

Clonidine (Answer A), an α_2-adrenoceptor agonist, may, in certain circumstances, cause some α_1-adrenoceptor stimulation. as well as rebound hypertension (when stopped) and is not advised in patients with pheochromocytoma.

Compared with doxazosin, phenoxybenzamine (Answer C) would likely provide superior control of hypertension. However, this benefit may be offset, as it may worsen sinus tachycardia in this patient.

Case 1 (continued)

After the patient is treated with metyrosine, her hypertension and sinus tachycardia improve, but she subsequently develops catecholamine-induced cardiomyopathy and is found to have a left ventricular ejection fraction of 30%. A cardiologist prescribes maximally tolerated dosages of goal-directed medical therapy, which includes her prior medication of metoprolol, 100 mg twice daily. Plasma metanephrines are measured, and normetanephrine demonstrates a further rise to 50 times the upper reference limit. She presents to the clinic with anxiety and palpitations and is found to have a heart rate of 120 beats/min and blood pressure of 115/85 mm Hg. Electrocardiography demonstrates a rhythm of sinus tachycardia. She is otherwise euvolemic.

Which of the following is the best next step to manage catecholamine-induced sinus tachycardia in this setting?

A. Add clonidine

B. Add ivabradine

C. Switch metoprolol succinate to bisoprolol

D. Switch metoprolol succinate to labetalol

Answer: B) Add ivabradine

In this circumstance, the patient presents with compensated heart failure for which she is already on goal-directed medical therapy and now has worsening norepinephrine-induced sinus tachycardia. In this situation, changing metoprolol succinate to bisoprolol (Answer C) would offer minimal benefit, as both are long-acting β-adrenoceptor–blocking agents. Additionally, switching metoprolol succinate to labetalol (Answer D) would not be advised, as it would offer minimal additional benefit and its β-adrenoceptor–blocking effect would not address the sinus tachycardia.

Clonidine (Answer A) should be avoided in patients with pheochromocytoma given the reasons stated above.

Ivabradine (Answer B) is a newer HCN (hyperpolarization-activated cyclic nucleotide-gated) channel inhibitor that can treat sinus tachycardia in patients with heart failure already on maximally tolerated doses of β-adrenoceptor blocking agents. Ivabradine acts solely on the sinoatrial node, which acts as the dominant pacemaker and is vital to heart-rate control.[24]

Case 2

A 34-year-old man presents to his primary care physician with swelling in the right side of his neck and coughing whenever he laughs. He has no symptoms or signs associated with catecholamine excess such as headache, sweating, flushing, palpitations, or elevated blood pressure. In the physician's office, his pulse rate is 61 beats/min and blood pressure is 138/60 mm Hg. Neck ultrasonography is performed, which identifies a 3.4 × 2.1 × 3.2-cm mass at the right carotid artery bifurcation.

Which of the following is the best next step in this patient's management?

A. Biochemical evaluation of plasma/urinary metanephrines
B. Genetic testing
C. Neck CT/MRI
D. Surgical consult
E. Whole-body imaging with CT/MRI

Answer: A) Biochemical evaluation of plasma/urinary metanephrines

The best step in the evaluation of a tumor at the carotid artery bifurcation is biochemical measurement of plasma/urinary metanephrines (Answer A). This patient had an elevated normetanephrine concentration (645 pg/mL [SI: 3.52 nmol/L]; reference range, 18-112 pg/mL [SI: 0.10-0.61 nmol/L]). Metanephrine concentrations were within the reference range. Therefore, a diagnosis of right carotid body paraganglioma was highly suspected.

Case 2 (continued)

Which of the following is the best next step in this patient's management?

A. α-Adrenoceptor blockade
B. Genetic testing
C. Neck CT/MRI
D. Surgical consult
E. Whole-body imaging with CT/MRI

Answer: A) α-Adrenoceptor blockade

The best next step in this patient's management is to appropriately block with α-adrenoceptor blockade (Answer A) before further imaging is performed.

Case 2 (continued)

The patient is started on phenoxybenzamine, 10 mg twice daily, which is then adjusted to 10 mg once daily after he reports fatigue, dizziness, and frequent episodes of hypotension following its initiation.

Which of the following is the best next step in this patient's management?

A. Genetic testing
B. Neck CT/MRI
C. Surgical consult
D. Whole-body imaging with CT/MRI
E. Whole-body imaging with ^{68}Ga-DOTATATE PET/CT

Answer: D) Whole-body imaging with CT/MRI

The best next step in management is to evaluate this patient with whole-body anatomic imaging with CT/MRI (Answer D). Because he has strikingly elevated normetanephrine not typically seen in head and neck paragangliomas, there is a high likelihood that a pheochromocytoma or paraganglioma is present outside of the head and neck region and/or that the primary tumor metastasized.

Case 2 (continued)

Neck CT confirms the location of a 2.5 × 2.1-cm tumor at the right carotid artery bifurcation (*arrow, figure 1A*), and abdominal CT reveals a 2.9 × 2.5-cm heterogeneous enhancing mass (*arrow, figure 1B*) in the left retroperitoneum along the left margin of the aorta.

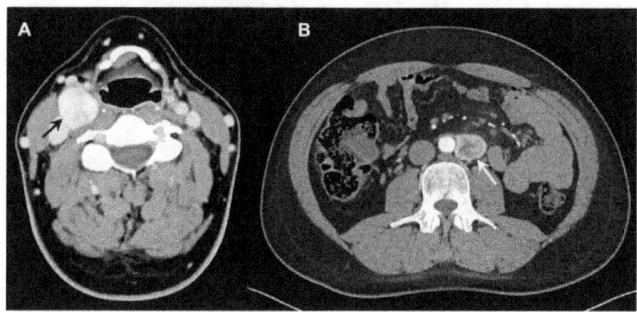

Figure 1. Select cross-sectional CT images of the neck (*panel A*) and abdomen (*panel B*).

No other tumors or metastases are identified. Notably, the myth of using adrenoceptor blockade in a patient with a catecholamine-producing pheochromocytoma before contrast CT is performed is not valid anymore because current contrast dyes do not provoke catecholamine release.

Which of the following is the best next step in this patient's management?

A. Genetic testing

B. Multidisciplinary tumor board discussion

C. Surgical consult

D. Whole-body imaging with ^{68}Ga-DOTATATE PET/CT

E. Whole-body imaging with ^{123}I-MIBG scintigraphy

Answer: D) Whole-body imaging with ^{68}Ga-DOTATATE PET/CT

Ga-68-DOTATATE PET/CT (Answer D) was performed and revealed 2 additional foci on the left side of the neck (*dotted and dashed arrows, figure 2 on 2A, 2B, and 2D*).

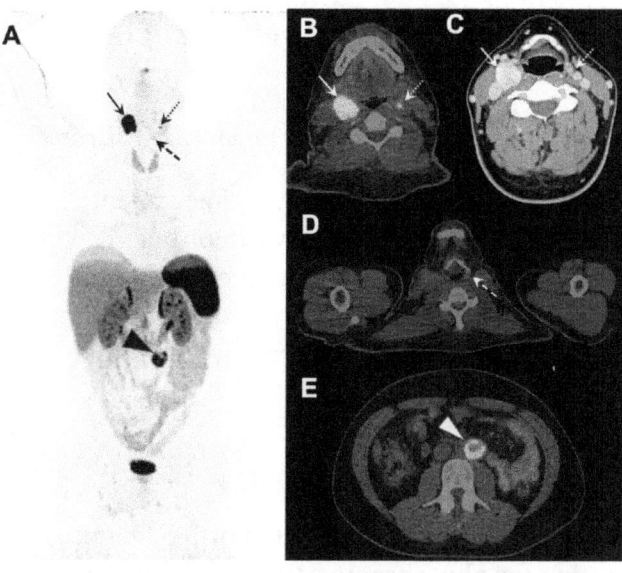

Figure 2. Whole-body (*panel A*) ^{68}Ga-DOTATATE PET/CT and select cross-sectional images (*panels B-E*). (Color—web and EPUB only)

One of these very small 2 additional foci is located at the left carotid artery bifurcation (*dotted arrows, figure 2A and 2B*), and its anatomic correlate is found retrospectively on CT (*dotted arrow, figure 2C*) following initial localization with ^{68}Ga-DOTATATE PET/CT. The second additional focus is located near the left hyoid bone (*dashed arrows, figure 2A and 2D*) whose anatomic correlate on CT cannot be found despite its known location on ^{68}Ga-DOTATATE PET/CT. Ga-68-DOTATATE PET/CT identifies a right carotid body tumor (*solid arrows, figure 2A, 2B, 2C*) and retroperitoneal paraganglioma (*arrowheads, figure 2A and 2E*), which are also demonstrated on CT (*figure 1*).

Case 2 (continued)

Which of the following is the best next step in this patient's management?

A. Genetic testing
B. ^{177}Lu-DOTATATE therapy due to ^{68}Ga-DOTATATE–avid lesions
C. Multidisciplinary tumor board discussion
D. Surgical consult
E. Whole-body imaging with ^{123}I-MIBG scintigraphy

Answer: C) Multidisciplinary tumor board discussion

The next step in this patient's management is to hold a multidisciplinary tumor board meeting (Answer C) consisting of physicians from endocrinology, surgery, oncology, nuclear medicine, and radiation oncology to discuss therapeutic options.

Case 2 (continued)

In this meeting, it is decided to order genetic testing for pheochromocytoma susceptibility genes and surgically resect the right carotid body and retroperitoneal paragangliomas. Further, additional foci (*dotted and dashed arrows, figure 2*) detected on ^{68}Ga-DOTATATE PET/CT do not require any intervention, as they are small and close follow-up at this stage is adequate.

How should surgery be approached?

A. First, resect the right carotid body paraganglioma and then the retroperitoneal paraganglioma
B. First, resect the retroperitoneal paraganglioma and then the right carotid body paraganglioma
C. Either paraganglioma can be resected first, and staged procedures are unnecessary
D. Both paragangliomas should be simultaneously resected in the same operative intervention

Answer: B) First, resect the retroperitoneal paraganglioma and then the right carotid body paraganglioma

In such a scenario, staged resection is critical to minimize potential morbidity. The retroperitoneal paraganglioma must be resected first (Answer B) due to the risk of perioperative hypertensive crisis and tachyarrhythmia, as this tumor is most likely the secretory source (less than 5% of head and neck paragangliomas produce norepinephrine/normetanephrine). After recovery from the first surgery, the right carotid body resection should be performed. Genetic testing before surgery did not reveal a pathogenic variant in any of the pheochromocytoma susceptibility genes. The patient underwent successful staged resection of his retroperitoneal paraganglioma first, and the right carotid body paraganglioma second.

Case 2 (continued)

What should be included in the follow-up of this patient in addition to history, physical examination, and heart rate/blood pressure measurements?

A. CT/MRI of the neck to monitor the unresected lesions
B. Whole-body CT/MRI in 3 to 6 months
C. Biochemical evaluation of plasma/urinary metanephrines in 3 to 6 months
D. ^{68}Ga-DOTATATE PET/CT
E. CT/MRI of the neck to monitor the unresected lesions and biochemical evaluation of plasma/urinary metanephrines in 3 to 6 months
F. Whole-body CT/MRI in 3 to 6 months and biochemical evaluation of plasma/urinary metanephrines in 3 to 6 months
G. Biochemical evaluation of plasma/urinary metanephrines in 3 to 6 months and ^{68}Ga-DOTATATE PET/CT

Answer: F) Whole-body CT/MRI in 3 to 6 months and biochemical evaluation of plasma/urinary metanephrines in 3 to 6 months

Both whole-body imaging with CT/MRI and biochemical evaluation of plasma/urinary metanephrines to detect recurrence and growth of the unresected lesions 3 to 6 months after surgery (Answer F) is recommended. Ga-68-DOTATATE PET/CT can be included for follow-up in patients with metastases or in patients with pathogenic variants in genes frequently associated with metastatic disease.[6]

Case 3

A 40-year-old woman has a 0.9-cm left adrenal mass incidentally discovered on CT (Hounsfield units = 18). She is in excellent health except for occasional palpitations and sweating, attributed to her high-stress occupation. Blood pressure and heart rate are in their respective reference ranges, as are plasma catecholamines, cortisol, and aldosterone. It is concluded that she does not have a pheochromocytoma. She is supposed to undergo spine surgery 2 months later.

Which of the following is the best next step in this patient's management?

A. Initiate adrenoceptor blockade before spine surgery

B. Measure plasma metanephrines

C. Proceed with functional imaging (PET) to better characterize the mass

D. Proceed with surgery as planned

Answer: B) Measure plasma metanephrines

Although more than 95% of pheochromocytomas produce catecholamines, only about 70% of these tumors release catecholamines into circulation due to efficient intratumoral metabolism of catecholamines into metanephrines and other metabolites. Furthermore, catecholamines are often released episodically from tumors, whereas metanephrines are released continuously. Moreover, elevated metanephrines measured by liquid chromatography–tandem mass spectrometry can detect tumors that are about 0.6 cm and larger, whereas elevated catecholamines can detect tumors that are 1.0 to 1.5 cm and larger. Thus, plasma metanephrines should be measured in this case (Answer B).

Case 3 (continued)

The patient was taken to the operating room, and after anesthesia was induced, she experienced severe hypertension (167/105 mm Hg) and tachycardia (119 beats/min). Surgery was canceled, and further evaluation for pheochromocytoma was recommended. Subsequent evaluation revealed an elevated plasma metanephrine concentration of 89 pg/mL (SI: 0.45 nmol/L) (upper reference limit = 61 pg/mL [0.31 nmol/L]) and confirmed the presence of a small left adrenal pheochromocytoma.

Which of the following is the best next step in this patient's management?

A. Initiate adrenoceptor blockade before spine surgery

B. Proceed with adrenal MRI to further characterize the mass

C. Proceed with functional imaging (PET) to better characterize the mass

Answer: A) Initiate adrenoceptor blockade before spine surgery

All patients with catecholamine-producing pheochromocytomas—regardless of whether catecholamines are elevated in plasma or urine—should be given adrenoceptor blockade (Answer A) as the first choice (rarely calcium-channel blockers can be used as monotherapy) before surgery based on an Endocrine Society clinical practice guideline and a position statement and consensus of the Working Group on Endocrine Hypertension of the European Society of Hypertension. Optimally, adrenoceptor blockade should be initiated 7 to 14 days before surgery. Treatment should also include a high-sodium diet and fluid intake to reverse catecholamine-induced blood volume contraction preoperatively to prevent severe hypotension after tumor removal. However, if surgery is planned for a later date, many experts recommend that all patients with catecholamine-producing tumors be given appropriate blockade at the initial diagnosis of these tumors.

Key Learning Points

- Pheochromocytomas are defined as catecholamine-producing (not as catecholamine-secreting) tumors. All pheochromocytomas have metastatic potential, and therefore the term "benign" should not be used. Tumor size matters, and all pheochromocytomas larger than 5 cm have a high metastatic potential.

- The following clinical features are significantly more prevalent in patients with rather than without pheochromocytoma: tachycardia, palpitations, lower BMI, pallor, sweating, tremor, and nausea.

- In patients with a higher likelihood of having pheochromocytoma (eg, an adrenal mass/incidentaloma or a genetic predisposition with typical clinical features), plasma metanephrines have a slightly better diagnostic value over urinary metanephrines. The measurement of plasma or urinary catecholamines is inferior to the measurement of plasma or urinary metanephrines. Urinary dopamine and 3-methoxytyramine have very limited value in the diagnosis of this tumor and are not recommended.

- Pheochromocytomas are mainly divided into 2 clinically relevant main clusters (1 [A and B] and 2). Cluster 1A tumors are well localized by ^{68}Ga-DOTATATE PET/CT, and cluster 1B and cluster 2 tumors are well localized by ^{18}F-fluorodopa PET/CT or ^{123}I-MIBG scintigraphy. All patients with suspected metastatic disease or head and neck paragangliomas should undergo ^{68}Ga-DOTATATE PET/CT.

- Adrenoceptor or other blockade to counteract catecholamine action on various organs should not only be used for surgery/tumor manipulation/anesthesia, but also as soon as the presence of a pheochromocytoma is proven. Pheochromocytomas can release excessive amounts of catecholamines in an unpredictable way at any time. A stepwise approach is recommended with adrenoceptor and other blockades (eg, calcium-channel blockers, HCN-channel blockers) in the treatment of tachyarrhythmias and hypertension.

- Systemic radiotherapies are not significantly affected by kidney function and can be used in patients with kidney insufficiency. Those radiotherapies, however, cause bone marrow suppression (HSA ^{131}I-MIBG to a higher degree than ^{177}Lu-DOTATATE) and catecholamine release (^{177}Lu-DOTATATE to a higher degree than HSA ^{131}I-MIBG). Therefore, their selection must be carefully considered in patients with abnormal bone marrow function and/or high metanephrine levels.

Acknowledgment

Thank you M. Nazari, A. Jha, J. Lenders, and L. Meuter for valuable comments and suggestions in the preparation of this chapter.

Funding

This study was funded by the National Institutes of Health (grant number Z1AHD008735) awarded to Karel Pacak. This work was supported by the Intramural Research Program of the National Institutes of Health, *Eunice Kennedy Shriver* National Institute of Child Health and Human Development.

Competing Interests

The author declares that there is no conflict of interest that could be perceived as prejudicing the impartiality of the research reported.

authorized under the domestic laws of the relevant country, subject to a paid-up, nonexclusive, irrevocable worldwide license to the United States in such copyrighted work to reproduce, prepare derivative works, distribute copies to the public and perform publicly and display publicly the work, and to permit others to do so.

References

1. Pacak K. New biology of pheochromocytoma and paraganglioma. *Endocr Pract.* 2022;28(12):1253-1269. PMID: 36150627

2. Eisenhofer G, Prejbisz A, Peitzsch M, et al. Biochemical diagnosis of chromaffin cell tumors in patients at high and low risk of disease: plasma versus urinary rree or deconjugated O-methylated catecholamine metabolites. *Clin Chem.* 2018;64(11):1646-1656. PMID: 30097498

3. Lenders JWM, Kerstens MN, Amar L, et al. Genetics, diagnosis, management and future directions of research of phaeochromocytoma and paraganglioma: a position statement and consensus of the Working Group on Endocrine Hypertension of the European Society of Hypertension. *J Hypertens.* 2020;38(8):1443-1456. PMID: 32412940

4. Eisenhofer G, Peitzsch M, Bechmann N, Huebner A. Biochemical diagnosis of catecholamine-producing tumors of childhood: neuroblastoma, pheochromocytoma and paraganglioma. *Front Endocrinol (Lausanne).* 2022;13:901760. PMID: 35957826

5. Remde H, Pamporaki C, Quinkler M, et al. Improved diagnostic accuracy of clonidine suppression testing using an age-related cutoff for plasma normetanephrine. *Hypertension.* 2022;79(6):1257-1264. PMID: 35378989

6. Taieb D, Hicks RJ, Hindie E, et al. European Association of Nuclear Medicine Practice Guideline/Society of Nuclear Medicine and Molecular Imaging Procedure Standard 2019 for radionuclide imaging of phaeochromocytoma and paraganglioma. *Eur J Nucl Med Mol Imaging.* 2019;46(10):2112-2137. PMID: 31254038

7. Nazari MA, Rosenblum JS, Haigney MC, Rosing DR, Pacak K. Pathophysiology and acute management of tachyarrhythmias in pheochromocytoma: JACC Review Topic of the Week. *J Am Coll Cardiol.* 2020;74:451-464. PMID: 32703516

8. Berends AMA, Kerstens MN, Lenders JWM, Timmers HJLM. Approach to the patient: perioperative management of the patient with pheochromocytoma or sympathetic paraganglioma. *J Clin Endocrinol Metab.* 2020;105(9):dgaa441. PMID: 32726444

9. Kantorovich V, Pacak K. A new concept of unopposed beta-adrenergic overstimulation in a patient with pheochromocytoma. *Ann Intern Med.* 2005;142(12 Pt 1):1026-1028. PMID: 15968023

10. Geroula A, Deutschbein T, Langton K, et al. Pheochromocytoma and paraganglioma: clinical feature-based disease probability in relation to catecholamine biochemistry and reason for disease suspicion. *Eur J Endocrinol.* 2019;181(4):409-420. PMID: 31370000

11. Martell N, Rodriguez-Cerrillo M, Grobbee DE, et al. High prevalence of secondary hypertension and insulin resistance in patients with refractory hypertension. *Blood Press.* 2003;12(3):149-154. PMID: 12875476

12. Eisenhofer G, Lenders J, Linehan W, Walther M, Goldstein D, Keiser H. Plasma normetanephrine and metanephrine for detecting pheochromocytoma in von Hippel-Lindau disease and multiple endocrine neoplasia type 2. *N Engl J Med.* 1999;340(24):1872-1879. PMID: 10369850

13. Peitzsch M, Novos T, Kaden D, et al. Harmonization of LC-MS/MS measurements of plasma free normetanephrine, metanephrine, and 3-methoxytyramine. *Clin Chem.* 2021;67(8):1098-1112. PMID: 33993248

14. Fishbein L, Leshchiner I, Walter V, et al. Comprehensive molecular characterization of pheochromocytoma and paraganglioma. *Cancer Cell.* 2017;31(2):181-193. PMID: 28162975

15. NGS in PPGL (NGSnPPGL) Study Group; Toledo RA, Burnichon N, et al. Consensus statement on next-generation-sequencing-based diagnostic testing of hereditary phaeochromocytomas and paragangliomas. *Nat Rev Endocrinol.* 2017;13(4):233-247. PMID: 27857127

16. Darr R, Nambuba J, Del Rivero J, et al. Novel insights into the polycythemia-paraganglioma-somatostatinoma syndrome. *Endocr Relat Cancer.* 2016;23(12):899-908. PMID: 27679736

17. Jha A, de Luna K, Balili CA, et al. Clinical, diagnostic, and treatment characteristics of *SDHA*-related metastatic pheochromocytoma and paraganglioma. *Front Oncol.* 2019;9:53. PMID: 30854332

18. Jha A, Patel M, Carrasquillo JA, et al. Sporadic primary pheochromocytoma: a prospective intraindividual comparison of six imaging tests (CT, MRI, and PET/CT Using (68)Ga-DOTATATE, FDG, (18)F-FDOPA, and (18)F-FDA). *AJR Am J Roentgenol.* 2022;218(2):342-350. PMID: 34431366

19. Jha A, Patel M, Carrasquillo JA, et al. Choice is good at times: the emergence of [(64)Cu]Cu-DOTATATE-based somatostatin receptor imaging in the era of [(68)Ga]Ga-DOTATATE. *J Nucl Med.* 2022;63(9):1300-1301. PMID: 35618479

20. Ellis RJ, Patel D, Prodanov T, Nilubol N, Pacak K, Kebebew E. The presence of SDHB mutations should modify surgical indications for carotid body paragangliomas. *Ann Surg.* 2014;260(1):158-162. PMID: 24169168

21. Jha A, Taieb D, Carrasquillo JA, et al. High-specific-activity (131)I-MIBG vs (177)Lu-DOTATATE targeted radionuclide therapy for metastatic pheochromocytoma and paraganglioma. *Clin Cancer Res.* 2021;27(11):2989-2995. PMID: 33685867

22. Jimenez C, Erwin W, Chasen B. Targeted radionuclide therapy for patients with metastatic pheochromocytoma and paraganglioma: from low-specific-activity to high-specific-activity iodine-131 metaiodobenzylguanidine. *Cancers (Basel).* 2019;11(7):1018. PMID: 31330766

23. Wolf KI, Santos JRU, Pacak K. Why take the risk? We only live once: the dangers associated with neglecting a pre-operative alpha adrenoceptor blockade in pheochromocytoma patients. *Endocr Pract.* 2019;25(1):106-108. PMID: 30289301

24. Malaza G, Brofferio A, Lin F, Pacak K. Ivabradine in catecholamine-induced tachycardia in a patient with paraganglioma. *N Engl J Med.* 2019;380(13):1284-1286. PMID: 30917266

Primary Aldosteronism: When and How to Test for It?

Adina F. Turcu, MD, MS. Division of Metabolism, Endocrinology, and Diabetes, University of Michigan, Ann Arbor, MI; Email: aturcu@umich.edu

Educational Objectives

After reviewing this chapter, learners should be able to:

- Identify candidates for primary aldosteronism (PA) screening.

- Interpret results of PA screening tests.

- Guide and interpret testing for PA diagnosis and subtyping.

Significance of the Clinical Problem

PA is highly prevalent among individuals with hypertension, but it is largely underrecognized. PA is a modifiable risk factor for cardiovascular and renal morbidity and mortality. At a minimum, screening for PA with simultaneous measurement of plasma aldosterone and renin should be pursued in patients with treatment-resistant hypertension; hypertension and hypokalemia (spontaneous or provoked by diuretics); and hypertension and adrenal nodules. While PA screening results are best interpreted in the absence of factors that can alter the renin-angiotensin-aldosterone system (RAAS), including a variety of antihypertensive medications, screening at the time of outpatient visits, without preceding preparations, often captures severe PA cases. An aldosterone-suppression test, with oral or intravenous salt loading, captopril, or fludrocortisone, typically follows positive screening results, to establish or exclude the diagnosis of PA. Selecting a confirmatory test is typically based on local resources and experience, feasibility, patient preference, and comorbidities. Following diagnosis confirmation, PA is subclassified as lateralized or bilateral based on adrenal vein sampling (AVS). Cross-sectional imaging can guide PA subtyping in patients younger than 35 years who have a solitary adrenal nodule. Patients with lateralized PA can be cured with unilateral adrenalectomy. Medical therapy incorporating a mineralocorticoid receptor antagonist is used in patients with PA who are not surgical candidates.

The complexity of PA testing and subtyping demands access to expertise and discourages broad implementation of PA screening. Where resources are lacking, a pragmatic approach would be to initiate a mineralocorticoid receptor antagonist in all patients with low-renin hypertension.

PA is a common cause of secondary hypertension, estimated to affect about 10% of individuals with hypertension, and more than 20% of those with apparent treatment-resistant hypertension.[1,2] PA is associated with higher renal and cardiovascular morbidity and mortality than equivalent primary hypertension.[3] Individuals with PA have higher rates of coronary artery disease,[4-6] atrial fibrillation,[4,6-8] stroke,[4,6,7] left ventricular hypertrophy and/or heart failure,[4,6,7] insulin resistance,[6,7] renal insufficiency, bone loss,[9] and depression and anxiety[10] than patients with primary hypertension with similar risk factors. PA-directed therapy can mitigate the excessive cardiovascular and renal risk.[6,11]

Expert guidelines recommend screening for PA in populations at risk, including those with treatment-resistant hypertension, hypertension and hypokalemia (either spontaneous or induced by diuretics), obstructive sleep apnea, or an adrenal mass.[12,13] Most patients at risk, however, are never tested for PA. For example, of patients with treatment-resistant hypertension seen across the US Veterans Health Administration or in referral academic centers, only approximately 3% were reportedly tested for PA.[14,15] In a retrospective population study conducted in Ontario, Canada, only 1.6% of adults with hypertension and hypokalemia underwent testing for PA.[16] Misperception regarding PA prevalence, complexity of testing and results interpretation, and clinic time constraints might be contributing to PA underdiagnosis.[17]

Practice Gaps

- Low awareness of PA prevalence and disease-specific complications.

- High complexity of PA diagnostic tests, prerequisites, and result interpretation.

- Lack of uniformity for PA testing and result interpretation.

- Limited access to expertise in PA diagnosis, subtyping, and treatment.

Discussion

PA Screening

The standard approach for PA screening consists of concomitant measurement of plasma or serum aldosterone and renin. Adjudicating the tandem aldosterone and renin as positive or negative PA screening hinges, however, on a number of variables, including assay and hormonal variability,[18] thresholds used, posture, time of the day, salt intake, comorbidities, and many medications (*table 1*). Ideally, aldosterone and renin measurements should be standardized and conducted in the absence of interfering medications. This approach, however, is not always feasible, due to logistical complexity and concern for complications. Given the wide availability and affordability of aldosterone and

renin assays, routine testing should be conducted, without concerns for interfering factors, as profound PA is often evident on circumstantial screening.[19] Retesting after medication adjustments can be considered if initial results are ambiguous, particularly if renin is not suppressed.

Table 1. Medications That Can Alter PA Screening Results

Medications	Effect on		
	Plasma aldosterone	Plasma renin	Aldosterone-to-renin ratio
Calcium-channel blockers	↔↓	↑	↓
ACE inhibitors and ARBs	↓	↑↑	↓
Potassium-sparing diuretic	↑	↑↑	↓
Potassium-wasting diuretic	↔↑	↑↑	↓
β-adrenergic receptor blockers	↓	↓↓	↑
Central α2 agonists	↓	↓↓	↑
Direct renin inhibitors	↔↓	↓↓	↑
Estrogens	↔	↓*	↑
NSAIDs	↓	↓↓	↑

Abbreviations: ACE, angiotensin-converting enzyme; ARBs, angiotensin II type 1 receptor blockers; NSAIDs, nonsteroidal anti-inflammatory drugs

* Only affects direct renin concentration assays, but not renin activity assays.

Reprinted with permission from Wannachalee T et al. *Curr Hypertens Rep*, 2022; 24(5): 123–132. © The Authors, under exclusive license to Springer Science+Business Media, LLC, part of Springer Nature.

Confirmatory Tests

A confirmatory test is recommended in most patients with positive PA screening results. Available confirmatory tests include oral or intravenous salt-loading tests, captopril challenge test, and fludrocortisone-suppression test, each with advantages and disadvantages (*table 2*).[20] Selecting a confirmatory test is often based on local resources and experience, but also on patient-related considerations, such as comorbidities and ensuing risk for complications.

Table 2. Confirmatory Tests for Primary Aldosteronism

Test	Procedure	Interpretation	Remarks
Recumbent saline infusion test	Intravenous infusion of 2 L of 0.9% saline over 4 hours in supine position	PAC >10 ng/dL: confirmed PA PAC 5-10 ng/dL: indeterminate PAC <5 ng/dL: PA unlikely	• Increased risk of volume overload and uncontrolled hypertension • Low sensitivity
Seated saline infusion test	Intravenous infusion of 2 liters of 0.9% saline over 4 hours in seated position	PAC >6 ng/dL: confirmed PA	• Increased risk of volume overload and uncontrolled hypertension • Higher sensitivity than recumbent saline infusion test
Oral salt-loading test	6 g/day of oral sodium intake for 3 consecutive days	24-hour urinary aldosterone >12 µg/24 h while 24-hour urinary sodium >200 mEq/24 h: confirmed PA	• Increased risk of volume overload and uncontrolled hypertension • False-negative in patients with kidney disease • Relies on patient's adherence
Captopril challenge test	Captopril, 25-50 mg	PAC suppressed by <30% and suppressed PRA: confirmed PA	• High false-negative rates
Fludrocortisone-suppression test	0.1 mg of oral fludrocortisone every 6 hours for 4 days with slow-released KCl and NaCl supplements	PAC >6 ng/dL and PRA <1 [ng / (mL × h)] on day 4 at 10:00 AM, and plasma cortisol at 10:00 AM less than at 07:00 AM: confirmed PA	• High sensitivity • Typically requires hospitalization • Increased risk of severe hypokalemia and/or uncontrolled hypertension

Abbreviations: PA, primary aldosteronism; PAC, plasma aldosterone concentration; PRA, plasma renin activity; KCl, potassium chloride; NaCl, sodium chloride.

Reprinted with permission from Wannachalee T et al. *Curr Hypertens Rep*, 2022; 24(5): 123–132. © The Authors, under exclusive license to Springer Science+Business Media, LLC, part of Springer Nature.

Confirmatory testing can be bypassed in patients with severe PA, as suggested by a plasma aldosterone concentration greater than 20 ng/dL (>554.8 pmol/L), suppressed renin (plasma renin activity <1 ng/mL per h or equivalent direct renin concentration), and hypokalemia, as well as in patients who do not have access to or are not candidates for AVS and/or adrenalectomy.

PA Subtyping

Most PA cases are sporadic and are caused by aldosterone-driver somatic pathogenic variants. Rare forms of familial PA are caused by a *CYP11B1/CYP11B2* chimeric gene (familial hyperaldosteronism type I or glucocorticoid-remediable aldosteronism) or by germline pathogenic variants in *CLCN2* (familial hyperaldosteronism type II), *KCNJ5* (familial hyperaldosteronism type III), *CACNA1H* (familial hyperaldosteronism type IV), or *CACNA1D* (primary aldosteronism with seizures and neurologic abnormalities, PASNA).

Sporadic PA is broadly subclassified into bilateral forms and unilateral (or lateralized) PA. Lateralized PA has been attributed mostly to solitary aldosterone-producing adenomas, but it can also be caused by unilateral adrenal hyperplasia or multifocal disease. Patients with lateralized PA benefit from unilateral adrenalectomy, while bilateral PA requires lifelong targeted therapy. Overall, the probability of lateralized PA increases with disease severity.[21] Because PA is often diagnosed in advanced stages, the prevalence of lateralized PA observed in referral centers roughly equals or exceeds that of bilateral PA. Nevertheless, it is likely that most milder, unrecognized PA cases are bilateral.

The role of cross-sectional imaging in identifying the PA source(s) is limited due to a high prevalence of nonfunctional adrenal nodules in the age group commonly diagnosed with PA (after the sixth decade of life), and also because PA can originate in aldosterone-producing micronodules.[22] Cross-sectional imaging findings are more informative in patients younger than 35 years, because nonfunctional adrenal incidentalomas are uncommon in this age group.[23]

AVS is endorsed by international expert guidelines as the standard-of-care for PA subclassification.[12] AVS is invasive, costly, and technically challenging, relying on expert interventional radiologists from referral centers. In addition, the procedure and data interpretation protocols are poorly harmonized among centers across the globe, resulting in differences in treatment recommendations.

To compare the hormonal output between the 2 adrenal veins (AV), the first step is to confirm that the catheters were correctly placed (*figure*), as indicated by the selectivity index. The selectivity index is computed as a ratio of cortisol at the catheter placement (AV)/peripheral cortisol concentration. Next, the cortisol-corrected aldosterone in each AV (aldosterone/cortisol) is used to compute the lateralization index, as a ratio, with the highest as the numerator (*figure*). In addition to the lateralization index, the contralateral suppression index evaluates the nondominant AV aldosterone contribution relative to the periphery. Contralateral suppression index using aldosterone either with or without correction to cortisol has been proposed. In principle, the higher the lateralization index and the lower the contralateral suppression index, the higher the confidence of lateralized PA. Contralateral

Figure. Adrenal vein sampling schematic representation and guide to result interpretation.

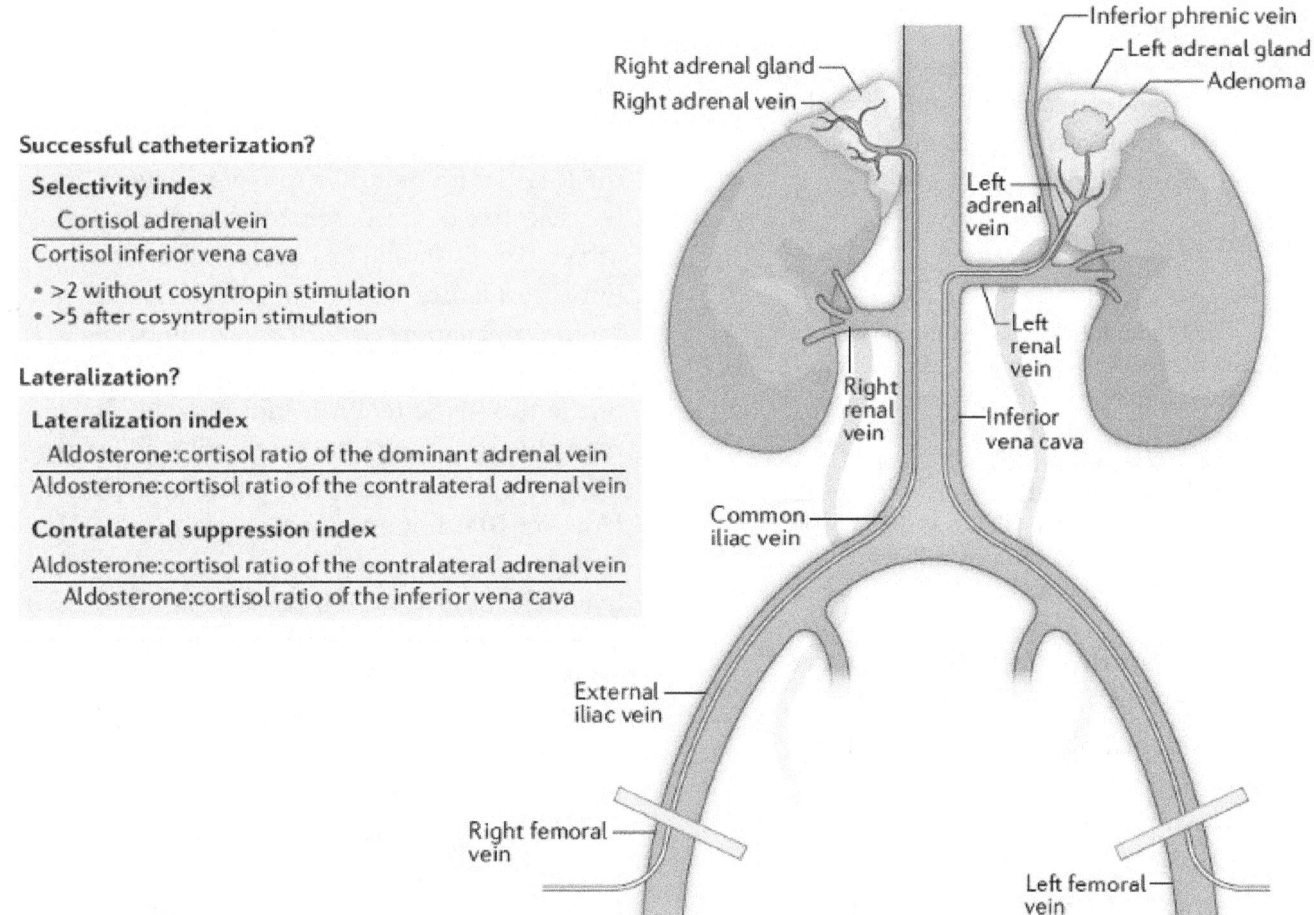

Reprinted from Turcu AF et al. Nat Rev Endocrinol, 2022; 18(11); 665–682. © Springer Nature Limited. (Color—web and EPUB only)

suppression, however, does not correlate well with postoperative outcomes. Occasionally, apparent bilateral aldosterone/cortisol suppression can be encountered. Such results might be due to immunoassay interference or to catheter positioning in a vein that bypasses an aldosterone-producing adenoma and have been reported more often in samples obtained without cosyntropin stimulation.

Clinical Case Vignettes

Case 1

A 77-year-old man is referred for evaluation of treatment-resistant hypertension after a recent transient ischemic attack. He also has a history of hypokalemia, obstructive sleep apnea, coronary artery disease, and prostate cancer (treated with prostatectomy 5 years ago).

On physical examination, his blood pressure is 163/88 mm Hg, pulse rate is 71 beats/min, and BMI is 31 kg/m².

His medications include lisinopril, 20 mg daily; amlodipine, 10 mg daily; metoprolol XL, 25 mg daily; spironolactone, 50 mg daily; and atorvastatin, 80 mg daily.

Laboratory test results:

> Serum sodium = 145 mEq/L (136-142 mEq/L)
> (SI: 145 mmol/L [136-142 mmol/L])
> Serum potassium = 3.3 mEq/L (3.5-5.0 mEq/L)
> (SI: 3.3 mmol/L [3.5-5.0 mmol/L])
> Serum creatinine = 1.06 mg/dL (0.6-1.1 mg/dL)
> (SI: 93.7 μmol/L [53.0-97.2 μmol/L])
> Serum aldosterone = 51.9 ng/dL (4-21 ng/dL)
> (SI: 1439.7 pmol/L [111.0-582.5 pmol/L])
> Plasma renin activity = 0.1 ng/mL per h
> (0.6-4.3 ng/mL per h)

Which of the following is the best next step in this patient's management?

A. Stop lisinopril, spironolactone, and metoprolol; start KCl, hydralazine, and doxazosin; and retest plasma aldosterone, renin, and metabolic panel in 4 to 6 weeks

B. Perform a confirmatory aldosterone-suppression test

C. Add KCl and discuss primary aldosteronism subtypes/AVS

Answer: C) Add KCl and discuss primary aldosteronism subtypes/AVS

This patient has several clinical and laboratory features suggestive of severe PA, including uncontrolled hypertension while being treated with 4 antihypertensive medications; hypokalemia, despite taking spironolactone and lisinopril; a high plasma aldosterone concentration; and undetectable renin activity.

Several medications, particularly antihypertensive agents, can alter the RAAS at various levels. Most such agents lead to renin elevation (*table 1*). Exceptions include β-adrenergic blockers, central agonists (eg, clonidine), renin inhibitors, and nonsteroidal anti-inflammatory drugs, which can lower renin activity. Additionally, estrogens increase angiotensinogen, and consequently renin concentrations decline to maintain normal angiotensin II levels and normal renin activity. Repeating PA screening after replacing medications that interfere with the RAAS with neutral antihypertensive agents (eg, selective α-adrenergic blockers, hydralazine, or verapamil) should be considered when initial results are indeterminate, particularly if renin is not suppressed. However, in patients with striking biochemical profiles, such as the one in this vignette, PA is indisputable. Thus, repeating screening after medication adjustments (Answers A) or conducting confirmatory tests (Answer B) is not necessary in this patient. He requires potassium supplementation to correct hypokalemia, followed by a discussion about PA subtyping and therapy options (Answer C).

Similarly, with PA screening and confirmatory testing, AVS is also preferably conducted in the absence of medications that interfere with the RAAS. However, in patients with difficult-to-control hypertension and/or hypokalemia, AVS can provide accurate results even in the presence of mineralocorticoid receptor antagonists, as long as renin is suppressed.[19]

Case 2

A 57-year-old man with type 2 diabetes mellitus, obesity, resistant hypertension, dyslipidemia, and intermittent hypokalemia is evaluated for a 2-cm left adrenal nodule found incidentally on abdominal CT without contrast. The nodule is homogeneous, with a density of –10 Hounsfield units on unenhanced images. The right adrenal gland is normal, without nodules or atrophy,

Laboratory test results obtained at 8 AM:

Plasma aldosterone = 32 ng/dL (4-21 ng/dL) (SI: 887.7 pmol/L [111.0-582.5 pmol/L])
Plasma renin activity = 0.1 ng/mL per h (0.6-4.3 ng/mL per h)
ACTH = 14 pg/mL (10-60 pg/mL) (SI: 3.1 pmol/L [2.2-13.2 pmol/L])
Cortisol = 13 µg/dL (5-25 µg/dL) (SI: 358.7 nmol/L [137.9-689.7 nmol/L])
DHEA-S = 72 µg /dL (20-299) (SI: 1.95 µmol/L [0.54-8.10 µmol/L])

Following a 1-mg overnight dexamethasone-suppression test:

Cortisol = 2.1 µg/dL (<1.8 µg/dL) (SI: 57.9 nmol/L [<49.7 nmol/L])
ACTH = <5 pg/mL (SI: <1.1 pmol/L)
Urinary cortisol = 33 µg/24 h (4-50 µg/24 h) (SI: 91.1 nmol/d [11-138 nmol/d])

The patient undergoes AVS after cosyntropin stimulation, which indicates lateralization of aldosterone excess to the right adrenal gland.

Which of the following is the best next step in this patient's management?

A. Left adrenalectomy

B. Right adrenalectomy

C. Medical treatment with spironolactone and reassess hypercortisolism in 6 to 12 months

D. Bilateral adrenalectomy

E. Medical treatment with ketoconazole

Answer: B) Right adrenalectomy

This patient with an adrenal incidentaloma has hormonal evidence of PA and an abnormal result following a 1-mg dexamethasone-suppression test. Mild ACTH-independent cortisol excess has been reported in up to 25% of patients with PA.[24] In contrast with PA, ACTH-independent cortisol excess is always associated with cortical nodules that are at least 1 cm in size, and cross-sectional imaging reliably indicates the source(s) of cortisol excess. ACTH-independent hypercortisolism arising from an adrenal nodule can lead to ACTH suppression, and, consequently, to decreased cortisol production from the opposite adrenal gland. Consequently, the aldosterone-to-cortisol ratio in the gland opposite to the cortisol-producing nodule becomes artificially higher, skewing the lateralization index. This can mask lateralized PA, or even indicate lateralization to the wrong gland. While lower clinical cure rates after unilateral adrenalectomy have been reported in patients with abnormal vs normal results on dexamethasone-suppression testing, mild hypercortisolism is thought to have little effect on aldosterone lateralization when AVS is conducted following cosyntropin stimulation.[25]

In this patient, the baseline ACTH and DHEA-S values are not suppressed, and the overnight 1-mg dexamethasone-suppression test result is minimally abnormal. Prolonged ACTH suppression can lead to atrophy of the adrenal cortex, but such findings are not present in this patient. Thus, the AVS results can be considered accurate, and right adrenalectomy can be offered to this patient (Answer B).

When AVS results are thought to be skewed by ACTH-independent cortisol excess (as suggested by suppressed baseline ACTH and/or DHEA-S, or by an atrophic contralateral adrenal gland on imaging), the clinical decision must consider the severity of PA and hypercortisolism in each individual patient. Initiating treatment with a mineralocorticoid receptor antagonist (Answer C) is a conservative approach, while surgery can be reconsidered following periodic reassessment of PA and cortisol excess severity.

In patients with overt ACTH-independent Cushing syndrome, surgical removal of the adrenal gland harboring the cortisol-producing adenoma should be pursued (thus, Answer A is incorrect). In such cases, surgery prioritizes cortisol over aldosterone excess, due to better medical treatment options available for PA.

All medical therapies available for Cushing syndrome have potential adverse effects and are reserved for inoperable cases. Inhibitors of enzymes required for cortisol synthesis (eg, ketoconazole [Answer E], metyrapone,

osilodrostat, and mitotane) or mifepristone (a progesterone and glucocorticoid-receptor antagonist) can be considered for patients with cortisol-producing tumors that cannot be treated or cured with surgery.

Bilateral adrenalectomy (Answer D) would remove the sources of adrenal hormone excess but would lead to lifelong hormonal replacement needs and risk of fatal adrenal crisis.

References

1. Kayser SC, Dekkers T, Groenewoud HJ, et al. Study heterogeneity and estimation of prevalence of primary aldosteronism: a systematic review and meta-regression analysis. *J Clin Endocrinol Metab.* 2016;101(7):2826-2835. PMID: 27172433

2. Brown JM, Siddiqui M, Calhoun DA, et al. The unrecognized prevalence of primary aldosteronism: a cross-sectional study. *Ann Intern Med.* 2020;173(1):10-20. PMID: 32449886

3. Monticone S, D'Ascenzo F, Moretti C, et al. Cardiovascular events and target organ damage in primary aldosteronism compared with essential hypertension: a systematic review and meta-analysis. *Lancet Diabetes Endocrinol.* 2018;6(1):41-50. PMID: 29129575

4. Murata M, Kitamura T, Tamada D, et al. Plasma aldosterone level within the normal range is less associated with cardiovascular and cerebrovascular risk in primary aldosteronism. *J Hypertens.* 2017;35(5):1079-1085. PMID: 28129245

5. Mulatero P, Monticone S, Bertello C, et al. Long-term cardio- and cerebrovascular events in patients with primary aldosteronism. *J Clin Endocrinol Metab.* 2013;98:4826-4833. PMID: 24057288

6. Hundemer GL, Curhan GC, Yozamp N, Wang M, Vaidya A. Cardiometabolic outcomes and mortality in medically treated primary aldosteronism: a retrospective cohort study. *Lancet Diabetes Endocrinol.* 2018;6(1):51-59. PMID: 29129576

7. Monticone S, Burrello J, Tizzani D, et al. Prevalence and clinical manifestations of primary aldosteronism encountered in primary care practice. *J Am Coll Cardiol.* 2017;69(14):1811-1820.

8. Rossi GP, Maiolino G, Flego A, et al. Adrenalectomy lowers incident atrial fibrillation in primary aldosteronism patients at long term. *Hypertension.* 2018;71(4):585-591. PMID: 28385310

9. Wu V-C, Chang C-H, Wang C-Y, et al. Risk of fracture in primary aldosteronism: a population-based cohort study. *J Bone Miner Res.* 2017;32(4):743-752. PMID: 27862274

10. Velema MS, de Nooijer AH, Burgers VWG, et al. Health-related quality of life and mental health in primary aldosteronism: a systematic review. *Horm Metab Res.* 2017;49(12):943-950. PMID: 29202493

11. Hundemer GL, Curhan GC, Yozamp N, Wang M, Vaidya A. Incidence of atrial fibrillation and mineralocorticoid receptor activity in patients with medically and surgically treated primary aldosteronism. *JAMA Cardiol.* 2018;3(8):768-774. PMID: 30027227

12. Funder JW, Carey RM, Mantero F, et al. The management of primary aldosteronism: case detection, diagnosis, and treatment: an Endocrine Society clinical practice guideline. *J Clin Endocrinol Metab.* 2016;101(5):1889-1916. PMID: 26934393

13. Whelton PK, Carey RM, Aronow WS, et al. 2017 ACC/AHA/AAPA/ABC/ACPM/AGS/APhA/ASH/ASPC/NMA/PCNA guideline for the prevention, detection, evaluation, and management of high blood pressure in adults: a

report of the American College of Cardiology/American Heart Association Task Force on Clinical Practice Guidelines. *Hypertension.* 2018;71(6):e13-e115. PMID: 29133356

14. Cohen JB, Cohen DL, Herman DS, Leppert JT, Byrd JB, Bhalla V. Testing for primary aldosteronism and mineralocorticoid receptor antagonist use among U.S. veterans: a retrospective cohort study. *Ann Intern Med.* 2021;174(3):289-297. PMID: 33370170

15. Jaffe G, Gray Z, Krishnan G, et al. Screening rates for primary aldosteronism in resistant hypertension a cohort study. *Hypertension.* 2020;75(3):650-659. PMID: 32008436

16. Hundemer GL, Imsirovic H, Vaidya A, et al. Screening rates for primary aldosteronism among individuals with hypertension plus hypokalemia: a population-based retrospective cohort study. *Hypertension.* 2022;79(1):178-186. PMID: 34657442

17. Mulatero P, Monticone S, Burrello J, Veglio F, Williams TA, Funder J. Guidelines for primary aldosteronism: uptake by primary care physicians in Europe. *J Hypertens.* 2016;34(11):2253-2257. PMID: 27607462

18. Yozamp N, Hundemer GL, Moussa M, et al. Intraindividual variability of aldosterone concentrations in primary aldosteronism. *Hypertension.* 2021;77(3):891-899. PMID: 33280409

19. Nanba AT, Wannachalee T, Shields JJ, et al. Adrenal vein sampling lateralization despite mineralocorticoid receptor antagonists exposure in primary aldosteronism. *J Clin Endocrinol Metab.* 2019;104(2):487-492. PMID: 33280409

20. Leung AA, Symonds CJ, Hundemer GL, et al. Performance of Confirmatory Tests for Diagnosing Primary Aldosteronism: a Systematic Review and Meta-Analysis. *Hypertension.* 2022;79(8):1835-1844. PMID: 35652330

21. Wannachalee T, Zhao L, Nanba K, et al. Three discrete patterns of primary aldosteronism lateralization in response to cosyntropin during adrenal vein sampling. *J Clin Endocrinol Metab.* 2019;104(12):5867-5876. PMID: 31408156

22. De Sousa K, Boulkroun S, Baron S, et al. Genetic, cellular, and molecular heterogeneity in adrenals with aldosterone-producing adenoma. *Hypertension.* 2020;75(4):1034-1044. PMID: 32114847

23. Wannachalee T, Caoili E, Nanba K, et al. The concordance between imaging and adrenal venous sampling varies with aldosterone-driver somatic mutation. *J Clin Endocrinol Metab.* 2020;105(10):e3628-e3637. PMID: 32717082

24. Arlt W, Lang K, Sitch AJ, et al. Steroid metabolome analysis reveals prevalent glucocorticoid excess in primary aldosteronism. *JCI Insight.* 2017;2(8). PMID: 28422753

25. O'Toole SM, Sze WC, Chung TT, et al. Low grade cortisol co-secretion has limited impact on ACTH-stimulated AVS parameters in primary aldosteronism. *J Clin Endocrinol Metab.* 2020;105(10):dgaa519. PMID: 32785656

Bilateral Adrenal Masses: Evaluation and Management

Stylianos Tsagarakis, MD, PhD. Department of Endocrinology and Diabetes, Evangelismos Hospital, Athens, Greece; Email: stsagara@otenet.gr

Educational Objectives

After reviewing this chapter, learners should be able to:

- Assess and evaluate patients with bilateral adrenal masses, particularly those that are incidentally discovered, which is the most common presentation.

- Manage patients presenting with hormonally active bilateral adrenal lesions, particularly those with autonomous cortisol secretion.

Significance of the Clinical Problem

Bilateral adrenal masses encompass a highly heterogeneous group of pathologies. The initial evaluation should aim to assess both the possibility of malignancy and hormonal secretory status. At the time of initial detection, due to the occasional coexistence of different entities, each lesion should be assessed individually to establish whether it is benign or malignant. A tumor density less than 10 Hounsfield units (HU) safely excludes malignancy. Hormonal evaluation includes testing for primary aldosteronism, pheochromocytoma, and cortisol excess. In case of hypercortisolism, ACTH independence must be confirmed. In patients with bilateral adrenal masses due to metastases, infiltrative lesions, or hemorrhage, adrenal hypofunction should be evaluated. Autonomous cortisol secretion in patients with bilateral lesions that are compatible with adenomas or hyperplasia is more common than in patients with unilateral lesions. In patients with hypercortisolism and radiologic appearance of primary bilateral macronodular adrenal hyperplasia (PBMAH), genetic causes and the presence of illegitimate receptors should be considered. The management of patients with bilateral adrenal adenomas or hyperplasia and autonomous cortisol secretion is individualized based on age, degree of cortisol autonomy, general condition, presence of cortisol-related comorbidities, and patient preference. If surgery is considered, unilateral adrenalectomy of the largest lesion is a reasonable option, compared with the debilitating outcome of bilateral adrenalectomy. Medical management is a compelling approach, but more studies are needed before it is implemented in routine practice.

Bilateral adrenal masses are discovered in different clinical settings. Most commonly, they are identified incidentally during thoracic/abdominal imaging performed for reasons unrelated to an adrenal disorder. Less frequently, adrenal masses are detected in patients with a suspected adrenal hormonal disorder or in patients undergoing imaging as part of a known malignancy. Adrenal masses are also detected in patients with genetic syndromes known to cause macronodular adrenal hyperplasia.

During the last 2 decades, we have witnessed a 10-fold increased detection of incidentally discovered adrenal masses, with up to 20% of them being bilateral lesions. The estimated prevalence of incidentally discovered bilateral adrenal masses in the general population is 0.3% to 0.6%.[1] Etiologies of bilateral adrenal masses vary widely. The most common causes are bilateral cortical adenomas,

PBMAH, and metastases, especially in patients with known extraadrenal malignancy. Bilateral adrenal masses do not necessarily represent the same entity in both adrenal glands. Coexistence of different causes is not uncommon, involving various combinations, such as adenoma, pheochromocytoma, cyst, myelolipoma, or even adrenocortical carcinoma or metastasis. In addition, causes of nodular adrenal hyperplasia secondary to ACTH stimulation (ACTH-dependent) should be considered. These causes mainly include congenital adrenal hyperplasia, Cushing disease, or ectopic ACTH secretion. A summary of the causes of bilateral adrenal masses is shown in the *box*.[2]

Box. Causes of Bilateral Adrenal Masses

Extraadrenal lesions
- Kidney, pancreas, and spleen lesions
- Technical artifacts

Adrenal lesions

Adrenal tumors and primary hyperplasias
- Bilateral macronodular adrenal hyperplasia
- Adenomas
- Pheochromocytomas
- Adrenocortical carcinoma

ACTH-dependent hyperplasia
- Cushing disease/ectopic ACTH Cushing syndrome
- Congenital adrenal hyperplasia
- Glucocorticoid resistance syndrome

Noncortical adrenal masses
- Metastasis
- Lymphoma
- Myelolipoma

Infections
- Tuberculosis
- Histoplasmosis
- Blastomycosis

Infiltrative
- Amyloidosis

Adrenal hemorrhage

Adapted from Vassiliadi DA et al. *Curr Opin Endocrinol Diabetes Obes,* 2020;27(3): 125-131. © Wolters Kluwer Health, Inc.

Evaluation of the diverse causes of bilateral adrenal masses is particularly challenging. Moreover, high rates of cortisol excess in the form of mild autonomous cortisol secretion require a thorough assessment of cortisol secretory status along with confirmation of ACTH independence. A substantial proportion of patients with bilateral adrenal masses in the form of bilateral macronodular hyperplasia carry germline pathogenic variants in the *ARMC5* gene. Thus, genetic testing and counseling should be recommended. Management of patients depends largely on the underlying diagnosis. For the most frequently encountered patients who present with autonomous cortisol secretion, various strategies of surgical and medical interventions are implemented.

Practice Gaps

- Although there is good evidence that a mass with a low density less than 10 HU is most likely benign, for higher-density, indeterminate adrenal masses, the most suitable imaging method to determine whether the mass is benign is still elusive.

- Assessment of autonomous cortisol secretion is largely based on the 1-mg dexamethasone-suppression test; caveats of this test are confounding factors for correct stratification of patients.

- Low levels of plasma ACTH with adrenal autonomy may overlap with cases of Cushing disease.

- Despite emerging evidence that autonomous cortisol secretion is a cardiometabolic risk factor associated with a higher mortality rate, there is a need for large, long-term confirmatory studies.

- In patients with autonomous cortisol secretion, outcomes from well-designed surgical intervention studies are required to define when and how to surgically treat these patients.

- Well-designed studies of medical treatment are needed.

- Selection criteria for genetic testing, as well as special guidance on the management of affected kindreds, are not well established.

- The reported recommendations and clinical guidelines in the literature have an overall low level of evidence.

Discussion

Radiologic Evaluation of Bilateral Adrenal Masses

As emphasized in the ESE/ENS@T guidelines,[3] due to the occasional coexistence of different entities, each lesion should be assessed separately. The imaging modality of choice, and the most widely validated, is CT, which provides information about the shape, size, invasion to adjacent structures, and density of the mass on noncontrast images. MRI is preferred when radiation exposure is of concern and provides similar information to unenhanced CT regarding fat content of the lesion(s). Overall, density of 10 HU or less on unenhanced CT safely excludes malignancy.[4] For all other lesions, most of which are likely benign, there is no consensus on the second-best additional imaging modality. If additional imaging is considered, FDG-PET/CT is preferred because it has the advantage that the risk of missing a malignant lesion is quite low. However, it is relatively expensive and, in many countries, is still not widely available. Some benign adrenal masses such as functional adenomas or pheochromocytomas may be FDG-positive. An alternative strategy for indeterminate lesions is to perform follow-up imaging in 6 to 12 months or even immediate surgery. Size has been traditionally associated with the risk of malignancy. Lesions measuring more than 4 cm (an arbitrary cutoff) are considered to harbor a significant likelihood of malignancy favoring surgical intervention.

Evaluation of Hormonal Status

In the most recent ESE/ENS@T guidelines update, it is suggested to approach bilateral adrenal masses according to the following 4-option schema based on imaging results: (1) bilateral (macronodular) hyperplasia, (2) bilateral adrenal adenomas, (3) 2 morphologically similar, but nonadenoma-like adrenal masses, (4) 2 morphologically different adrenal masses. This approach offers specific guidance for a more focused hormonal testing plan based on imaging phenotype. With this approach, some specific hormonal tests are restricted to a limited number of patients. For example, 17-hydroxyprogesterone is needed only in patients with bilateral hyperplasia, and testing for adrenal insufficiency is necessary only in patients with large and/or infiltrative bilateral masses (eg, lymphomas, metastases) or bilateral hemorrhage.

Hormonal excess in patients with bilateral adrenal masses may originate either from one of the lesions or bilaterally. Cushing syndrome, primary aldosteronism, and pheochromocytoma(s) may all be encountered.[1] The most common hormonal abnormality is mild cortisol excess, termed *autonomous cortisol secretion* (ACS) and is much more prevalent in patients with bilateral hyperplasia or adenomas than with unilateral adenomas.[5] Based on current recommendations, ACS is assessed by the 1-mg overnight dexamethasone-suppression test. Postdexamethasone cortisol values of 1.8 µg/dL or less (≤50 nmol/L) exclude ACS. Higher values are consistent with ACS. Additional tests, including measurement of midnight cortisol or 24-hour urinary free cortisol, may help to establish the degree of cortisol excess. In case of biochemical hypercortisolism, with or without clinical Cushing syndrome, measurement of ACTH levels is important, not only to support the diagnosis of ACS by demonstrating low or suppressed levels, but also to exclude ACTH dependence.[3] Occasionally, documenting ACTH independence may not be straightforward because ACTH levels may not be fully suppressed. The use of the dexamethasone-corticotropin-releasing hormone (CRH) test in these patients may lead to the erroneous diagnosis of ACTH-dependent Cushing syndrome, since a substantial number of patients may have positive responses.[6]

The term "autonomous" is used to describe ACTH independence from adrenal cortisol production, but in some cases, cortisol secretion is not truly autonomous. It may be regulated by ligands other than ACTH acting on illegitimate (ectopic or overexpressed eutopic), membrane G-protein–coupled receptors and/or by autocrine/paracrine loops.[7] Some authors recommend testing for the presence of aberrant G-protein–coupled receptors to identify patients who have specific receptors that would permit targeted medical treatment. The protocols comprise applying various stimuli such as a meal test, upright posture test, and LH-releasing hormone administration to document paradoxical cortisol responses. These tests are better conducted under dexamethasone suppression to avoid the confounding effects of inadvertent ACTH rise on cortisol secretion.

Genetics

Patients with bilateral adrenal masses consistent with PBMAH or pheochromocytomas may have germline pathogenic variants in various genes. Although PBMAH is most often sporadic, it is occasionally encountered in the context of hereditary familial tumor syndromes with both syndromic or isolated presentations.[8] Syndromic forms of PBMAH include multiple endocrine neoplasia type 1 (*MEN1* gene), familial adenomatous polyposis (*APC* gene), hereditary leiomyomatosis and renal cell cancer syndrome (*FH* gene), and McCune-Albright syndrome (*GNAS* gene). However, even in nonsyndromic cases, genetic factors are increasingly recognized. Germline pathogenic variants in the *ARMC5* gene are the most prevalent. Patients with pathogenic *ARMC5* variants typically have a more severe phenotype and more frequently develop signs of overt Cushing syndrome. The number of nodules correlates with the likelihood of a pathogenic germline *ARMC5* variant. Most recently, the genetic driver event that leads to PBMAH

associated with aberrant GIP-receptor expression (food-dependent Cushing syndrome) was linked to germline inactivating variants in the *KDM1A* gene.[7,8] Both *ARMC5* and *KDM1A* have been associated with other neoplasias, indicating that they represent new forms of multiple neoplasia syndromes: *ARMC5* pathogenic variants with meningiomas and *KDM1A* pathogenic variants with myelolipomas and multiple myeloma. Also, mild glucocorticoid receptor resistance due to heterozygous *NR3C1* pathogenic variants (the gene encoding the glucocorticoid receptor) have been reported in a proportion of patients with bilateral adrenal adenomas, more commonly in those with hypertension and low-normal potassium and aldosterone levels. In general, PBMAH is increasingly recognized to have a genetic predisposition and in such cases genetic testing and counseling should be offered to patients and their relatives. Bilateral pheochromocytomas are also often of genetic origin (*VHL*, *RET*, *SDHx*, *MAX*, *TMEM127*, *NF1*), and genetic testing for pheochromocytoma- and paraganglioma-associated genes is mandatory.

Management of Hormonally Active Lesions

As mentioned, patients with bilateral adrenal adenomas or PBMAH have a higher rate of mild autonomous cortisol secretion. In such patients, the ESE/ENS@T guidelines suggest individualization of specific treatment options based on age, sex, degree of cortisol autonomy, general condition, comorbidities, and patient preference.[3] If surgery is an option, bilateral adrenalectomy should be avoided in patients without clinical signs of overt Cushing syndrome. Compared with unilateral surgery, bilateral adrenalectomy is associated with higher morbidity. Patients who have bilateral adrenalectomy are dependent on lifelong adrenal replacement therapy and are at risk for life-threatening addisonian crises. In addition, glucocorticoid replacement is frequently suboptimal and cannot mimic the circadian profile of endogenous cortisol; this may result in persisting exposure to cortisol excess. A more reasonable approach, in selected patients, is unilateral adrenalectomy, which leads to clinical improvement of cortisol-related comorbidities.[9] Improvement, but not complete resolution, of biochemical markers of cortisol excess is achieved in most patients. Adrenal insufficiency, which is usually transient, occurs in about one-third of patients, despite the presence of a residual hyperplastic adrenal.

There is no indisputable criterion to determine which gland to remove. Excision of the largest adrenal was performed in most studies, based on observations that the size of the adrenal lesion correlates with the degree of cortisol excess. This is definitely true for patients with PBMAH. In contrast, patients with bilateral adenomas may need a more judicious approach. In the few studies that applied adrenal scintigraphy, the side of prevalent uptake was almost invariably on the side of the largest adrenal mass. Due to limited data, the utility of adrenal venous sampling is not well established. It is a cumbersome method, not widely available, with a less-than-optimal success rate and no clear criteria to document successful catheterization. According to the sparse available data, lateralization often coincides with the largest adrenal. If available, adrenal venous sampling is a reasonable choice in patients with equal-sized bilateral nodules to avoid removing a nonfunctional nodule and leaving the culprit lesion behind.[10]

Following unilateral adrenalectomy, some patients eventually require contralateral adrenalectomy due to recurrence of hypercortisolism. However, when bilateral completion surgery is potentially indicated, adrenal-sparing surgery might be considered, offering the opportunity to control hypercortisolism without the risk of adrenal crisis associated with complete bilateral adrenalectomy.[5] An alternative option in such patients is medical therapy with the same means (steroidogenesis inhibitors, glucocorticoid-receptor antagonists) used to treat patients with overt Cushing syndrome.[11] Although promising, this treatment option needs more studies, including larger patient numbers and more robust outcomes. In patients with bilateral pheochromocytomas, cortical-sparing surgery after preoperative treatment with α-adrenergic blockers is the most widely adopted option.

Clinical Case Vignettes
Case 1

During routine abdominal ultrasonography, a 52-year-old man is found to harbor a large left adrenal gland. Further testing with unenhanced abdominal CT shows a 4.6-cm mass in the left adrenal gland (density of 40 HU) and a 4.7-cm lesion in the right adrenal gland consisting of 2 components (the first is larger with density of 10 HU and the second is smaller with density of 20 HU) (*see image*). The patient is asymptomatic with no clinical stigmata of Cushing syndrome.

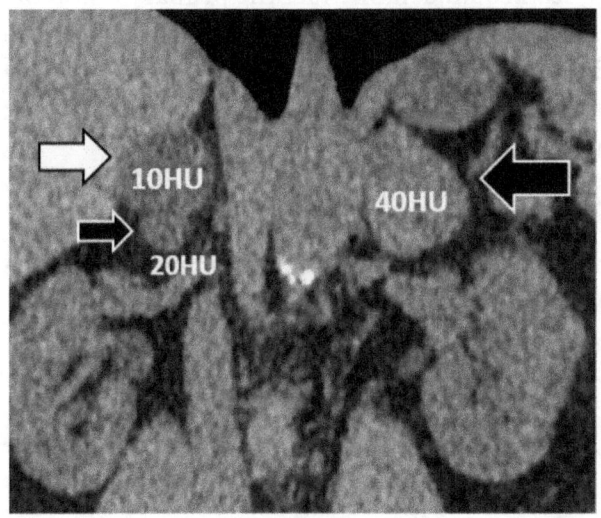

Which of the following is the best next step in this patient's evaluation?

A. Biopsy of the left adrenal lesion

B. FDG-PET

C. 1-mg dexamethasone-suppression test

D. MRI

E. Plasma free metanephrine measurement

Answer: E) Plasma free metanephrine measurement

This clinical vignette provides the unenhanced CT from a patient with incidentally discovered bilateral adrenal masses with different imaging characteristics. This is a good example of why each lesion should be individually assessed and characterized. Based on the unenhanced CT, the larger right adrenal mass of 10 HU is a benign lesion and most likely represents a benign adrenocortical adenoma. The 4.6-cm left adrenal mass with a density of 40 HU is indeterminate, and its characterization is of great importance. The third lesion is small, with a density of 20 HU, and is located in the right adrenal gland.

Further evaluation with MRI (Answer D) (although frequently recommended in most radiology reports) would not add any further information to that obtained from unenhanced CT.

FDG-PET (Answer B) could be useful, with a negative result excluding a malignant lesion. Also, if the indeterminate lesions were metastases, the scan could demonstrate the primary lesion or some additional lesion more accessible to perform a biopsy. However, FDG-PET may be positive in most functional lesions, so the functional status of the existing lesions should be assessed.

Not only is functionality part of the essential evaluation of all adrenal incidentalomas, but in some cases, the hormonal status may indicate the diagnosis. This is of particular relevance for pheochromocytomas, since they may mimic malignant tumors (high density on unenhanced CT, presence of necroses and/or calcifications, growth on repeated imaging). Measurement of plasma free metanephrines (Answer E) is the best next step in this patient's evaluation. In fact, biochemical testing documented abnormal plasma concentrations of fractionated metanephrines:

Metanephrine = 99 pg/mL (<88 pg/mL)
(SI: 0.50 nmol/L [<0.47 nmol/L])
Normetanephrine = 666 pg/mL (<162 pg/mL)
(SI: 3.64 nmol/L [<0.88 nmol/L])

These values are consistent with the diagnosis of a pheochromocytoma. Since most secretory pheochromocytomas are larger than 1.5 cm, the 4.6-cm, high-density left adrenal lesion is most likely a pheochromocytoma. Biopsy of the left

adrenal lesion (Answer A) is not only unnecessary but is contraindicated as it could precipitate a potentially lethal catecholamine crisis.

The 1-mg dexamethasone-suppression test (Answer C) has a place in this case. The low-density adenoma-like lesion in the right adrenal gland has a substantial probability of autonomous cortisol secretion. However, the diagnostic importance of elevated plasma free metanephrines surpasses the need for a dexamethasone-suppression test in this case.

The nature of the smaller lesion in the right adrenal gland (20 HU) is still indeterminate and this is important regarding the most appropriate surgical approach. Based on recent literature, the preoperative role of MIBG scintigraphy has been limited. However, in this patient, MIBG scintigraphy revealed uptake in both the left lesion and the small right lesion. Following phenoxybenzamine pretreatment, the patient underwent removal of both the left and right adrenal lesions. Pathology revealed a left PASS-score of 8 and a smaller right pheochromocytoma and a 5-cm right adrenocortical adenoma (Weiss: 1/9). Genetic testing with next-generation sequencing of pheochromocytoma-associated genes was negative.

Case 2

A 48-year-old woman undergoes abdominal CT to evaluate to abdominal discomfort. CT shows bilateral adrenal lesions: a 4-cm mass in the right adrenal (density of –2.5 HU) and a 2-cm mass in the left adrenal (density of 4.5 HU). The patient has obesity (BMI = 30 kg/m^2), hypertension treated with an angiotensin-converting enzyme inhibitor and diuretic, and diabetes mellitus. She has a history of osteoporosis and has been receiving bisphosphonates for the last 2 years. Cortisol after a 1-mg dexamethasone-suppression test is 5.3 μg/dL (SI: 146 nmol/L), urinary free cortisol excretion is normal, and ACTH is undetectable. The aldosterone-to-renin ratio is normal.

Which of the following is the most appropriate management?

A. Aggressive treatment of comorbidities

B. Bilateral adrenalectomy

C. Removal of the largest lesion

D. Testing to exclude bilateral adrenal pheochromocytomas

E. Watchful waiting with annual follow-up

Answer: C) Removal of the largest lesion

This clinical vignette deals with a case of bilateral adrenal masses with a benign imaging phenotype for which characterization of hormonal function is of primary importance. Both lesions have a density less than 10 HU. Recent studies have consistently shown the probability that an adrenal tumor with a density of 10 or less HU on unenhanced CT is a pheochromocytoma is close to zero.[12] Thus, it seems reasonable to not measure metanephrines (Answer D) to exclude a pheochromocytoma in this case.

On biochemical testing, the patient had an abnormal dexamethasone-suppression test result consistent with autonomous cortisol secretion with undetectable ACTH, indicating ACTH independence. The patient is young and has several cortisol-related comorbidities. According to published data, mostly from retrospective studies, nonsurgical approaches of such patients (watchful waiting [Answer E] or aggressive management of comorbidities [Answer A]) are usually associated with worsening of both biochemical and clinical features. A systematic review and meta-analysis including 26 studies and 584 patients with mild autonomous cortisol secretion showed that surgery improved hypertension and diabetes mellitus compared with outcomes associated with conservative follow-up.[13] Thus, despite the lack of robust evidence based on high-quality data, surgery is the most appropriate option in this 48-year-old patient.

Given that she has only mild hypercortisolism and not overt Cushing syndrome, bilateral adrenalectomy (Answer B) is not justified because the need for lifelong hydrocortisone replacement will convert the mild endogenous cortisol excess into chronic mild exogenous excess. Moreover, the patient will be prone to future addisonian crises. Unilateral adrenalectomy (Answer C) is the most appropriate option. Without adrenal venous sampling, the empirical removal of the largest adrenal lesion proves beneficial in most reported cases, and this was the scenario for this patient.[9,14]

Case 3

A 66-year-old woman with an 8-month history of fatigue and muscle aches undergoes abdominal CT, which shows bilateral adrenal masses: 9.5 cm on the right (density of 35 HU) and 9 cm on the left (density of 30 HU) (*see image*). The patient has obesity (BMI = 40 kg/m²) with recent weight loss and no stigmata of Cushing syndrome. Her blood pressure is 90/60 mm Hg.

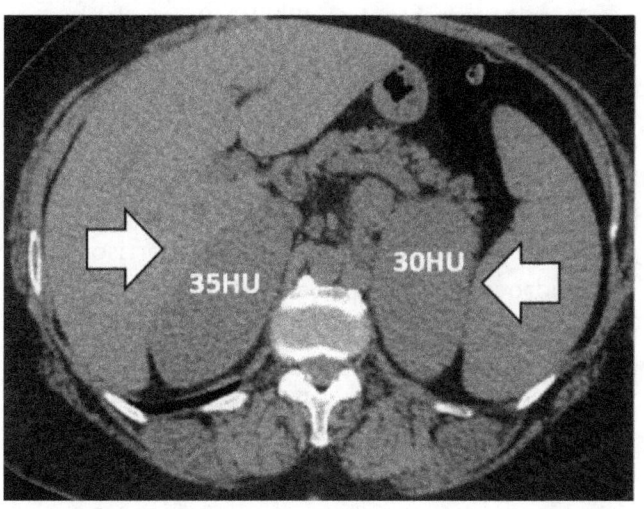

Which of the following is the most urgent hormonal assessment?

A. 1-mg dexamethasone-suppression test

B. 17-Hydroxyprogesterone

C. Plasma free metanephrines

D. Serum electrolytes

E. Urine steroid metabolomics

Answer: D) Serum electrolytes

The unenhanced CT shows 2 large bilateral adrenal masses with similar imaging characteristics that are not typical of an adenoma or hyperplasia. The 1-mg dexamethasone-suppression test (Answer A) and measurement of 17-hydroxyprogesterone (Answer B) are not relevant for this case. The high-density, large adrenal masses are most likely infiltrative lesions due to primary or secondary malignancy. The patient has an 8-month history of fatigue, muscle aches, and weight loss and is relatively hypotensive. This clinical setting along with the presence of what are most likely large infiltrative lesions on both adrenals raises the possibility of adrenal failure.

Laboratory test results, including serum electrolytes (Answer D):

> Sodium = 129 mEq/L (SI: 129 mmol/L)
> Potassium = 6.5 mEq/L (SI: 6.5 mmol/L)
> Morning cortisol = 4 μg/dL (SI: 110.5 nmol/L)
> ACTH = 240 pg/mL (SI: 52.8 pmol/L)
> Aldosterone = 2 ng/mL (SI: 55.5 pmol/L)
> Direct renin = >500 pg/mL (SI: >11.8 pmol/L)

These laboratory values are consistent with primary adrenocortical failure. The patient's condition greatly improved on hydrocortisone and fludrocortisone replacement therapy. Although in this clinical setting the possibility of bilateral pheochromocytomas is extremely unlikely, she underwent a left adrenal biopsy following laboratory testing documenting a normal plasma free metanephrine concentration (Answer C). Histology revealed a nonHodgkin B-cell lymphoma.

Urine steroid metabolomics (Answer E) is a promising tool for detecting a malignant "steroid fingerprint" in patients with adrenocortical carcinoma.[15] Bilateral adrenocortical carcinoma is rare. This clinical vignette illustrates prioritizing the need for adrenal insufficiency testing in all patients with bilateral adrenal masses and infiltrative characteristics on imaging.

Key Learning Points

- Bilateral adrenal masses represent a highly heterogeneous group of lesions that present many challenges in evaluation and management.

- Unenhanced abdominal CT is the most common imaging method used to detect and characterize adrenal masses and to help exclude an underlying adrenal malignancy.

- A thorough endocrine evaluation is required to detect cortisol excess and in special occasions to exclude pheochromocytoma, primary aldosteronism, congenital adrenal hyperplasia, or adrenal insufficiency.

- A substantial proportion of patients with macronodular adrenal hyperplasia on imaging harbor a germline pathogenic variant in the *ARMC5* tumor suppression gene, and therefore genetic testing is strongly recommended in this patient population.

- In case of cortisol excess, the decision to treat is based on the degree of cortisol excess and the presence of comorbidities. Currently, different forms of surgery represent the most widely elected treatment option. Medical therapy is emerging as an alternative option.

References

1. Bourdeau I, El Ghorayeb N, Gagnon N, Lacroix A. Management of endocrine disease: differential diagnosis, investigation and therapy of bilateral adrenal incidentalomas. *Eur J Endocrinol.* 2018;179(2):R57-R67. PMID: 29748231

2. Vassiliadi DA, Partsalaki E, Tsagarakis S. Approach to patients with bilateral adrenal incidentalomas. *Curr Opin Endocrinol Diabetes Obes.* 2020;27(3):125-131. PMID: 32209820

3. Fassnacht M, Arlt W, Bancos I, et al. Management of adrenal incidentalomas: European Society of Endocrinology Clinical Practice Guideline in collaboration with the European Network for the Study of Adrenal Tumors. *Eur J Endocrinol.* 2016;175(2):G1-G34. PMID: 27390021

4. Dinnes J, Bancos I, Ferrante di Ruffano L, et al. Management of endocrine disease: imaging for the diagnosis of malignancy in incidentally discovered adrenal masses: a systematic review and meta-analysis. *Eur J Endocrinol.* 2016;175(2):R51-R64. PMID: 27257145

5. Vassiliadi DA, Ntali G, Vicha E, Tsagarakis S. High prevalence of subclinical hypercortisolism in patients with bilateral adrenal incidentalomas: a challenge to management. *Clin Endocrinol (Oxf)*. 2011;74(4):438-444. PMID: 21175735

6. Vassiliadi DA, Tzanela M, Tsatlidis V, et al. Abnormal responsiveness to dexamethasone-suppressed CRH test in patients with bilateral adrenal incidentalomas. *J Clin Endocrinol Metab*. 2015;100(9):3478-3485. PMID: 26147608

7. Bertherat J, Bourdeau I, Bouys L, Chasseloup F, Kamenicky P, Lacroix A. Clinical, pathophysiologic, genetic and therapeutic progress in primary bilateral macronodular adrenal hyperplasia. *Endocr Rev*. [online ahead of print] PMID: 36548967

8. De Venanzi A, Alencar GA, Bourdeau I, Fragoso MC, Lacroix A. Primary bilateral macronodular adrenal hyperplasia. *Curr Opin Endocrinol Diabetes Obes*. 2014;21(3):177-184. PMID: 24739311

9. Perogamvros I, Vassiliadi DA, Karapanou O, Botoula E, Tzanela M, Tsagarakis S. Biochemical and clinical benefits of unilateral adrenalectomy in patients with subclinical hypercortisolism and bilateral adrenal incidentalomas. *Eur J Endocrinol*. 2015;173(6):719-725. PMID: 26330465

10. Johnson PC, Thompson SM, Adamo D, et al. Adrenal venous sampling for lateralization of cortisol hypersecretion in patients with bilateral adrenal masses. *Clin Endocrinol (Oxf)*. 2023;98(2):177-189. PMID: 36263687

11. Delivanis DA, Vassiliadi DA, Tsagarakis S. Current approach of primary bilateral adrenal hyperplasia. *Curr Opin Endocrinol Diabetes Obes*. 2022;29(3):243-252. PMID: 35621176

12. Gruber LM, Hartman RP, Thompson GB, et al. Pheochromocytoma Characteristics and Behavior Differ Depending on Method of Discovery. *J Clin Endocrinol Metab*. 2019;104(5):1386-1393. PMID: 30462226

13. Bancos I, Alahdab F, Crowley RK, et al. Therapy of endocrine disease: improvement of cardiovascular risk factors after adrenalectomy in patients with adrenal tumors and subclinical Cushing's syndrome: a systematic review and meta-analysis. *Eur J Endocrinol*. 2016;175(6):R283-R295. PMID: 27450696

14. Debillon E, Velayoudom-Cephise F-L, Salenave S, et al. Unilateral adrenalectomy as a first-line treatment of Cushing's syndrome in patients with primary bilateral macronodular adrenal hyperplasia. *J Clin Endocrinol Metab*. 2015;100(12):4417-4424. PMID: 26451908

15. Bancos I, Taylor AE, Chortis V, et al; ENSAT EURINE-ACT Investigators. Urine steroid metabolomics for the differential diagnosis of adrenal incidentalomas in the EURINE-ACT study: a prospective test validation study. *Lancet Diabetes Endocrinol*. 2020;8(9):773-781. PMID: 32711725

How Do I Workup a Woman With Androgen Excess?

Corrine Welt, MD. Division of Endocrinology, Metabolism and Diabetes, University of Utah, Salt Lake City, UT; Email: cwelt@genetics.utah.edu

Educational Objectives

After reviewing this chapter, learners should be able to:

- Identify the most likely diagnoses in women with androgen excess based on age and acuity of symptoms.

- Outline the diagnostic tests and expected results when evaluating women with androgen excess.

- Identify the best imaging modality for women with androgen excess based on hormone evaluation.

Significance of the Clinical Problem

Hyperandrogenism can be manifest by physical symptoms such as hirsutism or acne and irregular menstrual cycles or may only be detected by elevated androgen levels. The key components of the history include the age at presentation, rapidity of symptom development, menstrual cyclicity, medications, and supplement use. A tumor should be considered with rapid onset of hyperandrogenism and severe symptoms, including virilization. Physical examination requires vital signs, muscle assessment, and skin and genital exam. Blood testing includes testosterone and DHEA-S levels, along with targeted testing for rare disorders, as indicated by the history and physical exam. Imaging should begin with pelvic ultrasonography for elevated testosterone and CT with contrast for elevated DHEA-S. Rarely, FDG-PET, ovarian vein sampling, or adrenal vein sampling could be considered when a tumor is not apparent. Treatment is then targeted to the underlying cause.

Circulating androgens in women come from 2 main sources, the ovary and adrenal gland. The ovaries and adrenal glands contribute equal amounts of circulating testosterone to the circulation (*figure 1*). The remaining testosterone is derived from androstenedione, which is produced by both the ovaries and adrenal glands and is converted to testosterone in peripheral tissues. DHEA-S comes from the adrenal glands and is the best androgen to assess adrenal androgen production because it has a long half-life. Its level decreases in middle age, so age-based consideration is necessary. DHEA-S is less potent than testosterone, but it contributes to hyperandrogenic symptoms in women because overall testosterone levels are low.

Figure 1.

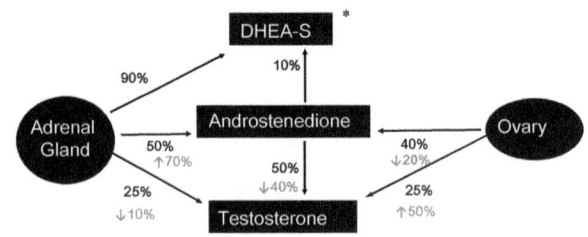

* Note: Additional hormone production due to peripheral conversion in adipose and muscle tissue.

Androgen contribution by the adrenal gland and ovary in premenopausal women (percentages noted in black) and the change in postmenopausal women (percentages noted in grey with arrows indicating change from premenopause to postmenopause).

Androgens have direct effects on the menstrual cycle by suppressing hypothalamic and pituitary secretion of GnRH, LH, and FSH and indirectly through aromatization to estradiol.[1] Androgens also have a role in ovarian function. Although they increase follicle recruitment at low levels, higher levels arrest follicle development. Optimal androgen concentrations are therefore required for ovarian follicle initiation, follicle growth, ovulation, and oocyte maturation.

Androgen excess is a common and distressing problem for women. The approach to the workup depends on the woman's age, severity of symptoms, and rapidity of presentation. Hirsutism is the most common presenting symptom. When the symptoms develop over an extended period, the possible causes are numerous, with polycystic ovary syndrome (PCOS) being the most common. Rapid and severe symptoms that include virilization are most likely to be caused by a tumor of the adrenal gland or ovary. Surgical resection is curative for tumors, while medical management is the mainstay for nontumorous causes.

Practice Gaps

- The breadth of causes for hyperandrogenism needs consideration.

- Incomplete laboratory testing.

- Imaging should be based on laboratory findings.

- What are the next steps when all imaging options fail?

Discussion

History and Physical Examination

The most important aspects when taking a history in women with hyperandrogenism are age, associated findings, and duration of symptoms. The top differential diagnoses change depending on these elements. The most common symptoms of hyperandrogenism are hirsutism, acne, alopecia, and menstrual irregularity. Virilization includes severe hirsutism (back, upper abdomen, and upper arms), male-pattern baldness, deepening of the voice, and clitoromegaly.

Hirsutism is defined as male-pattern terminal hair growth in a woman. The modified Ferriman-Gallwey score grades 9 androgen-sensitive areas on the quantity of hair growth and is useful for documentation. Scores range from 0 (absence of terminal hair) to 4 (fully covered). Abnormal total scores are as follows: ≥9 in Middle Eastern, Mediterranean, South Asian, and Hispanic women; ≥8 in Black women and European Caucasians; ≥7 in Southern Chinese women; ≥6 in South American women; and ≥2 in Han Chinese women.[2,3]

The typical pattern of hair loss in women with hyperandrogenism follows a male pattern with vertex thinning/balding. Male-pattern hair loss, or androgenic alopecia, is commonly associated with elevated levels of circulating androgens. Female-pattern hair loss usually occurs in the central scalp with preservation of the frontal hairline.[4] Elevated circulating androgens may or may not be associated.

Acne is promoted by androgens. Sebaceous glands are able to convert testosterone to dihydrotestosterone because they exhibit 5α reductase activity, contributing to an increased androgenic environment that promotes sebum formation.[5]

Menstrual irregularity and amenorrhea are common features, with the relationship to androgens described above. Documentation of age at menarche, menstrual cycle history, and use of any hormonal contraception that masks symptoms are important. In postmenopausal women, hyperandrogenism can lead to postmenopausal bleeding due to the increased conversion of testosterone to estrogen.

Differential Diagnosis

In premenopausal women with hyperandrogenism, the first step is to consider the complete differential (*figure 2*). All causes of irregular menses should be evaluated, such as thyroid disease, hyperprolactinemia, and primary ovarian insufficiency. Subsequently, all causes of hyperandrogenism need to be considered. Of note, elevated prolactin increases 3β-hydroxysteroid dehydrogenase activity and can itself cause hyperandrogenism.

PCOS is the most common endocrine disorder in reproductive-aged women, affecting approximately 10% of the population. Two of 3 Rotterdam criteria are required to achieve the diagnosis: (1) oligomenorrhea/amenorrhea, (2) clinical or biochemical hyperandrogenism, and/or (3) polycystic ovaries on ultrasonography, defined as 12 or more antral follicles measuring 2 to 9 mm in diameter and/or ovarian volume greater than 10 cm³.[6] However, it is a diagnosis of exclusion and all other causes of hyperandrogenism must be ruled out.

Nonclassic congenital adrenal hyperplasia (NCCAH) can look very similar to PCOS, presenting with menstrual irregularities and hyperandrogenism. The most common cause of NCCAH is 21-hydroxyase deficiency (P450c21) leading to increased 17-hydroxyprogesterone precursor available for the androgen pathway with increased production of androstenedione and testosterone. Unlike the classic form, NCCAH rarely manifests with cortisol deficiency.

Underlying diagnoses for hyperandrogenism presenting in postmenopausal women include ovarian hyperthecosis and androgen-producing tumors. Rapid onset (over months) of increased hair growth is concerning for an androgen-producing tumor, compared with PCOS (12 months vs 42 months in one study).[7] Ovarian hyperthecosis is a histologic diagnosis noted when there is the presence of nests of luteinized theca cells throughout the ovarian stroma. Affected postmenopausal women present with slow onset and progressive symptoms of hyperandrogenism. These women appear to have a history of PCOS prior to menopause. In severe cases, virilization can occur. Typical signs of insulin resistance are often present (acanthosis nigricans, skin tags, central obesity). Postmenopausal bleeding, due to endometrial hyperplasia from testosterone aromatization to estrogen, can also be a presenting symptom. Women often have elevated testosterone and estradiol concentrations with inappropriately low LH and FSH for a menopausal woman.

Figure 2. Algorithm outlining the workup for hyperandrogenism.

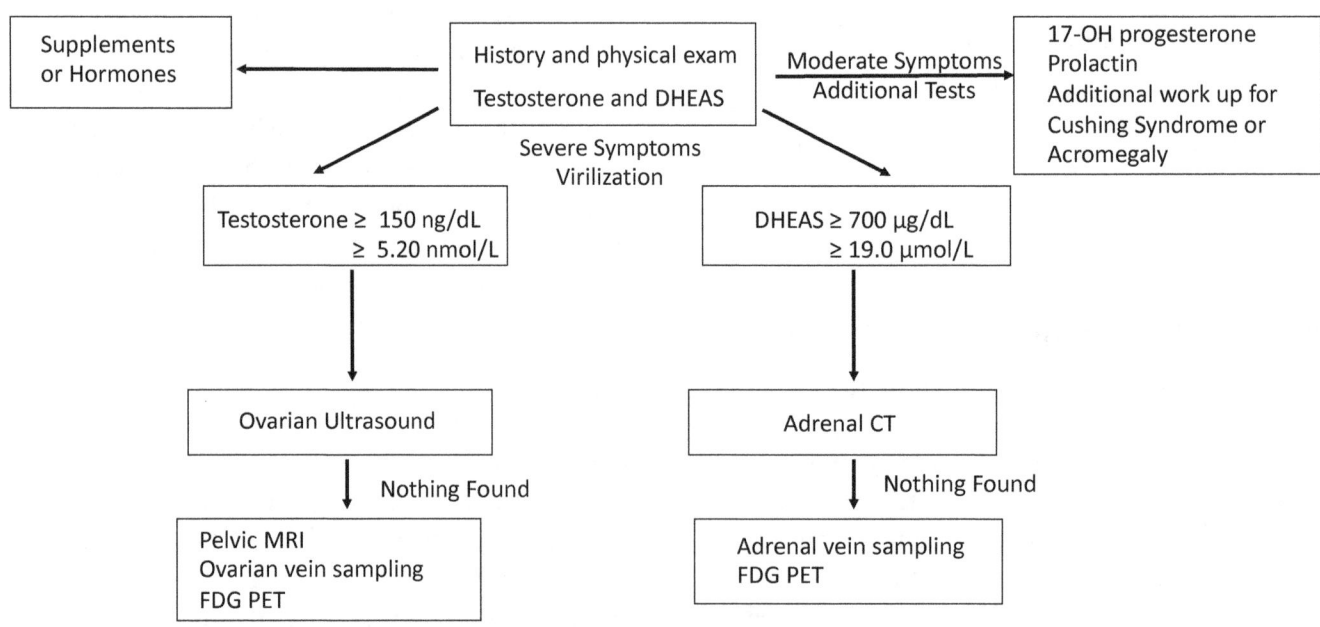

Note that the workup would be performed after testing for causes of irregular menses and amenorrhea (measurement of hCG, prolactin, TSH, and FSH).

In both premenopausal and postmenopausal women, a thorough drug history should be obtained to ensure there was no exposure to oral minoxidil, danazol, anticonvulsant agents, anabolic steroids, and exogenous androgens. These exogenous androgens can include transfer from a family member's prescription, DHEA supplements, bioidentical hormone creams/pills/pellets, hormone boosters, or antiaging cocktails supplied by wellness/antiaging clinics.

Finally, important clues to other underlying endocrine disorders should be considered in both premenopausal and postmenopausal women: signs of Cushing syndrome (purple striae, supraclavicular fullness, facial plethora, easy bruising) and acromegaly (enlarged jaw, macroglossia, and swollen hands/feet with an increase in shoe/ring size).

Laboratory Investigation

The laboratory investigation must assess both irregular menses and hyperandrogenism. Not all premenopausal women with hyperandrogenism have irregular menses, but in those that do, a pregnancy test should be performed. If negative, measurement of prolactin, FSH, and TSH should be evaluated to assess irregular menses. Then, causes of hyperandrogenism should be assessed with an early-morning 17-hydroxyprogesterone measurement (7-9 AM) in the follicular phase, testosterone, and DHEA-S. Cushing syndrome and acromegaly should be ruled out based on the presenting clinical symptoms and signs.

Total testosterone concentration is the most useful test for hyperandrogenism. Liquid chromatography–tandem mass spectrometry is the most reliable method to quantify testosterone in women. Direct radioimmunoassay and other immunoassays are sufficient to identify moderate to severe androgen excess (as is seen in tumors), but they often fail to detect mild elevations.[8] Free testosterone is most accurately measured by equilibrium dialysis and not immunoassay.[8] Low levels of SHBG can be used as an indirect marker of higher free testosterone levels. Of note, laboratory testing should not be performed until at least 3 months after stopping hormonal contraception of any type and in the absence of progestin-coated intrauterine devices. Hormones suppress endogenous androgens and make measurements inaccurate for clinical diagnostic purposes.

Assessing concentrations of androstenedione, DHEA, and DHEA-S is not part of the routine evaluation for hyperandrogenism. However, DHEA-S can be elevated in the settings of PCOS and adrenal tumors, and its measurement is expedient in the initial workup.[9] If the DHEA-S is 700 μg/dL or greater (≥19.0 μmol/L), an adrenal tumor should be ruled out. There are adrenal tumors that do not sulfate DHEA and adrenal steroid panels can be used to assess adrenal androgen production.[10]

Imaging

If the physical examination reveals virilization or the laboratory measurements document severe biochemical androgen excess (total testosterone by liquid chromatography–tandem mass spectrometry ≥150 ng/dL [≥5.2 nmol/L] in premenopausal women or ≥64 ng/dL [≥2.2 nmol/L] in postmenopausal women),[7] pelvic imaging should be the next step in evaluation. An ovarian source is the etiology in approximately 80% of cases.[7] Of note, imaging should not be performed until at least 3 months after stopping hormonal contraception of any type and in the absence of progestin-coated intrauterine devices. Hormones decrease the ovarian volume and make measurements inaccurate for clinical diagnostic purposes.

Due to lower cost, transvaginal ultrasonography with color Doppler should be first-line imaging. However, ovarian tumors are generally small (Leydig-cell tumors <3 cm) and isoechoic and are therefore easily missed by transabdominal ultrasonography. MRI is the best next step if pelvic ultrasonography is negative. Imaging with [18]FDG-PET is usually reserved for select cases.[11] Of note, ovarian hyperthecosis can be described on ultrasonography as a bilateral increase in ovarian size or a single ovarian nodule. Ultrasonography often reveals bilaterally enlarged, solid ovaries for the woman's stated age. Therefore, it is important to evaluate ovarian size compared with age-based references because ovaries that are normal in size compared with those of reproductive-aged women are likely enlarged (compared with normative data in postmenopausal women). In premenopausal women, ovaries may demonstrate an absence of small follicles on ultrasonography in addition to enlargement. Finally, the presence of 12 or more antral follicles and/or ovarian volume greater than 10 cm³ meet the Rotterdam criteria for PCOS.[6]

When pelvic imaging is negative or if androgen levels suggest an adrenal etiology (DHEA-S ≥700 µg/dL [19.0 µmol/L]), adrenal CT should be performed instead of ovarian ultrasonography. Adrenal CT should be performed with and without contrast, so that the Hounsfield units and absolute and relative washout can be calculated. If CT is contraindicated, MRI with measurement of chemical shift can be performed. In selected cases, ¹⁸FDG-PET/CT can also be considered as second-line imaging. Adrenal incidentalomas are common, especially in the postmenopausal age group. Adrenal imaging should therefore only be pursued if indicated by laboratory measurements. In the presence of an adrenal tumor, the woman should also be assessed for excess endogenous cortisol secretion.

Lastly, in the setting of severe hyperandrogenism, ovarian and adrenal vein sampling can be used when both pelvic and adrenal imaging are negative.[12] Right and left ovarian and adrenal veins are accessed and testosterone is measured to determine a left to right difference. This requires the skillset of a highly experienced interventional radiologist. Ovarian and adrenal vein sampling is useful in 2 scenarios: (1) in the premenopausal woman if preservation of fertility is desired and localization of 1 ovary for resection is required, and (2) in the postmenopausal woman with a small adrenal nodule but a suspected ovarian source.

Clinical Case Vignettes
Case 1

A 27-year-old woman is referred for hirsutism and an elevated 17-hydroxyprogesterone concentration. She notes irregular menses starting at menarche, with cycles every 45 to 60 days. Her last menses was 2 months ago. She reports hirsutism on her chin, lower abdomen, and upper thighs since age 18 years. Physical examination findings are notable for mild hirsutism, with a Ferriman-Gallwey score of 10. Her primary care physician ordered laboratory tests 1 month ago, prompting the consult.

Laboratory test results:

Testosterone = 81 ng/dL (8-86 ng/dL) (SI: 2.8 nmol/L [0.3-3.0 nmol/L])
DHEA-S = 115.1 µg/dL (104.1-457.6 µg/dL) (SI: 3.12 µmol/L [2.82-12.40 µmol/L])
17-Hydroxyprogesterone = 687 ng/dL (<200 ng/dL) (SI: 20.8 nmol/L [<6.1 nmol/L])

Which of the following is the best next step?

A. Perform a cosyntropin-stimulation test

B. Order adrenal CT

C. Order ovarian ultrasonography

D. Measure hCG

E. Determine free testosterone

Answer: D) Measure hCG

The patient has been having unprotected intercourse and is pregnant. Pregnancy is the most common cause of amenorrhea, and it should always be considered in women with amenorrhea and/or irregular menses. Thus, the best next step is to measure hCG (Answer D). In the current case, the last menses was 2 months ago; she likely ovulated 6 weeks ago and at the time of the blood draw by the primary care physician was 2 weeks pregnant. The case also brings up the point that in women with hyperandrogenism and irregular menses, the causes of irregular menses should be evaluated, including thyroid function, primary ovarian insufficiency, and hyperprolactinemia.

NCCAH is diagnosed based on an elevated 17-hydroxyprogesterone level, either at baseline or in response to cosyntropin. In the setting of pregnancy, hCG drives the corpus luteum to continue producing both hormones; therefore, 17-hydroxyprogesterone levels are high. When measuring 17-hydroxyprogesterone in women with irregular menses, it is important to check a concomitant progesterone level because the corpus luteum secretes progesterone and 17-hydroxyprogesterone, causing the 17-hydroxyprogesterone level to appear falsely elevated.

Adrenal CT (Answer B) should not be performed before a clear hormonal abnormality is identified.

Ovarian ultrasonography (Answer C) is not indicated in a patient with an elevated 17-hydroxyprogesterone level.

Free testosterone assays (Answer E) rely on the total testosterone assays to measure serum levels after separation of the free testosterone fraction. Thus, the testosterone levels are usually lower than accurately measured in these assays.

Case 2

A 33-year-old woman seeks evaluation for PCOS. She notes irregular menses since menarche at age 12 years. She gained 30 lb (13.5 kg) since high school but gained an additional 15 lb (6.8 kg) in the last year. Hirsutism developed in her 20s, requiring shaving of the chin once per week. She has no galactorrhea, visual changes, or headaches. She has been treated for depression.

On physical examination, her blood pressure is 118/85 mm Hg and BMI is 39.7 kg/m². She has hirsutism over her chin and acanthosis nigricans on her neck. She has dorsocervical fat and 4-mm violaceous striae on her abdomen.

Which of the following is the best test to order?

A. 24-Hour urinary free cortisol measurement

B. Adrenal CT

C. 17-Hydroxyprogesterone measurement

D. Cosyntropin-stimulation test

E. DHEA-S measurement

Answer: A) 24-Hour urinary free cortisol measurement

Although this patient has a long history of irregular menses and hirsutism, the additional symptoms of weight gain and depression and physical signs of striae and dorsal cervical adiposity should prompt a workup for Cushing syndrome with 24-hour urinary free cortisol measurement (Answer A).

Imaging (Answer B) should not be performed before a diagnosis is made.

NCCAH (Answer C) is a consideration in the workup for hyperandrogenism, but it would not be the first choice based on her symptoms.

A cosyntropin-stimulation test (Answer D) could be helpful to confirm NCCAH with an indeterminate morning 17-hydroxyprogesterone concentration (200-500 ng/dL).

DHEA-S levels (Answer E) are elevated in patients with Cushing disease, but it is not the test of choice in this scenario.

Case 3

A 68-year-old woman seeks evaluation for a 10-year history of hirsutism. She shaves her face daily, and she thinks the hirsutism has worsened over the last 3 years. Hair growth is also present over her chest, back, and upper arms. She has had no changes in her voice or libido. She had regular menses throughout her life until menopause at age 54 years. She has had 4 pregnancies.

She has a 20-year history of hypertension treated with lisinopril and a 10-year history of type 2 diabetes mellitus treated with metformin.

On physical examination, her blood pressure is 141/74 mm Hg and BMI is 35.3 kg/m². She has bitemporal balding and normal vocal intonation. Her Ferriman-Gallwey score is elevated at 17, and acanthosis nigricans is present on her neck. She has no supraclavicular or dorsocervical fat. She has no violaceous striae. Pelvic examination reveals a normal uterus and ovaries, but examination is limited by obesity.

Laboratory test results:

Hemoglobin A$_{1c}$ = 5.7% (4.0%-5.6%)
(SI: 39 mmol/mol [20-38 mmol/mol])
Prolactin = 10.7 ng/mL (4-30 ng/mL)
(SI: 0.46 nmol/L [0.17-1.30 nmol/L])
Sodium = 140 mEq/L (40-217 mEq/24 h)
(SI: 140 mmol/L [40-217 mmol/d])
Potassium = 3.9 mEq/L (17-77 mEq/24 h)
(SI: 3.9 mmol/L [17-77 mmol/d])
Testosterone = 154 ng/dL (8-60 ng/dL)
(SI: 5.34 nmol/L [0.3-2.1 nmol/L])
DHEA-S = 41 µg/dL (15-157 µg/dL)
(SI: 1.11 µmol/L [0.41-4.25 µmol/L])

Which of the following is the best diagnostic test to perform now?

A. 24-Hour urinary free cortisol measurement

B. 17-Hydroxyprogesterone measurement

C. Free testosterone measurement

D. Adrenal CT

E. Pelvic ultrasonography

Answer: E) Pelvic ultrasonography

In a postmenopausal woman with hirsutism since menopause and gradual worsening over 3 years, the differential diagnosis includes ovarian or adrenal tumors, exogenous androgen exposure, Cushing syndrome, and hyperthecosis. Testosterone is elevated and DHEA-S is normal, suggesting an ovarian source. Pelvic ultrasonography (Answer E) is the best diagnostic test. In this case, bilaterally enlarged heterogeneous ovaries were found, typical of hyperthecosis. Other causes of ovarian hyperandrogenism include ovarian tumors such as Sertoli-Leydig–cell and hilus-cell tumors.

These ovarian tumors would also be seen on pelvic ultrasonography.

Measuring free testosterone (Answer C) is unnecessary in this patient who has an elevated total testosterone level.

Androgen-secreting adrenal adenomas and carcinomas are marked by elevated DHEA-S and testosterone, which is not the case in this vignette. Therefore, adrenal CT (Answer D) is not necessary.

In longstanding NCCAH, signs of hyperandrogenism can worsen after menopause with increasing hirsutism or male-pattern hair loss. However, there should be a history of premature pubarche, irregular menses, hirsutism, or acne. Therefore, NCCAH is unlikely and measuring 17-hydroxyprogesterone (Answer B) is not necessary.

She has no signs of Cushing syndrome such as supraclavicular or dorsocervical fat or violaceous striae. Therefore, measuring 24-hour urinary free cortisol (Answer A) is not needed.

Key Learning Points

- A workup for hyperandrogenism should include a workup for general causes of irregular menses when present.

- Very elevated testosterone (≥150 ng/dL [≥5.2 nmol/L]) and DHEA-S (≥700 µg/dL [≥19.0 µmol/L]) indicate tumors of the ovary or adrenal, respectively.

- The best imaging modality is ovarian ultrasonography for elevated testosterone and adrenal CT for elevated DHEA-S.

References

1. Walters KA, Handelsman DJ. Role of androgens in the ovary. *Mol Cell Endocrinol.* 2018;465:36-47. PMID: 28687450

2. Afifi L, Saeed L, Pasch LA, et al. Association of ethnicity, Fitzpatrick skin type, and hirsutism: A retrospective cross-sectional study of women with polycystic ovarian syndrome. *Int J Womens Dermatol.* 2017;3:37-43. PMID: 28492053

3. Escobar-Morreale HF, Carmina E, Dewailly D, et al. Epidemiology, diagnosis and management of hirsutism: a consensus statement by the Androgen Excess and Polycystic Ovary Syndrome Society. *Hum Reprod Update.* 2012;18(2):146-170. PMID: 22064667

4. Carmina E, Azziz R, Bergfeld W, et al. Female pattern hair loss and androgen excess: a report from the Multidisciplinary Androgen Excess and PCOS Committee. *J Clin Endocrinol Metab.* 2019;104(7):2875-2891. PMID: 30785992

5. Makrantonaki E, Zouboulis CC. Testosterone metabolism to 5alpha-dihydrotestosterone and synthesis of sebaceous lipids is regulated by the peroxisome proliferator-activated receptor ligand linoleic acid in human sebocytes. *Br J Dermatol.* 2007;156(3):428-432. PMID: 17300229

6. Teede HJ, Misso ML, Costello MF, et al. Recommendations from the international evidence-based guideline for the assessment and management of polycystic ovary syndrome. *Hum Reprod.* 2018;33(9):1602-1618. PMID: 30052961

7. Sharma A, Kapoor E, Singh RJ, Chang AY, Erickson D. Diagnostic thresholds for androgen-producing tumors or pathologic hyperandrogenism in women by use of total testosterone concentrations measured by liquid chromatography-tandem mass spectrometry. *Clin Chem.* 2018;64:1636-1645. PMID: 30068692

8. Rosner W, Auchus RJ, Azziz R, Sluss PM, Raff H. Position statement: utility, limitations, and pitfalls in measuring testosterone: an Endocrine Society position statement. *J Clin Endocrinol Metab.* 2007;92(2):405-413. PMID: 17090633

9. Elhassan YS, Idkowiak J, Smith K, et al. Causes, patterns, and severity of androgen excess in 1205 consecutively recruited women. *J Clin Endocrinol Metab.* 2018;103(3):1214-1223. PMID: 29342266

10. Berke K, Constantinescu G, Masjkur J, et al. Plasma steroid profiling in patients with adrenal incidentaloma. *J Clin Endocrinol Metab.* 2022;107(3):e1181-e1192. PMID: 34665854

11. McCarthy-Keith DM, Hill M, Norian JM, Millo C, McKeeby J, Armstrong AY. Use of F 18-fluoro-D-glucose-positron emission tomography-computed tomography to localize a hilar cell tumor of the ovary. *Fertil Steril.* 2010;94(2):753.e11-e14. PMID: 20362283

12. Kaltsas GA, Mukherjee JJ, Kola B, et al. Is ovarian and adrenal venous catheterization and sampling helpful in the investigation of hyperandrogenic women? *Clin Endocrinol (Oxf).* 2003;59(1):34-43. PMID: 12807501

Adrenal Incidentalomas: Contemporary Evaluation and Management

William F. Young, Jr, MD, MSc. Division of Endocrinology, Diabetes, Metabolism, and Nutrition, Mayo Clinic, Rochester, MN; Email: wyoung@mayo.edu

Educational Objectives

After reviewing this chapter, learners should be able to:

- Use imaging characteristics to determine the likelihood that an adrenal incidentaloma is either malignant or a pheochromocytoma.

- Identify a framework for screening for hormonal hypersecretion in patients with adrenal incidentalomas.

- Describe management considerations for adrenal incidentalomas, including indications for surgery or monitoring.

Significance of the Clinical Problem

An adrenal incidentaloma is an adrenal mass discovered serendipitously by radiologic examination in the absence of symptoms or clinical findings suggestive of adrenal disease and 1 cm or more in diameter (ie, leaving no question that it really is a mass). The imaging characteristics of the incidentally discovered adrenal mass guide the clinician on both diagnostic evaluation and treatment. Imaging phenotypes are quite specific and predictive of underlying pathology. Unless another diagnosis is obvious (eg, pheochromocytoma), all patients with adrenal incidentaloma should be evaluated for subclinical glucocorticoid secretory autonomy (subclinical Cushing syndrome [CS]). If the unenhanced CT attenuation is 10 or more Hounsfield units (HU), biochemical testing for pheochromocytoma should be completed. Biochemical testing for primary aldosteronism should be performed in patients who present with either hypertension or hypokalemia. Surgical management should be considered in most patients with confirmed subclinical CS. In addition, surgery should be considered in patients with nonfunctioning, lipid-poor adrenal masses.

With increasing resolution of CT, specific attention from radiologists, and more careful prospective studies, the prevalence of adrenal incidentalomas increased from 0.6% in 1982[1] to 7.3% in patients under medical care in 2020.[2] In a recent report from China, at general health check-up, 25,356 volunteers had abdominal CT scans and 351 had adrenal tumors for a prevalence of 1.4%.[3] Prevalence increased with age: 0.28% in those younger than 35 years and 3.2% in those older than 65 years.[3]

In an epidemiologic study from Olmsted County, Minnesota, 1050 residents (1.5% of all CT scans) were found to have an adrenal incidentaloma[4]:

- 3.3% were malignant (neuroblastoma and adrenocortical cancer [ACC] in children and metastatic disease, lymphoma, and ACC in adults)

- 88% were adrenal adenomas:

- 1.1% had overt hormone excess (CS and primary aldosteronism)
  - 8.2% had confirmed subclinical CS
  - 12.4% had confirmed nonfunctioning adenomas
  - 66.4% were adrenal adenomas with unknown hormone status

- 0.8% were pheochromocytomas
- 7.8% were other benign tumors (myelolipoma > hematoma > cyst > calcification > ganglioneuroma, schwannoma > hemangioma, lymphangioma)

Practice Gaps

- Best management strategy for lipid-poor adrenal masses.
- Best management strategy for patients with subclinical CS.
- When to consider "prebiochemical pheochromocytoma."
- Lack of awareness of primary aldosteronism.

Discussion

The clinician should evaluate an adrenal incidentaloma for:

- **Functional status** with a history, physical examination, and hormonal assessment.
- **Malignant potential** based on imaging phenotype, size, growth, and history of extraadrenal malignancy.

The algorithm (*figure 1*) helps guide the evaluation of the patient with an adrenal incidentaloma.[5]

Hormonal Evaluation

Subclinical Cushing Syndrome

Unless another diagnosis is obvious (eg, pheochromocytoma), all patients should be evaluated for glucocorticoid secretory autonomy (referred to as *subclinical CS*) with measurement of dehydroepiandrosterone sulfate (DHEA-S) and corticotropin (ACTH). If the DHEA-S value is less than 40 µg/dL (<1.08 µmol/L), it is suspicious for subclinical CS, and an overnight 1-mg dexamethasone suppression-test (DST) should be performed.[6] If the DHEA-S value is greater than 100 µg/dL (>2.71 µmol/L), subclinical

Figure 1. Algorithm to evaluate incidentally discovered adrenal masses

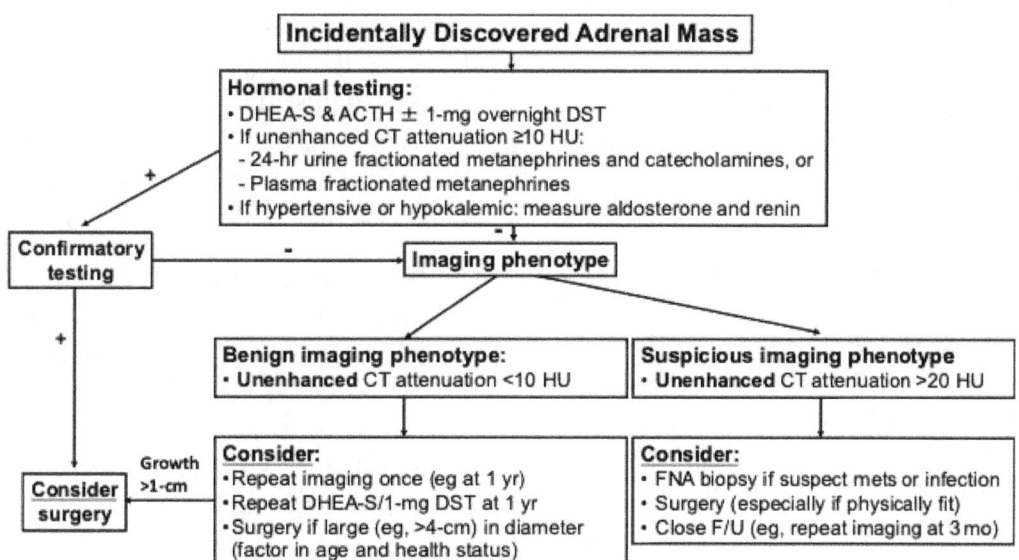

Abbreviations: ACTH, corticotropin; DHEA-S, dehydroepiandrosterone sulfate; DST, dexamethasone-suppression test; FNA, fine-needle aspiration; F/U, follow-up; HU, Hounsfield unit; mo, months. Adapted from Young WF Jr. N Engl J Med, 2007;356(6): 601-10. © Massachusetts Medical Society.

CS is very unlikely and an overnight DST can be avoided.[6] Due to the high false-positive rate with the 1-mg overnight DST, an abnormal result should be confirmed with an 8-mg overnight DST before considering surgical resection.[7] Because the blood cortisol concentration is never high in patients with subclinical CS, they do not filter much cortisol at the kidney and the 24-hour urinary free cortisol excretion tends to be low—a result that can confuse the clinician. It is the lack of cortisol drop in the afternoon and evening that leads to osteopenia/osteoporosis, hyperglycemia/diabetes mellitus, hypertension, hyperlipidemia, weight gain, insomnia, etc. It is as if the adrenal adenoma is dosing the patient with 4, 5, or 6 mg of prednisone equivalent every day—distributed evenly over 24 hours. Without intervention, the glucocorticoid secretory autonomy is not going to go away and can only get worse with time. In the era of laparoscopic adrenalectomy with expert endocrine surgeons, **consideration** should be given to treating with unilateral adrenalectomy in "all" (use common sense) of these patients who have confirmed autonomy on an 8-mg overnight DST.

Pheochromocytoma

If the unenhanced CT attenuation of an adrenal mass is less than 10 HU, it cannot be a pheochromocytoma and biochemical testing for this rare neoplasm should not be done. In a multicenter retrospective study of 533 patients with 548 histologically confirmed pheochromocytomas, among the 376 pheochromocytomas for which unenhanced CT attenuation data were available, 374 had an attenuation value greater than 10 HU (99.5%).[8] In the 2 exceptions (0.5%), the unenhanced CT attenuation was exactly 10 HU.[8] Thus, if the unenhanced CT attenuation is 10 or more HU, biochemical testing with plasma fractionated metanephrines or 24-hour urinary fractionated metanephrines and catecholamines is indicated.

Primary Aldosteronism

All patients with either hypertension or hypokalemia should be screened for primary aldosteronism by measurement of morning plasma aldosterone concentration and renin (either plasma renin activity or direct renin concentration). Positive case-detection testing cutoffs are plasma aldosterone concentration greater than 10 ng/dL (>277 pmol/L) and plasma renin activity less than 1 ng/mL per h or direct renin concentration less than 8 mU/L or below the lower limit of the reference range. If spontaneous hypokalemia is absent, a positive case-detection result should be followed up with confirmatory testing (eg, during a high-sodium diet, measure 24-hour urine excretion of aldosterone, sodium, and creatinine).[9]

Imaging Phenotype

Imaging phenotype refers to what an adrenal mass looks like on CT. On CT, the density of the image (black is less dense) is attributed to radiograph attenuation. The intracytoplasmic fat in adenomas results in low attenuation on unenhanced CT; nonadenomas have higher attenuation on unenhanced CT. The Hounsfield scale is a semiquantitative method of measuring radiograph attenuation. Typical precontrast values are −20 to −150 HU for adipose tissue and +20 to +150 HU for kidney. If an adrenal mass has an unenhanced CT attenuation less than 10 HU (ie, lipid rich), the likelihood that it is a benign adenoma (or other benign process such as myelolipoma) is nearly 100%. However, up to 30% of adenomas do not contain large amounts of lipid and may be indistinguishable from nonadenomas on unenhanced CT and are termed *lipid-poor adenomas*. Based on the unenhanced CT attenuation, adrenal masses can be divided into 3 categories:

1. When the unenhanced CT attenuation is less than 10 HU and the hormonal evaluation is normal, it is reasonable to recheck a CT or MRI 1 year later to be sure there was no error in the interpretation of the initial scan. Although the risk of an initially nonfunctioning adrenal adenoma to develop hyperfunction over time is low, I repeat DHEA-S measurement or the 1-mg overnight DST at the 1-year follow-up visit.

2. When the unenhanced CT attenuation is between 10 and 20 HU, it is indeterminant and follow-up should be individualized.

3. When the unenhanced CT attenuation is greater than 20 HU, the mass is considered lipid poor. Lipid poor adrenal masses are the landmines of adrenal disorders. Although lipid-poor adrenal masses may be benign, nonfunctional cortical adenomas, it can be difficult to make the distinction from more concerning diagnoses such as a small ACC and prebiochemical pheochromocytoma. Choosing nonsurgical management can carry clinically significant risk. After appropriate workup, most lipid-poor adrenal masses larger than 1.5 cm in diameter should be resected by an expert endocrine surgeon.

Adrenal Mass Size

The maximum diameter of the adrenal mass is predictive of malignancy. In a retrospective, single-center cohort of 4085 patients with adrenal tumors, 705 (17%) had adrenal masses measuring 4 cm or more in diameter. Of the 705 patients with adrenal masses greater than 4 cm in diameter, 216 (31%) were adrenocortical adenomas, 158 (22%) were pheochromocytomas, 116 (16%) were other benign adrenal tumors, 88 (13%) were ACCs, and 127 (18%) were other malignant tumors.[10] Thus, when greater than 4 cm in diameter, 53% of patients had either cancer or pheochromocytoma.[10] So, the 4-cm cutoff is an important one, but it should be ignored in patients with lipid-rich adrenal masses.

Typical Imaging Features

- **Benign adenomas** are round with homogeneous density, smooth contour, and sharp margination. They typically have low unenhanced CT attenuation values (<10 HU).

- **Pheochromocytomas** have increased attenuation on unenhanced CT (>20 HU), increased vascularity, and are inhomogeneous with cystic and hemorrhagic changes.

- **ACCs** typically have an irregular shape, inhomogeneous density because of central areas of low attenuation due to tumor necrosis, tumor microcalcifications, diameter usually greater than 4 cm, unilateral location, high unenhanced CT attenuation values (>20 HU), and inhomogeneous enhancement on CT with intravenous contrast administration.

- **Adrenal metastases** typically have an irregular shape and inhomogeneous nature, tendency to be bilateral, high unenhanced CT attenuation values (>20 HU), and enhancement with intravenous contrast on CT.

For those who like podcasts, I recently participated in the Curbsiders Internal Medicine Podcast on adrenal incidentalomas (https://thecurbsiders.com/episode-list January 16, 2023).

Clinical Case Vignettes
Case 1

A 71-year-old woman has a CT to investigate an abdominal wall hematoma. A 2.1 × 2.5-cm left adrenal mass is incidentally detected (*figure 2*). The unenhanced CT attenuation is 33.3 HU.

She is asymptomatic with no signs or symptoms of CS or pheochromocytoma. She has no history of cancer. She had an 8-year history of hypertension that is well-controlled with lisinopril, 20 mg daily. There is no history of hypokalemia.

Figure 2.

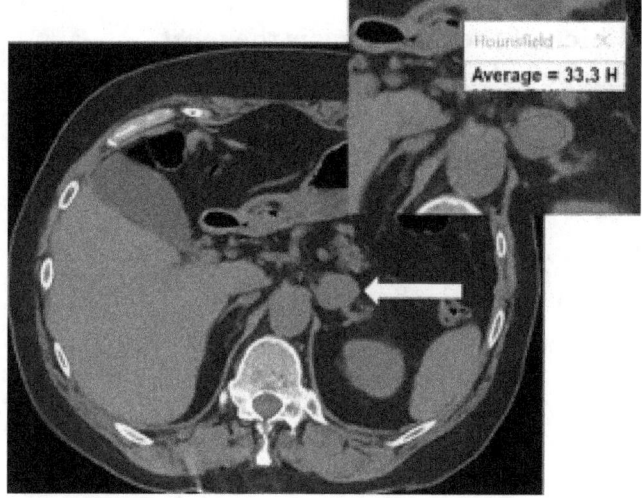

(Color—web and EPUB only)

The imaging phenotype of the adrenal mass in this patient is most consistent with which one of the following?

A. Benign cortical adenoma

B. Myelolipoma

C. Pheochromocytoma

D. Untreated congenital adrenal hyperplasia

E. Metastatic disease to the adrenal

Answer: C) Pheochromocytoma

Although the adrenal mass could be a lipid-poor adenoma (Answer A), most adrenal adenomas are lipid rich.

The CT image is not consistent with a myelolipoma (Answer B) because these tumors have areas of macroscopic fat with low unenhanced CT attenuation.

Untreated congenital adrenal hyperplasia (Answer D) usually has the CT appearance of bilaterally hyperplastic adrenal glands with or without myelolipomatous change.

This adrenal mass could represent metastatic disease to the adrenal (Answer E) because metastases are lipid poor; however, metastatic disease to the adrenal glands is usually bilateral and is found in patients with a known primary malignancy.

With all of those considerations and from the listed options, the unilateral lipid-poor adrenal mass in this patient has an imaging phenotype most consistent with pheochromocytoma (Answer C).

Case 1 (continued)

Which of the following is the most common clinical presentation of adrenal pheochromocytoma?

A. Paroxysmal hypertension

B. Adrenal incidentaloma

C. Found due to family or genetic testing

D. Symptomatic abdominal mass

E. Syncope

Answer: B) Adrenal incidentaloma

Before the year 2000, the most common clinical presentation of adrenal pheochromocytoma was hypertensive paroxysms (Answer A). However, with the wide-spread use of computed cross-sectional abdominal imaging, 60% pheochromocytomas are discovered incidentally on imaging performed for nonadrenal reasons (Answer B).

Although the frequency of diagnosing patients with pheochromocytoma by way of germline genetic testing and/or family screening (Answer C) is increasing, this mode of presentation represents less than 15% of all patients with pheochromocytoma going to surgery.

The diagnosis of pheochromocytoma based on the presentation of an abdominal mass (Answer D) is very rare.

Finally, although patients with pheochromocytoma can present with syncope (Answer E), it is not a common presentation.

ADDENDUM: Plasma fractionated metanephrines were diagnostic for a noradrenergic pheochromocytoma with a normetanephrine concentration of 4.6 nmol/L (normal, <0.9 nmol/L) and metanephrine concentration of 0.28 nmol/L (normal, <0.5 nmol/L). Following adrenergic blockade, the patient underwent laparoscopic left adrenalectomy, and pathology confirmed a 3 × 2.5 × 2-cm pheochromocytoma. Postoperative plasma fractionated metanephrines were normal. She had persistent hypertension that was treated with lisinopril. Germline genetic testing did not detect a pathogenic variant in a 14-gene panel. The patient will be followed with annual measurement of plasma fractionated metanephrines.

Case 2

A 56-year-old woman has a 3.4-cm incidentally discovered left adrenal mass that has an unenhanced CT attenuation of −16 HU (*figure 3*).

Figure 3.

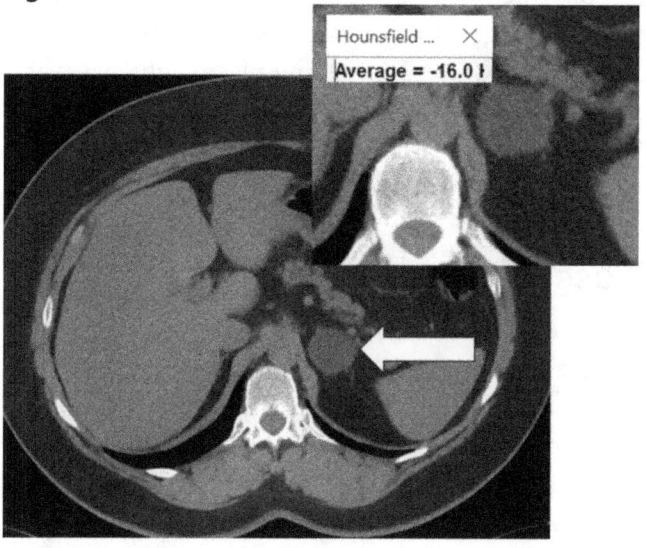

(Color—web and EPUB only)

She has no signs or symptoms of CS or pheochromocytoma. She has no history of hypertension or hypokalemia. She has obesity (BMI = 34 kg/m²) and has gained 20 lb (9 kg) over the past 3 years. She has osteoporosis treated with a bisphosphonate and hyperlipidemia treated with a statin. She is taking no other medications. Impaired fasting glucose has been noted over the past 5 years, and her hemoglobin A_{1c} level is 5.6% (normal, 4.0%-5.6%). The referring physician measures plasma fractionated metanephrines, which are abnormal with a normetanephrine concentration of 1.4 nmol/L (normal, <0.9 nmol/L) and metanephrine concentration of 0.25 nmol/L (normal, <0.5 nmol/L).

Which of the following is the best next diagnostic test in this patient?

A. Measurement of 24-hour urine fractionated metanephrines and catecholamines

B. Measurement of plasma aldosterone and renin

C. 1-mg overnight DST

D. Measurement of 24-hour urinary free cortisol

E. ^{123}I MIBG

Answer: C) 1-mg overnight DST

If the unenhanced CT attenuation of an adrenal mass is less than 10 HU, it cannot be a pheochromocytoma, and biochemical testing for this neoplasm is not indicated. The adrenal mass in this patient is lipid rich with an unenhanced CT attenuation of –16 HU; thus, further biochemical testing for pheochromocytoma (Answer A) or whole-body imaging (Answer E) is not indicated. Mild false-positive elevations in plasma normetanephrine are common.

The patient is normotensive and normokalemic, so testing for primary aldosteronism (Answer B) is not indicated.

She does not have clinical signs of CS, so measurement of 24-hour urinary free cortisol (Answer D) is not indicated. Twenty-four–hour urinary free cortisol excretion is a good test for clinical CS, but not for subclinical glucocorticoid secretory autonomy.

This patient does need a test for glucocorticoid secretory autonomy and, of the options listed, the 1-mg overnight DST (Answer C) is the best answer.

Case 2 (continued)

In addition to the 1-mg overnight DST, which of the following would be the most effective screening test for subclinical glucocorticoid secretory autonomy?

A. Serum DHEA-S measurement

B. Midnight salivary cortisol measurement

C. 24-Hour urinary free cortisol excretion

D. Corticotropin-releasing hormone–stimulation test

E. Cosyntropin-stimulation test

Answer: A) Serum DHEA-S measurement

Because subclinical CS is a disorder of low-level continuous cortisol secretion, the classic tests for clinical CS (eg, midnight salivary cortisol [Answer B] and 24-hour urinary free cortisol [Answer C]) cannot be used effectively to diagnose this disorder. The corticotropin-releasing hormone–stimulation test (Answer D) and the cosyntropin-stimulation test (Answer E) have not been used and would not be effective in detecting subclinical CS. DHEA-S measurement (Answer A), however, can be used to reflect long-term relative suppression of endogenous ACTH secretion. When the DHEA-S value is less than 40 μg/dL (<1.08 μmol/L), the patient may have subclinical CS. When the DHEA-S value is greater than 100 μg/dL (>2.71 μmol/L), subclinical CS is very unlikely.

ADDENDUM: The patient's baseline DHEA-S concentration was low at 22 μg/dL (0.6 μmol/L) (normal, 16-195 μg/dL [0.43-5.29 μmol/L]) and her ACTH concentration was low-normal at 15 pg/mL (3.3 pmol/L) (normal, 10-60 pg/mL [2.2-13.2 pmol/L]). The result of the 1-mg overnight DST was abnormal with a next-day serum cortisol concentration of 3.2 μg/dL (88.3 nmol/L) (normal <1.8 μg/dL [<50 nmol/L]). Glucocorticoid secretory autonomy was confirmed with an 8-mg overnight DST (the next-day serum cortisol concentration was 3.6 μg/dL (99.3 nmol/L) (normal <1 μg/dL [<27.6 nmol/L]). The patient was informed that the glucocorticoid secretory autonomy may be contributing to her weight gain, osteoporosis, hyperlipidemia, and impaired fasting glucose. In addition, it would not resolve on its own and the degree of autonomous cortisol secretion may increase over time. She elected to proceed with laparoscopic left adrenalectomy. Pathology showed a 3.5 × 3.2 × 2.8-cm adrenal adenoma. She was treated with perioperative corticosteroid coverage and went home on hydrocortisone, 20 mg in the morning and 10 mg in the afternoon. She was advised to taper the total dosage by 5 mg every 2 weeks until her dose was down to 15 mg every morning. At that point, she was followed every 6 weeks with a morning serum cortisol checked before she took her morning dose of hydrocortisone. Initially, the serum cortisol concentration was 1.8 μg/dL (50 nmol/L). She had moderate glucocorticoid withdrawal symptoms. The morning cortisol concentration slowly increased over the subsequent 4 months, at which time it was 11 μg/dL (303.5 nmol/L) and she was advised to discontinue hydrocortisone.[12] She was educated on the use of sick-day corticosteroid coverage to be initiated if needed over the subsequent 1 year after surgery. At her 1-year follow-up evaluation, she commented that her sleep (which she had not noted to be a problem prior to surgery) was markedly improved. She had lost 15 lb (6.8 kg). Her fasting plasma glucose was normal and her hemoglobin A_{1c} improved to 5.2%. She was very pleased with the outcome and her decision to pursue surgery.

Case 3

A 40-year-old man has an abdominal CT for nonadrenal reasons. A 1.6-cm, lipid-poor (39.1 HU) left adrenal nodule is incidentally detected. He is normotensive and normokalemic. He has no symptoms of adrenal hyperfunction and no history of a malignancy elsewhere. An axial image from the unenhanced CT scan is shown (*figure 4*).

Figure 4.

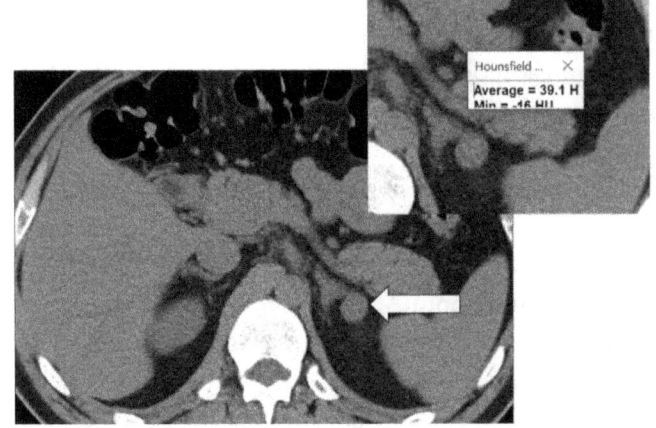

(Color—web and EPUB only)

Laboratory evaluation shows normal levels of plasma fractionated metanephrines, serum cortisol, 24-hour urinary free cortisol, and DHEA-S. Results of a 1-mg overnight DST are normal.

Which of the following is the best next step in the evaluation and management of this 1.6-cm left adrenal mass?

A. Left adrenalectomy

B. Abdominal MRI

C. No further evaluation or follow-up is needed

D. Follow-up CT in 3 months

E. Follow-up CT in 12 months

Answer: A) Left adrenalectomy

The best management approach to lipid-poor adrenal masses is controversial. Some adrenal experts (including this writer) are concerned that they may represent either an early ACC, "pre-ACC," or pre-biochemical pheochromocytoma and should either be resected (Answer A) or followed closely (Answer D, the second-best answer option). Typically, the findings on MRI (Answer B) do not add much to what was already learned from the noncontrast CT. Lipid-poor adrenal masses should either be resected or followed closely. Thus, recommending no further evaluation or follow-up (Answer C) is incorrect. In the setting of a lipid-poor adrenal mass, most clinicians would not wait 1 year (Answer E) before repeating the imaging.

Case 3 (continued)

Follow-up contrast-enhanced CT imaging is next completed at 4 years and then 5 years after the initial discovery of the lipid-poor left adrenal mass. The left adrenal mass is slightly larger at 1.8 cm (*figure 5, coronal views*). Hormonal testing is once again normal.

Which of the following is the best next step in the evaluation and management of this lipid-poor, 1.8-cm left adrenal mass that increased 2 mm in diameter over 5 years?

A. Left adrenalectomy

B. Abdominal MRI

C. Recommend no further evaluation or follow-up

D. Follow-up CT in 3 months

E. Follow-up CT in 5 years

Answer: A) Left adrenalectomy

Figure 5.

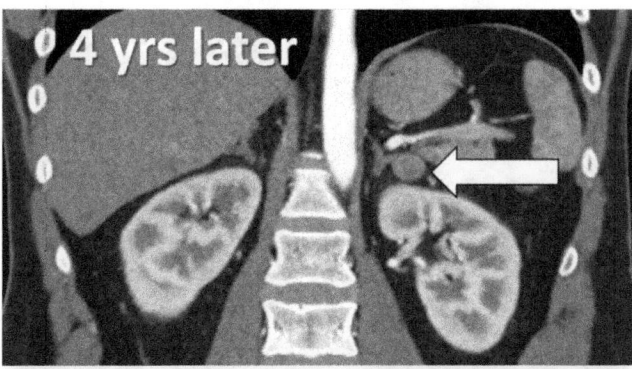

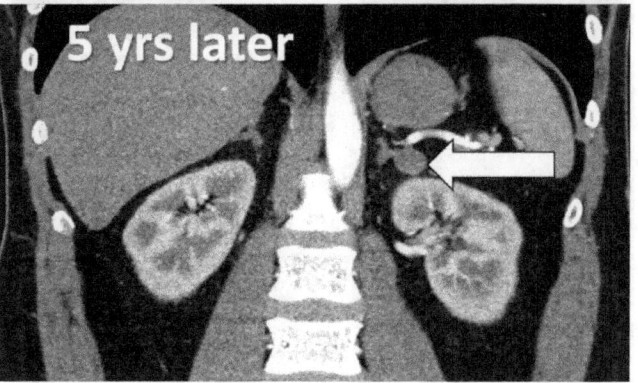

Lipid-poor adrenal masses are the landmines of adrenal disorders. After 5 years of relative stability, many clinicians would choose no further evaluation or follow-up (Answer C), and that would be an error. Some adrenal experts (including this writer) are concerned that lipid-poor adrenal masses may represent either an early ACC, "pre-ACC," or prebiochemical pheochromocytoma and should either be resected (Answer A) or followed closely (Answer D). Typically, the findings on MRI (Answer B) do not add much to what was already learned from noncontrast CT. In the setting of a lipid-poor adrenal mass, most clinicians would not wait 5 years (Answer E) before repeating the imaging, despite the relative stability over the previous 4 years.

ADDENDUM: Imaging 9 years after the initial CT scan demonstrated a markedly enlarged left adrenal mass and it proved to be ACC when resected. CT Imaging 11 years after the initial CT scan showed recurrent disease in the left adrenal bed (*figure 6, upper coronal image*) and diffuse hepatic metastases (*figure 6, lower coronal image*).

Figure 6.

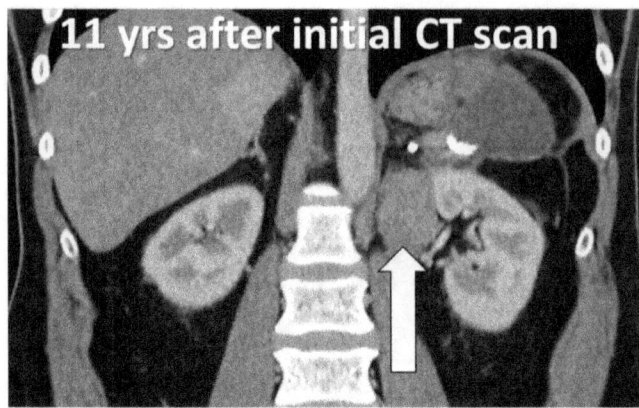

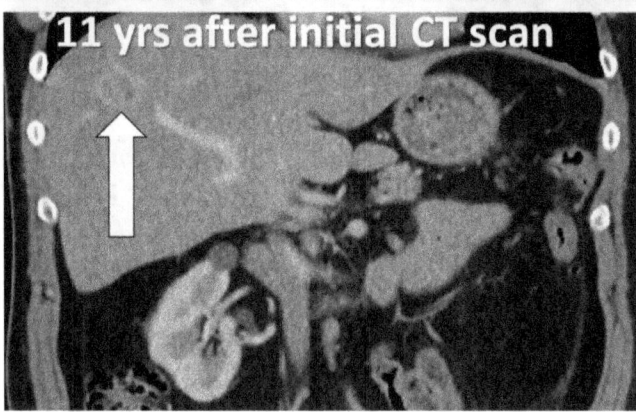

The patient underwent en bloc resection that included distal pancreatectomy, left hemicolectomy, and left nephrectomy. Intraoperative thermal ablation was used to treat 6 hepatic metastases. On pathology, metastatic ACC formed a 7.5 × 3.5 × 2.0-cm mass with additional multiple tumor deposits ranging in size between 1.0 and 2.5 cm. The patient died of metastatic ACC 14 years after the initial CT.

Key Learning Points

- The adrenal mass phenotype guides the clinician on both diagnostic evaluation and treatment—imaging phenotypes are quite specific and predictive of underlying pathology.

- Unless another diagnosis is obvious (eg, pheochromocytoma), all patients with adrenal incidentaloma should be evaluated for subclinical CS.

- If the unenhanced CT attenuation is 10 or more HU, biochemical testing for pheochromocytoma should be completed.

- Biochemical testing for primary aldosteronism should be performed in patients who present with either hypertension or hypokalemia.

- Surgical management should be considered in patients with confirmed (with an 8-mg overnight DST) subclinical CS.

- Surgical resection should be considered in patients with nonfunctioning, lipid-poor adrenal masses.

References

1. Glazer HS, Weyman PJ, Sagel SS, Levitt RG, McClennan BL. Nonfunctioning adrenal masses: incidental discovery on computed tomography. *AJR Am J Roentgenol.* 1982;139(1):81-85. PMID: 6979870

2. Reimondo G, Castellano E, Grosso M, et al. Adrenal incidentalomas are tied to increased risk of diabetes: findings from a prospective study. *J Clin Endocrinol Metab.* 2020;105(4):dgz284.

3. Jing Y, Hu J, Luo R, et al. Prevalence and characteristics of adrenal tumors in an unselected screening population: a cross-sectional study. *Ann Intern Med.* 2022;175(10):1383-1391. PMID: 36095315

4. Ebbehoj A, Li D, Kaur RJ, et al. Epidemiology of adrenal tumours in Olmsted County, Minnesota, USA: a population-based cohort study. *Lancet Diabetes Endocrinol.* 2020;8(11):894-902. PMID: 33065059

5. Young WF Jr. Clinical practice. The incidentally discovered adrenal mass. *N Engl J Med.* 2007;356(6):601-610. PMID: 17287480

6. Carafone LE, Zhang CD, Li D, et al. Diagnostic accuracy of dehydroepiandrosterone sulfate and corticotropin in autonomous cortisol secretion. *Biomedicines.* 2021;9(7):741. PMID: 34203283

7. Vanek C, Loriaux L. The 1 mg overnight dexamethasone suppression test: a danger to the adrenal gland? *Curr Opin Endocrinol Diabetes Obes.* 2022;29(4):403-405. PMID: 35799460

8. Canu L, Van Hemert JAW, Kerstens MN, et al. CT characteristics of pheochromocytoma: relevance for the evaluation of adrenal incidentaloma. *J Clin Endocrinol Metab.* 2019;104(2):312-318. PMID: 30383267

9. Young WF Jr. Diagnosis and treatment of primary aldosteronism: practical clinical perspectives. *J Intern Med.* 2019;285(2):126-148. PMID: 30255616

10. Iñiguez-Ariza NM, Kohlenberg JD, Delivanis DA, et al. Clinical, biochemical, and radiological characteristics of a single-center retrospective cohort of 705 large adrenal tumors. *Mayo Clin Proc Innov Qual Outcomes.* 2017;2(1):30-39. PMID: 302254430

11. Gandhi MM, Young WF, Williams PN, Watto MF. #377 Adrenal Incidentalomas with Dr. William Young. *The Curbsiders Internal Medicine Podcast.* Accessed April 27, 2023. https://thecurbsiders.com/episode-list.

12. Hurtado MD, Cortes T, Natt N, Young WF Jr, Bancos I. Extensive clinical experience: Hypothalamic-pituitary-adrenal axis recovery after adrenalectomy for corticotropin-independent cortisol excess. *Clin Endocrinol (Oxf).* 2018;89(6):721-733. PMID: 29968420

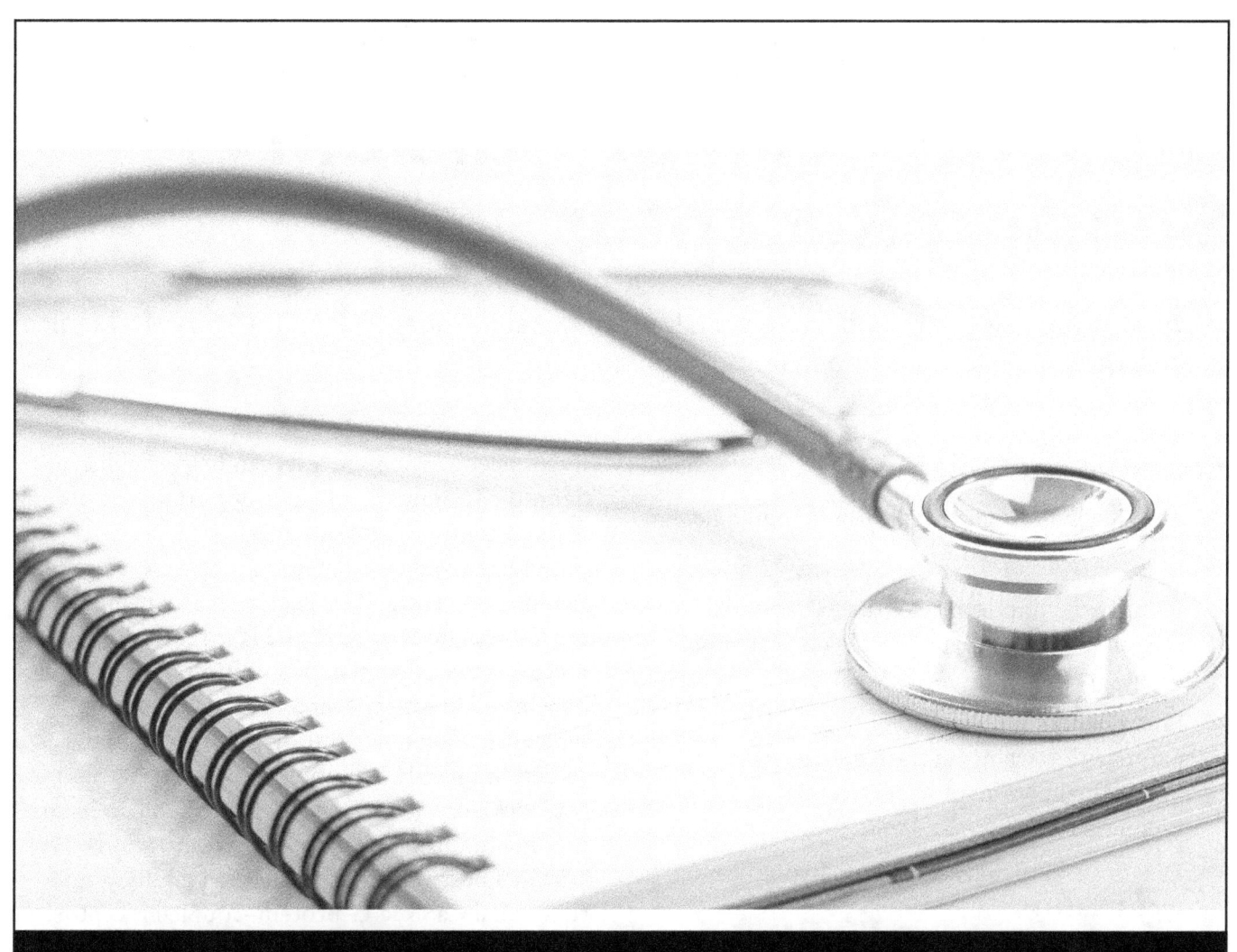

BONE AND MINERAL METABOLISM

Diseases Associated With the Extracellular Calcium-Sensing Receptor

Michael Mannstadt, MD. Endocrine Unit, Massachusetts General Hospital, Harvard Medical School, Boston, MA; Email: mannstadt@mgh.harvard.edu

Educational Objectives

After reviewing this chapter, learners should be able to:

- Identify the importance of the extracellular calcium-sensing receptor (CaSR) in calcium homeostasis.

- Illustrate the consequences of activating pathogenic variants in the *CASR* gene (autosomal dominant hypocalcemia type 1 [ADH1]).

- Diagnose familial hypocalciuric hypocalcemia type 1 (FHH1).

- Recommend management for ADH1 and FHH1.

Significance of the Clinical Problem

The CaSR plays a critical role in the maintenance of normal calcium levels. Pathogenic variants lead to several disorders with high penetrance. Loss-of-function *CASR* variants (found in FHH1) result in a decreased sensitivity of the CaSR to extracellular calcium. Extracellular calcium has a decreased ability to block PTH secretion. These pathogenic variants lead to hypercalcemia with inappropriately normal or mildly elevated PTH. However, FHH1 is a benign disorder and asymptomatic in most patients. The mirror image disorder, ADH1, is caused by activating *CASR* variants, resulting in the suppression of PTH and hypocalcemia. Genetic tests can help establish a definitive diagnosis, which is important for the management of these disorders.[1]

Parathyroid cells detect changes in extracellular calcium and adjust PTH secretion accordingly. If serum calcium is too low, PTH is released, which increases the calcium concentration in the blood by several different mechanisms. Conversely, when calcium concentrations are too high, the secretion of PTH is suppressed. This negative feedback loop allows the fine-tuned PTH release that maintains blood calcium concentrations within a narrow range. It relies on a fully functional CaSR, a G-protein–coupled receptor, which is highly expressed on the surface of parathyroid cells.

Activating and inactivating variants in the *CASR* gene disturb this negative feedback loop and lead to several diseases, including ADH1 and FHH1, respectively. The management of these diseases requires an in-depth understanding of their pathophysiology and the consequences of treatment.

Practice Gaps

- Knowledge of when to suspect and how to diagnose FHH1 and ADH1.

- Understanding the importance of avoiding parathyroid surgery in patients with FHH1.

- Identifying adverse outcomes in patients with ADH1 on conventional therapy.

Discussion

The CaSR is a G-protein–coupled receptor that plays a crucial role in regulating extracellular calcium concentrations.[2] The cloning of its gene (*CASR*) 30 years ago[3] allowed for extensive molecular studies of its function and the development of medical treatments such as positive allosteric modulators (eg, cinacalcet) for hyperparathyroid disorders.[4] The CaSR is expressed in various tissues, most highly in the parathyroid glands and kidneys. The functions of the CaSR in other tissues are subject to intense research but are beyond the scope of our discussion.[5] In the parathyroids, the CaSR detects changes in extracellular calcium levels; high calcium levels activate it, putting a brake on PTH secretion. When extracellular calcium levels are low, the brake on PTH secretion is released. Increased levels of PTH increase serum calcium, which, in turn, activates the CaSR, decreasing PTH secretion. This negative feedback loop with minute-to-minute regulation of PTH secretion keeps blood calcium levels within a tight physiological range. Pathogenic variants in the *CASR* gene can cause lifelong disruptions in this finely regulated homeostatic system. These disorders are described in more detail below.

The CaSR is also highly expressed in the kidneys, particularly in the thick ascending limb, where it contributes to the renal handling of calcium and magnesium.[6] Activation of the CaSR by elevated serum calcium decreases the reabsorption of calcium and magnesium, causing their increased excretion in the urine.

Loss-of-Function Pathogenic Variants

Familial Hypocalciuric Hypocalcemia Type 1

FHH1 is an inherited condition that results in elevated blood calcium levels. Individuals with FHH1 have heterozygous inactivating variants in the *CASR* gene that increase PTH levels for any given calcium level, leading to hypercalcemia and nonsuppressed PTH. In the kidneys, inactivating *CASR* variants lead to increased calcium reabsorption, resulting in low urinary calcium levels (hypocalciuria), which is characteristic of this disorder and different from primary hyperparathyroidism. Patients typically present with the incidental finding of mildly elevated serum calcium (often around 11 mg/dL [2.74 mmol/L]), mildly elevated PTH levels, mild hypermagnesemia, and low urinary calcium excretion. FHH1 is a benign disease with no significant adverse health effects or end-organ damage in most patients (pancreatitis might be an exception[7]). Confirming the diagnosis is important, as parathyroid surgery does not change the disease and should be avoided.

Neonatal Severe Hyperparathyroidism

Newborns with homozygous deletion of the *CASR* gene present with life-threatening hypercalcemia.[8] Emergency parathyroidectomy may be required. Some heterozygous pathogenic variants in *CASR* have been reported in patients with neonatal severe hyperparathyroidism.[5]

Gain-of-Function Pathogenic Variants

Autosomal Dominant Hypocalcemia Type 1

ADH1 is caused by heterozygous activating variants in the *CASR* gene resulting in low blood calcium levels.[9] In the parathyroid, the mutant CaSR puts a brake on PTH secretion even at low calcium levels. The inhibition of PTH secretion results in hypocalcemia and low but usually detectable circulating PTH concentrations. In the kidneys, the mutant CaSR leads to urinary calcium levels that are even higher than seen in the common form of hypoparathyroidism. The hypercalciuria leads to a high risk of nephrocalcinosis, nephrolithiasis, and chronic kidney disease in affected individuals, especially when treated with calcium and calcitriol. A recent analysis of 191 published patients with ADH1 found that 27% were asymptomatic at presentation, 32% had moderate symptoms, and 41% had severe symptoms (seizures).[10]

Because of this high risk for adverse renal outcomes, most experts recommend that asymptomatic patients should avoid treatment with calcium and calcitriol. Symptomatic patients can receive these 2 medications but at the lowest dosages possible. Oral calcilytics (negative allosteric modulators of the CaSR) hold promise for the treatment of patients with ADH1 and are currently in clinical trials.[11]

Bartter Syndrome V

Bartter syndrome V is a more severe form of ADH1; affected individuals present with renal salt wasting and hypokalemia, in addition to hypocalcemia and low PTH levels.[12]

Diagnosis

Diagnosing FHH1 or ADH1 by biochemical means only is difficult. A low calcium-to-creatinine clearance (<0.01) points to the presence of FHH1. A positive family history of FHH1 or ADH1 is another important clue for this disease. Genetic testing can confirm the diagnosis.

Antibodies to the CaSR

Rare cases of autoantibodies to the CaSR, either inactivating or activating, have been reported that lead to a clinical picture similar to FHH1 or ADH1, respectively.[5]

Clinical Case Vignettes

Case 1

A 21-year-old college athlete is evaluated in the emergency department for a possible concussion.

Laboratory test results:

Calcium = 11.0 mg/dL (8.5-10.5 mg/dL)
    (SI: 2.7 mmol/L [2.1-2.6 mmol/L])
PTH = 72 pg/mL (10-65 pg/mL)
    (SI: 72 ng/L [10-65 ng/L])
25-Hydroxyvitamin D = 19 ng/mL (20-80 ng/mL)
    (SI: 48 nmol/L [50-200 nmol/L])

Which of the following is the best next step?

A. Refer to a parathyroid surgeon

B. Replete vitamin D with 1000 units of vitamin D_3 daily

C. Measure serum and 24-hour urinary calcium and creatinine

D. Measure serum phosphate and magnesium

E. Measure DXA

Answer: C) Measure serum and 24-hour urinary calcium and creatinine

Primary hyperparathyroidism is unusual in young men and raises the possibility of a genetic form of hypercalcemia. FHH1 needs to be ruled out. Calculating the calcium-to-creatinine clearance ratio requires measuring 24-hour urinary calcium and creatinine (Answer C) and concomitant serum calcium and creatinine. A ratio less than 0.01 increases the likelihood that the patient has FHH1 as opposed to primary hyperparathyroidism.

The patient should not be referred to a parathyroid surgeon (Answer A) before FHH is ruled out.

Supplementing vitamin D (Answer B) will not improve the hypercalcemia.

Measuring phosphate and magnesium (Answer D) will not help in the diagnostic evaluation.

DXA (Answer E) is not indicated at this stage of the diagnostic workup.

Case 1 (continued)

His calcium-to-creatinine clearance ratio is 0.01. His dietary intake of calcium is about 1000 mg daily. He has no significant medial problems and is on no medications. His concussion is found to be mild, and he is discharged home.

Which of the following is the best next step?

A. Follow-up every 12 months in the endocrine clinic

B. Perform kidney ultrasonography for nephrocalcinosis

C. Perform a 24-hour urine stone profile

D. Recommend genetic testing

E. Check both of the patient's parents' serum calcium and albumin

Answer: D) Recommend genetic testing

If the patient has FHH, a "hands-off" approach is often possible; regular follow-up is not necessary in most patients, as it is a benign disease that typically does not need intervention.

There is no increased risk for nephrocalcinosis or nephrolithiasis; therefore, kidney ultrasonography (Answer B) or 24-hour urine stone profile (Answer C) is not needed.

A calcium-to-creatinine clearance ratio less than 0.01 is consistent with FHH; however, there are overlaps between the calcium-to-creatinine clearance ratio of patients with FHH and patients with primary hyperparathyroidism, especially in the range between 0.01 and 0.02. Genetic testing (Answer D) can help confirm the diagnosis and make the distinction between FHH1 (inactivating *CASR* variant, typically heterozygous), FHH2 (loss-of-function heterozygous variant in *GNA11* encoding the α-subunit of the G-protein G11), or FHH3 (heterozygous loss-of-function variant in the adapter protein AP2S1 encoded by the *AP2S1* gene). Pathogenic variant–specific testing can also help diagnose other affected family members and exclude the variant in unaffected family members. Pretest genetic counseling is recommended. Some companies offer genetic panel tests for hypercalcemia, which include all 3 FHH types and several other genes. A positive family history of PTH-dependent hypercalcemia is a strong predictor for the diagnosis of FHH, as it is the most common inherited form of hypercalcemia.

Knowing the parents' albumin-adjusted calcium (Answer E) might add information, but it is not the best choice here. Normal albumin-adjusted calcium of the parents does not rule out a de novo variant, which occurs in 10% to 20% of cases. Elevated calcium in one of the parents increases the likelihood for an inherited disease but does not rule out phenocopies and would still be followed by recommending genetic testing.

A known pathogenic heterozygous missense variant in the *CASR* gene was discovered in this patient, and the diagnosis of FHH1 was confirmed.

Case 2

A 28-year-old woman with a history of idiopathic hypoparathyroidism diagnosed 10 years ago seeks a second opinion. She presented with a seizure at age 18 years, was found to have profound hypocalcemia with inappropriately low PTH, received intravenous calcium, and was given a diagnosis of idiopathic hypoparathyroidism. She is prescribed calcium and calcitriol (unknown dosage) but has not taken them for years. She currently has mild tingling for hours at a time and often feels exhausted, with trouble concentrating.

Laboratory test results:

> Calcium = 7.2 mg/dL (8.5-10.5 mg/dL)
>   (SI: 1.8 mmol/L [2.1-2.6 mmol/L])
> PTH = 12 pg/mL (10-65 pg/mL) (SI: 12 ng/L
>   [10-60 ng/L])
> 25-Hydroxyvitamin D = 25 ng/mL (20-80 ng/mL)
>   (SI: 62 nmol/L [50-200 nmol/L])
> Phosphate = 4.5 mg/dL (2.6-4.5 mg/dL)
>   (SI: 1.45 mmol/L [0.84-1.45 mmol/L])
> Magnesium = 1.6 mg/dL (1.8-2.5 mg/dL)
>   (SI: 0.66 mmol/L [0.74-1.03 mmol/L])

Which of the following is the best next step?

A. Start calcitriol, 1 mcg daily

B. Start calcium, 1200 mg 3 times daily

C. Measure 24-hour urinary calcium

D. Start calcitriol, 0.25 mcg daily, and calcium, 500 mg 3 times daily

E. Start a thiazide diuretic

Answer: D) Start calcitriol, 0.25 mcg daily, and calcium, 500 mg 3 times daily

This patient has symptomatic and significant hypocalcemia that needs to be treated. Starting with 1 mcg of calcitriol appears to be too high. Large amounts of calcium (such as 1200 mg 3 times daily) should also be avoided as they are inconvenient and might cause large variations in serum calcium. 24-Hour urinary calcium monitoring is an important part of management of hypocalcemia, but this should be done once she is on a stable dosage of oral medications.

At this point, thiazides should not be added, as her urinary calcium excretion is not yet known.

Her urinary calcium is too high; simply increasing calcitriol or calcium or adding magnesium will not correct that.

Case 2 (continued)

She is taking her medications faithfully now. She currently has almost no symptoms, and her laboratory results are as follows:

> Calcium = 7.8 mg/dL (8.5-10.5 mg/dL)
>   (SI: 1.95 mmol/L [2.1-2.6 mmol/L])
> Phosphate = 4.2 mg/dL (2.6-4.5 mg/dL)
>   (SI: 1.36 mmol/L [0.84-1.45 mmol/L])
> Magnesium = 1.6 mg/dL (1.8-2.5 mg/dL)
>   (SI: 0.66 mmol/L [0.74-1.03 mmol/L])

Which of the following is the best next step?

A. Increase her calcitriol dosage to 0.75 mcg daily

B. Increase her calcium dosage to 600 mg 4 times daily

C. Add a thiazide diuretic

D. Check for glaucoma

E. Perform genetic testing and measure 24-hour urinary calcium and creatinine

Answer: E) Perform genetic testing and measure 24-hour urinary calcium and creatinine

Knowing whether the patient has ADH1 would change management. In ADH1, the lowest amount of calcium/calcitriol is used to avoid hypercalciuria, and she is currently asymptomatic. Before using thiazides to lower urinary calcium, 24-hour urinary calcium should be measured (Answer E). She has no symptoms of glaucoma, which makes testing for it not a priority.

Case 2 (continued)

Her genetic results come back positive for a pathogenic heterozygous activating variant in the *CASR* gene.

Her 24-hour urinary calcium excretion is 290 mg/24 h (<250 mg/24 h) (SI: 7.24 mmol/d [<6.24 mmol/d]).

Which of the following is the best next step?

A. Stop calcium and calcitriol

B. Start PTH

C. Start a thiazide diuretic

D. Measure urinary magnesium

Answer: C) Start a thiazide diuretic

Thiazide diuretics (Answer C) have been successfully used in patients with ADH1 to reduce urinary calcium excretion. Caution is warranted because of the potential to lower her serum magnesium further. Therefore, serum magnesium should be monitored after the start of the thiazide.

We successfully initiated treatment with calcium and calcitriol; stopping them now (Answer A) might risk recurrence of symptomatic hypocalcemia. Lowering calcium or calcitriol dosages can often be attempted.

PTH (Answer B) is currently not approved for patients with ADH1, but reports demonstrate that it can increase serum calcium and decrease urinary calcium and might be considered if lowering urinary calcium with other means is not successful.

Checking urinary magnesium (Answer D) would not help in her management.

Key Learning Points

- Distinguishing FHH1 from primary hyperparathyroidism involves family history, age of onset of disease, and determination of the calcium-to-creatinine clearance ratio, but only a genetic diagnosis is definitive.

- When clinical suspicion for FHH or ADH is present, genetic testing can confirm the diagnosis. Several companies offer panel testing, and some programs may even provide it for free.

- Parathyroidectomy should be avoided in patients with FHH because removing a parathyroid gland will not change the disease. All parathyroid cells express the mutant receptor, and the remaining parathyroid tissue will keep the extracellular calcium elevated.

- Treatment of patients with ADH1 should aim for the lowest possible amount of calcium supplementation and calcitriol to lessen the high risk of kidney calcifications.

References

1. Mannstadt M, Cianferotti L, Gafni RI, et al. Hypoparathyroidism: genetics and diagnosis. *J Bone Miner Res.* 2022;37(12):2615-2629. PMID 36375809
2. Leach K, Hannan FM, Josephs TM, et al. International Union of Basic and Clinical Pharmacology. CVIII. Calcium-sensing receptor nomenclature, pharmacology, and function. *Pharmacol Rev.* 2020;72(3):558-604. PMID: 32467152
3. Brown EM, Gamba G, Riccardi D, et al. Cloning and characterization of an extracellular Ca(2+)-sensing receptor from bovine parathyroid. *Nature.* 1993;366(6455):575-580. PMID: 8255296
4. Nemeth EF, Goodman WG. Calcimimetic and calcilytic drugs: feats, flops, and futures. *Calcif Tissue Int.* 2016;98(4):341-358. PMID: 26319799
5. Hannan FM, Kallay E, Chang W, Brandi ML, Thakker RV. The calcium-sensing receptor in physiology and in calcitropic and noncalcitropic diseases. *Nat Rev Endocrinol.* 2018;15(1):33-51. PMID: 30443043
6. Riccardi D, Valenti G. Localization and function of the renal calcium-sensing receptor. *Nat Rev Nephrol.* 2016;12(7):414-425. PMID: 27157444
7. Pearce SH, Wooding C, Davies M, Tollefsen SE, Whyte MP, Thakker RV. Calcium-sensing receptor mutations in familial hypocalciuric hypercalcaemia with recurrent pancreatitis. *Clin Endocrinol (Oxf).* 1996;45(6):675-680. PMID: 9039332
8. Vannucci L, Brandi ML. Familial hypocalciuric hypercalcemia and neonatal severe hyperparathyroidism. *Front Horm Res.* 2019;51:52-62. PMID: 30641521
9. Roszko KL, Bi RD, Mannstadt M. Autosomal dominant hypocalcemia (hypoparathyroidism) types 1 and 2. *Front Physiol.* 2016;7:458. PMID: 27803672
10. Roszko KL, Stapleton Smith LM, Sridhar AV, et al. Autosomal dominant hypocalcemia type 1: a systematic review. *J Bone Miner Res.* 2022;37(10):1926-1935. PMID: 35879818
11. Roberts MS, Gafni RI, Brillante B, Guthrie LC, Streit J, Gash D, et al. Treatment of autosomal dominant hypocalcemia type 1 with the calcilytic NPSP795 (SHP635). *J Bone Miner Res.* 2019;34(9):1609-1618. PMID: 31063613
12. Watanabe S, Fukumoto S, Chang H, et al. Association between activating mutations of calcium-sensing receptor and Bartter's syndrome. *Lancet.* 2002;360(9334):692-694. PMID: 12241879

Hypoparathyroidism: Case Management

Dolores Shoback, MD. University of California, San Francisco; Endocrine Research Unit, San Francisco Veterans Affairs Medical Center, San Francisco, CA; Email: dolores.shoback@ucsf.edu

Educational Objectives

After reviewing this chapter, learners should be able to:

- Construct the differential diagnosis of hypocalcemia and apply the principles to patient evaluation and care.

- Describe the natural history of hypocalcemia postoperatively after anterior neck surgery and evaluate and risk stratify patients postprocedure for acute vs chronic hypoparathyroidism (transient vs permanent).

- Evaluate patients with nonsurgical hypoparathyroidism for possible genetic etiologies and appreciate the likelihood of achieving a correct and definite diagnosis.

- Explain how to maximize conventional therapy for chronic hypoparathyroidism.

- Identify the complications of chronic hypoparathyroidism and describe available management guidelines to reduce disease complications.

- Describe treatments that are on the horizon in clinical trials that may change the way we manage hypoparathyroidism in the future.

Significance of the Clinical Problem

Chronic hypoparathyroidism is a condition that affects quality of life and key biochemical and physiologic parameters, despite efforts to control the disease and treat it as intensively and carefully as possible. This condition may ultimately contribute to increased mortality, although the data are not clear. Conventional therapy can control the biochemical parameters that are abnormal in this disease state, but it often does so at the expense of driving the urinary calcium to unwanted and high levels. These high levels of urinary calcium likely contribute directly to the propensity of patients with chronic hypoparathyroidism to experience kidney stones, kidney infections, nephrocalcinosis, and, over time, deterioration of kidney function (chronic kidney disease). Preservation of kidney function is a key goal in the long-term management of hypoparathyroidism, but we have not yet identified how to do this. We have not definitively identified the clinical risk factors that predispose patients with chronic hypoparathyroidism to kidney functional deterioration.

Guidelines for disease management have been proposed by the European Society for Endocrinology,[1] the First International Workshop on Chronic Hypoparathyroidism,[2] and the Second International Workshop.[3] These guidelines share many similar recommendations but do have some differences; all rest on a very limited evidence base. The shared evidence base includes modest high-quality/high-reliability data (trials and meta-analyses). Yet, with a rare disease such as this one, this is the norm, and patient care must still be directed by evaluating the best evidence available.

Over the last 20 years, studies have reported on the use of PTH in different forms in the treatment of chronic hypoparathyroidism as a "hormone replacement" strategy. These studies test the use of PTH(1-34), PTH(1-84), palopegteriparatide, and most recently a PTH/PTHrP peptide analogue (AZP3601).[4-7] Preliminary studies have also reported on the use of a calcium-sensing receptor (CASR) antagonist (calcilytic), encaleret, in the management of autosomal dominant hypocalcemia type 1 due to activating pathogenic variants in the *CASR* gene.[8] Thus, it is anticipated that the management of most patients with chronic hypoparathyroidism will differ in the future, compared with the traditional conventional management strategies that have been used in the past.

Chronic hypoparathyroidism is a rare disease, with approximately 77,000 to 115,000 affected individuals in the United States and with similar low rates of occurrence across multiple countries where surveys and estimates have been made.[9] For individuals with this condition, however, the disorder is often a central focus of their health care needs and lifestyle since the management of hypoparathyroidism may involve around-the-clock administration of medications and supplements, frequent office/clinic visits and laboratory monitoring, ongoing (sometimes daily) symptoms attributable to the disease, long-term complications of the disease and its therapy, and difficulties with maintaining a job and livelihood. Even with acceptable biochemical control of the disease, patients often experience symptoms and have a reduced quality of life by standard ways to assess that parameter.[10]

As noted above, kidney functional deterioration is a key concern for patients with chronic hypoparathyroidism. Conventional management reflected in the data from contemporary cohort studies[11-13] supports the idea that steady deterioration of kidney function and the occurrence of stones are common when patients with chronic hypoparathyroidism are compared with euparathyroid control participants. Thus, the protection of kidney function is a key clinical problem, and the prevention of renal/urologic morbidity is also critical. Improvement in quality of life is an added goal to address in clinical practice. The control and reduction of neuromuscular complications that often underpin the day-to-day symptomatology of chronic hypoparathyroidism (tetany, paresthesias, muscle cramping, weakness, etc) are key problems to address in the treatment of this disease.

Practice Gaps

- Lack of easy-to-use and well-tolerated calcium supplements.

- Insufficient knowledge about the best treatment schedules and calcium preparations to achieve steady calcium absorption in affected patients.

- Unclear understanding of who is at risk for kidney complications and how to prevent them.

- Weak evidence base pointing to effective therapies and targets for key parameters in chronic disease management and the factors that determine quality of life and symptom formation (calcium and/or PTH levels, the calcium x phosphate product, fluctuations in calcium, other concomitant disease states, etc).

Discussion

Diagnosis

The diagnosis of hypoparathyroidism should be straightforward. It is recommended that intact PTH, serum calcium, and albumin be measured and that laboratory testing be repeated over at least a 2-week period to confirm the diagnosis. In the postoperative case, the diagnosis of chronic hypoparathyroidism is confirmable if the surgery took place more than 12 months earlier.[3] The albumin-corrected serum calcium value should be below the lower limit of the normal range, and the plasma PTH value should be below the lower limit of normal or inappropriately low for the serum calcium concentration. Generally, the diagnosis is straightforward. In the acute setting of hospitalization in which intravenous fluids may be given or albumin is decidedly low, confirmation of hypocalcemia by an ionized calcium value can be helpful. Whether to measure ionized calcium is an individual decision based on its availability, the clinical circumstances and costs, and the reliability of the ionized calcium available. Serum magnesium should be measured and documented to be within the reference range, as it is well known that hypomagnesemia can lower serum calcium and reduce the ability of the parathyroid glands to produce PTH.

The differential diagnosis has its first branch point in determining whether the problem is postsurgical (75% of cases) or nonsurgical (25%). Almost any procedure on structures in the neck (thyroid, parathyroids, or larynx) can lead to postsurgical hypoparathyroidism. The natural history and epidemiology are well known.[10,14,15,20]

Therapy

Therapy for chronic hypoparathyroidism (*table*) can involve use of calcium and magnesium supplements, vitamin D supplements, activated vitamin D metabolites, thiazide diuretics, phosphate binders, and PTH.[14-16] The individualized regimens followed by each patient for optimization of their hypoparathyroid disease state must be that—optimized to the individual to gain control of symptomatology, reduce risk factors for complications, positively affect any complications present, help manage other comorbid conditions, and improve quality of life.

Management

Acute hypoparathyroidism with symptomatic hypocalcemia is generally addressed with intravenous calcium gluconate infusions tailored to restore an acceptable serum albumin-corrected calcium or ionized calcium level. In the acute setting, an ampule of intravenous calcium gluconate can be administered slowly over 10 to 20 minutes to achieve immediate increases in serum calcium. This can be repeated and should be done only with continuous electrocardiography monitoring in an emergency or intensive care unit

setting. Chronic calcium intravenous infusions can then be initiated, and the patient should be monitored closely with regular measurements of albumin-corrected total calcium or ionized calcium along with control of symptoms.

Chronic treatment of hypocalcemia is initiated with calcium supplements spread out over a 24-hour period to achieve steady levels of serum calcium and control of all symptoms. Treatment is begun at 500 mg elemental calcium given 2, 3, or 4 times daily orally. Should the degree of hypoparathyroidism and hypocalcemia be moderate to severe, then activated vitamin D analogues (calcitriol or alfacalcidol) may be started, usually once or twice daily (*table*). Once therapy is stabilized, symptoms are controlled, and laboratory tests indicate good levels of calcium in the blood, then urinary calcium levels are assessed, and further adjustments of calcium and activated vitamin D analogues are made. Eventually, thiazide diuretics may be started if urinary calcium targets are above sex-adjusted reference ranges.[1-3] Principles of management are well laid out in recent guidelines and management publications.[1-4,15,16]

Guidelines From the Second International Workshop on Hypoparathyroidism

These guidelines are summarized below and explained in detail elsewhere.[3] They are the most up-to-date guidelines available and use the GRADE methodology to calibrate the strength of evidence. There are 7 key graded recommendations as follows:

Recommendation 1
How should chronic hypoparathyroidism be diagnosed? (ungraded)

- Hypocalcemia + undetectable, low, or inappropriately normal PTH × 2 (2 weeks apart)

- Consider permanent if >12 months since surgery

Table. Therapy for Chronic Hypoparathyroidism

Name	Form	Dosage, route	Comments
Calcium supplements	Calcium carbonate (40% calcium by weight) Calcium citrate (21% calcium by weight)	Preparations of calcium carbonate contain: 200, 250, 500, or 600 mg elemental calcium; slow-release preparations are available Calcium citrate is available in tablets that contain as elemental calcium either 200, 250, 315, or 600 mg	Calcium carbonate achieves best absorption if it is given with meals; calcium citrate may be given at any time of the day Liquid formulations are available for calcium carbonate Health food stores and pharmacies may stock calcium-fortified drinks that enable patients to vary the means to take in sufficient calcium throughout the day
Magnesium supplements	Magnesium oxide Magnesium chloride Magnesium gluconate	400 mg (elemental magnesium = 241 mg/dose) 600 mg (elemental magnesium = 72 mg/dose) 1000 mg/5 mL solution (elemental magnesium = 54 mg/dose)	Sustained release preparations are preferred because magnesium is slowly absorbed. One-third the dose of sustained release preparations is absorbed with dosing. Can give 6 to 8 tablets (30 to 56 mEq [15 to 28 mmol]) in divided doses as the recommended/reasonable starting dose for patients with severe magnesium depletion. In patients with mild, asymptomatic hypomagnesemia, 2 to 4 tablets (10 to 28 mEq [5 to14 mmol]) daily is reasonable dose to start.[17-19] There is 119 mg of calcium in magnesium chloride tablets. Magnesium oxide, which is nonsustained and less bioavailable, more commonly causes diarrhea, which worsens the problem of magnesium wasting. Many patients with hypoparathyroidism without diarrhea and excessive losses are chronically treated with low dosages of magnesium oxide daily.
Vitamin D supplements	Cholecalciferol (D$_3$) Ergocalciferol (D$_2$)	Vitamin D replacement Oral doses of vitamin D to maintain vitamin D sufficiency and prevent vitamin D deficiency are recommended at individualized doses (typically 1000 to 4000 IU daily)	25-Hydroxyvitamin D levels should be monitored periodically to achieve target levels (either >20 ng/mL [>50 nmol/L] to prevent deficiency or >30 ng/mL [>75 nmol/L] to address insufficiency), recognizing that country- and region-specific targets are used at this time[1-3]
Vitamin D supplements	Cholecalciferol (D$_3$) Ergocalciferol (D$_2$)	High-dosage treatment with vitamin D 25,000 to 100,000 IU vitamin D$_2$ or vitamin D$_3$ per day orally may be given if activated vitamin D metabolites are not available or patient cannot tolerate	Higher dosages of ergocalciferol or cholecalciferol can be used to treat hypoparathyroidism[14] Serum 25-hydroxyvitamin D and calcium levels must be closely monitored because absorption varies and vitamin D intoxication can be difficult to predict and treat and should be avoided
Activated vitamin D metabolites	Calcitriol Alfacalcidol	Calcitriol, 0.25 mcg daily to doses of 2 or 3 mcg daily, given in divided doses Alfacalcidol is initiated at 0.5 mcg daily and titrated upward	Alfacalcidol is approximately one-half the potency of calcitriol[14]
Thiazide diuretic	Hydrochlorothiazide Chlorthalidone	Dosages of 12.5 mg to 100 mg daily for either of these diuretics may be used	Dosages of diuretics should be titrated upward gently with attention to serum sodium and potassium, as well as blood urea nitrogen (for dehydration) and serum creatinine. Urinary calcium, sodium, and creatinine should be monitored to achieve a therapeutic effect. Complications include hyponatremia, hypokalemia, dehydration/volume depletion, and orthostasis. Dietary salt restriction is an important adjunct to thiazide diuretic therapy to achieve urinary calcium lowering.
PTH therapy	Recombinant human PTH(1-34) or teriparatide off-label Recombinant human PTH(1-84)	20 mcg once or twice daily by subcutaneous injection 25, 50, 75, or 100 mcg daily by subcutaneous injection	This remains an off-label, non-FDA approved use of teriparatide. Due to the short half-life of teriparatide, efficacy is not strong. This compound is only available until the end of 2023 in the Special Use Program.

Recommendation 2
Avoid postsurgical hypoparathyroidism by avoiding parathyroid removal at surgery and autotransplant (ungraded)

Recommendation 3a
Serum calcium and PTH measurements done at an early time-point (12-24 hours) after thyroid surgery can indicate who will NOT develop hypoparathyroidism (*strong recommendation, moderate evidence*)

- If >10 pg/mL (12-24 hours after surgery), the chance of hypoparathyroidism is unlikely and there is no need to give calcium or vitamin D above the recommended daily allowance)

- If <10 pg/mL, most will still recover, but need attention and treatment

Recommendation 3b
Role of genetic testing in nonsurgical hypoparathyroidism (ungraded)

- Perform genetic testing if positive family history, syndromic features present, and the patient is younger than 40 years; if autoimmune features (autoimmune polyglandular syndrome type 1) are present, then test for *AIRE* pathogenic variants

Recommendation 4
What are the common symptoms and complications of hypoparathyroidism?
These were gathered from clinical surveys, and the percentage quoted is the median among studies reviewed.

- Cataract (17%)
- Nephrocalcinosis, nephrolithiasis (15%)
- Renal insufficiency (12%)
- Depression (12%)
- Infection (11%)
- Seizures (11%)
- Ischemic heart disease, arrhythmias (7%)

Recommendation 5
Recommended monitoring is based on expert clinician survey (*low quality*)

- Baseline kidney imaging

- Monitor serum calcium more frequently after change in regimen

- Serum creatinine, estimated glomerular filtration rate, calcium (either ionized or albumin-adjusted), serum magnesium, phosphate, *check every 3 to 12 months*

- 25-Hydroxyvitamin D, *check every 6 to 12 months*

- 24-hour urine for creatinine and calcium, *check every 6 to 24 months*

Notes: *These are graded as low-quality recommendations based on the practice of 70% of the respondents completing this at least 70% of the time. **For unstable patients: frequently measure serum calcium and phosphate as clinically indicated.

Recommendation 6
Conventional management (calcium, activated vitamin D) is first-line therapy (*weak recommendation, low quality*)
Ten individual recommendations on this topic:

- Aim for low-normal serum calcium concentration

- Alleviate symptomatic hypocalcemia while avoiding hypercalciuria

- Urinary calcium targets: women (<250 mg or < 6.25 mmol/24 h); men (<300 mg or <7.5 mmol/24 h)

- Avoid hyperphosphatemia

- Normalize serum magnesium and 25-hydroxyvitamin D levels

- Consider thiazide diuretic for elevated urinary calcium

- Consider PTH replacement for those whose disease is not responding or controlled on this regimen and for patients with malabsorption or poor adherence to oral medications or who are intolerant of large doses of calcium and active vitamin D; the guidelines propose that individuals with poor adherence or malabsorption or requiring high doses of conventional therapy (ie, elemental calcium >2 g/day or active vitamin D >2 mcg/day) may also benefit from PTH therapy

Recommendation 7

In pregnant women with hypoparathyroidism, the guidelines propose the following (ungraded):

- Aim to achieve serum calcium (ionized or albumin adjusted) in the mid- to low-normal range throughout pregnancy

- Aim to achieve serum phosphate, magnesium, and 25-hydroxyvitamin D levels in the normal range

- Closely monitor serum calcium (ionized or albumin-adjusted) every 3 to 4 weeks during pregnancy and lactation, with increased frequency in the months preceding and following parturition, as well as in the presence of symptoms of hypercalcemia or hypocalcemia.

- Work closely with the obstetrician to optimize pregnancy outcomes

- Coordinate with the pediatric team to ensure appropriate postnatal monitoring for transient neonatal hypocalcemia or hypercalcemia

- Avoid using thiazide diuretics and PTH or PTH analogues during pregnancy

Clinical Case Vignettes
Case 1

A 40-year-old man is wondering whether his treatment for hypoparathyroidism should be modified. At the age of 6 months, a left cervical neuroblastoma was diagnosed and resected, and he had radiation therapy. At age 15 years, the patient was found to have a thyroid mass. Papillary thyroid cancer was diagnosed, and he had a total thyroidectomy. He had 2 radioactive iodine treatments (^{131}I). In the last 10 years, he has had thyroglobulin monitoring, and his thyroglobulin levels are undetectable. After the thyroidectomy, he had acute and then chronic hypoparathyroidism with chronically low serum calcium and undetectable PTH. He says his ionized calcium is always more reliable that the albumin-corrected total calcium. He describes his symptoms as being "strong" for approximately 1 year and then asymptomatic for next 24 years.

He is currently doing well on the following regimen: elemental calcium, 1000 mg twice daily (250 mg tablets); vitamin D_3, 3000 IU once daily; calcitriol, 0.5 mcg twice daily; magnesium SR, 84 mg 3 tablets twice daily; and a multivitamin. He is taking 20 tablets for this condition alone.

Family history and other medical history are unremarkable.

On physical examination, he has a well-healed neck scar and negative Chvostek sign.

Date	Serum calcium	Albumin	Ionized calcium	Creatinine	PTH	Urinary calcium
6 months ago	9.9 mg/dL (SI: 2.5 mmol/L)	4.1 g/dL (SI: 41 g/L)	1.23 mmol/L	...	<3 pg/mL (SI:<3 ng/L)	...
Current	10.5 mg/dL (SI: 2.6 mmol/L)	4.0 g/dL (SI: 40 g/L)	1.32 mmol/L	1.25 mg/dL (SI: 110.5 µmol/L)	...	639 mg/24 h (SI:16.0 mmol/d)*

Reference ranges: serum calcium, 8.5-10.3 mg/dL (SI: 2.1-2.6 mmol/L); albumin, 3.5-5.0 g/dL (SI: 35-50 g/L); ionized calcium, 1.1-1.3 mmol/L; creatinine, 0.6-1.2 mg/dL (SI: 53.0-106.1 µmol/L); PTH, 15-65 pg/mL (SI: 15-65 ng/L); urinary calcium, <250 mg/24 h (SI: <6.3 mmol/d).

*First time this test was ever done.

Which of the following is the best first management step?

A. Decrease the calcium supplements

B. Decrease the magnesium supplements

C. Increase the calcitriol dosage

D. Both A and B

Answer: A) Decrease the calcium supplements

Of the answers provided, decreasing the calcium supplements (Answer A) is the best choice. The goal is to lower the filtered load of calcium to address the patient's marked hypercalciuria. This could also be accomplished by lowering the calcitriol dosage. It is a matter of personal choice but considering the eight 250-mg elemental calcium tablets per day he is taking currently, the regimen will be easier with a reduction in that dosing. The dosing of calcium and calcitriol should be titrated to achieve symptom control and reduce urinary calcium excretion. If urinary calcium does not reach the target range for men (<300 mg/24 h [<7.5 mmol/d]), a thiazide diuretic can be prescribed.

Case 1 (continued)

What monitoring should be recommended?

A. Retinal scan

B. Visual field testing

C. Kidney ultrasonography

D. Coronary artery calcium score

Answer: C) Kidney ultrasonography

Of the answers listed, kidney ultrasonography (Answer C) would be a good test to see if chronic hypercalciuria may have contributed to nephrocalcinosis and/or nephrolithiasis in this patient. Patients with longstanding hypoparathyroidism should also have vision testing (not visual fields) and a slit lamp examination for cataracts (not a retinal scan).

Case 1 (continued)

Should his management be changed to a form of PTH replacement and, if so, which formulation should be considered? Which of the following statements is true?

A. PTH(1-34); teriparatide can be used and dosed periodically as needed to balance out symptoms

B. PTH replacement is not needed, as he meets the criteria for successful treatment based on the Second International Workshop Guidelines

C. Long-acting forms of PTH not yet available would be an option to lower urinary calcium levels

D. Vitamin D analogue therapy should be stopped to decrease urinary calcium levels

Answer: C) Long-acting forms of PTH not yet available would be an option to lower urinary calcium levels

Data are supportive of long-acting PTH analogues as being capable of lowering urinary calcium values consistently (Answer C). However, these agents are not FDA approved. PTH(1-34) must be given twice daily to get the best biochemical responses (serum calcium stability), and even in this formulation, it usually does not improve severe hypercalciuria. Although stopping calcitriol might decrease urinary calcium in this patient, patients with such low PTH levels (in this case, undetectable), usually cannot tolerate just calcium supplements to treat hypoparathyroidism effectively. Calcitriol is generally needed. This patient does not meet biochemical parameters of good disease control as put forward by the Second International Workshop on disease management. Serum magnesium and 25-hydroxyvitamin D should also be measured.

Case 2

An 18-year-old woman is brought to the emergency department after an episode of loss of consciousness that was witnessed in a public place. Loss consciousness was preceded by palpitations.

She had no seizure activity, incontinence, or neurologic signs such as posturing or other changes. She is a healthy college student and has no history of thyroid or adrenal disease, diabetes mellitus, or candidiasis. She has no family history of endocrine disorders. She is taking no medications and she has had no prior surgeries.

She notes that over the past 2 to 3 years, she has had frequent eye twitching, cramping in her hands and legs, and tingling in her fingers about once a week. She has intermittent dizziness and lightheadedness upon awakening and generalized fatigue and weakness.

On physical examination, her temperature is 98.2°F (36.8°C), pulse rate is 74 beats/min, blood pressure is 118/62 mm Hg, respiratory rate is 14 breaths/min, and BMI is 25.6 kg/m². She has no neck scars or goiter. Findings on heart, lungs, skeletal, neurologic, and funduscopic examinations are normal. She has a strongly positive Chvostek sign.

Electrocardiography shows a prolonged QTc of 544 msec.

Laboratory test results:

> Calcium = 4.4 mg/dL (8.6-10.5 mg/dL)
> Albumin = 4.5 g/dL (3.4-4.8 g/dL)
> Ionized calcium = 0.52 mmol/L (1.12-1.32 mmol/L)
> Magnesium = 1.5 mg/dL (1.5-2.3 mg/dL)
> Phosphate = 7.8 mg/dL (2.4-4.5 mg/dL)
> Creatinine = 0.91 mg/dL (0.50-1.10 mg/dL)
> PTH = <6.3 pg/mL (repeated) (14-72 pg/mL)
> 25-Hydroxyvitamin D = 19.7 ng/mL (30-80 ng/mL)
> 1,25-Dihydroxyvitamin D = 33.2 pg/mL
>   (19.9-79.3 pg/mL)

No prior laboratory results are available.

The patient is admitted to the hospital for monitoring and treatment.

Which of the following is the best first step in treating her?

A. Establish an intravenous line and administer an infusion of calcium gluconate

B. Establish an intravenous line and administer intravenous calcitriol

C. Establish an intravenous line and administer parenteral PTH(1-34)

D. She does not need intravenous therapy as she has stable vital signs

Answer: A) Establish an intravenous line and administer an infusion of calcium gluconate

Although she is mentally compensated at the time of admission, she had a witnessed syncopal episode, which could have been a seizure or a cardiac event. She should be placed on telemetry. A screen for toxins should be done. She should be given intravenous calcium gluconate (Answer A) to titrate her serum ionized calcium to approximately 1.0 mmol/L and to control any neurologic or neuromuscular symptoms that emerge during observation. She needs inpatient therapy due to the presentation and the severity of her hypocalcemia. She should not be treated as an outpatient, as the risks are too high for decompensation and even death. She has not shown as yet that she needs parenteral PTH(1-34), and there are no formulations to give calcitriol intravenously in this situation. It is given intravenously after dialysis but generally not for the treatment of hypoparathyroidism.

Case 2 (continued)

She has undetectable intact PTH, which is verified by repeated testing, and her parents confirm that she has never had neck surgery (or any other surgery). Head CT shows basal ganglia calcifications.

What are the best next steps after starting treatment and stabilizing her serum ionized calcium levels?

A. Assess for signs of autoimmune disease by screening her for hypothyroidism and adrenal insufficiency

B. Measure serum copper and perform iron studies

C. Collect 24-hour urine for calcium and creatinine measurement

D. A and B

E. A and C

Answer: D) A and B

The best next steps are to assess for signs of autoimmune disease by screening her for hypothyroidism and adrenal insufficiency and measuring serum copper and performing iron studies because this will provide valuable information in the differential diagnosis of nonsurgical hypoparathyroidism.[14,15,20] Etiologies include hypermagnesemia or hypomagnesemia, magnesium excess, or magnesium depletion. She has a borderline/low-normal magnesium level, which could be contributing to the hypocalcemia and which should be gently repleted.[17] The magnesium level alone is not likely to be the cause of the dramatic hypocalcemia presentation. Other etiologies include autoimmune hypoparathyroidism, iron overload due to hemochromatosis, copper overload due to Wilson disease, radiation to the glands, multiple genetic etiologies, and idiopathic hypocalcemia. Genetic etiologies include autosomal dominant hypocalcemia type 1 and 2 due to activating pathogenic variants in the *CASR* gene and the *GNA11* gene, respectively; multiple syndromes that include hypoparathyroidism as a feature (DiGeorge, mitochondrial gene deletions and pathogenic variants, Kenny-Caffey, Kearns-Sayre, Sanjad-Sakati, HDR [hypoparathyroidism, deafness, and renal anomalies], and others); and isolated genetic causes for hypoparathyroidism (pathogenic variants in the *PTH* and *GCM2* genes).

Case 2 (continued)

Her care team is uncertain as to why she has a very low serum calcium level when she has normal levels of 25-hydroxyvitamin D and 1,25-dihydroxyvitamin D.

Which of the following is the best explanation for these tests?

A. 1,25-Dihydroxyvitamin D and PTH work synergistically to mobilize calcium from target tissues, and without PTH, 1,25-dihydroxyvitamin D is insufficient to maintain serum calcium on its own

B. Her 25-hydroxyvitamin D level should be brought closer to 30 ng/mL (75 nmol/L) to get its full effect

C. Her serum magnesium is blocking the interaction of the PTH that she does have with its receptor

D. Her phosphate level is preventing the effective production of PTH

Answer: A) 1,25-dihydroxyvitamin D and PTH work synergistically to mobilize calcium from target tissues, and without PTH, 1,25-dihydroxyvitamin D is insufficient to maintain serum calcium on its own

1,25-Dihydroxyvitamin D and PTH work synergistically to maintain serum calcium and phosphate homeostasis (Answer A). It is true that magnesium insufficiency blocks the secretion of PTH and blunts the actions of PTH on its target tissues (bone and kidney) through the PTH receptor, as the receptor needs magnesium as a cofactor to mediate signal transduction. However, this patient's magnesium level is most likely not low enough to implicate that mechanism. Her phosphate level is very high because the lack of PTH in her kidney removes the chance to excrete phosphate normally and it builds up. Even lowering her phosphate concentration will not restore secretion of PTH.

Case 2 (continued)

Further workup should include which of the following?

A. MRI to confirm basal ganglia calcifications

B. Eye examination to document presence or absence of cataracts

C. Electroencephalography

D. Genetic testing for nonsurgical causes of hypoparathyroidism

Answer: D) Genetic testing for nonsurgical causes of hypoparathyroidism

MRI is not needed. Basal ganglia calcifications are of uncertain significance and do not need repeated confirmation. Cataract documentation can be deferred and performed during outpatient evaluation. Genetic testing should be undertaken (Answer D). A full panel to look for genetic etiologies of this disease is worthwhile. She meets the Second International Workshop Guidelines for genetic testing because she is younger than 40 years.[3]

References

1. Bollerslev J, Rejnmark L, Marcocci C, et al; European Society of Endocrinology. European Society of Endocrinology clinical guideline: treatment of chronic hypoparathyroidism in adults. *Eur J Endocrinol.* 2015;173(2):G1-G20. PMID: 26160136

2. Brandi ML, Bilezikian JP, Shoback D, et al. Management of hypoparathyroidism: summary statement and guidelines. *J Clin Endocrinol Metab.* 2016;101(6):2273-2283. PMID: 26943719

3. Khan AA, Bilezikian JP, Brandi ML, et al. Evaluation and management of hypoparathyroidism summary statement and guidelines from the Second International Workshop. *J Bone Miner Res.* 2022;37(12):2568-2585. PMID: 36054621

4. Khan AA, Guyatt G, Ali DS, et al. Management of hypoparathyroidism. *J Bone Miner Res.* 2022;37(12):2663-2677. PMID: 36161671

5. Khan AA, Rejnmark L, Rubin M, et al. PaTH Forward: a randomized, double-blind, placebo-controlled phase 2 trial of TransCon PTH in adult hypoparathyroidism. *J Clin Endocrinol Metab.* 2022;107(1):e372-e385. PMID: 34347093

6. Khan AA, Rubin MR, Schwarz P, et al. Efficacy and safety of parathyroid hormone replacement with TransCon PTH in hypoparathyroidism: 26-week results from the phase 3 PaTHway Trial. *J Bone Miner Res.* 2023;38(1):14-25. PMID: 36271471

7. Mannstadt M, Clarke BL, Vokes T, et al. Efficacy and safety of recombinant human parathyroid hormone (1-84) in hypoparathyroidism (REPLACE): a double-blind, placebo-controlled, randomised, phase 3 study. *Lancet Diabetes Endocrinol.* 2013;1(4):275-283. PMID: 24622413

8. Roszko KL, Stapleton Smith LM, Sridhar AV, et al. Autosomal dominant hypocalcemia type 1: a systematic review. *J Bone Miner Res.* 2022;37(10):1926-1935. PMID: 35879818

9. Clarke BL. Epidemiology and complications of hypoparathyroidism. *Endocrinol Metab Clin North Am.* 2018;47(4):771-782. PMID: 30390812

10. Pasieka JL, Wentworth K, Yeo CT, et al. Etiology and pathophysiology of hypoparathyroidism: a narrative review. *J Bone Miner Res.* 2022;37(12):2586-2601. PMID: 36153665

11. Gosmanova EO, Chen K, Rejnmark L, et al. Risk of chronic kidney disease and estimated glomerular filtration rate decline in patients with chronic hypoparathyroidism: a retrospective cohort study. *Adv Ther.* 2021;38(4):1876-1888. PMID: 33687651

12. Gosmanova EO, Houillier P, Rejnmark L, Marelli C, Bilezikian JP. Renal complications in patients with chronic hypoparathyroidism on conventional therapy: a systematic literature review: renal disease in chronic hypoparathyroidism. *Rev Endocr Metab Disord.* 2021;22(2):297-316. PMID: 33599907

13. Swartling O, Evans M, Spelman T, et al. Kidney complications and hospitalization in patients with chronic hypoparathyroidism: a cohort study in Sweden. *J Clin Endocrinol Metab.* 2022;107(10):e4098-e4105. PMID: 35907259

14. Shoback D. Clinical practice. Hypoparathyroidism. *N Engl J Med.* 2008;359(4):391-403. PMID: 18650515

15. Gafni RI, Collins MT. Hypoparathyroidism. *N Engl J Med.* 2019;380(18):1738-1747. PMID: 31042826

16. Yao L, Li J, Li M, et al. Parathyroid hormone therapy for managing chronic hypoparathyroidism: a systematic review and meta-analysis. *J Bone Miner Res.* 2022;37(12):2654-2662. PMID: 36385517

17. Rosner MH, Ha N, Palmer BF, Perazella MA. Acquired disorders of hypomagnesemia. *Mayo Clin Proc.* 2023;98(4):581-596. PMID: 36872194

18. Van Laecke S. Hypomagnesemia and hypermagnesemia. *Acta Clin Belg.* 2019;74(1):41-47. PMID: 30220246

19. Hansen B-A, Bruserud Ø. Hypomagnesemia in critically ill patients. *J Intensive Care.* 2018;6:21. PMID: 29610664

20. Mannstadt M, Bilezikian JP, Thakker RV, et al. *Nat Rev Dis Primers.* 2017;3:17055. PMID: 28857066

Management of Bone Health in Breast Cancer Survivors

Joy Y. Wu, MD, PhD. Division of Endocrinology, Department of Medicine, Stanford University School of Medicine, Stanford, CA; Email: jywu1@stanford.edu

Educational Objectives

After reviewing this chapter, learners should be able to:

- Identify patients at risk for bone loss during breast cancer treatment.

- Select nonpharmacologic and pharmacologic options for prevention or reversal of bone loss associated with breast cancer treatment.

- Recognize the indications for adjuvant therapy in patients with breast cancer and survivors of breast cancer.

- Discuss the management of breast cancer bone metastases.

Significance of the Clinical Problem

Breast cancer affects approximately 1 in 8 women in their lifetime. Bone loss and increased fracture risk are common in women with breast cancer as a result of chemotherapy, premature menopause, endocrine therapy, and radiation therapy.[1]

Approximately 80% of breast cancers express the estrogen and/or progesterone receptor, and in these cases, endocrine therapy to lower estrogen levels is a common component of breast cancer therapy. Endocrine therapy includes selective estrogen receptor modulators (tamoxifen and raloxifene) that act as estrogen antagonists in the breast but partial agonists in bone and aromatase inhibitors (anastrozole, exemestane, letrozole) that prevent conversion of adrenal androgens to estrogens. Because the ovaries are the predominant source of estrogens prior to menopause, aromatase inhibitors cannot be used in premenopausal women without ovarian suppression by ovariectomy, irradiation, or treatment with GnRH agonists such as goserelin or leuprolide that suppress pituitary LH and FSH.

The effects of endocrine therapy on bone mass vary. Because tamoxifen acts as a partial agonist of the estrogen receptor in bone, tamoxifen decreases bone mineral density (BMD) slightly in premenopausal women[2] but increases BMD slightly in postmenopausal women.[3] Aromatase inhibitors may be recommended because of better efficacy and lower risk of endometrial cancer and thromboembolic events.[4] However, aromatase inhibitors cause more substantial declines in BMD, with the greatest effect in premenopausal women on aromatase inhibition with ovarian suppression.[5] While disease-free survival is higher with exemestane than with tamoxifen, so too is the risk of osteoporosis and fracture.[6]

Practice Gaps

- Patients with breast cancer and survivors of breast cancer are followed by oncologists who are already managing complex issues relating to cancer diagnosis and treatment, and who may not be aware of fracture risk screening and management recommendations.

- The safety of anabolic agents in patients with breast cancer has not been established.

- While antiresorptive medications have demonstrated benefit for various breast cancer–related indications, including treatment-induced bone loss, adjuvant therapy, and bone metastases, optimal dosing to maximize this benefit while minimizing risks such as osteonecrosis of the jaw and atypical fractures has not been established.

- Although the median survival of patients with metastatic breast cancer is increasing, the optimal management of bone metastases has not been established. Currently recommended dosing protocols result in high cumulative exposure to antiresorptive medications with increased risk of adverse effects.

Discussion

Lifestyle Recommendations

All patients starting endocrine therapy should be counseled on adequate intake of calcium (1000-1200 mg daily) and vitamin D (800-1000 IU daily). Patients should also be encouraged to undertake moderate exercise (average of 30 min daily), with a focus on strength training 2 to 3 times weekly.

Screening Recommendations

BMD measurement is recommended for postmenopausal women initiating endocrine therapy and for premenopausal women initiating aromatase inhibitor therapy with ovarian suppression.[7]

Risk factors for increased fracture risk in women with breast cancer beyond aromatase inhibitor therapy are similar to those for the general population: T-score less than −1.5, age older than 65 years, BMI less than 20 kg/m², family history of hip fracture, personal history of fragility fracture after age 50 years, corticosteroid use exceeding 6 months, rheumatoid arthritis, and cigarette smoking.[7]

The FRAX algorithm is an online tool for estimating fracture risk with or without BMD, incorporating age, BMI, and several risk factors for osteoporosis. However, it should be noted that FRAX is not designed for assessment of risk in patients with breast cancer and may underestimate the effect of endocrine therapy.

Treatment Recommendations

Pharmacologic therapy should be offered to those initiating endocrine therapy known to accelerate bone loss and who have a T-score less than −2.0 or have 2 or more of the following risk factors:

- Age >65 years
- T-score < −1.5
- Cigarette smoking (current or history of)
- BMI <20 kg/m²
- Family history of hip fracture
- Personal history of fragility fracture after age 50 years
- Oral glucocorticoid use >6 months

Oral and intravenous bisphosphonates and denosumab have been demonstrated to prevent cancer-induced bone loss in patients with breast cancer (Table 2 in reference 7). Based on available evidence, preferred agents include intravenous zoledronic acid (4 mg every 6 months) or subcutaneous denosumab (60 mg every 6 months).[7] Providers should be aware that abrupt cessation of denosumab is associated with rebound bone loss and increased risk of multiple vertebral fractures[8,9]; therefore, consolidation with bisphosphonate therapy is recommended.[10]

Patients with an initial T-score greater than −2.0 and no additional risk factors should have risk factors and BMD monitored at 1- to 2-year intervals. Pharmacologic therapy should be considered for an annual BMD decrease greater than 5% to 10%.[7]

Adjuvant Therapy

In postmenopausal women with breast cancer, adjuvant bisphosphonate therapy is associated with a modest improvement in overall survival. Therapeutic options with the strongest supporting data include oral clodronate (1600 mg daily for 2 to 3 years), oral ibandronate (50 mg daily for 3 years), or zoledronic acid (4 mg once every 6 months for 3 years or 4 mg once every 3 months for 2 years). Studies of adjuvant denosumab did not demonstrate consistent reduction of breast cancer recurrence in patients with early-stage breast cancer; therefore, the use of adjuvant denosumab is not recommended.[11]

Management of Bone Metastases

Bone is one of the most common sites for breast cancer metastases. Antiresorptive medications reduce skeletal-related events such as fractures and spinal cord compression.[12,13] In patients with evidence of bone destruction, treatment options include subcutaneous denosumab, 120 mg once every 3 to 4 weeks; intravenous pamidronate, 90 mg every 3 to 4 weeks; and intravenous zoledronic acid, 4 mg every 3 to 4 weeks or every 12 weeks. In patients with reduced creatinine clearance (<30 mL/min), denosumab is recommended.[14] The optimal duration of therapy has not been established. In most studies to date, follow-up has been limited to 24 to 36 months. However, since 1990, the median survival with metastatic breast cancer has improved from 20 months to 31 months.[15] Dosing regimens recommended for oncology indications are associated with a significantly higher incidence of osteonecrosis of the jaw than dosing regimens recommended for osteoporosis indications.[16] Again, denosumab at any dosing frequency should not be discontinued abruptly without bisphosphonate consolidation.

Clinical Case Vignettes

Case 1

A 58-year-old postmenopausal woman is diagnosed with early-stage invasive ductal carcinoma of the left breast. The tumor is positive for expression of estrogen and progesterone receptors and negative for expression of HER2. She has undergone lumpectomy and whole-breast radiation and is about to initiate treatment with exemestane, an aromatase inhibitor.

Which of the following is the most appropriate action?

A. Initiate treatment with oral alendronate, 70 mg weekly

B. Initiate treatment with subcutaneous denosumab, 60 mg every 6 months

C. Initiate treatment with subcutaneous teriparatide, 20 mcg daily

D. Perform DXA to measure BMD

E. Perform quantitative CT to measure BMD

Answer: D) Perform DXA to measure BMD

Postmenopausal women should be assessed for fracture risk, and DXA (Answer D) is the preferred screening method, not quantitative CT (Answer E). Pharmacologic therapy (Answers A, B, and C) is not indicated unless she is at increased risk for bone loss or fracture.

Case 1 (continued)

DXA scan reveals a lumbar spine T-score of −2.2.

Which of the following is NOT recommended for the management of bone loss during endocrine therapy?

A. Adequate calcium and vitamin D intake with regular exercise; no pharmacologic therapy indicated

B. Intravenous zoledronic acid, 4 mg every 6 months

C. Oral alendronate, 70 mg weekly

D. Subcutaneous denosumab, 60 mg every 6 months

E. Subcutaneous teriparatide, 20 mcg daily

Answer: E) Subcutaneous teriparatide, 20 mcg daily

The safety of anabolic therapy (Answer E) in patients with breast cancer is unknown, and thus, teriparatide is not recommended in this setting. All patients should be counseled on adequate calcium and vitamin D intake and regular exercise (Answer A). Because this patient's T-score is lower than −2.0, pharmacologic therapy with an antiresorptive medication (Answers B, C, and D) is recommended.

Case 1 (continued)

Which of the following could be offered as adjuvant therapy for breast cancer in this patient?

A. Intravenous zoledronic acid, 4 mg every 6 months

B. Oral alendronate, 70 mg weekly

C. Oral ibandronate, 150 mg monthly

D. Oral risedronate, 35 mg weekly

E. Subcutaneous teriparatide, 20 mcg daily

Answer: A) Intravenous zoledronic acid, 4 mg every 6 months

In postmenopausal women, adjuvant bisphosphonate therapy is associated with modest improvement in overall survival. The strongest data support the use of intravenous zoledronic acid (Answer A); oral clodronate, 1600 mg daily; or oral ibandronate, 50 mg daily (thus Answers B, C, and D are incorrect). The safety of anabolic therapy (Answer E) has not been demonstrated in breast cancer.

Case 2

A 43-year-old premenopausal woman with early-stage breast cancer has undergone mastectomy and chemotherapy. Screening DXA reveals a lumbar spine T-score of −0.9. She has no significant risk factors for bone loss. She is planning to initiate treatment with ovarian suppression and anastrozole.

Which of the following is the most appropriate management plan?

A. Counsel the patient on adequate calcium and vitamin D intake and regular exercise and repeat DXA in 1 year

B. Counsel the patient on adequate calcium and vitamin D intake and regular exercise and repeat DXA at age 50 years

C. Recommend intravenous zoledronic acid, 4 mg every 6 months

D. Recommend subcutaneous denosumab, 60 mg every 6 months

E. Recommend tamoxifen, 20 mg daily

Answer: A) Counsel the patient on adequate calcium and vitamin D intake and regular exercise and repeat DXA in 1 year

This patient does not meet indications for pharmacologic treatment (Answers C, D, and E) but is at high risk for significant bone loss with ovarian suppression and aromatase inhibition. She should therefore be offered repeated DXA in 1 to 2 years (Answer A, not Answer B) to assess for interval bone loss, which may be substantial.

Case 3

A 67-year-old woman is diagnosed with metastatic breast cancer including bony involvement.

Which of the following is NOT a recommended treatment regimen in this setting?

A. Intravenous pamidronate, 90 mg every 3 to 4 weeks

B. Intravenous zoledronic acid, 4 mg every 3 to 4 weeks

C. Intravenous zoledronic acid, 4 mg every 12 weeks

D. Subcutaneous denosumab, 60 mg every 6 months

E. Subcutaneous denosumab, 120 mg every 3 to 4 weeks

Answer: D) Subcutaneous denosumab, 60 mg every 6 months

Of these answer options, only subcutaneous denosumab, 60 mg every 6 months (Answer D) is *not* recommended by the American Society for Clinical Oncology as a management option for metastatic breast cancer with bony involvement.

Key Learning Points

- Breast cancer treatment is associated with increased risk of bone loss and fracture.

- Tamoxifen is associated with a moderate decrease in BMD in premenopausal women and a moderate increase in BMD in postmenopausal women.

- Aromatase inhibition and ovarian suppression are associated with significant bone loss and increased fracture risk.

- Patients at risk for bone loss from breast cancer treatment should be offered bone density screening with DXA if available.

- Patients at risk for bone loss from breast cancer treatment should be counseled on exercise and adequate intake of calcium and vitamin D.

- Antiresorptive medications are effective for the prevention and treatment of breast cancer treatment–related bone loss.

- Bisphosphonates may be indicated for adjuvant therapy in postmenopausal women with breast cancer.

- Antiresorptive medications decrease skeletal adverse events in breast cancer bone metastases, but at high cumulative doses, they are associated with increased risk of osteonecrosis of the jaw and atypical fractures.

References

1. Chen Z, Maricic M, Bassford TL, et al. Fracture risk among breast cancer survivors: results from the Women's Health Initiative Observational Study. *Arch Intern Med.* 2005;165(5):552-558. PMID: 15767532

2. Sverrisdottir A, Fornander T, Jacobsson H, von Schoultz E, Rutqvist LE. Bone mineral density among premenopausal women with early breast cancer in a randomized trial of adjuvant endocrine therapy. *J Clin Oncol.* 2004;22(18):3694-3699. PMID: 15365065

3. Eastell R, Adams JE, Coleman RE, et al. Effect of anastrozole on bone mineral density: 5-year results from the anastrozole, tamoxifen, alone or in combination trial 18233230. *J Clin Oncol.* 2008;26(7):1051-1057. PMID: 18309940

4. Early Breast Cancer Trialists' Collaborative Group (EBCTCG). Aromatase inhibitors versus tamoxifen in early breast cancer: patient-level meta-analysis of the randomised trials. *Lancet.* 2015;386(10001):1341-1352. PMID: 26211827

5. Gralow JR, Biermann JS, Farooki A, et al. NCCN Task Force feport: bone health in cancer care. *J Natl Compr Canc Netw.* 2013(11 Suppl 3):S1-S50; quiz S51. PMID: 23997241

6. Pagani O, Regan MM, Walley BA, et al; TEXT and SOFT Investigators; International Breast Cancer Study Group. Adjuvant exemestane with ovarian suppression in premenopausal breast cancer. *N Engl J Med.* 2014;371(2):107-118. PMID: 24881463

7. Hadji P, Aapro MS, Body J-J, et al. Management of aromatase inhibitor-associated bone loss (AIBL) in postmenopausal women with hormone sensitive breast cancer: joint position statement of the IOF, CABS, ECTS, IEG, ESCEO IMS, and SIOG. *J Bone Oncol.* 2017;7:1-12. PMID: 28413771

8. Bone HG, Bolognese MA, Yuen CK, et al. Effects of denosumab treatment and discontinuation on bone mineral density and bone turnover markers in postmenopausal women with low bone mass. *J Clin Endocrinol Metab.* 2011;96(4):972-980. PMID: 21289258

9. Cummings SR, Ferrari S, Eastell R, et al. Vertebral fractures after discontinuation of denosumab: a post hoc analysis of the randomized placebo-controlled FREEDOM trial and its extension. *J Bone Miner Res.* 2018;33(2):190-198. PMID: 29105841

10. Everts-Graber J, Reichenbach S, Ziswiler HR, Studer U, Lehmann T. A single infusion of zoledronate in postmenopausal women following denosumab discontinuation results in partial conservation of bone mass gains. *J Bone Miner Res.* 2020;35(7):1207-1215. PMID: 31991007

11. Eisen A, Somerfield MR, Accordino MK, et al. Use of adjuvant bisphosphonates and other bone-modifying agents in breast xancer: ASCO-OH (CCO) guideline update. *J Clin Oncol.* 2022;40(7):787-800. PMID: 35041467

12. Kohno N, Aogi K, Minami H, et al. Zoledronic acid significantly reduces skeletal complications compared with placebo in Japanese women with bone metastases from breast cancer: a randomized, placebo-controlled trial. *J Clin Oncol.* 2005;23(15):3314-3321. PMID: 15738536

13. Stopeck AT, Lipton A, Body J-J, et al. Denosumab compared with zoledronic acid for the treatment of bone metastases in patients with advanced breast cancer: a randomized, double-blind study. *J Clin Oncol.* 2010;28(35):5132-5139. PMID: 21060033

14. Van Poznak C, Somerfield MR, Barlow WE, et al. Role of bone-modifying agents in metastatic breast cancer: an American Society of Clinical Oncology-Cancer Care Ontario Focused Guideline Update. *J Clin Oncol.* 2017;35(35):3978-3986. PMID: 29035643

15. Caswell-Jin JL, Plevritis SK, Tian L, et al. Change in survival in metastatic breast cancer with treatment advances: meta-analysis and systematic review. *JNCI Cancer Spectr.* 2018;2(4):pky062. PMID: 30627694

16. Khan AA, Morrison A, Hanley DA, et al; International Task Force on Osteonecrosis of the Jaw. Diagnosis and management of osteonecrosis of the jaw: a systematic review and international consensus. *J Bone Miner Res.* 2015;30(1):3-23. PMID: 25414052

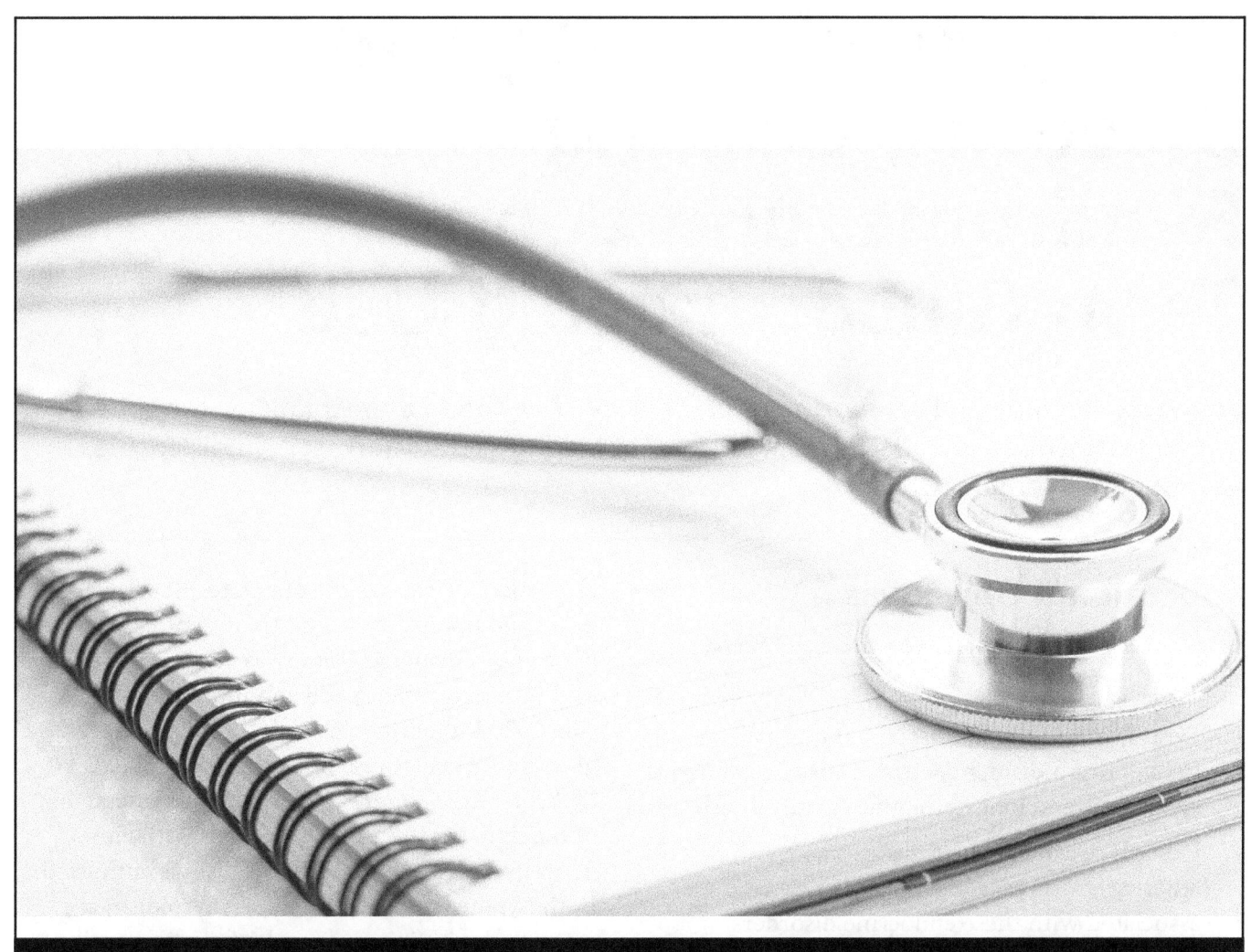

CARDIOVASCULAR ENDOCRINOLOGY

Dyslipidemia in Thyroid Diseases, Cushing Syndrome, and Long-Term Glucocorticoid Use

Connie B. Newman, MD. Department of Medicine, Division of Endocrinology, Diabetes and Metabolism, New York University School of Medicine, New York, NY; Email: connie.newman@nyulangone.org

Educational Objectives

After reviewing this chapter, learners should be able to:

- Describe lipid and lipoprotein abnormalities in hypothyroidism, hyperthyroidism, Cushing syndrome, and long-term glucocorticoid use.

- Describe cardiovascular diseases and atherosclerotic cardiovascular disease risk associated with these endocrine disorders.

- Summarize results of studies of thyroid hormone replacement in patients with overt hypothyroidism, subclinical hypothyroidism, and overt hyperthyroidism.

- Apply this knowledge to management of dyslipidemia in patients with hypothyroidism and hyperthyroidism, Cushing syndrome, and long-term use of glucocorticoids above replacement dosages.

Significance of the Clinical Problem

Hypothyroidism is associated with elevations in LDL cholesterol (LDL-C), apolipoprotein B, and triglycerides, and treatment of hypothyroidism has been shown to reduce these parameters.

Hyperthyroidism has the opposite effect on lipids and lipoproteins, and treatment of hyperthyroidism has been shown to increase LDL-C, triglycerides, and apolipoprotein B. The 2020 Endocrine Society clinical practice guideline, *Management of Dyslipidemia in Patients with Endocrine Disorders*, recommends assessment of the lipid profile after the patient with either hypothyroidism or hyperthyroidism is euthyroid. Both hypothyroidism and hyperthyroidism are associated with increased risk of cardiovascular diseases, which could be related to the disease and/or the associated dyslipidemia.

Cortisol increases synthesis of fatty acids and triglycerides in the liver, and chronic cortisol excess increases lipogenesis and storage of fat in adipose tissue. Cushing syndrome is associated with increased LDL-C and triglycerides, as well as diabetes mellitus, hypertension, and central obesity. All these factors increase cardiovascular disease risk. In patients with persistent Cushing syndrome, evaluation of the lipid profile is recommended, and treatment with a statin is suggested if LDL-C is above 70 mg/dL (>1.8 mmol/L).

Long-term use of glucocorticoids with a dosage that exceeds that recommended for replacement may be associated with elevations in triglycerides and LDL-C. Assessment and treatment of lipids and other cardiovascular disease risk factors is important.

Hormones affect many pathways in lipoprotein metabolism and therefore endocrine diseases may be associated with dyslipidemia. Treatment of the endocrine disease has been shown to improve the lipid profile. Hypothyroidism is estimated to occur in 5% of the population, with an additional 5% untreated. Endocrinologists, internists, and family physicians are likely to have patients with hypothyroidism in their practice. Practitioners must understand that in a patient with hypothyroidism, hypercholesterolemia is secondary to the thyroid disease and will improve as thyroid hormone is replaced. Patients with hyperthyroidism may have LDL-C levels that appear appropriate, but when patients become euthyroid, LDL-C and triglycerides will be higher.

Hypercortisolemia also affects lipoprotein metabolism. Patients with Cushing syndrome may have higher LDL-C and triglycerides, compared with values in the pre-Cushing period. Importantly, patients with Cushing syndrome have an estimated 2-fold increase in mortality, and increased risk of various cardiovascular diseases. The Endocrine Society 2020 guideline, *Lipid Management in Patients with Endocrine Disorders*, recommends obtaining a lipid profile in all patients with Cushing syndrome and suggests reducing LDL-C with a statin if the LDL-C concentration is above 70 mg/dL (>1.81 mmol/L), regardless of cardiovascular risk score.

Practice Gaps

- Lack of knowledge of management of dyslipidemia in patients with endocrine diseases.

- Insufficient time to read clinical practice guidelines.

- Late adopters of recommendations in guidelines.

- Lipid management in Cushing syndrome is a low priority.

Discussion

Hypothyroidism and Hyperthyroidism

Thyroid hormones affect lipoprotein metabolism by complex mechanisms. Thyroid hormones increase free fatty acids by lipolysis of adipose tissue and dietary fat, increased uptake of free fatty acids by the liver, and hepatic synthesis of VLDL. In addition, thyroid hormones regulate the LDL receptor and increase the activity of enzymes in the cholesterol metabolism pathway. These enzymes include hepatic lipase, cholesteryl ester protein (CETP), and lecithin cholesterol acyltransferase (LCAT). Changes in lipids and lipoproteins are shown in *table 1*.

Hypothyroidism
Lipids and Lipoproteins
Studies have reported hypothyroidism in 1.4% to 13% of patients with high cholesterol. In 2014, a chart review of more than 4000 patients with newly diagnosed hyperlipidemia reported that 3.0% of them had TSH elevations above 5.0 mIU/L and 1.7% had TSH elevations above 10.0 mIU/L. In overt hypothyroidism, LDL-C and apolipoprotein B may be increased (due to increased activity of hydroxymethyl glutaryl coenzyme-A [HMG-CoA] reductase and upregulation of the LDL receptor). Metabolism of fatty acids may be reduced, leading to increased triglycerides.

Table 1. Changes in LDL-C, HDL-C, Triglycerides, and Apolipoprotein B in Thyroid Disorders

Disorder	LDL-C	HDL-C	TG	Apo B
Overt hypothyroidism	No change or increased	Normal or increased	Normal or increased	No change or increased
Subclinical hypothyroidism	No change or increased	Normal or decreased	Normal or increased	No change or increased
Overt hyperthyroidism	Decreased	Normal or decreased	Normal or increased	No change or decreased

Abbreviations: LDL-C, low-density lipoprotein cholesterol; HDL-C, high-density lipoprotein cholesterol; TG, triglycerides; Apo B, apolipoprotein B.

In patients with subclinical hypothyroidism (TSH 4.0-10.0 mIU/L), total cholesterol and LDL-C may be increased, although the change in LDL-C is less than that seen with overt hypothyroidism. Triglycerides may be normal or increased and HDL-C is usually in the range considered to be normal for men and women.

Cardiovascular Disease

Overt hypothyroidism is associated with increased risk of coronary heart disease and congestive heart failure. Data on coronary heart disease in patients with subclinical hypothyroidism are inconsistent.

Management

In patients with hyperlipidemia (elevation of cholesterol and/or triglycerides), overt hypothyroidism should be considered and ruled out before treatment with lipid-lowering medications. This is a recommendation of the 2020 Endocrine Society Guideline and is supported by high-quality clinical trial data. In patients with hypothyroidism, the lipid profile should be repeated, and the need for lipid-lowering medications assessed, when the patient is euthyroid (after thyroid hormone replacement).

For patients with subclinical hypothyroidism (TSH <10.0 mIU/L) and hyperlipidemia, treatment with levothyroxine to reduce cholesterol and/or triglycerides is not standard practice because clinical trials have failed to show a benefit in symptoms and/or quality of life. However, a 2020 meta-analysis by Kotwal et al of lipid and lipoprotein data from studies in patients with subclinical hypothyroidism found significant reduction in LDL-C, which can be considered a benefit. These data provide evidence for the suggestion in the 2020 Endocrine Society guideline that thyroid hormone replacement be considered as a means of reducing LDL-C in adults with subclinical hypothyroidism.

The 2020 report by Kotwal et al describe results of a meta-analysis of more than 70 studies of patients with overt and subclinical hypothyroidism. Levothyroxine treatment, in comparison with placebo or no treatment, was associated with reduction in total cholesterol, LDL-C, and triglycerides (*table 2*). In 55 studies of 2305 patients with overt hypothyroidism who were treated with levothyroxine, the mean baseline LDL-C concentration was 168.8 mg/dL (4.37 mmol/L) and was reduced by 41.1 mg/dL (1.06 mmol/L), which represents 24% of the baseline LDL-C. Mean triglyceride concentrations were 147.3 mg/dL (1.66 mmol/L) before replacement. With levothyroxine, triglycerides were reduced by 27.3 mg/dL (0.31 mmol/L), which represents 18.5% of the baseline value. In 79 studies of subclinical hypothyroidism in 4588 patients, mean LDL-C at baseline was 139.5 mg/dL (3.61 mmol/L), and with levothyroxine treatment LDL-C was reduced by 11.1 mg/dL (0.29 mmol/L), which represents 8% of baseline.

Table 2. Lipid Changes in Patients With Overt Hypothyroidism Who Are Euthyroid After Levothyroxine Treatment[a]

Measurement	Mean baseline	Change from baseline	Percentage change from baseline	Number of studies
Total cholesterol	260 mg/dL (SI: 6.73 mmol/L)	58 mg/dL (SI: 1.50 mmol/L)	22%	72
LDL-C	169 mg/dL (SI: 4.38 mmol/L)	41 mg/dL (SI: 1.06 mmol/L)	24%	55
HDL-C	54 mg/dL (SI: 1.40 mmol/L)	4 mg/dL (SI: 0.10 mmol/L)	7%	57
Triglycerides	147 mg/dL (SI: 1.66 mmol/L)	27 mg/dL (SI: 0.31 mmol/L)	18%	60

[a]Data derived from Kotwal A, Cortes T, Genere N, et al. Treatment of thyroid dysfunction and serum lipids: a systematic review and meta-analysis. *J Clin Endocrinol Metab.* 2020;105(12):dgaa672.

Hyperthyroidism

Lipids and Lipoproteins

Thyroid hormone increases cholesterol metabolism (thus, reducing LDL-C levels) by stimulation of the gene for LDL receptor synthesis and upregulation of the LDL receptor. In overt hyperthyroidism that is not transient, total cholesterol, LDL-C, apolipoprotein B, apolipoprotein A, and lipoprotein (a) are reduced. Triglycerides may be normal and HDL-C unchanged or decreased (*table 1*).

Management

In patients with untreated overt hyperthyroidism, LDL-C levels increase as the patient becomes euthyroid. Therefore, the lipid profile should be reassessed after the patient is euthyroid. In the 2020 meta-analysis of 31 studies of 938 patients with overt hyperthyroidism, the mean LDL-C concentration before treatment was 89.2 mg/dL (2.31 mmol/L), and after treatment with either thyroidectomy, antithyroid medications, or radioactive iodine, the mean LDL-C concentration increased by 31 mg/dL (0.80 mmol/L). HDL-C (mean = 46.5 mg/dL [1.20 mmol/L]) significantly increased by 5.5 mg/dL (0.14 mmol/L), while triglycerides, which were 110 mg/dL (1.24 mmol/L) at baseline, did not significantly change. Significant increases in apolipoprotein A, apolipoprotein B, and lipoprotein (a) were observed in 12, 13, and 10 studies, respectively, after patients were euthyroid.

In 3 studies of patients with subclinical hyperthyroidism, mean LDL-C did not significantly increase after the patients became euthyroid. However, repeating the lipid profile when the patient is euthyroid is reasonable.

Thyroid Disease and the Heart

Hypothyroidism may be associated with congestive heart failure. In elderly persons and those with atherosclerotic cardiovascular disease, thyroid hormone replacement should be prescribed in small increments. Hyperthyroidism is associated with atrial fibrillation, which disappears in about two-thirds of patients after treatment.

Cushing Syndrome

Lipids and Lipoproteins

The effects of hypercortisolemia on lipids and lipoproteins and adipose tissue are complex and incompletely understood. Hypercortisolemia stimulates hepatic synthesis and secretion of VLDL. In addition, high cortisol stimulates lipoprotein lipase activity, leading to lipolysis and uptake of fatty acids and glycerol in adipose tissue, especially in the visceral area. Lipid and lipoprotein changes (*table 3*) include normal or increased LDL-C, increased triglycerides, and normal or decreased HDL-C.

The prevalence of dyslipidemia in persons with Cushing syndrome is difficult to determine because of varying definitions of cutoff points for dyslipidemia. Estimates of dyslipidemia prevalence range from 38% to 71%. Factors affecting the lipid profile are severity and duration of exposure to excess cortisol and the presence of diabetes and visceral adiposity.

Cardiovascular Disease Risk

Persons with Cushing syndrome have increased rates of mortality and cardiovascular and cerebrovascular morbidity. A cohort study in Denmark of 343 patients with Cushing syndrome (median age at diagnosis 43.8 years) and 34,300

Table 3. Changes in Total Cholesterol, LDL-C, HDL-C, and Triglycerides in Endogenous and Exogenous Hypercortisolemia

Disorder	Total Cholesterol	LDL-C	HDL-C	TG
Cushing syndrome	Increased	No change or increased	Normal or decreased	Increased
Long-term glucocorticoid therapy	No change or increased	No change or increased	Normal or increased	Normal or increased

Abbreviations: LDL-C, low-density lipoprotein cholesterol; HDL-C, high-density lipoprotein cholesterol; TG, triglycerides.

control participants found increased total mortality during 12 years of follow-up (unadjusted hazard ratio, 2.3; 95% CI, 1.8-2.9). With adjustments for baseline characteristics, the hazard ratio was 1.6 (95% CI, 1.3-2.1). These patients also had increased risk for acute myocardial infarction (hazard ratio, 2.6; 95% CI, 1.5-4.7), stroke (hazard ratio, 2.0; 95% CI, 1.3-3.2), and venous thromboembolism (hazard ratio 2.6; 95% CI, 1.5-4.7). Increased cardiovascular risk was documented even 3 years before diagnosis. Patients considered cured after adrenal or pituitary surgery continued to have increased risk for mortality, stroke, and myocardial infarction more than 1 year after the surgery. These data are consistent with those in other studies.

Management

The long-term cardiovascular risk in patients with Cushing syndrome, even in those "cured," suggests the importance of managing cardiovascular risk factors: dyslipidemia, diabetes mellitus, hypertension, and obesity. Patients in remission after treatment of Cushing syndrome may or may not have improvement in dyslipidemia and other risk factors.

In adults with Cushing syndrome, assessment of the lipid profile at diagnosis and periodically thereafter identifies patients with dyslipidemia. The Endocrine Society 2020 guideline suggests consideration of statin treatment (in addition to lifestyle therapy) in adults with persistent Cushing syndrome and an LDL-C concentration above 70 mg/dL (>1.81 mmol/L). The target is LDL-C and the aim is to reduce atherosclerotic cardiovascular disease risk regardless of the actual risk score. However, in patients with limited life expectancy, statins and other lipid-lowering therapies may not be appropriate. It is also important to control other risk factors for atherosclerotic cardiovascular disease.

In patients with cured Cushing syndrome, cardiovascular risk assessment and treatment of dyslipidemia should be the same as in the general population.

Long-Term Glucocorticoid Therapy

Lipids and Lipoproteins

Long-term glucocorticoid therapy with dosages above those used for replacement may be associated with dose-dependent increases in total cholesterol, LDL-C, and triglycerides, although studies have found inconsistent results. One study of glucocorticoid replacement in patients with hypopituitarism found that dosages of hydrocortisone above 20 mg daily were associated with higher LDL-C and triglycerides compared with dosages below 20 mg daily. The effects of long-term glucocorticoid therapy on the lipid profile are dependent on the dosage, route of administration, duration of therapy, underlying medical illnesses, and concomitant medications.

Cardiovascular Disease Risk

Observational studies have shown that long-term glucocorticoid therapy is associated with increased risk of cardiovascular disease and stroke, with the risk of heart failure higher than the risk of ischemic heart disease. A longitudinal cohort study using medical records of 87,794 adults (mean age, 56 years) with immune-mediated inflammatory diseases (including rheumatoid arthritis, polymyalgia, giant-cell arteritis, systemic lupus erythematosus), who had a mean duration since diagnosis of 9.6 years, reported that the estimated cumulative risk of all-cause cardiovascular disease increased from 1.5% when steroids were not used, to 3.8% for a daily prednisolone dosage equivalent, to less than 5.0 mg and to 9.1% for daily dosages above 25 mg.

Management

We do not have data to determine the optimal dosage of glucocorticoids for replacement or long-term use (for inflammatory or other diseases). The health care provider should aim to minimize risk of atherosclerotic cardiovascular disease by evaluating for and treating cardiovascular risk factors. Treatment of these risk factors (including LDL-C and triglycerides) according to guidelines is important. In an adult with a low to moderate 10-year atherosclerotic cardiovascular disease risk (5%-7.5%), a discussion about the added risk associated with long-term glucocorticoid therapy, and the possibility of adding statin therapy to lifestyle measures, may be helpful. In patients for whom glucocorticoid treatment is being considered, the clinician should choose the lowest dosage that will be effective.

Clinical Case Vignettes

Case 1

A 52-year-old man is referred for management of newly diagnosed hypothyroidism. He reports feeling increasingly fatigued over the past year, and he initially attributed this to aging. He also noticed increased swelling of his eyelids causing drooping, challenges with his vision, and constipation.

Two weeks ago, his primary care physician prescribed levothyroxine, 50 mcg daily. He does not take any other medications. He does not smoke cigarettes. He drinks 3 to 4 glasses of beer on the weekends. He has never had chest pain or shortness of breath. His grandparents lived into their 90s. His father is treated for high blood pressure and his mother does not take any medication.

On physical examination, his blood pressure is 128/92 mm Hg and pulse rate is 54 beats/min. His height is 73 in (185.4 cm) and weight is 182 lb (82.6 kg) (BMI = 24.0 kg/m^2). His waist circumference 39 in (99.1 cm). He has significant periorbital edema. The thyroid gland is estimated to be twice normal size and is firm, mobile, and nontender. He has delayed relaxation phase of reflexes and mild edema of the ankles.

Laboratory test results:

> TSH = 88.0 mIU/L (0.5-5.0 mIU/L)
> Free T$_4$ = 0.2 ng/dL (0.7-1.9 ng/dL) (SI: 2.57 pmol/L [9.00-24.5 pmol/L])
> Total cholesterol = 320 mg/dL (SI: 8.29 mmol/L)
> LDL-C = 208 mg/dL (SI: 5.39 mmol/L)
> HDL-C = 62 mg/dL (SI: 1.61 mmol/L)
> Triglycerides = 250 mg/dL (SI: 2.83 mmol/L)

Which of the following is the best interpretation of this patient's lipid and lipoprotein values?

A. High HDL-C
B. Hypertriglyceridemia
C. Primary hypercholesterolemia
D. Secondary hypercholesterolemia

Answer: D) Secondary hypercholesterolemia

When a patient has high cholesterol, LDL-C, and TSH, hypercholesterolemia is usually caused by the thyroid disease and is therefore termed secondary (Answer D). With thyroid hormone treatment, total and LDL-C will decrease.

The term primary hypercholesterolemia (Answer C) refers to elevations in cholesterol that are genetically determined (monogenic or polygenic), rather than acquired.

This patient's triglycerides appear elevated (Answer B); however, his blood was drawn when he was not fasting and the test must be repeated on a fasting sample. Hypothyroidism may be associated with elevations in triglycerides as well as cholesterol. Triglycerides may be reduced with thyroid hormone treatment. In a meta-analysis of 60 studies of patients with overt hypothyroidism, mean triglyceride levels were reduced by 27.3 mg/dL (0.31 mmol/L).

HDL-C concentrations in men are considered normal if greater than 40 mg/dL (>1.04 mmol/L). Values less than 40 mg/dL (<1.04 mmol/L) are considered low. However, in estimating atherosclerotic cardiovascular disease risk, the most critical lipoprotein to consider is LDL-C, regardless of whether HDL-C is above normal or "high." This patient's HDL-C concentration may be related to hypothyroidism, and with thyroid hormone replacement it will likely decrease by 2.5 to 5.5 mg/dL (0.06 to 0.14 mmol/L).

Case 1 (continued)

In addition to increasing this patient's levothyroxine dosage, which of the following medications should be started now?

A. Ezetimibe

B. Fibrate

C. PCSK9 inhibitor

D. Statin

E. No additional therapy now

Answer E) No additional therapy now

This patient has overt hypothyroidism, with elevated TSH and low free T_4. The hypothyroidism may be longstanding. Lipid and lipoprotein changes due to hypothyroidism can include increased total cholesterol, HDL-C, LDL-C, and triglycerides. While this patient's LDL-C concentration is above 200 mg/dL (>5.18 mmol/L), statin therapy (Answer D) is not appropriate at this time, because as hypothyroidism is treated, the LDL-C level will fall. A lipid panel must be repeated when the patient is euthyroid. The absence of other risk factors, the lack of cardiac symptoms, and the history of longevity in his family suggest that the patient may not have high cardiovascular disease risk. Thus, no additional therapy (Answer E) is recommended now.

PCSK9 inhibitors (Answer C) are generally used in patients taking statins when LDL-C requires further reduction. This patient is not taking a statin and does not require lipid-lowering therapy now.

Fibrates (Answer B) may be used to treat moderate hypertriglyceridemia in patients with increased triglycerides despite diet or diet and a statin. Generally, such patients have a triglyceride concentration above 500 mg/dL (>5.65 mmol/L). The combination of a statin and a fibrate may increase the risk of myopathy. There is no reason to use a fibrate in this patient. It is not clear that triglycerides are elevated, and even if they are elevated, treatment of hypothyroidism could normalize his triglyceride level. Further, if triglycerides remain elevated when the patient is euthyroid, the next step would be diet, followed by diet plus a statin.

Ezetimibe (Answer A) is a cholesterol absorption inhibitor that reduces LDL-C by about 18%. It is not indicated for this patient now. After he is euthyroid, the treatment of choice for inappropriately elevated LDL-C is a statin.

Case 2

A 50-year-old woman is referred for management of persistent hypercortisolemia due to Cushing syndrome. She was in good health until 2 years ago. At that time, she noticed weight gain of 45 lb (20.5 kg), with noticeable increase in abdominal weight, acne, and bruising. MRI showed an 11-mm pituitary mass, determined to be a pituitary adenoma after surgery. Visual fields were normal. Fasting blood glucose was elevated, with a hemoglobin A_{1c} value of 7.5% (58 mmol/mol). After transsphenoidal surgery, 24-hour urinary cortisol excretion was 200 µg/24 h (552 nmol/d) (reference range, 10-100 µg/24 h [27.6- 276.0 nmol/d]). The pituitary tumor was not seen on repeated MRI. Extensive evaluation did not reveal ectopic ACTH or an adrenal tumor.

Family history is notable for myocardial infarction in her father at age 70 years and hypertension in her mother.

Medications are metformin, 1000 mg twice daily, and ketoconazole, 200 mg twice daily.

On physical examination, her blood pressure is 145/85 mm Hg. Her height is 64 in (162.6 cm), and weight is 170 lb (77.1 kg) (BMI = 29.2 kg/m²). She has moonlike facies, central deposition of fat, and bruises on her legs.

Laboratory test results (sample drawn 1 month ago while fasting):

> Total cholesterol = 240 mg/dL (SI: 6.22 mmol/L)
> LDL-C = 115 mg/dL (SI: 2.98 mmol/L)
> HDL-C = 45 mg/dL (SI: 1.17 mmol/L)
> Triglycerides = 400 mg/dL (SI: 4.52 mmol/L)
> Urinary cortisol = 125 µg/24 h (SI: 345 nmol/24 h)

Calculated 10-year atherosclerotic cardiovascular disease risk using the Pooled Cohort Equation is 4.5%.

Which of the following is the best interpretation of the lipid and lipoprotein values?

A. All values are appropriate for this patient

B. Elevation in triglycerides only

C. HDL-C is normal

D. LDL-C is inappropriately high for a patient with persistent Cushing syndrome; triglycerides are above the upper limit of normal

E. LDL-C is optimal for level of atherosclerotic cardiovascular disease risk

Answer: D) LDL-C is inappropriately high for a patient with persistent Cushing syndrome, triglycerides are above the upper limit of normal

This patient has persistent Cushing syndrome after surgery with continued elevation of cortisol on ketoconazole, 200 mg twice daily. Cushing syndrome is associated with elevated triglycerides, increased LDL-C, and the presence of other risk factors for cardiovascular disease such as diabetes mellitus and hypertension. This patient's LDL-C concentration (115 mg/dL [2.98 mmol/L]) is considered inappropriately high for a patient with Cushing syndrome (Answer D).

Triglycerides are elevated (Answer B), but as discussed above, LDL-C is also inappropriately high for a patient with Cushing syndrome.

In women, an HDL-C value greater than 50 mg/dL (>1.30 mmol/L) is considered normal. This patient has an HDL-C value of 45 mg/dL (1.17 mmol/L), which is low, not normal (Answer C) for a woman.

Persistent Cushing syndrome is associated with increased risk for atherosclerotic cardiovascular disease, in part because of associated risk factors such as dyslipidemia, diabetes, and hypertension. An LDL-C value of 115 mg/dL (2.98 mmol/L) is inappropriately high for the level of atherosclerotic cardiovascular disease risk in this patient. The Endocrine Society 2020 guideline, Lipid Management in Endocrine Disorders, suggests that lipid-lowering therapy be considered in patients with Cushing syndrome if the LDL-C concentration is above 70 mg/dL (>1.81 mmol/L).

As discussed, this patient's triglycerides are elevated, HDL-C is low, and LDL-C is inappropriate (thus, Answer A is incorrect).

Case 2 (continued)

Which of the following is the best next step in this patient's management?

A. Add semaglutide, 0.25 mg once weekly

B. Discontinue ketoconazole and order another fasting lipid panel

C. Order a lipid panel and schedule another visit in 3 months

D. Recommend diet and exercise

E. Recommend diet, exercise, and statin therapy

Answer: E) Recommend diet, exercise, and statin therapy

This patient has chronic hypercortisolism (due to Cushing syndrome), type 2 diabetes, and possibly hypertension. Cushing syndrome is associated with increased risk of atherosclerotic cardiovascular disease, which is the most common cause of death in persons with Cushing syndrome. The 2020 Endocrine Society guideline recognizes the increased risk of cardiovascular disease in patients with persistent Cushing syndrome and suggests management of lipids, regardless of the cardiovascular risk score, with lifestyle modification and appropriate lipid-lowering medication (Answer E).

Diet and exercise (Answer D) should be recommended, but a statin is also needed to reduce atherosclerotic cardiovascular disease risk.

Rather than discontinue ketoconazole (Answer B), consideration should be given to increasing the dosage to further reduce cortisol levels.

Ordering a lipid panel and scheduling another visit in 3 months (Answer C) could be done but would delay treatment of atherosclerotic cardiovascular disease risk.

Semaglutide, 0.25 mg weekly (Answer A), is the starting dosage for this medication in adults with diabetes. In this patient, diabetes is adequately controlled with metformin, and the addition of semaglutide would not be appropriate.

Case 2 (continued)

Which of the following is the best treatment of this patient's dyslipidemia?

A. Eicosapentaenoic acid ethyl ester

B. Fenofibrate

C. Niacin

D. Statin

E. Statin plus fenofibrate

Answer: D) Statin

Persistent or untreated Cushing syndrome enhances atherosclerotic cardiovascular disease risk. The 2020 Endocrine Society guideline on management of lipids in patients with endocrine disorders suggests statin treatment (Answer D) as adjunct to diet and exercise in adults with persistent Cushing syndrome to reduce cardiovascular risk, regardless of the cardiovascular risk score. Statins lower LDL cholesterol and triglycerides in patients with Cushing syndrome.

Fenofibrate (Answer B) is generally used for patients with triglyceride concentrations greater than 500 mg/dL (>5.65 mmol/L) who require further reduction beyond that provided by diet and exercise and a statin, or in patients who cannot tolerate a statin.

The statin plus fenofibrate combination (Answer E) would be inappropriate in this patient and may increase the risk of myopathy.

Niacin (Answer C) lowers LDL-C, but it is not often used because of adverse effects and lack of cardiovascular benefit in randomized controlled trials. Niacin may worsen glycemic control in patients with diabetes.

Eicosapentaenoic acid ethyl ester (Answer A) is not indicated in this patient. This medication is indicated as adjunct to statin therapy to reduce cardiovascular disease in patients with atherosclerotic cardiovascular disease or diabetes mellitus and 2 additional risk factors who have triglyceride concentrations of 150 mg/dL or greater (≥1.70 mmol/L).

Case 2 (continued)

Which of the following statins and dosage would be most appropriate for treating this patient?

A. Atorvastatin, 20 mg daily

B. Atorvastatin, 80 mg daily

C. Lovastatin, 40 mg daily

D. Rosuvastatin, 10 mg daily

E. Simvastatin, 40 mg daily

Answer: D) Rosuvastatin, 10 mg daily

Ketoconazole is a strong inhibitor of cytochrome P450 3A4 (CYP 3A4), and when taken with statins that are metabolized by CYP 3A4, it increases the risk of myopathy (unexplained muscle pain or weakness accompanied by marked elevations in creatine kinase). Rosuvastatin (Answer D), which is metabolized by cytochrome P450 2C9, would be the best choice. CYP 3A4 has only a minor role in the metabolism of rosuvastatin.

Simvastatin (Answer E), lovastatin (Answer C), and, to a lesser extent, atorvastatin (Answers A and B), are metabolized by cytochrome P450 3A4 (CYP3A4). Concomitant administration of moderate or strong inhibitors of CYP3A4, such as ketoconazole, increases plasma levels of these statins and increases the risk of myopathy.

Case 3

A 55-year-old woman is referred because of elevated triglycerides. She has a history of severe asthma, which has been controlled in the past 3 months by the addition of oral prednisone, 10 mg orally daily. She has hypertension controlled by valsartan. She reports that her diet is balanced and low in saturated fat. She does not smoke cigarettes. She drinks 2 glasses of wine a week.

On physical examination, her temperature is 98.4°F (36.9°C) and blood pressure is 135/80 mm Hg. Her height is 64 in (162.6 cm), and weight is 134 lb (60.8 kg) (BMI = 23.0 kg/m²). Waist circumference is 33 in (83.8 cm).

On review of symptoms, she reports a sore throat and moderate abdominal pain that began 2 days ago.

Laboratory test results (sample drawn while fasting):

Total cholesterol = 195 mg/dL (SI: 5.05 mmol/L)
LDL-C = 80 mg/dL (SI: 2.07 mmol/L)
HDL-C = 55 mg/dL (SI: 1.42 mmol/L)
Triglycerides = 300 mg/dL (SI: 3.39 mmol/L)

Which of the following statements is true?

A. Her degree of triglyceride elevation is associated with increased risk of pancreatitis

B. Her HDL-C is low

C. If she continues to take prednisone, 10 mg daily, the steroid will likely contribute to increased risk of cardiovascular disease

D. She has very high cardiovascular disease risk because of long-term glucocorticoid treatment

E. Statin treatment is recommended to reduce triglycerides

Answer: C) If she continues to take prednisone, 10 mg daily, the steroid will likely contribute to increased risk of cardiovascular disease

This patient may develop very high cardiovascular disease risk if prednisone is continued long-term (Answer C). The patient has been taking prednisone for a short time (3 months) (thus, Answer D is incorrect).

An HDL-C value of 55 mg/dL (1.42 mmol/L) in a woman is in the reference range (thus, Answer B is incorrect).

This patient's triglyceride concentration is 300 mg/dL (3.39 mmol/L). Triglyceride levels of 500 mg/dL or higher (≥5.65 mmol/L) are associated with increased risk of pancreatitis (thus, Answer A is incorrect). Often triglyceride values are greater than 1000 mg/dL (>11.30 mmol/L) in patients who develop pancreatitis.

A triglyceride concentration of 300 mg/dL (3.39 mmol/L) may respond to lifestyle measures (nutrition, physical activity). In this patient, it is also possible that discontinuation of prednisone or reduction in the dosage will reduce triglyceride levels. Statin therapy is not indicated now to treatment hypertriglyceridemia in this patient (thus, Answer E is incorrect).

Key Learning Points

- Before treating hypercholesterolemia, rule out hypothyroidism.

- Reassess the lipid profile after treatment of hypothyroidism and hyperthyroidism when the patient is euthyroid.

- In adults with persistent Cushing syndrome, consider statin therapy regardless of the atherosclerotic cardiovascular disease risk score.

- In adults taking long-term glucocorticoid therapy (at a dosage greater than a replacement dosage), assess the lipid profile and atherosclerotic cardiovascular disease risk score. In patients with a calculated 10-year risk score (using the American College of Cardiology/American Heart Association ASCVD risk calculator) of 5% to 7.5%, consider statin treatment.

References

1. Arnaldi G, Scandali VM, Trementino L, Cardinaletti M, Appolloni G, Boscaro M. Pathophysiology of dyslipidemia in Cushing's syndrome. *Neuroendocrinology.* 2010;92(Suppl 1):86-90. PMID: 20829625

2. Cappola AR, Desai AS, Medici M, et. Al. Thyroid and cardiovascular disease, research agenda for enhancing knowledge, prevention, and treatment. *Circulation.* 2019;139:2892-2909. PMID: 31081673

3. Collet T-H, Bauer DC, Cappola AR, et al; Thyroid Studies Collaboration. Thyroid antibody status, subclinical hypothyroidism, and the risk of coronary heart disease: an individual participant data meta-analysis. *J Clin Endocrinol Metab.* 2014;99(9):3353-3362. PMID: 24915118

4. Dekkers OM, Horvath-Puho E, Jorgensen JO, et al. Multisystem morbidity and mortality in Cushing's syndrome: a cohort study. *J Clin Endocrinol Metab.* 2013;98(6):2277-2284. PMID: 23533241.

5. Duntas LH, Brenta G. A renewed focus on the association between thyroid hormones and lipid metabolism. *Front Endocrinol (Lausanne).* 2018;9:511. PMID: 30233497

6. Filipsson, H, Monson JP, Koltowska-Haggstrom M, Mattsson A, Johannsson G. The impact of glucocorticoid replacement regimes on metabolic outcome and comorbidity in hypopituitary patients. *J Clin Endocrinol Metab.* 2006;91(10):3954-3961. PMID: 16895963

7. Kotwal A, Cortes T, Genere N, et al. Treatment of thyroid dysfunction and serum lipids: a systematic review and meta-analysis. *J Clin Endocrinol Metab.* 2020;105(12):dgaa672. PMID: 32954428

8. Mason RL, Hunt HM, Hurxthal L. Blood cholesterol values in hyperthyroidism and hypothyroidism—their significance. *N Engl J Med.* 1930;203(26):1273-1278.

9. Newman CB, Blaha MJ, Boord JB, et al. Lipid management in patients with endocrine disorders: an Endocrine Society clinical practice guideline. *J Clin Endocrinol Metab.* 2020;105(12):1-70. PMID: 32951056

10. Pearce EN. Update in lipid alterations in subclinical hypothyroidism. *J Clin Endocrinol Metab.* 2012;97(2):326-333. PMID: 22205712

11. Pujades-Rodriguez M, Morgan AW, Cubbon RM, Wu J. Dose-dependent oral glucocorticoid cardiovascular risks in people with immune-mediated inflammatory diseases: a population-based cohort study. *PLoS Med.* 2020;17(12):e1003432. PMID: 33270649

12. Rodondi N, den Elzen WP, Bauer DC, et al; Thyroid Studies Collaboration. Subclinical hypothyroidism and the risk of coronary heart disease and mortality. *JAMA.* 2020;304(12):1365-1374. PMID: 20858880

13. Souverein PC, Berard A, Van Staa TP, et al. Use of oral glucocorticoids and risk of cardiovascular and cerebrovascular disease in a population based case-control study. *Heart.* 2004;90(8):859-865. PMID: 15253953

14. Willard DL, Leung AM, Pearce EN. Thyroid function testing in patients with newly diagnosed hyperlipidemia. *JAMA Intern Med.* 2014;174(2):287-289. PMID: 24217672

Lipid Management in Patients With Diabetes Mellitus

Lisa R. Tannock, MD. Division of Endocrinology, Diabetes, and Metabolism, University of Kentucky, Lexington, KY; Email: Lisa.Tannock@uky.edu

Educational Objectives

After reviewing this chapter, learners should be able to:

- Recommend escalation of lipid-lowering therapy for patients at high risk of atherosclerotic cardiovascular disease (ASCVD).

- Manage ASCVD risk in patients with type 1 or type 2 diabetes mellitus.

- Identify ASCVD risk-enhancing factors.

Significance of the Clinical Problem

It is generally well understood that patients with diabetes are at increased risk for ASCVD. However, the management of these patients remains challenging, in part related to the frequent need for multiple medications to lower risk and the complexity of various guidelines. Furthermore, most clinical research has focused on patients with type 2 diabetes, making it more confusing for providers to know how to address risk in patients with type 1 diabetes. In this session, we will review the escalation of lipid-lowering therapy for patients at high risk, discuss lipid-lowering therapy for patients with type 1 or type 2 diabetes, and use recognition of ASCVD risk-enhancing factors to guide therapeutic decisions.

Diabetes is commonly recognized as an ASCVD risk factor, and most guidelines clearly support use of statin therapy for adults with diabetes, typically for those aged 40 years and older. However, despite the use of statin therapy, many patients remain at high ASCVD risk and additional lipid-lowering therapy should be considered. In addition, there is often confusion about how to assess ASCVD risk in patients younger than 40 years and in those with type 1 diabetes, as well as how to recognize and consider risk-enhancing factors to guide therapeutic decisions. This session will discuss case vignettes that address these areas.

Practice Gaps

- Understanding when to add lipid-lowering therapy in addition to statins.

- Managing ASCVD risk in patients with diabetes younger than 40 years.

- Managing ASCVD risk in patients with type 1 diabetes.

Discussion

Primary Prevention of ASCVD in Patients With Diabetes Aged 40 to 75 Years

It is generally well recognized that adults with diabetes aged 40 to 75 years should be on statin therapy to reduce their ASCVD risk. For primary prevention, use of at least moderate-intensity statin therapy is recommended. However, the guidelines have varied over time about whether to use on-statin LDL-cholesterol levels to guide further decision-making, including consideration of additional lipid-lowering medications. For patients with diabetes who have high ASCVD risk, many guidelines recommend achieving LDL-cholesterol concentrations less than 70 mg/dL

(<1.81 mmol/L) to reduce their risk. While use of high-intensity statin monotherapy will achieve this target in some patients, others may require the use of additional lipid-lowering agents, such as ezetimibe or PCSK9 inhibitors. Currently, use of ezetimibe is recommended as the best second-line therapy due to cost-effectiveness, although PCSK9 inhibitors are more potent.[1]

Secondary Prevention of ASCVD in Patients With Diabetes

For patients with diabetes who have known ASCVD, newer guidelines recommend LDL-cholesterol reduction of at least 50% and an LDL-cholesterol target less than 55 mg/dL (<1.42 mmol/L),[2] which will often require combination lipid-lowering therapy to achieve. The addition of ezetimibe and/or a PCSK9 inhibitor is frequently needed.

Primary Prevention of ASCVD in Patients With Diabetes Younger Than 40 Years

Few trials have addressed the use of statin or other lipid-lowering therapy in patients younger than 40 years. However, efficacy studies clearly demonstrate that regardless of age, statins lower LDL cholesterol. Age is such a contributor to ASCVD risk that for most patients younger than 40, the goal is not reducing their 10-year risk of an ASCVD event but rather reducing their lifetime risk. An analogy with "pack-years of smoking" is appropriate: atherosclerotic risk is related to both degree of LDL-cholesterol elevation (equivalent to number of packs of cigarettes smoked per day) and the duration of LDL-cholesterol elevation (equivalent to duration of smoking). Emerging evidence suggests that statin users have lower lifetime risk of ASCVD events than nonusers and that initiation of statin therapy at younger ages is cost-effective.[3]

ASCVD Prevention in Patients With Type 1 Diabetes

Most randomized controlled trials investigating lipid-lowering therapy have included patients with diabetes, but most of these studies either do not report type 1 vs type 2 diabetes or have not included patients with type 1 diabetes. The Heart Protection Study, a large secondary prevention study, reported outcomes on 615 individuals with type 1 diabetes and 5348 individuals with type 2 diabetes and found a similar, albeit not significant, risk reduction with statin therapy when comparing patients with type 1 and type 2 diabetes.[4] A meta-analysis of studies evaluating patients with diabetes in statin trials found that statin use was effective in LDL-cholesterol lowering and cardiovascular disease outcomes in patients with type 1 diabetes.[5] The Endocrine Society guidelines suggest use of statin therapy in patients who have had type 1 diabetes for more than 20 years, who have type 1 diabetes and microvascular complications, or who are 40 years or older.[6]

Risk-Enhancing Factors

The American Heart Association/American College of Cardiology 2018 lipid guidelines included the recognition of risk-enhancing factors as indications to consider statin therapy. Risk-enhancing factors include family history of premature ASCVD, metabolic syndrome, chronic kidney disease, history of preeclampsia or premature menopause (defined as occurring in women younger than 40 years), chronic inflammatory disorders, and high-risk ethnic groups.[1] The presence of 1 or more of these factors in patients who are calculated to be at intermediate risk can guide towards use of statin therapy. In patients with diabetes (both type 1 and type 2), the Endocrine Society guidelines use presence of chronic kidney disease to suggest statin therapy, regardless of age.[6] Based on evidence that increased weight gain with intensification of insulin therapy identifies patients with type 1 diabetes at increased ASCVD risk, the Endocrine

Society also recommends statin therapy for those patients with obesity and type 1 diabetes.

Clinical Case Vignettes

Case 1

A 58-year-old man was diagnosed with diabetes 4 years ago when he presented to the emergency department with chest pain. He had not seen a physician in many years. At that time, type 2 diabetes was diagnosed with a hemoglobin A_{1c} value of 9.4% (79 mmol/mol). He also had coronary artery disease and underwent 3-vessel coronary artery bypass grafting. He has established care with a primary care physician and was recently referred to endocrinology for further evaluation.

He has never smoked cigarettes. He is unsure whether he has ever had high blood pressure, but he has been on lisinopril since his bypass surgery. He never knew his father, and there is no cardiac disease on his mother's side of the family. He has 2 children who are in their 20s and healthy.

He has been on metformin and premixed insulin for 4 years. His hemoglobin A_{1c} values have ranged from 7.7% to 8.4% (61-68 mmol/mol). His medications include gabapentin; aspirin; atorvastatin, 40 mg daily; metformin; and 70/30 insulin, 24 units twice daily.

He has a sedentary office job and does not exercise. He has no concerns other than mild peripheral neuropathy.

On physical examination, his blood pressure is 126/72 mm Hg and pulse rate is 72 beats/min and regular. His height is 71 in (180.3 cm), and weight is 240 lb (108.9 kg) (BMI = 33.5 kg/m²). Examination findings are unremarkable. Specifically, no xanthomas are noted.

Laboratory test results (sample drawn while fasting and on statin therapy):

    Total cholesterol = 171 mg/dL (<200 mg/dL [optimal]) (SI: 4.43 mmol/L [<5.18 mmol/L])
    HDL cholesterol = 33 mg/dL (>60 mg/dL [optimal]) (SI: 0.85 mmol/L [>1.55 mmol/L])
    LDL cholesterol = 82 mg/dL (<100 mg/dL [optimal]) (SI: 2.12 mmol/L [<2.59 mmol/L])

    Triglycerides = 280 mg/dL (<150 mg/dL [optimal]) (SI: 3.16 mmol/L [<1.70 mmol/L])
    Hemoglobin A_{1c} = 8.2% (4.0%-5.6%) (66 mmol/mol [20-38 mmol/mol])
    TSH = 1.8 mIU/L (0.5-5.0 mIU/L)

Which of the following is the best next step?

A. Add a fibrate

B. Add a PCSK9 inhibitor

C. Add ezetimibe

D. Change from atorvastatin to rosuvastatin, 40 mg daily

E. Increase the atorvastatin dosage to 80 mg daily

Answer: B) Add a PCSK9 inhibitor

This patient has stable ASCVD and is on a high-potency statin (atorvastatin, 40 mg daily). A fasting lipid panel was appropriately obtained, and it documents an LDL-cholesterol value of 82 mg/dL (2.12 mmol/L). Thus, per guidelines, additional lipid-lowering therapy is indicated. Current guidelines recommend an LDL-cholesterol concentration less than 70 mg/dL (<1.81 mmol/L) (American Heart Association/American College of Cardiology guidelines)[1] or even less than 55 mg/dL (<1.42 mmol/L) (American Diabetes Association guidelines).[2] Either maximizing the atorvastatin dosage (Answer E) or changing to rosuvastatin (Answer D) is a reasonable option and should lead to additional LDL-cholesterol lowering but may not achieve the target value less than 70 mg/dL (<1.81 mmol/L), and almost certainly would not achieve the more aggressive goal of less than 55 mg/dL (<1.42 mmol/L). To make the best choice, one must understand the relative impact of different dosages of different statins. Increasing this patient's atorvastatin dosage to 80 mg daily would be expected to modestly lower LDL cholesterol further (up to approximately 5%),[7] but this would not likely achieve the goal of less than 70 mg/dL (<1.81 mmol/L). Similarly, comparing atorvastatin, 40 mg daily, with rosuvastatin, 40 mg daily, one would expect greater LDL-cholesterol lowering with rosuvastatin (50% to 60% lowering with rosuvastatin vs 40% to 50% lowering with atorvastatin, compared with baseline, pre-statin therapy values), but this may not achieve the LDL-cholesterol target less than 70 mg/dL (<1.81 mmol/L) and would be very unlikely to achieve a value less than 55 mg/dL (<1.42 mmol/L). Thus, while both are reasonable options, they are unlikely to be sufficient to achieve targets.

Although this patient has elevated triglycerides, and triglycerides are a risk factor for ASCVD, to date there is little to no evidence to support fibrate plus statin therapy for ASCVD risk reduction.[8] Thus, the addition of a fibrate (Answer A) is not the best next step. In general, the addition of a fibrate to statin therapy should be used when triglycerides are so elevated that there is concern for pancreatitis risk, whereas if the main concern is ASCVD risk, the focus should be on LDL-cholesterol lowering. While not offered as an option in this vignette, there is a randomized controlled trial that did show ASCVD benefit from the addition of icosapent ethyl to statins,[9] and this could be an option for this patient.

Most guidelines recommend the addition of other nonstatin lipid-lowering drugs to achieve an LDL-cholesterol concentration less than 70 mg/dL (<1.81 mmol/L), or even less than 55 mg/dL (<1.42 mmol/L) in patients at high risk. Due to cost-effectiveness analyses, the addition of ezetimibe (Answer C) is preferred over the addition of PCSK9 inhibitors (Answer B). The addition of ezetimibe would be expected to achieve a further 20% to 25% LDL-cholesterol lowering, and thus should be sufficient to achieve target value less than 70 mg/dL (<1.81 mmol/L), but is unlikely to achieve the more aggressive target less than 55 mg/dL (<1.42 mmol/L). However, the addition of a PCSK9 inhibitor would be expected to lead to up to 50% additional LDL-cholesterol lowering, and it would clearly get to either target. Of note, the use of PCSK9 inhibitors is often limited by insurance challenges, and they are also injectable drugs, which can cause some patient resistance to their use.

While not addressed in this case vignette, providers are encouraged to consider other therapies with established ASCVD outcomes benefit in patients such as this. For example, the addition of a GLP-1 receptor analogue or use of a SGLT-2 inhibitor would be expected to both provide further glycemic improvement, as well as reduce his ASCVD risk, and either is a reasonable option to consider in cases similar to this.

Case 2

A 36-year-old woman has recently moved to the area and presents to establish care. Type 1 diabetes was diagnosed at age 8 years after she presented in diabetic ketoacidosis. She had several episodes of diabetic ketoacidosis in her teens and early 20s that she attributes to rebellion and denial about her diabetes diagnosis. She has recently become much more accepting of her diabetes, and her hemoglobin A_{1c} values in the past 5 years have ranged from 6.7% to 7.7% (50-61 mmol/mol). She began using insulin pump therapy 8 years ago, and for the past 3 years she has used closed-loop insulin pump technology. She has never smoked cigarettes. She has been told her blood pressure was too high for her diabetes, but it is now controlled with lisinopril. She has struggled with her weight most of her life and notes that she gained about 20 lb (9.1 kg) when she began using insulin pump therapy, which coincided with her improved glycemic control. She has no family history of premature cardiovascular disease, although both of her grandfathers died of cardiac issues in their early 70s.

Her only medications are insulin via pump therapy and lisinopril.

On physical examination, her blood pressure is 126/72 mm Hg. Her height is 66 in (167.6 cm), and weight is 198 lb (89.8 kg) (BMI = 32.0 kg/m²). Examination findings are normal.

Laboratory test results (sample drawn while fasting):

Total cholesterol = 170 mg/dL (<200 mg/dL [optimal]) (SI: 4.40 mmol/L [<5.18 mmol/L])
HDL cholesterol = 52 mg/dL (>60 mg/dL [optimal]) (SI: 1.35 mmol/L [>1.55 mmol/L])
LDL cholesterol = 82 mg/dL (<100 mg/dL [optimal]) (SI: 2.12 mmol/L [<2.59 mmol/L])
Triglycerides = 180 mg/dL (<150 mg/dL [optimal]) (SI: 2.03 mmol/L [<1.70 mmol/L])

Hemoglobin A_{1c} = 6.8% (4.0%-5.6%) (51 mmol/mol [20-38 mmol/mol])

TSH = 1.2 mIU/L (0.5-5.0 mIU/L)

Estimated glomerular filtration rate = 57 mL/min per 1.73 m² (>60 mL/min per 1.73 m²)

Which of the following is the best next step?

A. Counsel on reducing dietary fat intake

B. Discuss fibrate therapy now

C. Discuss statin therapy now

D. Recommend a statin starting at age 40 years

E. Recommend both a statin and an oral contraceptive

Answer: C) Discuss statin therapy now

The main consideration in this vignette is the patient's ASCVD risk given her young age but long history of diabetes and presence of some early diabetes-related complications. The ASCVD risk calculator cannot estimate her 10-year ASCVD risk because of her age, but her lifetime ASCVD risk is 50%. Based on her age, many physicians would not recommend lipid-lowering therapy now, and most guidelines would only recommend statin therapy if she had additional (classic) ASCVD risk factors, such as hypertension, cigarette smoking, family history, etc. However, emerging evidence suggests that duration of diabetes, presence of chronic kidney disease, and excessive weight gain with intensive insulin therapy all indicate higher ASCVD risk,[2,10,11] and statin therapy has been shown to reduce this risk. Epidemiologic studies demonstrate that individuals with type 1 diabetes have a lower life expectancy than matched control participants without diabetes, especially for women, and which correlates to age at diagnosis of type 1 diabetes.[10] This patient was diagnosed prior to age 10, which was the group with the largest impact of life years lost. In follow-up from the DCCT/EDIC study, those who gained the most weight with intensification of insulin therapy had a higher risk for cardiovascular disease events than those who gained minimal weight.[11] Finally, the presence of microvascular complications of diabetes, including retinopathy or chronic kidney disease, appears to identify individuals at higher risk and thus those for whom statin therapy should be considered. The Swedish national registry compared survival in patients with type 1 diabetes who used lipid-lowering therapy (97% of whom used statins) with survival in those who did not use lipid-lowering therapy and found improved survival in statin users.[12] Thus, this patient is likely at increased risk due to these risk-enhancing factors, and statin therapy should be discussed (Answer C). Deferring statin therapy until she is 40 (Answer D) is acceptable, but it denies her the benefit of early intervention. While most randomized controlled ASCVD trials have only enrolled older adults with high-risk conditions, emerging evidence suggests that early intervention with lipid-lowering therapy provides greater benefit, at minimal risk of harm and very low cost.

A common consideration for women in this age group is the risk of pregnancy. The US FDA initially designated statins as pregnancy category X, meaning contraindicated. However, this label was removed in 2021. There is relatively little literature to guide use of statins in pregnancy. Animal studies demonstrate teratogenic effects, but often at much higher dosages than those used in humans. An uncontrolled case series published in 2004 reported 31 adverse outcomes in 214 pregnancies with verified statin exposure.[13] There is an accumulating literature based on case cohort series demonstrating the relative safety of statins in pregnancy.[14,15] At this point, there is not enough evidence to recommend the use of statins in pregnancy, but perhaps less fear when an unplanned pregnancy occurs in a statin user, and current FDA guidance describes that statins are safe to use in women who are not pregnant but may become pregnant. This patient is already on lisinopril, an agent clearly contraindicated in pregnancy. Thus, reviewing with her that both lisinopril and the statin should be discontinued if she plans a pregnancy is reasonable, but a valuable therapy should not be denied simply because she is of reproductive age. There is no need to mandate an oral contraceptive (Answer E) in order to prescribe a statin; the choice of contraceptive agent should be a separate discussion with this patient.

While her triglycerides are modestly elevated, there is little to no evidence that fibrate therapy (Answer B) would reduce her ASCVD risk, whereas statin therapy would. Certainly, counseling her on a healthy lifestyle, including decreased dietary fat consumption (Answer A) is appropriate but misses the point that a statin now could help reduce her lifetime risk.

Key Learning Points

- For patients with diabetes and established ASCVD, consider combination lipid-lowering therapy to target an LDL-cholesterol concentration less than 70 mg/dL (<1.81 mmol/L) or even less than 55 mg/dL (<1.42 mmol/L).

- When escalating lipid-lowering therapy, start with the highest dosage tolerated on a high-intensity statin, then add ezetimibe and/or a PCSK9 inhibitor to achieve the LDL-cholesterol target.

- For patients with type 1 diabetes, consider their age, duration of diabetes, and presence of risk-enhancing factors to guide initiation of statin therapy.

- For women of reproductive age, do not withhold lipid-lowering therapy simply based on pregnancy potential.

References

1. Grundy SM, Stone NJ, Bailey AL, et al. 2018 AHA/ACC/AACVPR/AAPA/ABC/ACPM/ADA/AGS/APhA/ASPC/NLA/PCNA guideline on the management of blood cholesterol: a report of the American College of Cardiology/American Heart Association Task Force on Clinical Practice Guidelines. *J Am Coll Cardiol.* 2019;73(24):e285-e350. PMID: 30423393

2. ElSayed NA, Aleppo G, Aroda VR, et al; American Diabetes Association. 10. Cardiovascular disease and risk management: *standards of care in diabetes—2023. Diabetes Care.* 2023;46(Suppl 1):S158-S190. PMID: 36507632

3. Kohli-Lynch CN, Bellows BK, Zhang Y, et al. Cost-effectiveness of lipid-lowering treatments in young Adults. *J Am Coll Cardiol.* 2021;78(20):1954-1964. PMID: 34763772

4. Collins R, Armitage J, Parish S, Sleigh P, Peto R; Heart Protection Study Collaborative Group. 2MRC/BHF Heart Protection Study of cholesterol-lowering with simvastatin in 5963 people with diabetes: a randomised placebo-controlled trial. *Lancet.* 2003;361(9374):2005-2016. PMID: 12814710

5. Cholesterol Treatment Trialists' (CTT) Collaborators; Kearney PM, Blackwell L, Collins R, et al. Efficacy of cholesterol-lowering therapy in 18,686 people with diabetes in 14 randomised trials of statins: a meta-analysis. *Lancet.* 2008;371(9607):117-125. PMID: 18191683

6. Newman CB, Blaha MJ, Boord JB, et al. Lipid management in patients with endocrine disorders: an Endocrine Society clinical practice guideline. *J Clin Endocrinol Metab.* 2020;105(12):dgaa674. PMID: 32951056

7. Jones P, Kafonek S, Laurora I, Hunninghake D. Comparative dose efficacy study of atorvastatin versus simvastatin, pravastatin, lovastatin, and fluvastatin in patients with hypercholesterolemia (the CURVES study). *Am J Cardiol.* 1998 Mar 1;81(5):582-7. PMID: 9514454

8. ACCORD Study Group; Ginsberg HN, Elam MB, Lovato LC, et al. Effects of combination lipid therapy in type 2 diabetes mellitus. *N Engl J Med.* 2010;362(17):1563-1574. PMID: 20228404

9. Bhatt DL, Steg PG, Miller M, et al; REDUCE-IT Investigators. Cardiovascular risk reduction with icosapent ethyl for hypertriglyceridemia. *N Engl J Med.* 2019;380(1):11-22. PMID: 30415628

10. Rawshani A, Sattar N, Franzén S, et al. Excess mortality and cardiovascular disease in young adults with type 1 diabetes in relation to age at onset: a nationwide, register-based cohort study. *Lancet.* 2018;392(10146):477-486. PMID: 30129464

11. Purnell JQ, Braffett BH, Zinman B, et al; DCCT/EDIC Research Group. Impact of excessive weight gain on cardiovascular outcomes in type 1 diabetes: results from the Diabetes Control and Complications Trial/Epidemiology of Diabetes Interventions and Complications (DCCT/EDIC) Study. *Diabetes Care.* 2017;40(12):1756-1762. PMID: 29138273

12. Hero C, Rawshani A, Svensson AM, et al. Association between use of lipid-lowering therapy and cardiovascular diseases and death in individuals with type 1 diabetes. *Diabetes Care.* 2016;39(6):996-1003. PMID: 27208327

13. Edison RJ, Muenke M. Mechanistic and epidemiologic considerations in the evaluation of adverse birth outcomes following gestational exposure to statins. *Am J Med Genet A.* 2004;131(3):287-298. PMID: 15546153

14. Bateman BT, Hernandez-Diaz S, Fischer MA, et al. Statins and congenital malformations: cohort study. *BMJ.* 2015;350:h1035. PMID: 25784688

15. Chang J-C, Chen Y-J, Chen I-C, Lin W-S, Chen Y-M, Lin C-H. Perinatal outcomes after statin exposure during pregnancy. *JAMA Netw Open.* 2021;4(12):e2141321. PMID: 34967881

Evidence-Based, Practical Approach to Primary Aldosteronism

Jun Yang, MBBS, PhD. Hudson Institute of Medical Research, Clayton, Victoria, Australia; Email: Jun.yang@hudson.org.au

Educational Objectives

After reviewing this chapter, learners should be able to:

- Explain the importance of a timely diagnosis of primary aldosteronism (PA).

- Identify factors that can cause false-positive or false-negative screening tests for PA.

- Explain the tests required to diagnose PA and its subtypes.

- Treat PA to optimize both biochemical and clinical outcomes.

Significance of the Clinical Problem

PA, characterized by autonomous aldosterone production from the adrenal glands, is a common but underdiagnosed form of secondary hypertension. An accurate diagnosis is important because PA is associated with an increased risk of heart disease, stroke, and atrial fibrillation compared with risks in patients with blood pressure–matched essential hypertension. The clinical features of PA can vary from asymptomatic hypertension to resistant hypertension, with hypokalemia and adrenal adenomas being present in some patients. It is often impossible to distinguish PA from essential hypertension without a blood test for case detection. The recommended test is the aldosterone-to-renin ratio (ARR),

which is calculated from the plasma aldosterone concentration (PAC) and plasma renin activity (PRA) or renin concentration (DRC) (typically low or suppressed). An ARR that is elevated above a laboratory-specific threshold represents a positive screening test that is followed by confirmatory testing, and then subtyping to determine whether the aldosterone excess is from one adrenal gland (unilateral disease) or both (bilateral disease). Unilateral disease can be cured with laparoscopic adrenalectomy, while bilateral disease can be effectively treated with mineralocorticoid receptor antagonists such as spironolactone to achieve normalization of serum potassium (if previously low), renin, and blood pressure.

PA is the most common endocrine cause of hypertension, yet it is widely underdiagnosed in both primary and tertiary care settings.[1] When first described in 1955 by Jerome W. Conn, features such as resistant hypertension and hypokalemia were considered hallmarks of the condition. However, more recent data have demonstrated that PA may be detected in patients with any degree of hypertension and most have a normal serum potassium concentration.[2] It is estimated that 4% to 14% of treatment-naïve hypertensive patients in primary care and up to 30% of those with resistant hypertension may have this condition.[3-6]

Early detection is crucial, as undiagnosed and untreated primary aldosteronism is associated with increased cardiovascular, renal, and metabolic morbidity and mortality related specifically to the effect of aldosterone excess on the mineralocorticoid receptor in a range of target tissues.[7] Furthermore, treatment outcomes are better in younger patients with a shorter duration of disease. The early detection of PA crucially depends on the measurement of aldosterone and renin. However, studies around the world have demonstrated that hypertensive patients are rarely tested for primary aldosteronism, be it in primary care or tertiary care.[8-10]

Importantly, PA can be effectively treated with mineralocorticoid receptor antagonists to specifically block the detrimental effects of aldosterone excess. Furthermore, unilateral aldosterone-producing adrenal adenomas (APAs) can be resected, which may lead to a surgical cure. Targeted treatment can mitigate many of the cardiovascular complications associated with primary aldosteronism, especially if instituted early in the disease course.[11] Given that 1.2 billion people are currently living with hypertension, a conservative prevalence estimate of 5% suggests that 60 million have PA but few are actually aware of their diagnosis. Missed or belated diagnoses represent missed opportunities to improve patient outcomes and reduce the burden of disease associated with uncontrolled hypertension and aldosterone-mediated tissue injury.

Practice Gaps

- Clinicians do not routinely test for PA in patients with hypertension, even in those with high-risk features such as hypokalemia or resistant hypertension.

- PAC and DRC, which are the screening tests for PA, are not accurately interpreted in patients who take interfering medications such as diuretics, ACE inhibitors, angiotensin II receptor blockers, or oral contraceptive pills.

- Decisions regarding surgery or medical treatment are made purely on the basis of adrenal imaging even though adrenal vein sampling (AVS) is the current gold standard for distinguishing between unilateral and bilateral subtypes of PA.

- Targeted medical treatment (eg, spironolactone) for PA should be titrated to achieve an unsuppressed PRA or DRC; unsuppressed renin indicates adequate dosage.

Discussion

Primary Aldosteronism is Common but Underdiagnosed

PA is common, although prevalence estimates are variable. A systematic review of 39 studies in hypertensive adults conducted before 2012 reported prevalence ranging between 3.2% and 12.7% in primary care settings and between 1% and 29.8% in hypertension referral centers.[3] More recent prevalence studies in primary care settings in Italy, China, and Australia described similar figures of 4% to 14%.[4-6] Despite a high prevalence documented in research studies, PA is rarely diagnosed in the real world due to a lack of screening. In a population-based cohort study from Alberta, Canada, only 0.7% of 1.1 million adults with hypertension were screened for PA.[8] Even among people with clinical characteristics strongly suggestive of PA, such as those with hypertension and hypokalemia, or resistant hypertension, less than 2% were screened.[9,10,12]

Screening for Primary Aldosteronism Requires Careful Interpretation of Aldosterone and Renin

The Endocrine Society PA management guidelines recommend case detection for PA using the ARR in the following groups[13]:

- Sustained blood pressure >150/100 mm Hg on 3 measurements obtained on different days, or drug-resistant hypertension (blood pressure >140/90 mm Hg despite treatment with 3 antihypertensive medications), or controlled hypertension (blood pressure <140/90 mm Hg) on 4 or more antihypertensive medications

- Hypertension and spontaneous or diuretic-induced hypokalemia

- Hypertension with adrenal incidentaloma

- Hypertension and obstructive sleep apnea

- Hypertension and a family history of early-onset hypertension or cerebrovascular accident at a young age (<40 years)

- All hypertensive first-degree relatives of patients with PA

There is a push for PA testing to be done in all hypertensive patients, preferably from the onset of hypertension prior to the initiation of antihypertensive medications. This approach should ensure the early detection of disease, prevention of cumulative end-organ damage, and reduced risk of missing the diagnosis. However, this approach has not yet been adopted by current hypertension guidelines.

To screen for PA, the ARR is the recommended test[13] on the basis that isolated measurements of either PAC, DRC, or PRA show broad overlap between normal patients and those with PA. Despite its routine use, there are laboratory-based analytical issues with the measurement of ARR. In particular, both DRC and PRA may be subject to cryoactivation if the sample is stored on ice, which may lead to a false-negative ARR. Hence, appropriate sample handling and processing are important for an accurate result.

The accurate interpretation of the ARR also requires assessment of antihypertensive medications. Most commonly prescribed antihypertensive agents, including diuretics, ACE inhibitors, angiotensin II receptor blockers, mineralocorticoid receptor antagonists, and dihydropyridine calcium-channel blockers, can all increase renin or decrease aldosterone and cause a false-negative ARR. β-Adrenergic blockers can decrease renin and cause a false-positive ARR. If safe to do so, these medications should be switched to noninterfering agents such as verapamil, prazosin, moxonidine, and/or hydralazine for blood pressure control during the diagnostic process. If medication switching is not safe, then the results should be interpreted accordingly. A low or suppressed renin, even with a normal ARR, should be considered abnormal in the setting of diuretic, angiotensin II receptor blocker, or ACE inhibitor use. In women who take the oral contraceptive pill, another form of contraception should be used during testing, especially if the baseline ARR is positive, as the pill can falsely increase the ARR.

The recommended ARR thresholds vary among laboratories, depending on their analytical methods, and are associated with different test sensitivity and specificity.[14] In the absence of an international consensus, it is most practical to use the local threshold.

Confirming the Diagnosis With Dynamic Testing

Due to the dynamic nature of aldosterone and renin, positive screening tests are often followed by confirmatory testing designed to suppress aldosterone production. Confirmatory testing is not required in patients with florid PA, as reflected by a high PAC (>20 ng/dL [>550 pmol/L]), suppressed renin (PRA <1 ng/mL per h or DRC <2.5 mU/L), and hypokalemia.

Available confirmatory tests include salt-loading tests (oral or intravenous), captopril-challenge test, and fludrocortisone-suppression test. Each has advantages and disadvantages, and the choice is typically based on local resources and center experience. In the last 3 years, the seated saline-suppression test has surpassed the traditional recumbent saline-suppression test as the favored confirmatory test, with superior sensitivity and increased convenience for the patient.[15] PAC greater than 163 pmol/L (measured by LC/MS-MS) or 170 pmol/L (measured by immunoassay) following 2 L saline infusion over 4 hours is considered diagnostic of PA.[16] Oral salt loading conducted at home for 3 consecutive days averts the cost of diagnostic centers, but poses a high risk to patients with severe hypertension and/or cardiovascular comorbidities. Urinary aldosterone excretion greater than 10 to 12 mcg/24 h (27-33 nmol/d) along with urinary sodium greater than 180 to 200 mmol/d is diagnostic of PA.

Subtyping for Optimal Treatment

PA is a heterogeneous collection of conditions, which most commonly include unilateral APA and bilateral adrenal hyperplasia. Rarely, PA may be caused by aldosterone-producing adrenocortical carcinoma (<1%). The importance of accurate subtyping lies in the possibility of surgical cure for unilateral types of PA, whereas bilateral PA requires lifelong treatment with mineralocorticoid antagonists. AVS is the current gold standard for subtyping PA, as adrenal imaging with CT or MRI may miss small APAs or misdiagnose nonfunctioning adrenal adenomas. Even in patients younger than 40 years, a unilateral adrenal adenoma may not represent an APA.[17] Measurement of the cortisol concentration in both adrenal veins compared with the concentration in the peripheral vein enables assessment of adrenal vein cannulation success, while comparison of the aldosterone-to-cortisol ratio in the 2 adrenal veins determines lateralization. However, AVS may not always be available or successful. Other tools for subtyping include ^{11}C-metomidate PET/CT and predictive algorithms based on clinical, biochemical, and radiologic characteristics.[18]

PA occurs as a sporadic form in most cases, but it is familial in approximately 5% of patients. Young patients with PA or those with a family history of hypertension and early stroke should be tested for familial forms of hyperaldosteronism. In familial hyperaldosteronism type 1, also known as glucocorticoid-remediable aldosteronism, the diagnosis can be reliably made by genetic testing for a hybrid gene variant composed of 11β-hydroxylase gene regulatory sequences and aldosterone synthase gene coding sequences. Other genetic forms can be screened for by dedicated next-generation sequencing panels.[19]

Targeted Treatment of PA

Laparoscopic adrenalectomy is indicated for unilateral APA and leads to biochemical cure in 83% to 100% of patients. Mineralocorticoid receptor antagonist therapy, most commonly with spironolactone, is indicated for patients with bilateral adrenal disease, patients who are not surgical candidates, or those who prefer medical treatment. Adverse effects of spironolactone, especially at dosages greater than 50 mg daily, include gynecomastia, mastodynia, reduced libido, and menstrual disturbances. Eplerenone is an alternative mineralocorticoid receptor antagonist if spironolactone is poorly tolerated, but it is less potent and has a short half-life, thus requiring twice-daily dosing. Amiloride (an epithelial sodium channel blocker) can also lower blood pressure and normalize plasma potassium but may be less accessible than mineralocorticoid receptor antagonists. The medications should be up-titrated to normalize not just serum potassium and blood pressure, but also renin concentration or renin activity. The reduction in cardiovascular risk is only observed in patients whose renin is unsuppressed (PRA >1 ng/mL per h) with adequate mineralocorticoid receptor antagonist dosing.[20]

A therapeutic trial of a mineralocorticoid receptor antagonist may be beneficial if: (1) the patient has a positive ARR but access to a specialist for confirmatory testing is not possible or (2) the patient has a negative ARR, or does not have access to an ARR test, but has moderate to severe or resistant hypertension.

Clinical Case Vignettes

Case 1

A 48-year-old man has a blood pressure of 156/98 mm Hg on routine testing. Hypertension is confirmed on 24-hour blood pressure monitoring. He has no other cardiovascular risk factors. Perindopril is initiated with the later addition of amlodipine; however, his blood pressure remains elevated at greater than 140/90 mm Hg despite maximal up-titration of both medications. At this stage, his primary care physician orders assessment of ARR. His PAC is 35 ng/dL (968 pmol/L), while his DRC is 35 mU/L with a normal ARR of 27 (<70).

Which of the following is the best next step?

A. Add a third antihypertensive medication

B. Advise salt reduction

C. Recheck PAC and DRC after 1 week

D. Switch perindopril and amlodipine to verapamil and prazosin and recheck PAC and DRC after 4 weeks

E. Switch perindopril and amlodipine to verapamil and prazosin and recheck PAC and DRC after 1 week

Answer: D) Switch perindopril and amlodipine to verapamil and prazosin and recheck PAC and DRC after 4 weeks

Commonly prescribed antihypertensive medications can affect aldosterone and renin concentrations. This patient is taking 2 medications which can increase renin, decrease aldosterone, and cause a falsely low ARR. In particular, ACE inhibitors, angiotensin II receptor blockers, and diuretics can increase the renin concentration to well above the normal range. Hence, having a normal DRC of 35 mU/L while on interfering medications may not be an accurate result. It takes more than 2 weeks for the effect to wash out, so the best course of action is to change the perindopril and amlodipine to alternative noninterfering agents such as verapamil and prazosin and recheck PAC and DRC after 4 weeks (Answer D).

If investigations have already been completed, then adding a third agent for blood pressure control (Answer A) would be appropriate, but it is too early to add one at this stage.

Salt reduction (Answer B) is always helpful for blood pressure control, but it can cause a false-negative screening result. Hence, it would be best to save dietary changes to after the investigations are completed.

Rechecking PAC and DRC in 1 week (Answer C) would be reasonable if the patient were not taking interfering medications.

Switching medications and rechecking within 1 week (Answer E) does not allow enough time to washout the effects of perindopril and amlodipine.

The patient's DRC dropped to 3.1 mU/L following the medication switch, and the ARR increased to 318. The patient was eventually found to have a unilateral APA and was cured surgically.

Case 2

A 33-year-old woman was found to have a blood pressure of 160/100 mm Hg on routine examination at age 30 years. She was otherwise well, with a BMI of 20 kg/m². On amlodipine, 10 mg daily, her average blood pressure has been 130/86 mm Hg. Following a switch to verapamil 180 mg daily, she underwent full workup for secondary hypertension. Laboratories findings were PAC of 12.4 ng/dL (344 pmol/L), DRC of 2 mU/L, and an elevated ARR of 172 (<70). Her potassium concentration has always been normal (>4 mmol/L) with normal kidney function. A saline-suppression test (in the supine position) confirmed the diagnosis of PA with a post-saline PAC of 6.5 ng/dL (179 pmol/L), while adrenal CT demonstrated a 13-mm, lipid-rich, left-sided adrenal adenoma. Result from a 1-mg dexamethasone-suppression test was normal.

Which of the following is the best step in her management?

A. Refer to an endocrine surgeon for left adrenalectomy

B. Repeat adrenal imaging with MRI

C. Refer for AVS

D. Repeat the saline-suppression test in a seated position

E. Monitor her condition given her well-controlled blood pressure

Answer: C) Refer for AVS

For young people with hyperaldosteronism and a unilateral adrenal adenoma, some centers have suggested that it is appropriate to proceed directly to surgery without AVS. However, more recent literature suggests that nonfunctioning adrenal adenomas are just as common in young people as they are in elderly people.[21] Even people younger than 40 years may have bilateral disease despite the presence of a unilateral adenoma, especially if they do not present with florid hyperaldosteronism (ie, suppressed DRC, high PAC, and hypokalemia). Hence, to enhance the certainty of lateralization, AVS is recommended (Answer C).

Referral to an endocrine surgeon for removal of the left adrenal adenoma (Answer A) may lead to unnecessary surgery.

An adrenal-protocol, contrast-enhanced CT is the best way to image the adrenal gland, although MRI (Answer B) can be used if there are contraindications to CT.

Given the abnormal supine saline-suppression test, it is not necessary to repeat the confirmatory test (Answer D).

It is also not appropriate to just observe (Answer E) given her young age and significant hypertension.

Case 2 (continued)

AVS successfully demonstrates lateralization of aldosterone excess to the right side prior to stimulation with cosyntropin, with an aldosterone-to-cortisol ratio of 15 in the right adrenal vein, 0.7 in the left adrenal vein, and 0.4 in the peripheral vein. There is complete loss of lateralization after cosyntropin administration, with an aldosterone-to-cortisol ratio of 2.5 in the right, 2.3 in the left, and 0.8 in the periphery.

Which of the following is the best step now?

A. Refer to an endocrine surgeon for right adrenalectomy

B. Prescribe spironolactone for medical treatment, if not planning pregnancy

C. Monitor her condition

D. Repeat AVS

Answer: B) Prescribe spironolactone for medical treatment, if not planning pregnancy

The use of cosyntropin-stimulation during AVS has led to increased rates of successful adrenal vein cannulation but also decreased lateralization indices. Published data demonstrate that the complete loss

of lateralization after cosyntropin is associated with lack of surgical cure.[22] Hence, commencing treatment with a common mineralocorticoid receptor antagonist, spironolactone, is the most appropriate course of action, assuming the patient is not planning pregnancy (Answer B), rather than referring for unilateral adrenalectomy (Answer A).

Monitoring (Answer C) is not sufficient given the diagnosis of PA.

AVS does not need to be repeated (Answer D) if successful the first time.

The patient is now taking spironolactone, 37.5 mg daily, as monotherapy and has achieved normal blood pressure and DRC.

Case 3

A 69-year-old man has a blood pressure of 167/102 mm Hg despite dual therapy with telmisartan, 80 mg daily, and amlodipine, 10 mg daily. His antihypertensive medications are changed to verapamil, 180 mg daily, and moxonidine, 400 mcg every night, to facilitate screening for PA. An elevated ARR (PAC = 15.5 ng/dL [560 pmol/L]; DRC = 2 mU/L) is documented and PA is diagnosed by the seated saline-suppression test. Serum potassium is consistently within the normal range. Adrenal CT reveals bilateral lipid-rich adrenal nodules, while AVS demonstrates bilateral aldosterone secretion. Spironolactone, 25 mg daily, is added to his treatment regimen. Eight weeks later, his blood pressure is 143/95 mm Hg, serum potassium is 4.8 mmol/L, and DRC is 4 mU/L.

Which of the following is the best adjustment to his antihypertensive medications?

A. Increase spironolactone dosage to 37.5 mg daily to achieve a higher DRC

B. Increase verapamil dosage to 180 mg twice daily to further reduce blood pressure

C. Change verapamil and moxonidine back to telmisartan and amlodipine

D. Continue to monitor without changing any medications or dosages

E. Change spironolactone to eplerenone

Answer: A) Increase spironolactone dosage to 37.5 mg daily to achieve a higher DRC

A retrospective study of patients with PA who were treated with mineralocorticoid receptor antagonists found that cardiovascular risk reduction only occurred in patients who took sufficient doses to unsuppress their PRA more than 1 ng/mL per h. Hence, in the absence of complete normalization of renin, the dose of spironolactone should be up-titrated until renin is fully unsuppressed (Answer A). Once the dose of spironolactone is optimized, other medications can then be changed to achieve blood pressure control (Answers B and C).

Monitoring without any change (Answer D) is less appropriate than Answer A given the residual poor blood pressure control.

It is unnecessary to change from spironolactone in the absence of adverse effects (Answer E).

Case 3 (continued)

Four months after the dosage adjustment, the patient's blood pressure decreased to 125/68 mm Hg with a serum potassium concentration of 4.9 mmol/L and DRC of 25 mU/L (within normal range). He feels well and has no adverse effects on spironolactone, 37.5 mg daily.

Which of the following is the best step regarding his antihypertensive medications?

A. Increase spironolactone dosage to achieve a higher DRC

B. Increase verapamil dosage to 180 mg twice daily to further reduce blood pressure

C. Gradually wean off verapamil and/or moxonidine depending on blood pressure

D. Continue to monitor without changing any medications or dosages

E. Change spironolactone to eplerenone

Answer: C) Gradually wean off verapamil and/or moxonidine depending on blood pressure

Now that the optimal dosage of spironolactone has been reached on the basis of a normal DRC and blood pressure is well controlled, it is reasonable to gradually decrease the dosages of other antihypertensive medications (Answer C). Monotherapy may or may not be sufficient to maintain normal blood pressure and regular blood pressure monitoring is required while weaning other medications. If additional blood pressure control is needed after stopping verapamil and moxonidine, it may be best to add a more conventional antihypertensive agent such as an ACE inhibitor or angiotensin II receptor blocker.

It is not necessary to aim for a high DRC (Answer A) or to reduce blood pressure further (Answer B) if already within target.

Monitoring without changing medications (Answer D) may result in unnecessary pill burden, and there is no need to change to eplerenone (Answer E) if spironolactone is well tolerated.

Key Learning Points

- PA, characterized by autonomous aldosterone secretion from the adrenal glands, is a common but underdiagnosed form of secondary hypertension.

- An accurate diagnosis is important because PA is associated with increased risk of heart disease, stroke, and atrial fibrillation compared with risk associated with blood pressure–matched essential hypertension.

- It is often impossible to distinguish PA from essential hypertension without measuring PAC and DRC.

- An ARR that is elevated above a laboratory-specific threshold represents a positive screening result, which is followed by confirmatory testing and then subtyping using AVS to determine if the aldosterone excess is from 1 adrenal gland (unilateral disease) or both (bilateral disease).

- Unilateral disease can be cured with laparoscopic adrenalectomy, while bilateral disease can be effectively treated with mineralocorticoid receptor antagonists such as spironolactone to achieve normalization of serum potassium (if previously low), renin (important to check), and blood pressure.

References

1. Libianto R, Fuller PJ, Young MJ, Yang J. Primary aldosteronism is a public health issue: challenges and opportunities. *J Hum Hypertens*. 2020;34(7):478-486. PMID: 32341439

2. Turcu AF, Yang J, Vaidya A. Primary aldosteronism - a multidimensional syndrome. *Nat Rev Endocrinol*. 2022;18(11):665-682. PMID: 36045149

3. Käyser SC, Dekkers T, Groenewoud HJ, et al. Study heterogeneity and estimation of prevalence of primary aldosteronism: a systematic review and meta-regression analysis. *J Clin Endocrinol Metab*. 101(7):2826-2835. PMID: 27172433

4. Monticone S, Burrello J, Tizzani D, et al. Prevalence and clinical manifestations of primary aldosteronism encountered in primary care practice. *J Am Coll Cardiol*. 2017;69(14):1811-1820. PMID: 28385310

5. Xu Z, Yang J, Hu J, et al. Primary aldosteronism in patients in China with recently detected hypertension. *J Am Coll Cardiol*. 2020;75(16):1913-1922. PMID: 32327102

6. Libianto R, Russell GM, Stowasser M, et al. Detecting primary aldosteronism in Australian primary care: a prospective study. *Med J Aust*. 2022;216(8):408-412. PMID: 35218017

7. Monticone S, D'Ascenzo F, Moretti C, et al. Cardiovascular events and target organ damage in primary aldosteronism compared with essential hypertension: a systematic review and meta-analysis. *Lancet Diabetes Endocrinol*. 2018;6(1):41-50. PMID: 29129575

8. Liu Y-Y, King J, Kline GA, et al. Outcomes of a specialized clinic on rates of investigation and treatment of primary aldosteronism. *JAMA Surg*. 2021;156(6):541-549. PMID: 33787826

9. Cohen JB, Cohen DL, Herman DS, Leppert JT, Byrd JB, Bhalla V. Testing for primary aldosteronism and mineralocorticoid receptor antagonist use among U.S. Veterans: a retrospective cohort study. *Ann Intern Med*. 2021;174(3):289-297. PMID: 33370170

10. Hundemer GL, Imsirovic H, Vaidya A, et al. Screening rates for primary aldosteronism among individuals with hypertension plus hypokalemia: a population-based retrospective cohort study. *Hypertension*. 2022;79(1):178-186. PMID: 34657442

11. Lin X, Ullah MHE, Wu X, et al. Cerebro-cardiovascular risk, target organ damage, and treatment outcomes in primary aldosteronism. *Front Cardiovasc Med*. 2021;8:798364. PMID: 35187110

12. Jaffe G, Gray Z, Krishnan G, et al. Screening rates for primary aldosteronism in resistant hypertension. *Hypertension*. 2020;75(3):650-659. PMID: 32008436

13. Funder JW, Carey RM, Mantero F, et al. The management of primary aldosteronism: case detection, diagnosis, and treatment: an Endocrine Society clinical practice guideline. *J Clin Endocrinol Metab*. 2016;101(5):1889-1916. PMID: 26934393

14. Ariens J, Horvath AR, Yang J, Choy KW. Performance of the aldosterone-to-renin ratio as a screening test for primary aldosteronism in primary care. *Endocrine*. 2022;77(1):11-20. PMID: 35622194

15. Stowasser M, Ahmed AH, Cowley D, et al. Comparison of seated with recumbent saline suppression testing for the diagnosis of primary aldosteronism. *J Clin Endocrinol Metab*. 2018;103(11):4113-4124. PMID: 30239841

16. Thuzar M, Young K, Ahmed AH, et al. Diagnosis of primary aldosteronism by seated saline suppression test-variability between immunoassay and HPLC-MS/MS. *J Clin Endocrinol Metab*. 2020;105(3):dgz150. PMID: 31676899

17. Gkaniatsa E, Sakinis A, Palmér M, Muth A, Trimpou P, Ragnarsson O. Adrenal venous sampling in young patients with primary aldosteronism. Extravagance or irreplaceable? *J Clin Endocrinol Metab*. 2021;106(5):e2087-e2095. PMID: 33507307

18. Wu X, Senanayake R, Goodchild E, et al. [^{11}C]metomidate PET-CT versus adrenal vein sampling for diagnosing surgically curable primary aldosteronism: a prospective, within-patient trial. *Nat Med*. 2023;29(1):190-202. PMID: 36646800

19. Fernandes-Rosa FL, Boulkroun S, Fedlaoui B, et al. New advances in endocrine hypertension: from genes to biomarkers. *Kidney Int*. 2023;103(3):485-500. PMID: 36646167

20. Hundemer GL, Curhan GC, Yozamp N, Wang M, Vaidya A. Cardiometabolic outcomes and mortality in medically treated primary aldosteronism: a retrospective cohort study. *Lancet Diabetes Endocrinol*. 2018;6(1):51-59. PMID: 29129576

21. Jing Y, Hu J, Luo R, et al. Prevalence and characteristics of adrenal tumors in an unselected screening population: a cross-sectional study. *Ann Intern Med*. 2022;175(10):1383-1391. PMID: 36095315

22. Chee NYN, Abdul-Wahab A, Libianto R, et al. Utility of adrenocorticotropic hormone in adrenal vein sampling despite the occurrence of discordant lateralization. *Clin Endocrinol (Oxf)*. 2020;93(4):394-403. PMID: 32403203

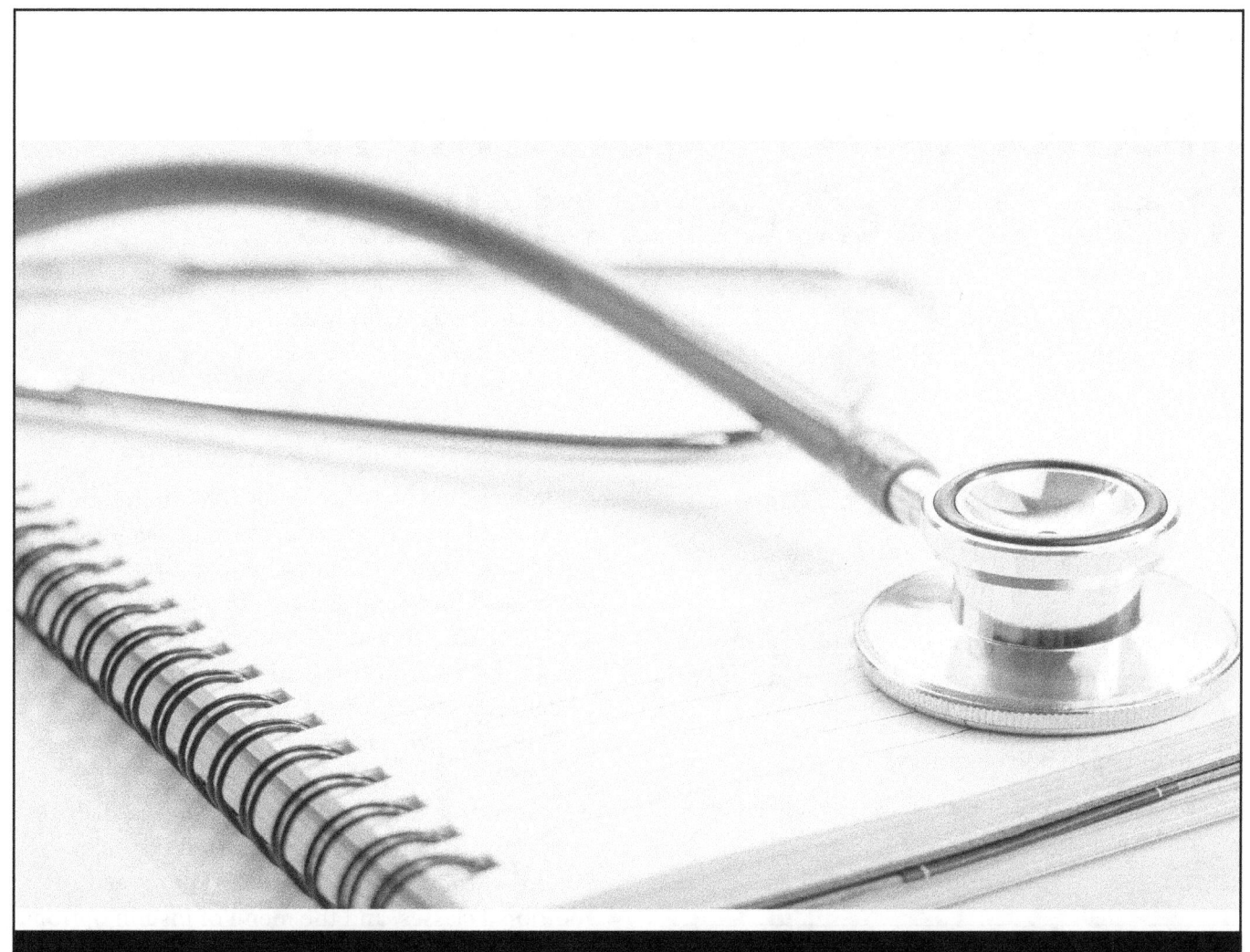

DIABETES MELLITUS AND GLUCOSE METABOLISM

An Evidence-Based Medication Algorithm for Type 2 Diabetes Mellitus

Howard B. A. Baum, MD. Division of Diabetes, Endocrinology, and Metabolism, Department of Medicine, Vanderbilt University Medical Center, Nashville, TN; Email: howard.baum@vumc.org

Educational Objectives

After reviewing this chapter, learners should be able to:

- Develop a treatment algorithm for type 2 diabetes mellitus treatment that is consistent with the evidence base.

- Avoid futile polypharmacy.

- Explain the role of insulin as type 2 diabetes mellitus progresses.

Significance of the Clinical Problem

The proliferation of noninsulin agents for treatment of type 2 diabetes simultaneously creates opportunities and responsibilities. We now have a variety of drugs that allows us to tailor treatment based on patient preferences, a balancing of benefits and adverse effects, and cost. Given numerous treatment options, published guidelines allow the clinician broad discretion in choosing diabetes medications. What we must avoid is the temptation to use most or all of these drugs in every patient. In addition, because diabetes is a disease characterized by progressive insulin deficiency, insulin is a virtually inevitable part of the treatment regimen for patients with longstanding type 2 diabetes. As endocrinologists, it is our responsibility in recommending pharmacologic treatment to understand the efficacy of noninsulin agents and not to label insulin, the most potent drug class in our armamentarium, as a treatment to be avoided.

Using data regarding efficacy of pharmacologic agents alone or in combination, we can employ an evidence-based treatment algorithm to treat type 2 diabetes as the disease progresses.

In 1994, 2 classes of pharmacologic agents were available for the treatment of type 2 diabetes in the United States, sulfonylureas and insulin. Since that time, agents have been approved in 10 additional classes, and the menu of insulin options has expanded to include analogues from the ultra–rapid-acting to the ultra–long-acting. While the array of drugs gives clinicians more tools and obviates a one-size-fits-all approach, the large number of available medications makes developing appropriate treatment algorithms exceedingly complex.

The American Diabetes Association (ADA) and European Association for the Study of Diabetes (EASD) recently published an updated consensus statement for management of type 2 diabetes.[1] This publication recognizes the need to individualize care and describes pathways for those with chronic kidney disease and cardiac risk. The statement advises the sequential addition of noninsulin agents when treatment goals are not met, without taking into account the specific hemoglobin A_{1c} level of the patient or the efficacy of the medication. The illustration of various treatment pathways indicates that the patient can be prescribed as many as 5 noninsulin agents in addition to metformin before moving to insulin. No trials have evaluated the efficacy of any diabetes medication when added as the fourth, fifth, or sixth drug.

While data are available regarding the effectiveness of diabetes medications, there are no guideline-level algorithms to help the clinician prioritize these agents. Clinicians should be prescribing regimens that are effective and efficient, avoiding futile polypharmacy, but currently must do so with limited published guidance.

Practice Gaps

- Published guidelines on pharmacologic management of type 2 diabetes recognize the need for adding medications as the disease progresses, but do not take into account the hemoglobin A_{1c}–lowering efficacy of medications nor the degree of the patient's hemoglobin A_{1c} elevation. This leaves clinicians to make therapeutic decisions without expert guidance.

- Insulin is an almost inevitable component of type 2 diabetes treatment assuming disease course of moderate to long duration. Published guidelines do not offer clear recommendations as to the appropriate timing of insulin implementation.

- Phenotyping for precision medicine approaches.

Discussion
Historical Context of Diabetes Guidelines

In 1995, the US regulatory authorities added metformin to sulfonylureas as the only noninsulin agents available for diabetes management. Later in the 1990s, α-glucosidase inhibitors, thiazolidinediones, and glinides were introduced, followed in 2005 by pramlintide and the

GLP-1 receptor agonist exenatide, adding potential complexity to diabetes management. In 2006, the ADA and EASD published a consensus which nonetheless was straightforward.[2] The consensus prioritizes metformin as the initial treatment for diabetes and allows for use of sulfonylureas, thiazolidinediones, and insulin, advising against use of the other agents.

The discovery that GLP-1 receptor agonists and SGLT-2 inhibitors (first introduced in 2013) afford cardiovascular and renal protection for high-risk groups added substantial complexity to medication selection.[3-5] Later versions of the ADA and EASD consensus take these factors into account, and also recognize that avoidance of hypoglycemia and cost, and desire for weight loss, are factors in choosing a treatment regimen. As we adopt a more holistic approach to patient-centered care beyond hemoglobin A_{1c} lowering alone, weight loss in particular has become increasingly emphasized as an essential component of comprehensive diabetes care. Weight loss as a factor in choosing treatment has gained increasing interest, especially because we have drugs that can facilitate that goal. In developing treatment approaches it is also important to consider social determinants of health. This includes access to care, expense of medications, and complexity of care that may exceed the personal and financial resources of some patients. These challenges have resulted in an understandably complex map for pharmacologic treatment recommendations, exemplified by the 2022 consensus statement.[1] The advantage of this approach is that it introduces numerous factors that must be considered in prescribing treatment and gives the clinician broad discretion in choosing pharmacologic agents, including insulin. The challenges are that the hemoglobin A_{1c}–lowering potential for noninsulin drugs is described only qualitatively (very high, high, intermediate) and that, in providing choice for patients and clinicians, there is no limit depicted for the number of drugs that could be described for a single patient, and the place of insulin in the progression is not clear.

Principles Guiding Medication Selection in Type 2 Diabetes

The foundation of diabetes management is lifestyle modification. Implementation of appropriate diet and exercise is essential to the success of any diabetes treatment plan. Because diabetes is a progressive disease characterized by worsening β-cell function over time, we ultimately need to use medications beyond the initial prescription for most patients. A critical consideration in the stepwise addition of diabetes medication is to take into account the hemoglobin A_{1c}–lowering potency of the medication being considered and the distance of the patient's hemoglobin A_{1c} from goal. In meta-analyses, the impact of add-on therapy is modest for oral agents and is in the range of 0.4% to 0.7% in combination with metformin or when added to metformin + sulfonylurea.[6,7] The effect of GLP-1 receptor agonists, particularly semaglutide, is more robust as add-on treatment, with hemoglobin A_{1c} lowering over 1.3%.[4] Tirzepatide—a dual glucose-dependent insulinotropic polypeptide and GLP-1 receptor agonist—demonstrates more significant hemoglobin A_{1c} lowering when added to metformin, but because of the relative novelty of the drug, its performance as assessed in meta-analyses of add-on treatment is not yet known.

The Glycemia Reduction in Type 2 Diabetes (GRADE) trial evaluated the effectiveness of glucose-lowering medications added to metformin.[8] The medications studied were insulin glargine, liraglutide, glimepiride, and sitagliptin. Over a 5-year mean follow-up, 71% of the participants exceeded the target hemoglobin A_{1c} of less than 7.0% (<53 mmol/mol). Insulin and liraglutide performed marginally better than the other agents, but the failure rates for each agent were similar: insulin glargine, 67%; liraglutide, 68%; glimepiride, 71%; and sitagliptin, 72%. SGLT-2 inhibitors, semaglutide, and tirzepatide were unavailable at the time of randomization.

Insulin, the most potent diabetes treatment, shows variable hemoglobin A_{1c}–lowering capacity as add-on therapy depending on the nature of the study and the mode of insulin administration. The pivotal study for the introduction of insulin glargine demonstrates a 1.6% average hemoglobin A_{1c} decline when basal insulin is added to 1 or 2 baseline oral medications (metformin and/or sulfonylurea).[9] In meta-analyses, the impact of basal insulin is smaller, around 0.8%, likely due to the inclusion of studies without forced insulin titration.[7]

Approach to Treatment

Along with comprehensive lifestyle management, metformin has long been recommended as the initial pharmacologic treatment for type 2 diabetes. Metformin's low cost, weight neutrality, lack of associated hypoglycemia, and long track record of safety continue to make it a good first choice. For those patients with higher hemoglobin A_{1c} values at presentation or a strong desire for weight loss, a GLP-1 or GIP/GLP-1 receptor agonist are reasonable alternatives based on the performance of these agents in clinical trials. For patients with symptomatic hyperglycemia at presentation—hemoglobin A_{1c} greater than 10.0% (>86 mmol/mol), for example—introduction of insulin is reasonable, especially if there is even a remote concern for type 1 diabetes. As new recommendations place particular emphasis on managing complications of diabetes rather than hemoglobin A_{1c} alone, pioglitazone should be considered as a first-line treatment for patients with nonalcoholic steatohepatitis based on data suggesting benefit of pioglitazone for this condition.[10] For patients with a hemoglobin A_{1c} value more than 2% above target, initial combination treatment can be considered since metformin alone is unlikely to achieve goal, but often even modest lifestyle modification introduced at the outset may provide a significant complementary effect.

When the hemoglobin A_{1c} exceeds the target on a single agent, consideration of a second agent should be based on the degree of hemoglobin A_{1c} elevation and the potency of the agent contemplated. If the hemoglobin A_{1c} is 2% or more above target, GLP-1 or GIP/GLP-1 receptor agonists and insulin are the only medications likely to get the patient to goal. If the patient is already on a GLP-1 agent, metformin could be added to mitigate insulin dosage and weight gain, but would be unlikely to be sufficient on its own. For hemoglobin A_{1c} elevations less than 2% above goal, data indicate that GLP-1 receptor agonists are the best choice based on meta-analyses and GRADE.[6,8] Based on its higher potency, tirzepatide is also an option here. Other agents have been shown to produce a less than 1% drop in hemoglobin A_{1c}, although patients might display individual variation in response. Options to consider in ascending order of potency are DPP-4 inhibitors, SGLT-2 inhibitors, sulfonylureas, and thiazolidinediones. Decisions can be based on potency, cost, potential adverse effects, and patient preference.

If a patient does not have success on 2 noninsulin agents, a third can be considered if the hemoglobin A_{1c} is within 1% to 1.5% of the target, assuming a GLP-1 receptor agonist is already in place. There might be a bit more leeway if a GLP-1 agent has not yet been used. Otherwise, initiation of insulin is appropriate.

For patients with albuminuric chronic kidney disease or heart failure, SGLT-2 inhibitor therapy should be considered early. One could consider these as first-line agents, but given their low potency, it is more likely that this would need to be started in combination with metformin (if glomerular filtration rate allows). Similarly, for those with coronary artery disease, a GLP-1 receptor agonist (not yet tirzepatide given the absence of cardiac safety data) or SGLT-2 inhibitor should be included early. Note that the trials demonstrating cardiac benefit for these agents included patients with preexisting heart disease. The studies also included patients at high risk for cardiac events due to underlying kidney disease.[3-5] There is not yet evidence of a protective effect of these medicines for patients at usual risk of adverse cardiac outcomes. Both classes can ultimately be included in the treatment protocol based on the need for hemoglobin A_{1c} lowering. Some early data suggest that the cardioprotective aspect of these drugs may be additive, but the data are not conclusive.[11] In the absence of clear evidence of benefit, there is no strong recommendation to introduce, say, a SGLT-2 inhibitor for a patient with coronary artery disease without congestive heart failure already on a GLP-1 receptor agonist unless needed for additional hemoglobin A_{1c} lowering. Other considerations are similar to those of patients without these high-risk conditions.

Clinical Case Vignettes
Case 1

A 58-year-old woman with 8 years of type 2 diabetes is transferring her care after moving from another city. She has been taking metformin, 1000 mg twice daily; glimepiride, 4 mg once daily; and semaglutide, 0.5 mg subcutaneously weekly, which she tolerates well. She has a history of coronary artery disease with a stent placement, but no congestive heart failure. She has no nephropathy although she is on a prophylactic antibiotic regimen for recurrent urinary tract infections. Her point-of-care hemoglobin A_{1c} measurement today is 6.7% (50 mmol/mol).

Which of the following is the best next step for her diabetes regimen?

A. Stop glimepiride and add linagliptin to mitigate hypoglycemia and avoid excess cardiac risk

B. Leave the regimen as is

C. Add empagliflozin due to her cardiac history

D. Increase the semaglutide dosage

E. Change metformin to extended release

Answer: B) Leave the regimen as is

This patient has excellent diabetes control on triple noninsulin treatment. While other sulfonylureas have been implicated in promoting cardiac ischemia, glimepiride and linagliptin were shown to be equivalent with regard to cardiac risk in the CAROLINA trial.[12]

We do not yet have convincing data that addition of a SGLT-2 inhibitor to a GLP-1 receptor agonist adds significant cardiac risk reduction in the absence of congestive heart failure, and the patient is at risk for SGLT-2 inhibitor adverse effects due to frequent urinary tract infections.

While the semaglutide dosage could be increased to lower weight a bit further, this issue is not mentioned in the case, and raising the dosage increases the chance of gastrointestinal intolerance, which is not an issue currently. Similarly, the main reason to switch to metformin extended release is gastrointestinal intolerance, which is not the case.

Case 2

A 63-year-old woman with more than 20 years of type 2 diabetes is referred by her internist. Her hemoglobin A_{1c} level has been in the 8.8% to 9.2% range (73-77 mmol/mol) for the last year on a regimen of metformin, 1000 mg twice daily, and semaglutide, 1 mg subcutaneously weekly. She has no kidney or vascular complications. She takes alendronate for osteoporosis. She has been advised to start insulin but is fearful of hypoglycemia, having witnessed that in her uncle when she was a girl.

Which of the following is the best advice?

A. Start insulin degludec at 10 units and titrate based on fasting glucose values

B. Switch from semaglutide to tirzepatide

C. Increase the semaglutide dosage to 2 mg subcutaneously weekly

D. Add pioglitazone

E. Add sitagliptin

Answer: A) Start insulin degludec at 10 units and titrate based on fasting glucose values

After 20 years of diabetes, this patient's insulin deficiency has progressed, and her hemoglobin A_{1c} level is significantly above goal. Insulin (Answer A) is the only agent that can lower hemoglobin A_{1c} below 7.0% (<53 mmol/mol). It is conceivable that basal insulin will be insufficient and that prandial insulin may be required. By using degludec with its smooth pharmacokinetics, she can be reassured

that her risk of severe hypoglycemia will be low compared with the risk associated with regimens predating analogues. Tirzepatide is more potent than semaglutide at maximum dosage, but only by 0.5% of hemoglobin A_{1c}, if one uses the studies of each drug individually in the absence of a comparison trial. Similarly, increasing the semaglutide dosage would yield a modest change. Pioglitazone might yield a hemoglobin A_{1c} drop approaching 1%, but this is insufficient, and this medication may increase her fracture risk. Sitagliptin is much too weak.

Case 3

A 42-year-old man with a 6-year history of type 2 diabetes presents for follow-up. He did well initially, modifying his diet, introducing exercise, and taking maximum dosage metformin. He lost about 20 lb (9 kg), but his BMI is still 31 kg/m². His hemoglobin A_{1c} has been creeping up in the last year, but he has resisted adding medication, attributing the change to work stress and the need to attend better to his diet. Despite trying to address these issues, his hemoglobin A_{1c} is now 8.5% (69 mmol/mol). He has no diabetes complications.

Which of the following is the best advice?

A. Visit once again with the dietician to help get him back on track

B. Add a sulfonyulrea

C. Change metformin to metformin/empagliflozin combination and add a sulfonylurea

D. Add insulin

E. Add a GLP-1 receptor agonist

Answer: E) Add a GLP-1 receptor agonist

Periodic visits for diabetes education have been shown to improve hemoglobin A_{1c}, and it is reasonable for him to get a refresher, but this is unlikely to lower hemoglobin A_{1c} sufficiently. The GRADE trial showed that the preferred second agents after metformin for durability of effect are GLP-1 receptor agonists and insulin. In this instance, his hemoglobin A_{1c} is at a level that allows him to get to goal with a GLP-1 receptor agonist (Answer E) while perhaps losing additional weight, rather than gaining weight, and avoiding hypoglycemia. The triple combination could conceivably work, but it is unnecessarily complex. A sulfonylurea is too weak. This admittedly straightforward case makes the point that the degree of hemoglobin A_{1c} lowering needed is a critical guide to advancing therapy.

Key Learning Points

- Using data regarding the potency of glucose-lowering agents for type 2 diabetes, the clinician can implement an evidence-based approach to medication selection as the condition progresses.

- There are no data indicating the efficacy of diabetes medications when added as a fourth drug in a regimen.

- It is not yet established that all patients with coronary artery disease should be treated with both a GLP-1 receptor agonist and SGLT-2 inhibitor.

- Clinicians should not hesitate to prescribe insulin when this most potent agent in our armamentarium becomes necessary to achieve hemoglobin A_{1c} goals.

References

1. Davies MJ, Aroda VR, Collins BS, et al. Management of hyperglycemia in type 2 diabetes, 2022. A consensus report by the American Diabetes Association (ADA) and the European Association for the Study of Diabetes (EASD). *Diabetes Care.* 2022;45(11):2753-2786. PMID: 36148880

2. Nathan DM, Buse JB, Davidson MB, et al. Management of hyperglycemia in type 2 diabetes: a consensus algorithm for initiation and adjustment of therapy. *Diabetes Care.* 2006;29(8):1963-1972. PMID: 16873813

3. Zinman B, Wanner C, Lachin JM, et al. Empagliflozin, cardiovascular outcomes, and mortality in type 2 diabetes. *N Engl J Med.* 2015;373(22):2117-2128. PMID: 26378978

4. Marso SP, Bain SC, Consoli A, et al; SUSTAIN-6 Investigators. Semaglutide and cardiovascular outcomes in patients with type 2 diabetes. *N Engl J Med.* 2016;375(19):1834-1844. PMID: 27633186

5. Perkovic V, Jardine MJ, Neal B, et al; CREDENCE Trial Investigators. Canagliflozin and renal outcomes in type 2 diabetes and nephropathy. *N Engl J Med.* 2019;380(24):2295-2306. PMID: 30990260

6. Tsapas A, Avergerinos I, Karagiannis T, et al. Comparative effectiveness of glucose-lowering drugs for type 2 diabetes: a systematic review and network meta-analysis. *Ann Intern Med.* 2020;173(4):278-286. PMID: 32598218

7. Zaccardi F, Dhalwani NN, Dales J, et al. Comparison of glucose-lowering agents after dual therapy failure in type 2 diabetes: a systematic review and network meta-analysis of randomized controlled trials. *Diabetes Obes Metab.* 2018;20(4):985-997. PMID: 29205774

8. The GRADE Research Study Group, Nathan DM, Lachin JM, et al. Glycemia reduction in type 2 diabetes—glycemic outcomes. *N Engl J Med.* 2022;387(12):1063-1074. PMID: 36129996

9. Riddle MC, Rosenstock J, Gerich J. The treat-to-target trial. Randomized addition of glargine or human NPH insulin to oral therapy of type 2 diabetic patients. *Diabetes Care.* 2003;26(11):3080-3086. PMID: 14578243

10. Zhao YM, Zhao W, Wang H, Zhao Y, Bu H, Takahashi H. Pioglitazone on nonalcoholic steatohepatitis: a systematic review and meta-analysis of 15 RCTs. *Medicine.* 2022;101(46):e31508. PMID: 36401449

11. Clegg LE, Penland RC, Bachina S, et al. Effects of exenatide and open-label SGLT2 inhibitor treatment, given parallel or sequentially, on mortality and cardiovascular and renal outcomes in type 2 diabetes: insights from the EXSCEL trial. *Cardiovasc Diabetol.* 2019;18(1):138-149. PMID: 31640705

12. Rosenstock J, Kahn SE, Johansen OE, et al; CAROLINA Investigators. Effect of linagliptin vs glimepiride on major adverse cardiovascular outcomes in patients with type 2 diabetes. The CAROLINA randomized clinical trial. *JAMA.* 2019;322(12):1155-1166. PMID: 31536101

Management of Untoward Metabolic Effects of Psychotropic Medications

Susanne U. Miedlich, MD. University of Rochester Medical Center, Department of Medicine, Division of Endocrinology, Rochester, New York; Email: susanne_miedlich@urmc.rochester.edu

Educational Objectives

After reviewing this chapter, learners should be able to:

- Explain how mental illness and psychotropic medications promote obesity, metabolic syndrome, and type 2 diabetes mellitus (T2DM) and why this is important to know.

- Identify patients on psychotropic medications who are at risk for obesity, metabolic syndrome, and T2DM.

- Implement strategies to prevent and treat obesity, metabolic syndrome, and T2DM in patients on psychotropic medications.

Significance of the Clinical Problem

Mental health problems are common, and so are prescriptions of psychotropic medications. Psychotropic medications improve mental health, but they can also mediate adverse effects, including weight gain, metabolic syndrome, and T2DM.

People with serious mental illness, for instance, have a high cardiovascular morbidity and mortality, which is at least in part attributed to second-generation antipsychotic medication (SGA) use and their mediation of weight gain and hyperglycemia. In addition, socioeconomic deprivation, limited access to health care, low motivation, and adverse health behaviors contribute to cardiometabolic morbidity and mortality.

This chapter lays out how to positively impact both physical and mental health outcomes in this high-risk patient population by choosing psychotropic medications wisely, by identifying cardiometabolic risk factors early, by using incretin analogues ± SGLT-2 inhibitors early to treat obesity and T2DM, and last, but not least, by improving access to and integrating health care for people with mental illness.

As of 2020, about 1 in 5 adults in the United States had a mental illness, about one-quarter of these had a serious mental illness (SMI).[1] The highest rates of mental illness were reported in young adults aged 18 to 25 years. Most notably, people with SMI (which includes schizophrenia, schizoaffective or bipolar disorder) die at much younger ages than people without SMI, most often from cardiovascular causes.[2]

Proposed mediators of these adverse health outcomes are high rates of obesity, T2DM, and hypertension, as well as cigarette smoking and social deprivation.[3,4] Psychotropic medications, specifically SGAs, are highly effective in promoting lasting improvements in mental and physical health in people with SMI.[5] At the same time, they have been directly implicated as mediators of adverse cardiometabolic outcomes.[4,6] Olanzapine and clozapine, for instance, often cause hyperphagia, weight gain, insulin resistance, and hyperglycemia, thus promoting obesity and T2DM.[7] Psychotropic medication use has also been associated with sedentary behavior in people with SMI.[8] In addition, autonomous motivation is low in people with SMI[9,10] and may contribute to adverse health behaviors. Low income, low educational level, poor diet quality (and limited access to healthy foods), and limited access to health care further shape the risk for obesity and T2DM in people with chronic mental illness.[11-13]

Prescriptions of SGAs are increasing. At a large pharmacy for patients with SMI at the University of Rochester Medical Center, prescriptions of SGAs almost doubled between 2014 and 2020 (unpublished data). In addition, off-label use of SGAs has increased and so have their adverse metabolic effects.[14]

What about antidepressant medications? Antidepressant medication use is common[15] and can also lead to weight gain and potentially T2DM, although the evidence is not as consistent across different antidepressants compared to the evidence for SGAs. Specifically, amitriptyline, paroxetine, and mirtazapine have been associated with weight gain.[16] As a class, antidepressants have been associated with a 20% increased risk of T2DM (corrected for depression and BMI).[17]

In this context, it is notable that people on various psychotropic medications and/or with SMI tend to benefit less from lifestyle intervention programs in terms of weight loss and diabetes prevention.[18-20]

Practice Gaps

- The risk of cardiometabolic morbidity and mortality is high in people with mental illness, especially in people with SMI. Psychotropic medications, particularly SGAs, are highly effective in improving mental health, but they also contribute to adverse cardiometabolic outcomes.

- Studies of lifestyle interventions in people with mental illness are limited and report only modest improvements in cardiometabolic markers.

- Poverty, limited access to health care, poor diet habits (which are at least in part due to limited access to healthy foods), high rates of cigarette smoking, depression, and low motivation

further add to an adverse cardiometabolic risk profile in people with mental illness.

- Studies demonstrating efficacy and safety of diabetes medications that can improve cardiometabolic outcomes, such as GLP-1 receptor agonists and SGLT-2 inhibitors, are extremely scarce or nonexistent in patients with chronic mental illness and/or patients who are treated with psychotropic medications.

Discussion

How should one approach a patient with chronic mental illness on a psychotropic medication? The following discussion proposes strategies for (1) choosing a specific psychotropic medication from a cardiometabolic perspective, (2) identifying and addressing cardiometabolic risk factors, (3) screening for obesity and T2DM, (4) treating obesity and T2DM, and (5) optimizing health care delivery to people with chronic mental illness.

How to Choose a Psychotropic Medication From a Cardiometabolic Perspective

Adverse metabolic effects of SGAs are attributed to their antagonism of histaminergic (H1), serotonergic (mainly 5HT2c) and dopaminergic (D2) receptors, as well as anticholinergic effects as elegantly demonstrated in animal studies and further corroborated in human studies.[21] Accordingly, the choice of a specific SGA should be carefully weighed based on the mental health symptomatology, as well as cardiometabolic risk factors and/or comorbidities. From a cardiometabolic viewpoint, it is important to note that patients switching to olanzapine or clozapine gain over 4.4 lb (2 kg) of weight. These medications should therefore be reserved for patients for whom alternative medications fail.[22] Alternative medications with a more favorable metabolic adverse effect profile are aripiprazole or ziprasidone. Patients switching to aripiprazole or ziprasidone lose about 4.4 lb (2 kg).[22] A switch to aripiprazole also leads to significant improvements in lipids, most notably in total cholesterol and triglyceride levels.[22] A switch to amisulpride, lurasidone, paliperidone, risperidone, or quetiapine does not affect weight or other cardiometabolic markers, although respective studies are limited.[22]

Based on these data, in a patient with or at risk for obesity and T2DM, aripiprazole and/or ziprasidone should be preferred over other SGAs whenever possible. That said, olanzapine and clozapine are undoubtedly superior to these medications and are often necessary to effectively control psychotic symptoms in people with SMI. The combination of olanzapine with samidorphan, an opioid antagonist, may serve as a valuable alternative for patients who are at risk for or have obesity and T2DM for whom treatment with another SGA has failed. The addition of samidorphan does not affect antipsychotic efficacy of olanzapine; it does, however, mitigate weight gain.[23]

With antidepressants, high-affinity antagonism of central histamine H1 receptors may contribute to weight gain seen with selective serotonin-reuptake inhibitors (SSRIs).[16] Noradrenergic stimulation (serotonin-norepinephrine-reuptake inhibitors [SNRIs]), while promoting weight loss, may promote hyperglycemia.[24] The atypical antidepressant bupropion deserves special attention here: it is FDA-approved for depression, smoking cessation, and in combination with naltrexone for treatment of obesity. Bupropion treatment alone or in combination with naltrexone, an opioid antagonist such as samidorphan, can promote 3% to 6% weight loss and has also been shown to prevent SGA-induced weight gain in small studies.[25,26]

Identify and Address Patient-Related Risk Factors

Compared with use in the general population, cigarette smoking, alcohol use, and substance use are dramatically increased in people with SMI, and cessation rates are lower.[27] That said, the reasons for lower cessation rates may not be low motivation but lack of promoting smoking cessation and reduced access to smoking cessation programs.[27] In fact, smoking cessation leads to improved mental health in people with SMI. Behavioral interventions and pharmacotherapy targeting smoking cessation in people with SMI are effective, although data are limited.[27]

Poor lifestyle habits have been reported in people with chronic mental illness. Specifically, people with SMI when compared with control participants tend to eat more, they also eat less healthy overall (diet high in carbohydrates and refined sugars, and low in fruit and vegetables—a finding that may be owed at least in part to limited access to healthy foods.[11] In addition, our own observations in patients with SMI on SGAs revealed that poor diet habits correlated with higher fasting glucose and triglyceride levels.[28] As previously mentioned, behavioral intervention studies in people with SMI demonstrate modest weight reductions (about 6.6 lb [3 kg]) without significant improvements in glycemic or lipid markers.[20] Greater weight loss is achieved when the intervention is started at initiation of SGA therapy, emphasizing the importance of timely action.[29] A lifestyle coaching study focusing on physical activity goals failed to show improvements in weight, lipid, or glycemic markers.[30]

In summary, addressing cigarette smoking, alcohol use, and substance use in patients with chronic mental illness has the potential to prevent adverse physical health outcomes and may improve mental health outcomes. Detailed assessments of diet habits and providing dietary guidance, ideally at initiation of SGA therapy, has the potential to identify and assist patients with or at risk for metabolic syndrome and T2DM. Lifestyle interventions can produce modest weight loss, pharmacologic interventions should be considered early.

Screening for Obesity, Prediabetes, and T2DM

Screening for prediabetes and diabetes with hemoglobin A_{1c} or fasting glucose alone can miss a substantial number of patients when compared with oral glucose tolerance testing.[31,32]

For instance, in studies of patients on various antipsychotic medications, hemoglobin A_{1c} screening alone misses most patients with diabetes compared with oral glucose tolerance testing.[28,33] Based on these results, Mitchell and colleagues propose a 2-step screening approach, starting with hemoglobin A_{1c} measurements, followed by oral glucose tolerance testing for patients with a hemoglobin A_{1c} value of 5.7% or greater (≥39 mmol/mol).[33] Per our own observations, a diagnosis of either prediabetes or diabetes by hemoglobin A_{1c} is associated with significantly higher waist-to-hip ratios, triglyceride concentrations, C-reactive protein concentrations, and insulin resistance,[28] further emphasizing that interventions should be put in place when hemoglobin A_{1c} levels are in the prediabetes range. Screening for obesity and diabetes should begin at least 3 months after starting an SGA and then be performed annually.[6]

Treating Obesity, Prediabetes, and T2DM

The above noted observations of adverse metabolic effects of SGAs, as well as limited success of behavioral interventions in people with SMI, emphasize the need for early pharmacologic interventions. For patients on SGAs, metformin should be considered when prediabetes is diagnosed. An incretin analogue, and specifically semaglutide or tirzepatide (pending FDA approval for obesity for tirzepatide), would be obvious choices for patients on SGAs with obesity ± prediabetes, as these medications have the potential to mediate weight loss and prevent diabetes to an extent that approaches bariatric surgery results.[34,35] Unfortunately, these medications are expensive and often excluded from medical insurance plans.

According to the current American Diabetes Association guidelines,[36] patients newly diagnosed with T2DM should be started on either a GLP-1 receptor agonist or an SGLT-2 inhibitor if they are at high risk for cardiovascular disease (age >55 years, 2+ risk factors) or have preexisting cardiovascular disease, independent of metformin use. Considering the high rates of obesity, hypertension, and cigarette smoking in people with SMI, treatment with either a GLP-1 receptor agonist or an SGLT-2 inhibitor should therefore be considered for most patients at the time of T2DM diagnosis.

With all that said, data demonstrating efficacy and safety of GLP-1 receptor agonists or SGLT-2 inhibitors in patients with SMI treated with SGAs who also have T2DM are extremely sparse.

Studies using metformin in patients on SGAs who have obesity but not T2DM show weight loss between 2.2 and 13.2 lb (1-6 kg) and small hemoglobin A_{1c} reductions.[37,38] Studies using GLP-1 receptor agonists in patients on SGAs show slightly more robust weight loss and hemoglobin A_{1c} reductions.[39]

We do not know if these benefits apply to patients on SGA with T2DM. Our own retrospective cohort study of patients with obesity and T2DM who were treated with SGAs showed an average weight loss of 15.4 lb (7 kg) and hemoglobin A_{1c} reductions of about 1% in patients treated with a GLP-1 receptor agonists but weight gain in patients on alternative regimens.[40] These findings are reassuring but clearly need confirmation in larger, prospective trials.

In preclinical studies of cigarette smoking, alcohol, and substance use, GLP-1 receptor agonists have also shown promise in alleviating addiction disorders.[41] If confirmed in clinical trials, that would make GLP-1 receptor agonists clearly superior to alternative regimens, especially for patients with SMI who smoke cigarettes.

What about SGLT-2 inhibitors? The risk of congestive heart failure is significantly increased in people with schizophrenia.[42] SGLT-2 inhibitors have been shown to be superior to metformin in preventing heart failure admissions when used as first-line therapy for T2DM in the general population.[43] It therefore makes sense to consider a SGLT-2 inhibitor as first-line treatment for T2DM in patients with SMI, particularly in those with schizophrenia. That said, efficacy and safety of SGLT-2 inhibitors in patients on SGAs have not been demonstrated. Why is that important? Both SGAs, but also SGLT-2 inhibitors, have been associated with an increased risk of diabetic ketoacidosis (0.1%-0.3%). Risk factors for diabetic ketoacidosis in the setting of clozapine therapy, for instance, are Black race and short duration of clozapine and other medication use, including diabetes medications.[44] As for SGLT-2 inhibitors, low insulin levels, surgery, infection, diet changes, and alcohol use are among the most common risk factors for diabetic ketoacidosis.[45] Taken together, because of a high risk of heart failure in patients with schizophrenia, an SGLT-2 inhibitor should be considered as first-line treatment of T2DM. However, in the presence of concurrent SGA therapy, high vigilance is recommended regarding an increased risk of diabetic ketoacidosis, especially in ethnic minorities and in the setting of acute illness. SGLT-2 inhibitors should also promote modest weight reductions, although we do not know if this is true for patients on SGAs.

Similar to patients on SGAs, patients with T2DM on antidepressants have not been specifically studied regarding specific strategies targeting weight and glycemic control. In a retrospective cohort study, we confirmed superiority of GLP-1 receptor agonists in mediating weight loss in patients on antidepressant medications but noted overall blunted glycemic improvements, a finding that was independent of the treatment strategy used.[46] Another retrospective cohort study showed blunted weight loss following GLP-1 receptor agonist initiation in patients on citalopram, escitalopram, or bupropion (<2.2 lb [<1 kg]). Glycemic outcomes were not reported (>60% of patients had T2DM).[47] It remains to be seen whether newer incretin analogues such as semaglutide or tirzepatide or combinations of incretin analogues and SGLT-2 inhibitors prove more effective for glycemic and weight control in patients on antidepressant medications.

Optimizing Health Care Delivery in Patients With Mental Illness

As previously mentioned, adverse health behaviors, socioeconomic deprivation, and limited access to health care are moderators of adverse health outcomes in people with mental illness.[12,13,48] Specifically, rates of T2DM screening (hemoglobin A_{1c}) are lower, while hospital admissions are higher in people with mental illness than in those without.[49] Integrated or co-located specialty care within primary care settings has the potential to reverse or mitigate adverse health outcomes and successfully engage patients with mental illness. In fact, integrated care is cost-effective and associated with increased patient satisfaction, emotional well-being, and improved diabetes outcomes in patients with mental illness.[50,51] While it may not be feasible or cost-effective to create specifically tailored, integrated care settings and programs for all people with chronic mental illness, an interdisciplinary and personalized approach to patient care should always be the goal. It should include continuous communications between patients, care managers, social workers, and health care providers to best support this high-risk and often very complex patient population.

Clinical Case Vignettes
Case 1

A 25-year-old Black man with schizophrenia controlled on olanzapine is referred for advice regarding management of T2DM. He was recently admitted to the hospital with diabetic ketoacidosis and was discharged on conventional insulin therapy (insulin NPH/insulin lispro 70/30 twice daily). His BMI is 40 kg/m². Currently, his fasting glucose values are between 140 and 160 mg/dL (7.8-8.9 mmol/L), and predinner glucose values are between 180 and 200 mg/dL (10.0-11.1 mmol/L).

Which of the following is the best strategy for his diabetes care?

A. Switch to basal-bolus insulin therapy and increase total daily insulin by 10%

B. Add metformin

C. Add an SGLT-2 inhibitor

D. Stop mixed insulin and start basal insulin and a GLP-1 receptor agonist

Answer: D) Stop mixed insulin and start basal insulin and a GLP-1 receptor agonist

This patient likely has ketosis-prone diabetes. Introduction of olanzapine triggered weight gain, hyperglycemia, and eventually diabetic ketoacidosis. Upon resolution of hyperglycemia, his β-cell function is expected to improve significantly, allowing for implementation of non-insulin treatment strategies. Since he also has class III obesity, a strategy to target both diabetes and weight control is preferred, ideally with semaglutide or tirzepatide (Answer D).

While switching to basal-bolus insulin therapy (Answer A) is certainly a reasonable approach, it is expected to further weight gain and place the patient at risk for hypoglycemia.

Metformin (Answer B) and SGLT-2 inhibitors (Answer C) are alternative non-insulin treatment options, but they would likely mediate only modest weight loss. Furthermore, the patient's recent history of diabetic ketoacidosis precludes consideration of an SGLT-2 inhibitor.

Case 2

A 51-year-old woman seeks advice regarding obesity. She is concerned about continued weight gain and describes food cravings triggered by negative emotions that she cannot control. Her medical history is notable for depression, hypertension, and asthma. She is taking paroxetine, chlorthalidone, and budesonide/formoterol.

On physical examination, her BMI is 32 kg/m². She has a round face, central obesity, and white striae on her abdomen.

Laboratory test results:

Hemoglobin A_{1c} = 5.8% (40 mmol/mol)
Midnight salivary cortisol, normal (2 measurements)

Which of the following is the best next step in this patient's care?

A. Refer her to a structured lifestyle program

B. Add bupropion/naltrexone after a discussion with her mental health care team

C. Start metformin

Answer: B) Add bupropion/naltrexone after a discussion with her mental health care team

This patient struggles with emotional eating, a scenario in which bupropion/naltrexone (Answer B) may be particularly helpful. Bupropion may also replace paroxetine for treatment of depression. Paroxetine is an SSRI that has been associated with weight gain. Of further interest in this patient's case, a study comparing personalized vs randomized obesity treatment based on specific phenotypic patient characteristics (personalized treatments: reduced satiation → phentermine/topiramate; reduced satiety → GLP-1 receptor agonist; emotional eating → bupropion/naltrexone; low metabolic rate → phentermine/strength training) noted an average weight loss of 16% in patients treated with the personalized approach based on above features, compared with only in 9% in patients with randomly selected treatment.[52]

While referral to a structured lifestyle program (Answer A) should always be recommended, there is concern regarding its efficacy to promote weight loss and prevent T2DM in this patient on an SSRI who struggles with emotional eating. In addition, prior studies of lifestyle interventions (Diabetes Prevention Program [DPP]) demonstrated less weight loss and no effect on diabetes prevention in patients on antidepressants.[18]

Metformin (Answer C) has been shown to prevent progression to diabetes in patients on antidepressants, although it would be expected to be less effective in producing weight loss than bupropion/naltrexone.

Case 3

A 45-year-old man is referred for newly diagnosed T2DM. His medical history is notable for bipolar disorder, chronic obstructive pulmonary disease (he smokes cigarettes, 1 pack daily), hypertension, and recent hospital admission for heart failure. Medications are aripiprazole, venlafaxine, hydrochlorothiazide, tiotropium, and albuterol.

On physical examination, BMI is 30 kg/m² and blood pressure is 139/85 mm Hg.

His hemoglobin A_{1c} value is 6.5% (48 mmol/mol).

In addition to smoking cessation and a lifestyle program, which of the following should be recommended?

A. Metformin

B. GLP-1 receptor agonist

C. SGLT-2 inhibitor

Answer: C) SGLT-2 inhibitor

A lifestyle program (such as the DPP) is expected to mediate modest weight loss in this patient. Together with smoking cessation, it should definitely be recommended. In patients with SMI, more frequent sessions that are tailored to the specific patient are suggested to promote lasting lifestyle changes. However, pharmacologic therapy should be implemented at this time as well. Based on this patient's recent hospital admission for heart failure, therapy with an SGLT-2 inhibitor (Answer C) should be considered first-line therapy for T2DM to prevent future admissions for heart failure, as well as to reduce his risk for major cardiovascular events.[36]

A GLP-1 receptor agonist (Answer B) would also be expected to reduce his risk for adverse cardiovascular outcomes, although it would not affect his risk for heart failure admissions.[36] Adding a GLP-1 receptor agonist would be a great second choice for this patient if needed, especially for weight control.

While metformin (Answer A) used to be the first-line treatment choice for patients newly diagnosed with diabetes and may also mediate modest weight loss, any benefit in reducing adverse cardiovascular events would likely be delayed. Metformin would also not be expected to reduce his risk of hospital admission for heart failure.[36]

Key Learning Points

- Identify patients with mental illness who are at risk for obesity, T2DM, and adverse cardiovascular outcomes.

- Support patients with mental illness by facilitating access to lifestyle and smoking cessation programs.

- Prevent obesity ± prediabetes by critically choosing psychotropic medications. In addition to lifestyle programs, consider incretin analogues and metformin early for the treatment of obesity ± prediabetes in patients on SGAs.

- Treat T2DM first-line with incretin analogues and SGLT-2 inhibitors. Beware of a possibly increased risk of diabetic ketoacidosis with SGLT-2 inhibitors in patients who are also treated with SGAs.

References

1. Substance Abuse and Mental Health Services Administration. *Key substance use and mental health indicators in the United States: Results from the 2021 National Survey on Drug Use and Health.* (HHS Publication No. PEP22-07-01-005, NSDUH Series H-57). Center for Behavioral Health Statistics and Quality Services Administration. 2022. Available at: https://www.samhsa.gov/data/report/2021-nsduh-annual-national-report

2. Olfson M, Gerhard T, Huang C, Crystal S, Stroup TS. Premature mortality among adults with schizophrenia in the United States. *JAMA Psychiatry.* 2015;72(12):1172-1181. PMID: 26509694

3. Goff DC, Sullivan LM, McEvoy JP, et al. A comparison of ten-year cardiac risk estimates in schizophrenia patients from the CATIE study and matched controls. *Schizophr Res.* 2005;80(1):45-53. PMID: 16198088

4. Osborn DP, Hardoon S, Omar RZ, et al. Cardiovascular risk prediction models for people with severe mental illness: results from the prediction and management of cardiovascular risk in people with severe mental illnesses (PRIMROSE) research program. *JAMA Psychiatry.* 2015;72(2):143-151. PMID: 25536289

5. Correll CU, Solmi M, Croatto G, et al. Mortality in people with schizophrenia: a systematic review and meta-analysis of relative risk and aggravating or attenuating factors. *World Psychiatry.* 2022;21(2):248-271. PMID: 35524619

6. De Hert M, Detraux J, van Winkel R, Yu W, Correll CU. Metabolic and cardiovascular adverse effects associated with antipsychotic drugs. *Nat Rev Endocrinol.* 2011;8(2):114-126. PMID: 22009159

7. Ballon JS, Pajvani U, Freyberg Z, Leibel RL, Lieberman JA. Molecular pathophysiology of metabolic effects of antipsychotic medications. *Trends Endocrinol Metab.* 2014;25(11):593-600. PMID: 25190097

8. Vancampfort D, Firth J, Schuch FB, et al. Sedentary behavior and physical activity levels in people with schizophrenia, bipolar disorder and major depressive disorder: a global systematic review and meta-analysis. *World Psychiatry.* 2017;16(3):308-315. PMID: 28941119

9. Barch DM, Yodkovik N, Sypher-Locke H, Hanewinkel M. Intrinsic motivation in schizophrenia: relationships to cognitive function, depression, anxiety, and personality. *J Abnorm Psychol.* 2008;117(4):776-787. PMID: 19025225

10. Silverstein SM. Bridging the gap between extrinsic and intrinsic motivation in the cognitive remediation of schizophrenia. *Schizophr Bull.* 2010;36(5):949-956. PMID: 20064900

11. Teasdale SB, Ward PB, Samaras K, et al. Dietary intake of people with severe mental illness: systematic review and meta-analysis. *Br J Psychiatry.* 2019;214(5):251-259. PMID: 30784395

12. Bradford DW, Kim MM, Braxton LE, Marx CE, Butterfield M, Elbogen EB. Access to medical care among persons with psychotic and major affective disorders. *Psychiatr Serv.* 2008;59(8):847-852. PMID: 18678680

13. Kaufman EA, McDonell MG, Cristofalo MA, Ries RK. Exploring barriers to primary care for patients with severe mental illness: frontline patient and provider accounts. *Issues Ment Health Nurs.* 2012;33(3):172-180. PMID: 22364429

14. Stogios N, Smith E, Bowden S, et al. Metabolic adverse effects of off-label use of second-generation antipsychotics in the adult population: a systematic review and meta-analysis. *Neuropsychopharmacology.* 2022;47(3):664-672. PMID: 34446830

15. Pratt LA, Brody DJ, Gu Q. Antidepressant use among persons aged 12 and over: United States, 2011-2014. *NCHS Data Brief.* 2017(283):1-8. PMID: 29155679

16. Salvi V, Mencacci C, Barone-Adesi F. H1-histamine receptor affinity predicts weight gain with antidepressants. *Eur Neuropsychopharmacol.* 2016;26(10):1673-1677. PMID: 27593622

17. Salvi V, Grua I, Cerveri G, Mencacci C, Barone-Adesi F. The risk of new-onset diabetes in antidepressant users - A systematic review and meta-analysis. *PLoS One.* 2017;12(7):e0182088. PMID: 28759599

18. Rubin RR, Ma Y, Marrero DG, et al. Elevated depression symptoms, antidepressant medicine use, and risk of developing diabetes during the diabetes prevention program. *Diabetes Care.* 2008;31(3):420-426. PMID: 18071002

19. Daumit GL, Dickerson FB, Wang NY, et al. A behavioral weight-loss intervention in persons with serious mental illness. *N Engl J Med.* 2013;368(17):1594-1602. PMID: 23517118

20. Gierisch JM, Nieuwsma JA, Bradford DW, et al. Pharmacologic and behavioral interventions to improve cardiovascular risk factors in adults with serious mental illness: a systematic review and meta-analysis. *J Clin Psychiatry.* 2014;75(5):e424-e440. PMID: 24922495

21. Cernea S, Dima L, Correll CU, Manu P. Pharmacological management of glucose dysregulation in patients treated with second-generation antipsychotics. *Drugs.* 2020;80(17):1763-1781. PMID: 32930

22. Siskind D, Gallagher E, Winckel K, et al. Does switching antipsychotics ameliorate weight gain in patients with severe mental illness? A systematic review and meta-analysis. *Schizophr Bull.* 2021;47(4):948-958. PMID: 33547471

23. Jawad MY, Alnefeesi Y, Lui LMW, et al. Olanzapine and samidorphan combination treatment: A systematic review. *J Affect Disord.* 2022;301:99-106. PMID: 35007644

24. Hennings JM, Schaaf L, Fulda S. Glucose metabolism and antidepressant medication. *Curr Pharm Des.* 2012;18(36):5900-5919. PMID: 22681169

25. Gadde KM, Xiong GL. Bupropion for weight reduction. *Expert Rev Neurother.* 2007;7(1):17-24. PMID: 17187492

26. Greenway FL, Fujioka K, Plodkowski RA, et al. Effect of naltrexone plus bupropion on weight loss in overweight and obese adults (COR-I): a multicentre, randomised, double-blind, placebo-controlled, phase 3 trial. *Lancet.* 2010;376(9741):595-605. PMID: 20673995

27. Sharma R, Gartner CE, Hall WD. The challenge of reducing smoking in people with serious mental illness. *Lancet Respir Med.* 2016;4(10):835-844. PMID: 27707462

28. Miedlich S, Akinbowale C, Sahay P, et al. Poor diet habits, depression and low physical activity correlate with cardiometabolic risk markers in persons with severe mental illness on second-generation antipsychotic medications. *J Endocr Society.* 2022;6(Suppl 1):A422-A423.

29. Teasdale SB, Ward PB, Rosenbaum S, Samaras K, Stubbs B. Solving a weighty problem: systematic review and meta-analysis of nutrition interventions in severe mental illness. *Br J Psychiatry.* 2017;210(2):110-118. PMID: 27810893

30. Speyer H, Jakobsen AS, Westergaard C, et al. Lifestyle interventions for weight management in people with serious mental illness: a systematic review with meta-analysis, trial sequential analysis, and meta-regression analysis exploring the mediators and moderators of treatment effects. *Psychother Psychosom.* 2019;88(6):350-362. PMID: 31522170

31. Cowie CC, Rust KF, Byrd-Holt DD, et al. Prevalence of diabetes and high risk for diabetes using A1C criteria in the U.S. population in 1988-2006. *Diabetes Care.* 2010;33(3):562-568. PMID: 20067953

32. Meijnikman AS, De Block CEM, Dirinck E, et al. Not performing an OGTT results in significant underdiagnosis of (pre)diabetes in a high risk adult Caucasian population. *Int J Obes (Lond).* 2017;41(11):1615-1620. PMID: 28720876

33. Mitchell AJ, Vancampfort D, Manu P, et al. Which clinical and biochemical predictors should be used to screen for diabetes in patients with serious mental illness receiving antipsychotic medication? A large observational study. *PLoS One.* 2019;14(9):e0210674. PMID: 31513598

34. Davies M, Faerch L, Jeppesen OK, et al. Semaglutide 2.4 mg once a week in adults with overweight or obesity, and type 2 diabetes (STEP 2): a randomised, double-blind, double-dummy, placebo-controlled, phase 3 trial. *Lancet.* 2021;397(10278):971-984. PMID: 33667417

35. Jastreboff AM, Aronne LJ, Ahmad NN, et al. Tirzepatide Once Weekly for the Treatment of Obesity. *N Engl J Med.* 2022;387(3):205-216. PMID: 35658024

36. ElSayed NA, Aleppo G, Aroda VR, et al. 9. Pharmacologic approaches to glycemic treatment: standards of care in diabetes-2023. *Diabetes Care.* 2023;46(Suppl 1):S140-S157. PMID: 36507650

37. Siskind DJ, Leung J, Russell AW, Wysoczanski D, Kisely S. Metformin for clozapine associated obesity: a systematic review and meta-analysis. *PLoS One.* 2016;11(6):e0156208. PMID: 27304831

38. Taylor J, Stubbs B, Hewitt C, et al. The effectiveness of pharmacological and non-pharmacological interventions for improving glycaemic control in adults with severe mental illness: a systematic review and meta-analysis. *PLoS One.* 2017;12(1):e0168549. PMID: 28056018

39. Horska K, Ruda-Kucerova J, Skrede S. GLP-1 agonists: superior for mind and body in antipsychotic-treated patients? *Trends Endocrinol Metab.* 2022;33(9):628-638. PMID: 35902330

40. Perlis LT, Lamberti JS, Miedlich SU. Glucagon-like peptide analogs are superior for diabetes and weight control in patients on antipsychotic medications: a retrospective cohort study. *Prim Care Companion CNS Disord.* 2020;22(1):19m02504. PMID: 32027785

41. Klausen MK, Thomsen M, Wortwein G, Fink-Jensen A. The role of glucagon-like peptide 1 (GLP-1) in addictive disorders. *Br J Pharmacol.* 2022;179(4):625-641. PMID: 34532853

42. Correll CU, Solmi M, Veronese N, et al. Prevalence, incidence and mortality from cardiovascular disease in patients with pooled and specific severe mental illness: a large-scale meta-analysis of 3,211,768 patients and 113,383,368 controls. *World Psychiatry.* 2017;16(2):163-180. PMID: 28498599

43. Shin H, Schneeweiss S, Glynn RJ, Patorno E. Cardiovascular outcomes in patients initiating first-line treatment of type 2 diabetes with sodium-glucose cotransporter-2 inhibitors versus metformin. *Ann Intern Med.* 2022;175(12):W155. PMID: 36534995

44. Nihalani ND, Tu X, Lamberti JS, et al. Diabetic ketoacidosis among patients receiving clozapine: a case series and review of socio-demographic risk factors. *Ann Clin Psychiatry.* 2007;19(2):105-112. PMID: 17612850

45. Bonora BM, Avogaro A, Fadini GP. Sodium-glucose co-transporter-2 inhibitors and diabetic ketoacidosis: An updated review of the literature. *Diabetes Obes Metab.* 2018;20(1):25-33. PMID: 28517913

46. Gonzalez CL, Azim S, Miedlich SU. GLP-1 analogs are superior in mediating weight loss but not glycemic control in diabetic patients on antidepressant medications: a retrospective cohort study. *Prim Care Companion CNS Disord.* 2021;23(5):20m02868. PMID: 34507389

47. Durell N, Franks R, Coon S, Cowart K, Carris NW. Effect of antidepressants on glucagon-like peptide-1 receptor agonist-related weight loss. *J Pharm Technol.* 2022;38(5):283-288. PMID: 36046348

48. Druss BG, Zhao L, Von Esenwein S, Morrato EH, Marcus SC. Understanding excess mortality in persons with mental illness: 17-year follow up of a nationally representative US survey. *Med Care.* 2011;49(6):599-604. PMID: 215771183

49. Druss BG, Zhao L, Cummings JR, Shim RS, Rust GS, Marcus SC. Mental comorbidity and quality of diabetes care under Medicaid: a 50-state analysis. *Med Care.* 2012;50(5):428-433. PMID: 22228248

50. Lemmens LC, Molema CC, Versnel N, Baan CA, de Bruin SR. Integrated care programs for patients with psychological comorbidity: A systematic review and meta-analysis. *J Psychosom Res.* 2015;79(6):580-594. PMID: 26354890

51. Chwastiak LA, Luongo M, Russo J, et al. Use of a mental health center collaborative care team to improve diabetes care and outcomes for patients with psychosis. *Psychiatr Serv.* 2018;69(3):349-352. PMID: 29191136

52. Acosta A, Camilleri M, Abu Dayyeh B, et al. Selection of antiobesity medications based on phenotypes enhances weight loss: a pragmatic rrial in an obesity clinic. *Obesity (Silver Spring).* 2021;29(4):662-671. PMID: 33759389

Challenges in the Diagnosis and Management of Hypoglycemia

Mary Elizabeth Patti, MD. Research and Clinic Divisions, Joslin Diabetes Center, Boston, MA; Email: Mary.elizabeth.patti@joslin.harvard.edu

Educational Objectives

After reviewing this chapter, learners should be able to:

- Illustrate the challenges of identifying causes of hypoglycemia.

- Illustrate the challenges of localizing sources of insulin production.

- Learn about medications that can increase risk for hypoglycemia.

- Identify risk factors for postprandial hypoglycemia after upper gastrointestinal surgery.

- Identify range of sensor glucose values in the healthy population and limitations of continuous glucose monitoring (CGM) in diagnosis.

Significance of the Clinical Problem

Hypoglycemia in individuals without diabetes often poses a diagnostic challenge for the endocrinologist, and it is an underrecognized but highly significant clinical problem for affected individuals. Determining whether hypoglycemia is present, whether it is the cause of the patient's symptoms, and identifying the cause of hypoglycemia is essential to guide formulation of an effective treatment plan.

Mild adrenergic and cholinergic symptoms are nonspecific and may be caused by hypoglycemia but also by altered gastric emptying ("dumping syndrome"), cardiac dysrhythmias, hypotension, anxiety, and other disorders. Severe (level III) hypoglycemia can be distressing and impair safety, especially when associated with neuroglycopenia and hypoglycemia unawareness. Hypoglycemia associated with neuroglycopenia mandates full endocrine workup to rule out systemic illness or medications associated with hypoglycemia, to rule out insulinoma or other tumors contributing to hypoglycemia, and to define the underlying pathophysiology to guide effective therapy. A common cause of hypoglycemia increasingly encountered in clinical practice is hypoglycemia after bariatric or other upper gastrointestinal surgeries. For a comprehensive review of this condition and approaches to diagnosis and treatment, please see previously published reviews.[1,2]

In otherwise healthy individuals, diagnostic evaluation of confirmed hypoglycemia should be aimed at (1) ruling out autonomous insulin or insulin-like hormone production by an insulinoma or other tumor, (2) identifying medications and concurrent medical conditions that can cause or worsen hypoglycemia, and (3) identifying functional alterations in glucose and insulin dynamics that contribute to reactive hypoglycemia after bariatric or other upper gastrointestinal surgical procedures (e.g., gastric bypass, sleeve gastrectomy, and fundoplication).

Practice Gaps

- Due to nonspecific and sometimes mild nature of hypoglycemia symptoms, diagnosis of hypoglycemia is often delayed for several years.

- It is often challenging to fulfill the Whipple triad in clinical practice. Nevertheless, this remains an essential goal in the diagnostic process.

- Even when hormonal analysis indicates inappropriately high insulin secretion at the time of hypoglycemia, localization of an insulinoma is often challenging.

Discussion

Challenges in the Diagnosis of Hypoglycemia

What Should Be Defined as Hypoglycemia?
Step 1 in the evaluation of hypoglycemia should be to verify the Whipple triad. This concept provides a useful framework to be certain that hypoglycemia is truly present, that it is the cause of the patient's symptoms, and that symptoms respond to treatments that raise glucose levels. Unfortunately, achieving this in clinical practice is often very challenging.

What Concentration of Venous Glucose Is Considered Abnormal?
Given the inaccuracies of capillary and CGM-derived glucose values, venous plasma glucose remains the gold standard for diagnosis of hypoglycemia. Level 1 hypoglycemia is defined as glucose concentration less than 70 mg/dL (<3.9 mmol/L), level 2 less than 54 mg/dL (<3.0 mmol/L), and level 3 (severe) as alterations in physical or mental status requiring the assistance of others.

What If Obtaining a Venous Sample Is Not Possible?
Verifying that low plasma glucose is present at the time of spontaneous symptoms is challenging, as patients with severe hypoglycemia are often unable to get to a laboratory safely for a blood draw before treating. If venous sampling has not been successful, capillary glucose measurements together with symptom/food/activity logs may provide some information, but the clinician needs to be sure that capillary sampling is not falsely low due to improper technique or peripheral vasoconstriction (eg, Raynaud syndrome).

Can CGM Be Used to Diagnose Hypoglycemia?
Given the false-positive rates for low sensor glucoses with current CGM devices, sensor glucose data should not be used to diagnose hypoglycemia. A study of CGM in healthy individuals provided important perspectives about what is normal based on sensor glucose.[3] Healthy individuals had 1.1% of sensor glucose values less than 70 mg/dL (<3.9 mmol/L), but time below 54 mg/dL (<3.0 mmol/L) was rare (<0.2%). However, 28% of healthy individuals had at least 1 "event" with sensor glucose under 54 mg/dL for at least 15 minutes. These events were more likely to occur during the first 2 days of sensor wear, implicating technology-related issues. Compression-related artifactual low sensor glucose may also complicate interpretation of nocturnal readings. Thus, it is important not to diagnose hypoglycemia on the basis of a few low sensor readings in an otherwise healthy, asymptomatic patient, as these may be part of the normal range of interstitial readings using the available technology. However, masked CGM, together with symptom/food/activity log, can be helpful to identify patterns of glycemic excursions in patients with established hypoglycemia. If CGM or capillary glucose levels are normal at the time of symptoms, this may also help to rule out hypoglycemia as the cause of patient symptoms.

How Can We Identify Causes of Hypoglycemia in Adults?
There are many suggested frameworks for establishing differential diagnosis. In my clinical practice, I usually consider whether the individual is ill-appearing or healthy-appearing (*box*). In this chapter, we will consider evaluation in the healthy-appearing outpatient.

Box. Causes of Hypoglycemia

Ill-appearing patient	Healthy-appearing patient
Medications	**Endogenous hyperinsulinism**
• Insulin and secretagogues	• Insulinoma
• Other medications	• Functional β-cell disorders (often postprandial)
• Medication errors	• Postbariatric (Roux-en-Y gastric bypass, sleeve gastrectomy)
• Total parenteral nutrition	• Postfundoplication
• Ethanol	• Other esophageal/gastric surgery
Critical illness	• Early type 2 diabetes or type 1 diabetes
• Hepatic, renal, cardiac failure	• Noninsulinoma pancreatogenous hyperinsulinemia (NIPHS)
• Liver disease	• Rapid gastric emptying and gastrointestinal dysmotility
• Impaired clearance of insulin	**Autoimmune hypoglycemia**
• Inadequate glycogen stores	• Antibodies to insulin, IR
• Inadequate gluconeogenesis	**Medications:**
• Portosystemic shunts	• Insulin secretagogues, SSRI/SNRI, tramadol, gabapentin, others
• Sepsis	• Ethanol, marijuana
• Malaria	• Medication errors or surreptitious ingestion
Hormone deficiency	**Miscellaneous:**
• Cortisol (adrenal insufficiency)	Adrenal insufficiency
• Glucagon, epinephrine, GH	Autonomic dysfunction
Non–islet-cell tumor – IGF-2, IGF-1, large tumor burden	Pancreas/islet transplant
Malnutrition	Fructose intolerance
	Ackee and unripe lychee fruit intake
	Rare: pathogenic variants in IR, GK, MCT, potassium channels (long QT), mitochondrial disease, and other congenital disorders

Adapted from Cryer PE et al. *J Clin Endocrinol Metab*, 2009; 94(3): 709–728. © The Endocrine Society.

History remains the essential component of the evaluation. What are the symptoms—adrenergic, cholinergic, neuroglycopenia? *Neuroglycopenia mandates full evaluation!* Have you required assistance of others? Have you had upper gastrointestinal surgery? If so, what type, and how long ago? Do symptoms occur in the fasting state, after meals, after activity, during nocturnal hours?

This information may help guide your evaluation, but remember that *insulinoma-related hypoglycemia does not occur only in the fasting state.* Insulinoma-related hypoglycemia occurs exclusively in the postprandial state in 6% of patients and in both fasting and postprandial states in 21%.[4] Moreover, insulinoma can occur in patients who have had gastrointestinal surgery! Personal and family history of multiple endocrine neoplasia syndromes and hypoglycemia should be noted. All medications and supplements should be reviewed, and any history of recent corticosteroid use (including topical/inhaled/injected) should be ascertained.

Once hypoglycemia has been confirmed, laboratory testing should be used to rule out other diagnoses, such as adrenal disease (eg, morning cortisol measurement), noninsulinoma tumor (eg, IGF-2 measurement), and autoimmune hypoglycemia (antibodies to insulin). Overall glycemia should also be assessed (hemoglobin A_{1c} measurement).

How Do We Determine If Excess Insulin Is Causing the Hypoglycemia?

In an ideal world, venous blood samples for glucose, insulin, C-peptide, and proinsulin would be obtained at the time of spontaneous hypoglycemia. However, spontaneous hypoglycemia does not usually occur within close proximity to the clinical laboratory, and delay in treatment to allow travel to a laboratory setting may not be safe. Thus, assessment of insulin secretion in response to fasting is often used to determine if insulin can be appropriately suppressed during fasting or whether insulin secretion remains inappropriately nonsuppressed, as with an insulinoma. If the patient has a family member who can assist with monitoring, fasting can sometimes be started at home in the late afternoon and continued overnight, with continued monitoring in the clinical setting by trained staff for up to a total of 24 hours. If this does not induce hypoglycemia, or if outpatient monitoring is not deemed feasible or safe, hospital admission may be required. Fasting should continue until hypoglycemia is achieved (venous glucose <45 mg/dL), neuroglycopenia develops, or the total fast duration is 48 to 72 hours. A critical venous blood sample should be obtained for measurement of glucose, insulin, C-peptide, proinsulin, and β-hydroxybutyrate, and antidiabetes medication should be screened. Full suppression of insulin, C-peptide, and proinsulin levels and increases in β-hydroxybutyrate indicate appropriate response to fasting. By contrast, if insulin levels are not fully suppressed, this suggests either endogenous insulin production from insulinoma or sulfonylureas (both with elevated C-peptide, distinguishable with sulfonylurea screen), or exogenous insulin administration (undetectable C-peptide). Proinsulin levels can be helpful as some tumors secrete predominantly proinsulin. If exogenous insulin administration is suspected, but insulin levels are not elevated, specific insulin assays that can detect insulin analogues should be performed. Online nomograms can help with interpretation.

Additional information about insulin action can be obtained from analysis of β-hydroxybutyrate, which will remain suppressed if insulin action is ongoing despite fasting, and by glycemic response to injection of glucagon (1 mg) at the end of the fast. A rise in glucose greater than 25 mg/dL at 30 minutes implicates presence of glycogen, consistent with inappropriate insulin action during the fast. A rise in glucose less than 25 mg/dL at 30 minutes postglucagon suggests that the fast has depleted glycogen stores, consistent with appropriate suppression of insulin action during the fast. If insulin action is present, but insulin and C-peptide levels are not diagnostic, proinsulin should be measured, as some insulinomas secrete predominantly proinsulin.

If a patient has predominantly postprandial hypoglycemia, there are no consistent guidelines or standards for interpreting provocative testing. Consuming food that typically provokes hypoglycemia, or a mixed-meal test, may be considered. Given that some insulinomas only cause hypoglycemia in the postprandial state, fasting testing should still be considered if clinical suspicion is high.

If Insulin Is Not Suppressed During Fasting, How Do We Localize the Insulinoma?

Contrast CT and MRI can be first steps for imaging. If these are negative, endoscopic ultrasonography by an experienced gastroenterologist provides enhanced sensitivity.[5] Additional options (rarely needed) include DOTATATE (somatostatin analogue) imaging and selective arterial calcium-stimulation testing (requiring an experienced interventional radiologist).

Therapies for Hypoglycemia

Treatment options are determined by the diagnosis. Insulinomas or non–islet-cell tumors require surgical resection. Other causes of reactive hypoglycemia are typically managed with medical nutrition therapy to reduce intake of simple carbohydrates and acarbose to limit glycemic stimulus for insulin secretion. Additional dietary and medication strategies for the management of postbariatric hypoglycemia are reviewed elsewhere.[1]

Irrespective of diagnosis, strategies to improve safety are important. Patients—especially those with hypoglycemia unawareness—should have access to home glucose monitoring and CGM to test glucose in high-risk situations (eg, before driving), but insurance coverage is currently woefully inadequate. Patients should always have treatment options with them, including glucose tablets/gel/food and should be advised to wear medical identification tags. Family members and patients should be instructed in the use of glucagon preparations. Supplemental cornstarch, a very complex carbohydrate, should be considered.

Clinical Case Vignettes

Case 1

A 62-year-old man is referred for evaluation of possible hypoglycemia. He has had random plasma glucose values in the range of 50 to 60 mg/dL (2.8-3.3 mmol/L) on routine laboratory testing over the last 5 years. Further evaluation was not performed because the patient reported no symptoms and low glucose values were attributed to high leukocyte count from chronic lymphocytic leukemia diagnosed 13 years earlier (white blood cell count, 25,000-30,000/μL). Recent routine laboratory testing revealed a glucose value of 49 mg/dL (2.7 mmol/L). Home glucose monitoring was initiated, which documented capillary glucose levels ranging from 42 to 119 mg/dL (2.3-6.6 mmol/L), with low values often occurring in late afternoon. Flash glucose monitoring revealed 45% of sensor glucose under 70 mg/dL and 1% under 54 mg/dL.

The patient is referred for evaluation of hypoglycemia and to determine whether this is true or artifactual hypoglycemia.

Which of the following factors can contribute to artifactual hypoglycemia?

A. Poor tissue perfusion (Raynaud syndrome, shock, sepsis, severe vascular disease, severe acidosis) when capillary glucose is measured

B. Inaccuracy of CGM

C. Delayed blood processing (separation of serum/plasma from red/white blood cells), especially in patients with high levels of leukocytes or red blood cells, elevated viscosity, or trypanosomiasis

D. All of the above

Answer: D) All of the above

Both red and white blood cells metabolize glucose. As long as serum/plasma remains in contact with these cells, glucose concentration can be reduced by 5% to 7% per hour. Since glycolysis in white blood cells can be even higher, marked artifactual lowering of glucose can occur in the setting of pathologic leukocytosis (as with leukemia, lymphoma), especially if samples are not separated quickly and are allowed to remain at room temperature. Fluoride present in gray blood collection tubes inhibits glycolysis, but this may not be adequate in patients with severe leukocytosis. Serum separator tubes that have been immediately centrifuged may be used for reproducible plasma glucose determinations for as long as 4 days, even at room temperature. Hyperviscosity (eg, Waldenstrom macroglobulinemia, other myeloma, and monoclonal gammopathy of undetermined significance) can also be associated with artifactual hypoglycemia.

CGM technology has rapidly evolved over the past decade. Mean absolute relative difference (MARD) is widely used to report accuracy of CGM in individuals with diabetes. However, accuracy at low glucose levels is lower, with both low sensitivity to detect hypoglycemia (44%) and high rates of falsely low glucose levels (7%) recently reported in a pediatric hyperinsulinemia population using current CGM technology.[6] Unfortunately, the use of personal CGM, even in patients without diabetes, is increasing, potentially resulting in another cause of "pseudohypoglycemia."

Case 1 (continued)

Upon detailed history, the patient reports an increase in longstanding excessive sweating, also attributed to chronic lymphocytic leukemia, and occasional dizziness. His wife notes some slowness in thinking, tendency to "eat a lot of sugar," and increased anxiety around eating times, with improvement after meals. His family history is negative for multiple endocrine neoplasia type 1 or hypoglycemia.

Physical examination findings are notable for massive splenomegaly, but no other masses.

After an overnight fast of 14 hours, venous plasma glucose measured immediately in the clinic setting is 51 mg/dL (2.8 mmol/L), with some sweating and slow speech noted. Concurrent hormonal analysis:

Insulin = 18.2 μIU/mL (3-19 μIU/mL)
C-peptide = 8.63 ng/mL (1.1-4.2 ng/mL)
β-Hydroxybutyrate = 0.1 mmol/L
Insulin antibodies, undetectable

Which of the following is the best next step?

A. Proceed with a 72-hour fast

B. Insulin levels are normal, so recommend no further evaluation, as this is likely artifactual hypoglycemia

C. Measure proinsulin levels and order imaging for localization of possible insulinoma vs noninsulinoma pancreatogenous hypoglycemia syndrome

D. Advise him to continue to eat sweets

Answer: C) Measure proinsulin levels and order imaging for localization of possible insulinoma vs noninsulinoma pancreatogenous hypoglycemia syndrome

Given that his glucose concentration was 51 mg/dL (2.8 mmol/L) after an overnight fast, in association with inappropriately high insulin levels, further fasting testing is not required. Proinsulin levels were elevated at 110 pmol/L (<19 pmol/L), further confirming hyperinsulinism. Imaging was ordered to determine whether insulin excess was related to insulinoma or noninsulinoma pancreatogenous hyperinsulinemia syndrome (Answer C), a rare disorder usually causing hypoglycemia in the postprandial state.

Case 1 (continued)

CT reveals a 1.8-cm well-circumscribed rounded nodule with enhancement along the inferior margin of the distal body/tail of the pancreas. MRI evaluation suggests this is an accessory spleen. DOTATATE scan is negative. Endoscopic ultrasonography reveals fatty infiltration of the pancreas but no mass. He is referred to our institution for further evaluation. Repeat endoscopic ultrasonography shows an intrapancreatic lymph node, which is biopsied; pathology is consistent with lymphatic tissue. An additional lesion is seen and thought to be a splenule. Given that imaging has been inconclusive despite documented inappropriate insulin secretion, and patient is thought to be high risk for blind exploratory surgery, a selective arterial calcium-stimulation test is performed to localize the source of the excessive insulin secretion. Arteriography does not reveal a tumor. Insulin levels obtained from the hepatic vein after injection of calcium into vessels supplying the pancreas are shown in the table. C-peptide levels are similar in pattern.

Time after calcium injection	Superior mesenteric artery	Gastro-duodenal artery	Proximal splenic artery	Distal splenic artery
0 sec	13	13	17	22
30 sec	14	26	104	266
60 sec	10	30	188	498
90 sec	11	28	152	404
120 sec	7	28	161	234

Insulin values presented in μIU/mL.

What do these results indicate?

A. Noninsulinoma pancreatogenous hyperinsulinemia syndrome

B. Insulinoma outside of the pancreas

C. Insulinoma in the head of the pancreas

D. Insulinoma in the tail of the pancreas

E. Increased blood flow through splenic artery due to splenomegaly

Answer: D) Insulinoma in the tail of the pancreas

Insulin levels were markedly stimulated by injection of calcium into the distal splenic artery, suggesting insulinoma in the tail of the pancreas (Answer D). The patient underwent laparoscopic surgery. Splenectomy was required for adequate visualization. The tumor was identified in the tail of the pancreas, adjacent to an accessory spleen. Distal pancreatectomy was performed. Hypoglycemia resolved after brief, mild hyperglycemia in the postoperative period. Pathology confirmed insulinoma. Results of multiple endocrine neoplasia type 1 genetic testing were negative.

Take-home points:

- If you suspect pseudohypoglycemia, measure plasma glucose in a laboratory setting where you can be assured that sample processing is rapid and appropriate. This may need to be done several times, and in the setting of the factors associated with the prior low glucose values (eg, fasting).

- Do not rely on CGM for diagnosis of hypoglycemia for several reasons: (1) healthy people have sensor glucose levels less than 70 mg/dL and (2) CGM can give falsely low glucose levels, not verified by capillary or venous glucose.[3] Adrenergic and cholinergic symptoms of hypoglycemia are often nonspecific, so low sensor glucose at the time of symptoms does not necessarily indicate that hypoglycemia is the cause of those symptoms. To achieve the Whipple triad, symptoms occurring with documented low glucose (preferably venous, possibly capillary) and relief with treatment to raise glucose must be documented.

- One study using CGM in asymptomatic, metabolically healthy individuals with normal BMI demonstrated that 96% of all readings were between 70 and 140 mg/dL, with only 1.1% of values less than 70 mg/dL (<3.9 mmol/L) and rarely values below 54 mg/dL (<3.0 mmol/L) (<0.2%).[3] However, 28% of healthy individuals had

at least 1 "event" with sensor glucose under 54 mg/dL for at least 15 minutes. Given these data, it is important to encourage patients to test glucose with capillary glucose to verify low sensor glucose, especially during the first 1 to 2 days after sensor application.

- If insulin and C-peptide levels are not 100% clear, be sure to measure proinsulin levels at the same time. Do not forget that other measures of insulin action can be helpful, especially during a fast. If insulin metabolic effect is present, insulin will repress lipolysis and ketogenesis; thus, β-hydroxybutyrate should be low after a prolonged fast if insulin action is present. Likewise, response to glucagon at the end of a prolonged fast can help discriminate between low insulin action (glycogen depleted, low response to glucagon) or high insulin action (glycogen still present, higher response to glucagon).

- If the biochemistry is clear, but imaging is not, keep pursuing imaging options, or consider sending the patient to exploratory surgery by an experienced surgeon, with intraoperative ultrasonography.

- Future imaging options may include GLP-1 receptor agonist imaging, given that insulinoma cells express abundant GLP-1 receptors on their surface.[7]

Case 2

A 54-year-old man with a 19-year history of type 2 diabetes mellitus well controlled on metformin and thiazolidinediones presents with episodic postprandial hypoglycemia. Symptoms began 1 month following acute myocardial infarction, with both adrenergic and neuroglycopenic symptoms typically occurring within 1 hour after meals if meals were delayed, and in response to exercise, with no fasting or nocturnal episodes. He began consuming additional carbohydrate snacks prior to exercise to prevent hypoglycemia and treated symptoms successfully with glucose tablets. Symptoms were attributed to initiation of lifestyle modifications after the myocardial infarction, including dietary restriction and increased physical activity, which had resulted in a 24-lb (10.9-kg) weight loss. Despite withdrawal of metformin and thiazolidinedione therapy, hypoglycemia persists.

The patient reports he does not use insulin, other diabetes medications, or supplements. He has no personal history of hypoglycemia, including during episodic dieting. In retrospect, over the past year, he noted that during a long shift at work without meals, he would feel "grumpy" and eat candy for relief, and a random glucose measurement 6 months previously was 66 mg/dL (3.7 mmol/L) (on metformin and rosiglitazone). His family history is negative for hypoglycemia or multiple endocrine neoplasia but is positive for type 2 diabetes, obesity, and pancreatic adenocarcinoma.

On physical examination, his BMI is 28 kg/m^2, blood pressure is normal, and he has mild abdominal obesity. He has no hyperpigmentation, vitiligo, acanthosis, hepatomegaly, or abdominal masses. Home glucose monitoring demonstrates fasting glucose of 70 to 90 mg/dL (3.9-5.0 mmol/L) and 2-hour postprandial glucose of 44 to 60 mg/dL (2.4-3.3 mmol/L). Continuous glucose monitoring reveals that 27% of all sensor glucose values are less than 70 mg/dL (<3.9 mmol/L), including midnocturnal (12-2 AM) and afternoon (2-4 PM) values.

Overnight fasting is not successful in inducing hypoglycemia.

Which of the following is the best next step in this patient's evaluation?

A. Extended fasting in a monitored setting

B. Glucose tolerance testing

C. Continue to follow over time

D. Tell the patient nothing is wrong as he does not have any fasting hypoglycemia

Answer: A) Extended fasting in a monitored setting

An extended overnight fasting evaluation (Answer A) was conducted in the office setting under close observation. After a 15-hour fast, the patient was noted to have some sweating and decreased cognitive function.

Laboratory test results:

Plasma glucose = 50 mg/dL
Inappropriate insulin secretion, insulin = 36 μIU/mL
C-peptide = 4.4 ng/dL
Proinsulin = 310 pmol/L
β-Hydroxybutyrate, inappropriately low
Insulin antibodies, negative
Free T$_4$, normal
Prolactin, normal
Cortisol, normal
Calcium, normal
PTH, normal
Chromogranin A, normal

MRI revealed a 1-cm mass in the head of the pancreas, near the superior mesenteric artery. The mass was resected using robot-assisted minimally invasive central pancreatectomy. Pathologic examination findings were consistent with a well-differentiated, 0.9-cm insulinoma, grade 1 of 3 (World Health Organization classification), with focal low-grade pancreatic intraepithelial neoplasia (PanIN1). Insulin staining was diffusely positive. Postoperatively, glucose increased to diabetes-range levels, requiring reinstitution of metformin and ultimately both prandial and basal insulin.

Take-home messages:

- Insulinoma can rarely occur in patients with type 2 diabetes. Insulinoma should be suspected if progressive hypoglycemia persists after withdrawal of diabetes medications.

- Although we always think of insulinoma causing hypoglycemia in the fasting state, insulinoma-related hypoglycemia can be exclusively postprandial in 6%, both fasting and postprandial in 21%, and only fasting in 73%.[4]

- Given day-to-day variability in glucose metabolism, repeated testing may be required to attain hypoglycemia sufficient for diagnostic testing.

Case 3

A 41-year-old woman with a BMI of 44 kg/m² undergoes sleeve gastrectomy. Her postoperative course is complicated by cardiac arrest due to polymorphic ventricular tachycardia and prolonged QT interval (as long as 576 msec). Several weeks after surgery, the patient develops episodic headache, sweatiness, shakiness, and nightmares, despite following a diet of low–glycemic index foods. In retrospect, she notes that similar symptoms of headache, sweating, confusion, and lightheadedness began in her 20s, and symptoms were relieved by food. Workup was not performed at that time. She began to gain weight, and weight-loss efforts, including diet and exercise, resulted in more symptoms.

Capillary glucose readings are initiated, and values are as low as 33 mg/dL (1.8 mmol/L) at the time of symptoms, largely in the postprandial state. Clinical and laboratory analysis does not suggest non–insulin-mediated causes of hypoglycemia, such as malnutrition, kidney and liver disease, adrenal disease, or sepsis.

Due to the severity of hypoglycemia and recent cardiac arrest, the patient is hospitalized for a diagnostic fast to assess insulin secretion and its suppressibility with fasting. Blood glucose values decrease progressively with fasting, with nadir value of 52 mg/dL (2.9 mmol/L) at 46 hours of fasting with associated headache, sweating, shakiness, and slowed thinking. The fast is terminated due to mild neuroglycopenia and concerns for safety if glucose continues to fall, given her recent cardiac arrest.

Concurrent laboratory test results:

Insulin = 1.9 μIU/mL (2.0-19.6 μIU/mL)
C-peptide = 0.54 ng/mL (0.80-3.85 ng/mL)
Proinsulin = <7.5 pmol/L (≤18.8 pmol/L)
β-Hydroxybutyrate = 2.5 mmol/L
Glucagon = 73 pg/mL (8-57 pg/mL)

Glucose rises minimally to 67 mg/dL (3.7 mmol/L) after administration of 1 mg glucagon, consistent with depletion of glycogen stores during fasting. Together, these results are consistent with lack of autonomous insulin secretion in the fasting state, confirming the clinical pattern of largely prandial insulin secretion.

Which of the following should be considered?

A. She has an atypical insulinoma with predominantly postprandial insulin secretion

B. She has postbariatric hypoglycemia and should be treated with medical nutrition therapy and addition of acarbose

C. She could have a genetic long QT syndrome that could be contributing to both polymorphic ventricular tachycardia and hypoglycemia

Answer: C) She could have a genetic long QT syndrome that could be contributing to both polymorphic ventricular tachycardia and hypoglycemia

Suppression of insulin secretion during the diagnostic fast, along with an increase in β-hydroxybutyrate and reduced response to glucagon, suggests that insulin metabolic effect is not present during fasting.

Hypoglycemia occurring within weeks of bariatric surgery is highly atypical, as most patients with typical forms of postbariatric hypoglycemia present between 1 and 3 years postoperatively. Thus, individuals who develop hypoglycemia early postoperatively (eg, <6-12 months) should have aggressive evaluation for other causes of hypoglycemia.

Given the coexistence of hypoglycemia and prolonged QT interval in this patient (also subsequently found in her daughter), we considered an underlying genetically determined long QT syndrome as a potential contributor to her hypoglycemia. Genetic testing revealed a pathogenic variant in the *KCNQ1* gene, which encodes subunits of the voltage-gated potassium channels ($K_v7.1$) and ($K_v11.1$) that are expressed in both cardiomyocytes and pancreatic β cells. Patients with loss-of-function pathogenic variants in *KCNQ1* or *KCNH1* have longer QT, lower serum glucose and potassium levels, and increases in postprandial GLP-1 and insulin secretion.[8] For this patient, therapeutic goals to reduce the risk of recurrent arrhythmia included avoidance of medications that prolong the QT interval, as well as prevention of both hypokalemia and hypoglycemia. Medical nutrition therapy was aimed at reducing postprandial glycemic spikes that could stimulate insulin secretion and increase risk for subsequent hypoglycemia after meals. Given the potential for hypoglycemia-related arrhythmia, low-dosage diazoxide was prescribed at bedtime to reduce nocturnal hypoglycemia, and CGM was provided to help the patient recognize possible impending hypoglycemia and treat before severe hypoglycemia developed.

Take-home message:

- Patients with a history of long QT syndrome may have reactive hypoglycemia. Any patient considering bariatric surgery who has a personal history or family history of long QT syndrome should be fully evaluated to exclude hypoglycemia. Risk-to-benefit ratio of surgery should be extensively discussed, as bariatric surgery is likely to further increase postprandial GLP-1 and insulin secretion, thus increasing the risk of severe hypoglycemia and further prolongation of the QT interval.

Case 4

A 41-year-old woman with a BMI of 38 kg/m² is planning gastric bypass and is referred by her surgeon for advice regarding whether surgery should be performed due to potential hypoglycemia. Since her early 20s, the patient has noted symptoms of lightheadedness, shakiness, palpitations, sweating, and difficulty concentrating that are relieved by eating within 15 minutes. Symptoms do not occur in the fasting state and are more likely to occur several hours after eating or after activity, especially in the afternoon. Symptoms are more frequent during periods of dieting. There is no history of neonatal hypoglycemia. Family history is notable for similar symptoms in her mother (never evaluated), and she has no findings consistent with multiple endocrine neoplasia type 1.

Five years earlier, the patient had seen an endocrinologist and was provided a home glucose meter. Her minimum capillary glucose concentration was 59 mg/dL (3.3 mmol/L) at the time of weakness, 1.5 hours after a meal. The patient was told she had reactive hypoglycemia and was advised to follow a low–glycemic index diet. Further evaluation was not pursued.

Current medications include long-term fluoxetine for mild depression.

Physical examination reveals central adiposity and no acanthosis or lipodystrophy.

Laboratory test results (sample collected after an overnight fast):

Hemoglobin A_{1c} = 5.0%
Glucose = 85 mg/dL
Insulin = 8 μIU/mL
C-peptide = 2 ng/mL
Cortisol, normal
Insulin antibodies, undetectable

Which of the following medications has/have been associated with hypoglycemia?

A. Antidepressants, including SSRI, SNRI, MAO-I classes

B. Marijuana

C. Gabapentin

D. Tramadol

E. All of the above

Answer: E) All of the above

Beyond insulin, sulfonylureas, and meglitinides, multiple drugs can aggravate hypoglycemia,[9] including SSRIs. SNRIs, gabapentin, and tramadol. Ethanol can promote hypoglycemia via inhibition of gluconeogenesis, and marijuana has been associated with increased risk of hypoglycemia.

Case 4 (continued)

Which of the following is the best recommendation?

A. Proceed with gastric bypass

B. Recommend sleeve gastrectomy instead of bypass

C. Explain that studies have shown that hypoglycemia following bariatric surgery is more common in those individuals who report a history of hypoglycemia symptoms preoperatively, even if it was not evaluated. Given that postbariatric hypoglycemia can be quite severe, refractory to treatment in some patients, and not completely reversible, recommend against surgery at this time.

Answer: C) Explain that studies have shown that hypoglycemia following bariatric surgery is more common in those individuals who report a history of hypoglycemia symptoms preoperatively, even if it was not evaluated. Given that postbariatric hypoglycemia can be quite severe, refractory to treatment in some patients, and not completely reversible, recommend against surgery at this time.

A recent analysis of a longitudinal cohort of more than 2000 patients who had bariatric surgery revealed that the greatest single risk factor for self-reported postoperative hypoglycemia was preoperative hypoglycemia (Answer C).[10] In addition, patients without diabetes preoperatively who were taking SSRIs or SNRIs were more likely to report postoperative hypoglycemia.

Although mechanisms of action may differ somewhat, hypoglycemia occurs after both gastric bypass and sleeve gastrectomy with similar frequency. A recent study demonstrated that glycemic patterns in patients with hypoglycemia after Roux-en-Y gastric bypass include postprandial glucose "spikes" followed by rapid drop to hypoglycemia levels. Patients with hypoglycemia after sleeve gastrectomy have lower-magnitude glycemic spikes but similar nadir glucose levels.[11]

Case 4 (continued)

The patient is disappointed with this advice. However, after conversing with others she had met online in postbariatric hypoglycemia support groups, she appreciates the potential severity of postbariatric hypoglycemia and the lack of complete resolution after reversal surgery.[12] The bariatric surgeon concurs with the plan to pursue medical therapy for obesity instead.

Which of the following is the best next step?

A. Pursue complete evaluation for hypoglycemia, including evaluation of current glycemic pattens and consideration of both fasting and mixed-meal testing

B. Enroll in a comprehensive weight-loss program, including medical nutrition therapy and activity

C. After completion of hypoglycemia evaluation, consider gradual GLP-1 receptor agonist therapy with careful observation for possible aggravation of hypoglycemia during therapy

D. All of the above

Answer: D) All of the above

Substantive data are lacking regarding the efficacy and safety of GLP-1 receptor agonists in the management of obesity in individuals with reactive hypoglycemia (including postbariatric hypoglycemia). Use of these agents might initially seem to be counterintuitive given that high levels of GLP-1 are characteristic of the postprandial hormonal response in postbariatric hypoglycemia[1] and data regarding use of GLP-1 receptor antagonists to reduce hypoglycemia are promising.[13] However, it is possible that GLP-1 receptor agonists may also improve reactive hypoglycemia in postbariatric hypoglycemia, potentially via slowing gastric emptying and/or sustained occupancy of the GLP-1 receptor, limiting surges in *endogenous* GLP-1 action and insulin secretion after meals and reducing glycemic variability. One study compared 5 different approaches to postbariatric hypoglycemia[14] and found no significant impact of liraglutide 1.2 mg in glycemic or insulin response to a mixed meal. (By contrast, both acarbose and octreotide were successful in reducing hypoglycemia.) Liraglutide did yield improvements in CGM-derived indices of both hyperglycemia and hypoglycemia. Additional data are largely derived from small case reports.[15]

Experience in our patient population with reactive hypoglycemia has demonstrated variable response, with some patients experiencing improvement and some patients noting increased frequency and severity of hypoglycemia. Given the paucity of data thus far, we recommend that patients be fully evaluated before consideration of GLP-1 receptor agonist therapy, and that patients should be carefully monitored during initiation and dosage escalation. Moreover, we do not advocate use of GLP-1 receptor agonists until fasting hypoglycemia and autonomous insulin secretion (insulinoma) have been fully excluded, as GLP-1 receptors are highly expressed on the surface of insulinomas.

Key Learning Points

- Insulinoma may present with only postprandial hypoglycemia.

- Despite improvements in localization of insulinoma, including endoscopic ultrasonography, selective arteriography and calcium-stimulated venous sampling by an experienced interventional radiologist may still be required in some patients.

- If the history and clinical scenario indicate that insulin action is likely to be the cause of hypoglycemia, use multiple strategies—beyond just insulin and C-peptide levels—to assess metabolic response to hypoglycemia and determine if insulin action is playing a role: (1) ketogenic response to fasting, (2) response to glucagon at the end of a prolonged fast, and (3) measurement of proinsulin levels. This is especially important if insulin values are not clearly diagnostic.

- Hypoglycemia in patients with type 2 diabetes persisting despite withdrawal of antihyperglycemic medications should be fully evaluated to rule out autonomous insulin secretion and rare coexisting insulinoma.

- Pseudohypoglycemia has long been recognized to be caused by delayed processing of blood samples, especially in those individuals with high leukocyte counts, or by peripheral vasoconstriction resulting in falsely low capillary glucose. This term may now also be applied to erroneous results from CGM (often patient-initiated). Nevertheless, true hypoglycemia needs to be ruled out by repeated analysis of venous glucose levels with appropriate processing.

- Multiple medications can increase the severity of hypoglycemia.

- Patients who are considering bariatric surgery for obesity should be asked about history of hypoglycemic symptoms. Even if these symptoms were not formally evaluated in the past, prior symptoms are the dominant clinical risk factor identified to date for postbariatric hypoglycemia. Given that reversal of bariatric surgery is usually incomplete and may not resolve hypoglycemia, instead consider use of lifestyle and dietary modifications, and (reversible) medications to treat obesity in these patients. If GLP-1 receptor agonists are chosen, careful follow-up will be required to ensure that hypoglycemia does not worsen.

- Long QT syndrome may be associated with hypoglycemia.

References

1. Salehi M, Vella A, McLaughlin T, Patti M-E. Hypoglycemia after gastric bypass surgery: current concepts and controversies. *J Clin Endocrinol Metab.* 2018;103(8):2815-2826. PMID: 30101281

2. Sandoval DA, Patti ME. Glucose metabolism after bariatric surgery: implications for T2DM remission and hypoglycaemia. *Nat Rev Endocrinol.* 2023;19(3):164-176. PMID: 36289368

3. Shah VN, DuBose SN, Li Z, et al. Continuous glucose monitoring profiles in healthy nondiabetic participants: a multicenter prospective study. *J Clin Endocrinol Metab.* 2019;104(10):4356-4364. PMID: 31127824

4. Placzkowski KA, Vella A, Thompson GB, et al. Secular trends in the presentation and management of functioning insulinoma at the Mayo Clinic, 1987-2007. *J Clin Endocrinol Metab.* 2009;94(4):1069-1073. PMID: 19141587

5. Kann PH. Is endoscopic ultrasonography more sensitive than magnetic resonance imaging in detecting and localizing pancreatic neuroendocrine tumors? *Rev Endocr Metab Disord.* 2018;19(2):133-137. PMID: 30267296

6. Worth C, Dunne MJ, Salomon-Estebanez M, et al. The hypoglycaemia error grid: a UK-wide consensus on CGM accuracy assessment in hyperinsulinism. *Front Endocrinol (Lausanne).* 2022;13:1016072. PMID: 36407313

7. Christ E, Wild D, Ederer S, et al. Glucagon-like peptide-1 receptor imaging for the localisation of insulinomas: a prospective multicentre imaging study. *Lancet Diabetes Endocrinol.* 2013;1(2):115-122. PMID: 24622317

8. Hylten-Cavallius L, Iepsen EW, Wewer Albrechtsen NJ, et al. Patients with long-QT syndrome caused by impaired hERG-encoded K(v)11.1 potassium channel have exaggerated endocrine pancreatic and incretin function associated with reactive hypoglycemia. *Circulation.* 2017;135(18):1705-1719. PMID: 28235848

9. Murad MH, Coto-Yglesias F, Wang AT, et al. Clinical review: drug-induced hypoglycemia: a systematic review. *J Clin Endocrinol Metab.* 2009;94(3):741-745. PMID: 19088166

10. Fischer LE, Wolfe BM, Fino N, et al; LABS Investigators. Postbariatric hypoglycemia: symptom patterns and associated risk factors in the Longitudinal Assessment of Bariatric Surgery study. *Surg Obes Relat Dis.* 2021;17(10):1787-1798. PMID: 34294589

11. Lee CJ, Clark JM, Egan JM, et al. Comparison of hormonal response to a mixed-meal challenge in hypoglycemia after sleeve gastrectomy vs gastric bypass. *J Clin Endocrinol Metab.* 2022;107(10):e4159-e4166. PMID: 35914520

12. Arora I, Patti ME. Can reversal of RYGB also reverse hypoglycemia? *Mol Metab.* 2018;9:1-3. PMID: 29371089

13. Craig CM, Lawler HM, Lee CJE, et al. PREVENT: a randomized, placebo-controlled crossover trial of avexitide for treatment of postbariatric hypoglycemia. *J Clin Endocrinol Metab.* 2021;106(8):e3235-e3248. PMID: 33616643

14. Ohrstrom CC, Worm D, Hojager A, et al. Postprandial hypoglycaemia after Roux-en-Y gastric bypass and the effects of acarbose, sitagliptin, verapamil, liraglutide and pasireotide. *Diabetes Obes Metab.* 2019;21(9):2142-2151. PMID: 31144430

15. Llewellyn DC, Ellis HL, Aylwin SJB, et al. The efficacy of GLP-1RAs for the management of postprandial hypoglycemia following bariatric surgery: a systematic review. *Obesity (Silver Spring).* 2023;31(1):20-30. PMID: 36502288

Effective Use of Telehealth in Outpatient Endocrine Care

Varsha Vimalananda, MD, MPH. Center for Healthcare Organization and Implementation Research (CHOIR), Bedford VA Medical Center, Bedford, Massachusetts; Section of Endocrinology, Diabetes, and Nutrition, Boston University Chobanian & Avedisian School of Medicine, Boston, MA; Email: varsha.vimalananda@va.gov

Stephanie Crossen, MD, MPH. Division of Pediatric Endocrinology, University of California Davis Children's Hospital, Sacramento, CA; Center for Health and Technology, University of California Davis, Sacramento, CA; Email: scrossen@ucdavis.edu

Educational Objectives

After reviewing this chapter, learners should be able to:

- Identify the benefits and limitations of using telehealth (video and audio-only encounters) for outpatient endocrine care.

- Evaluate when telehealth may be an appropriate and effective modality for specific endocrine patient scenarios.

- Summarize the current state, future outlook, and available resources related to telehealth policy and reimbursement.

Significance of the Clinical Problem

The COVID-19 pandemic and associated changes in health care policy led to an explosion in use of video and audio-only telehealth for outpatient care. Telehealth offers increased access to and flexibility in endocrine care for patients who do not require a hands-on physical examination or procedure. In these cases, use of telehealth can avoid the drawbacks of in-person visits, including time, cost, and infection exposure. Endocrinology was one of the highest adopters of telehealth, and use persists to a significant degree in our specialty now 3 years after the onset of the US public health emergency. This chapter will provide information to guide clinicians in effective use of telehealth for endocrine care.

Evidence accumulated from prepandemic and postpandemic periods suggests that telehealth is highly convenient for patients and can help to facilitate individualized and person-centered care. However, population-level data demonstrate an ongoing "digital divide" that makes telehealth less accessible for many demographic groups. Other barriers to optimal telehealth use include a need for evidence-based clinical guidance, establishment of ideal telehealth workflows and staffing models, and a still-early body of research to support ongoing improvements to telehealth quality. In addition, payors have chosen to adopt widely varying policies for reimbursement of video and audio-only encounters. At the time of this writing, the US public health emergency is set to expire in May 2023. While some progress has been made to establish permanent changes that support telehealth, other policies are rapidly changing.

Against this complicated backdrop, clinicians have had to draw on their own judgment to define when telehealth is and is not an appropriate modality for care in a given circumstance. The Endocrine Society, in response to this challenge, published a policy perspective that describes 5 major domains to be considered in concert for each patient encounter. These include clinical factors, patient factors, the patient-clinician relationship, clinician factors, and the health care setting. A mix of telehealth and in-person visits can be used over time, with an evaluation at each visit about the best approach for subsequent care. Patient preference should be considered as part of this decision-making.

This chapter will review what is known about the benefits and limitations of telehealth for outpatient endocrine care, offer guidance based on the Endocrine Society Policy Perspective for how clinicians may determine when it is appropriate to employ telehealth, and provide an overview of current and future policies that are likely to impact telehealth use moving forward. While the term *telehealth* can refer to a broad range of technology-supported care modalities, this chapter will focus specifically on synchronous video and audio-only (telephone) encounters between patients and clinicians in an outpatient setting.

Practice Gaps

- Persistent patient-level inequities in access to necessary infrastructure and skills (eg, broadband internet, devices, digital literacy).

- Inconsistent clinician training and practice in use of telehealth for care delivery.

- Lack of established workflows that engage clinical staff to support telehealth encounters.

- A limited body of research from which to identify best practices, benefits, and limitations of telehealth in various scenarios.

- Variability (across locations and time) in telehealth reimbursement policies, hindering consistent investment by health systems.

Discussion

While telehealth had been used in a few settings prior to the COVID-19 pandemic, legislation passed in the United States as part of the pandemic PHE loosened multiple reimbursement-,

licensing-, and HIPAA-related telehealth restrictions, which led to skyrocketing use.[1] In the early part of the pandemic, telehealth accounted for 30% of outpatient visits among commercially insured and Medicare Advantage enrollees, and endocrinology emerged as one of the medical specialties with the highest proportion of visits conducted by telehealth.[2] This high use of telehealth in endocrinology—particularly diabetes care—was also noted internationally.[3] This is likely because endocrine care is especially well-suited to telehealth, relying more heavily on history and test results in most cases than on hands-on physical examination and procedures.

Evidence on Benefits and Limitations of Telehealth

The dramatic increase in telehealth at the start of the pandemic created a large body of observational data about access and use, which added to a smaller body of research about outcomes such as satisfaction and efficacy. Observational studies in a wide variety of populations confirmed lower use of telehealth among older patients and patients with public insurance, minority race or ethnicity, or non-English language preferences. These disparities held true in comparisons of telehealth vs in-person care,[4] as well as video vs audio-only encounters,[5] and appeared to stem from underlying inequities in access to smartphone and internet technology,[6] as well as digital literacy.[7]

In parallel to population studies documenting disparities in telehealth access, multiple publications from pre- and post-COVID have demonstrated its utility in improving health outcomes and patient-reported outcomes for individuals with endocrine conditions, particularly diabetes mellitus. Telehealth use has been associated with improvements in visit frequency, satisfaction, patient engagement and self-efficacy, and glycemic control among patients with diabetes,[8,9] including for communities experiencing geographic access barriers or negative social determinants of health.[10]

The available evidence thus suggests that telehealth may be beneficial for a broader population than has been able to access it to date. However, data remain limited and heterogeneous, with uncertainty whether findings from one population and intervention can be reliably translated to another. Just as "in-person care" cannot be deemed broadly effective or ineffective, telehealth is a care modality that can be used effectively or ineffectively in a variety of situations, and extensive research will be needed to evaluate its many potential applications.

Appropriate Use of Telehealth for Outpatient Endocrine Care

Endocrinologists in practice are at the front line of determining whether a particular patient visit should be conducted in-person or via telehealth, but the determination is not straightforward.[11] There is a shortage of empiric data or clinical practice guidelines to inform such decision-making. In response to this gap, in 2022 the Endocrine Society published a policy perspective that offers guidance to clinicians on appropriate use of telehealth.[12] The piece also offers strategies to support high-quality endocrine care via telehealth and identifies areas for future research.

The perspective was developed among a panel of 9 US academic endocrinologists with relevant expertise. The panel defined appropriate use as that which promotes high-quality care as defined by the Institute of Medicine: patient-centered, equitable, safe, effective, timely, and efficient.[13] Literature search and group discussion were used to develop 5 domains that should be considered in determining whether telehealth would be an appropriate option in a given scenario. The perspective outlines how the 5 domains—clinical factors, patient factors, the patient-clinician relationship, clinician factors, and the health care setting—can influence the effectiveness of telehealth encounters, and how this, in turn, can affect the overall quality of endocrine care. The *figure* lists the domains with considerations for each, and how they may influence the choice of visit modality.

Guide to Appropriate Use of Telehealth Visits for Endocrine Care

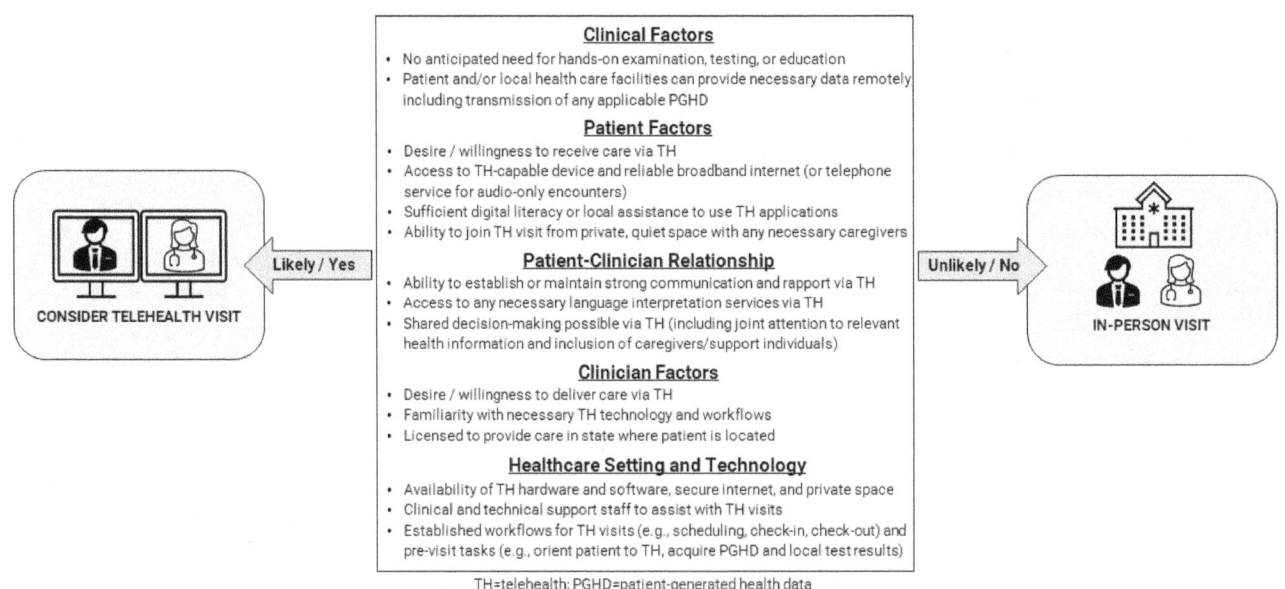

Reprinted from Vimalananda VG et al. J Clin Endocrinol Metab, 2022; 107(11): 2953-2962. © The Endocrine Society.

Several key points should be noted:

- Considerations for each domain must be weighed in the context of the other domains, for each patient.

- This evaluation needs to happen at each visit—a telehealth visit at one point may need to be followed by an in-person visit, or vice versa.

- Telehealth care can involve, at the extremes, all telehealth or all in-person care, but using a combination of modalities over time can provide a high degree of flexibility to adapt to changing priorities.

- If the patient prefers one care modality and clinical concerns can be feasibly, adequately, and safely addressed through that care modality, then patient preference should be weighted strongly.

- The panel did not reach consensus about the absolute appropriateness of telehealth or in-person visits for specific endocrine conditions, since appropriateness is judged in the context of all 5 domains. Clinicians and patients need to work together to weigh the relative importance of competing priorities in the different domains over time.

Clinicians can modify their practices in several ways to deliver high-quality endocrine care via telehealth (*see table*).

Strategies to support high-quality endocrine care via telehealth
Use a combination of in-person and telehealth care
• Complete required assessments or testing at sites close to patient's home when possible.
• Allow multidisciplinary care team members to engage patient via different modalities as appropriate.
• Mix telehealth and in-person visits as part of a longitudinal care plan via shared decision-making process.
• Conclude each visit with careful consideration of optimal care modality for next encounter.

Anticipate and address patient needs related to telehealth
• Establish practice criteria for use of audio-only and video telehealth.
• Allow patients the flexibility to change modality of scheduled visit if needed.
• Proactively assess need for language interpretation services before telehealth encounters.
• Clarify expectations with patient that telehealth will require a private, quiet, safe location for visit.
• Facilitate previsit outreach by clinic support staff to assist with technology and sharing of pertinent patient-generated health data.
• Engage caregivers to participate in visits and/or support patient's use of necessary technology.
Develop personal best practices and skills specific to telehealth
• Ensure private, quiet space from which to deliver care, with adequate and secure broadband access.
• Strengthen relationships over telehealth through building skills in remote engagement and trust-building.
• Become familiar with telehealth hardware, software, clinical workflows, and licensing requirements.
• Develop strong relationships and norms for bidirectional communication with referring clinicians.
• Participate in telehealth training within endocrinology fellowship programs and professional conferences.
Promote health system processes that optimize the telehealth experience and access
• Adopt telehealth platforms with advanced features such as screen sharing and electronic health record integration, and that support broad access, including availability in multiple languages.
• Leverage clinical and information technology staff to support telehealth workflows and improve efficiency of virtual care.
• Advocate for policies that expand access and affordability of telehealth.

Reprinted from Vimalananda VG et al. *J Clin Endocrinol Metab*, 2022; 107(11): 2953-2962. © The Endocrine Society.

Policy and Reimbursement in the United States

As endocrinologists look to optimize their use of telehealth, they must keep in mind the applicable government and payor policies, which are currently in flux. At a national level, the Centers for Medicare and Medicaid Services currently allow video care for Medicare recipients only for specific services and under certain circumstances. As of fall 2022, Medicaid programs in every state will reimburse for video visits, although many also impose restrictions on eligible providers, services, or originating sites.[14] The patient's home is currently permitted as an originating site for telehealth in 36 states and the District of Columbia; in addition, audio-only visits are covered by Medicaid in 34 states and the District of Columbia. However, these policies do not always translate to coverage by commercial payors. At the time of this writing, only 24 states carry laws requiring payment parity for telehealth by commercial insurance plans, and many of these laws are written to expire in 2024 or 2025. In addition, state medical licensure laws remain highly variable regarding the delivery of telehealth across state lines. Thus far, 37 states and the District of Columbia have joined the Interstate Medical Licensure Compact to enable cross-state licensing for physicians,[15] while several other states have developed processes to grant limited telehealth licenses. One of the best sources for up-to-date information about these and other telehealth policies is the Center for Connected Health Policy, which can be accessed online at https://www.cchpca.org/.

Clinical Case Vignettes

Case 1

An 84-year-old woman has well-controlled type 2 diabetes mellitus with stage 3 chronic kidney disease and mild nonproliferative diabetic retinopathy. Her medications for glycemic control include metformin, 500 mg twice daily; insulin glargine, 12 units daily; and once-weekly semaglutide, 1 mg subcutaneously. Her most recent hemoglobin A_{1c} measurement, 2 months after a hospital admission for a urinary tract infection, was 9.2% (77 mmol/mol). This represents a change from her usual values, which tend to run between 7.0% and 8.0% (53-64 mmol/mol). She is scheduled for her regular in-person visit with her endocrinologist. The day before her appointment, she calls to say she feels unwell and cannot come in.

How could telehealth be leveraged to provide effective care in this case?

Upon receiving the patient's call, the clinic staff asked whether she would be interested in converting to a video appointment, if the endocrinologist felt it would be appropriate. The patient said that she would like to do that and would arrange for her daughter to join and help with the logistics. The clinic staff sent a message to the endocrinologist through the electronic health record asking if a video telehealth visit would be appropriate.

The endocrinologist weighed several factors. She had seen the patient in person for more than 10 years and was confident that she would be able to converse effectively over video. She would have liked to examine the patient for any evidence of new infection, but decided that it was better to evaluate over video rather than wait until the patient felt well enough to come in. The patient's daughter was available to assist with the technology, help share blood glucose monitoring data, and coordinate any care needed locally. The endocrinologist had a functional telehealth workflow and lived in the same state as the patient, so was not hindered by policies limiting cross-state care. The scheduled appointment was converted from in-person to video.

Fifteen minutes before the scheduled appointment, clinic staff called the patient, who was with her daughter. The staff member guided the family through the process of connecting to the video visit, so everything was ready at the scheduled appointment time.

During the visit, the endocrinologist was able to ascertain that the patient had not been feeling herself since hospital discharge. Her daughter reported that she seems slightly confused at times and wobbly on her feet. The daughter read out recent blood glucose values, which were all elevated. She showed the medications to the endocrinologist over video, and the patient demonstrated correct injection technique. However, the patient was vague about whether she was remembering to take her medications regularly.

The endocrinologist was concerned about a persistent urinary tract infection or other process causing hyperglycemia and altered mental status. She asked the patient's daughter if they had local care available, and the daughter said it was no problem to have her evaluated at urgent care locally. The daughter was also able to ensure that the patient would take her medications as prescribed until her mental status improved. The endocrinologist asked for an update following that visit and scheduled an in-person visit in 3 weeks.

Notes: In this situation, the endocrinologist switched from in-person to video telehealth because the patient was too sick to come in person. This strategy enabled timely assessment, visual review of medications and injection technique, and involvement of a caregiver. This evaluation facilitated a necessary in-person workup for concurrent illness by another clinician at a location close to the patient's home.

Case 2

A 42-year-old otherwise healthy man has a history of autoimmune hypothyroidism and a 1.2-cm TI-RADS 4 thyroid nodule. He has been on a stable levothyroxine dosage for 3 years and has no problems with adherence. A recent TSH measurement in preparation for this visit was within the target range. He is scheduled for a video telehealth appointment, but at the time of the appointment, he is unable to get his camera to work.

How could telehealth be leveraged to provide effective care in this case?

The endocrinologist determined that video evaluation was not possible and proceeded with audio-only care. His level of clinical concern is low given that the patient's condition has been stable and that his recent TSH value was within the target range. He called the patient on the phone to review the results and ascertained that he felt well and had no concerns about his thyroid disease. The endocrinologist prefers to see his patients in person at least annually, and the patient agrees to attending the next visit in person.

Notes: In this situation, audio-only care was appropriate because of the low clinical complexity, stability of the patient's condition, and availability of lab results. Physical examination was not needed to determine whether a dosage change was needed. At the time of the phone visit, the appropriate modality of care for the subsequent visit was determined and was largely based on the endocrinologist's preference for at least 1 annual in-person evaluation.

Case 3

A 5-year-old girl is referred to endocrinology for precocious puberty. Her mother first noticed breast growth 4 months ago. The patient's primary care provider could not tell on examination whether this was true glandular tissue or fatty tissue associated with recent weight gain. She ordered LH, FSH, and estradiol measurements, which came back below the laboratory's reference ranges for the adult assays. The closest pediatric endocrinologist is a 4-hour drive from the patient's hometown (although in the same state). When contacted to schedule the appointment, the patient's mother requests a video visit because she does not want to take an entire day off work for this consultation, especially since her daughter's lab work was normal. The appointment is scheduled as a telehealth encounter.

How could telehealth be leveraged to provide effective care in this case?

The endocrinologist noted this new patient appointment on her schedule on the morning of the visit and provided feedback to her staff that due to the referral diagnosis (precocious puberty), this should have been an in-person appointment, so that a physical examination could be performed. The staff apologized but explained that the child could not come in person that day (because she lived 4 hours away) and new appointments were booked out 3 months. Given that the endocrinologist thought that the child should be evaluated as soon as possible, she elected to continue with the video visit.

The patient and her mother joined the visit from their car, which was parked outside the child's school. The endocrinologist attempted to establish a rapport with them over video using open-ended questions, attentive listening, and warm facial expressions. She did not perform any visual examination of sensitive body areas because the patient was not in a private space. She explained that the lab work previously completed was not definitive and that without examining the patient in-person, she could not provide an answer about whether the child is in precocious puberty. She explained the typical workup, causes, risks, and treatment considerations for the diagnosis. She then elicited the family's preferences.

The patient's mother expressed an initial preference to do further diagnostic testing (eg, LH, FSH, and estradiol measurement using more sensitive pediatric assays) locally to avoid travel. However, after learning that even normal results could necessitate additional evaluation at the endocrine center (eg, leuprolide-stimulation testing) and that an in-person examination might eliminate the need for the child to have additional blood draws, she opted to schedule an in-person visit with the endocrinologist. Because the child was an established patient at that point, she was scheduled in a follow-up slot that was available in 2 weeks. The follow-up visit focused on the examination and discussion of next steps, since the history and diagnostic discussion took place during the video session.

Notes: This case highlights how telehealth can be used to advance care, even in circumstances that are not ideal. Factors in several domains—such as the need for a physical exam (clinical), the lack of established patient-clinician rapport (relationship), and the endocrinologist's preference (clinician)—would have favored an in-person encounter, but patient and health care factors led it to be scheduled as telehealth. The clinician then had to adapt her practice to provide timely care. Thanks to her efforts, the video consultation enabled an exchange of essential information and shared decision-making that resulted in a safe and effective care plan.

Case 4

A 20-year-old man with longstanding type 1 diabetes mellitus is transferring colleges and will be moving temporarily to another part of the state. He typically has excellent glycemic control, but at the last visit, his hemoglobin A_{1c} level had risen to 8.1% (65 mmol/mol) due to competing time demands and less attention to glucose management between meals. He was subsequently started on a hybrid closed-loop system and has not been seen back since then. He calls to inform his endocrinologist that he is moving and would like to continue in her care, but he will not be able to attend his next appointment, which is scheduled for the following month. He asks whether they can delay his next visit until the following summer, which is 6 months in the future.

How could telehealth be leveraged to provide effective care in this case?

The endocrinologist knew that the patient was motivated and tech-savvy and felt he would be able to navigate the remote data-sharing and video applications necessary to make telehealth possible. They had worked together for several years, so had an established rapport. She did not think that he should go another 6 months without a visit, since he had a rising hemoglobin A_{1c} level and recently started a new automated insulin delivery system. She asked if he would like to change his next appointment to telehealth and outlined the steps he would need to take (downloading several apps and sharing his diabetes device data to the clinic) to make this possible. He agreed, and the clinic staff reached out to assist him with this process. The appointment went well, and together the patient and his endocrinologist made a plan to continue quarterly video visits with an in-person annual visit each summer (when he is home from college) for an in-depth physical examination and recommended screening tests.

Notes: This case illustrates an ideal scenario for telehealth use. The patient and clinician have an established rapport, the patient has sufficient technology access and digital literacy to share patient-generated health data prior to the visits, and it is clinically safe and appropriate to have remote quarterly visits with an annual in-person examination.

Key Learning Points

- Telehealth is likely to remain a major modality for delivery of outpatient endocrine care, requiring endocrinologists to become comfortable with its use and reimbursement considerations.

- Appropriate use of telehealth for a given visit should be determined based on patient preference, as well as considerations within the 5 domains: clinical factors, patient factors, the patient-clinician relationship, clinician factors, and the health care setting.

- Clinicians may be able to modify some aspects of their typical practice to render a telehealth visit appropriate when it would not have been so otherwise.

- Future work is needed to develop the research base about telehealth in endocrinology, standardize clinician and trainee education in telehealth, and strengthen policies that promote widespread and equitable access to clinically appropriate telehealth.

References

1. Mehrotra A, Chernew ME, Linetsky D, Hatch H, Cutler DM, Schneider EC. *The Impact of the COVID-19 Pandemic on Outpatient Visits: Changing Patterns of Care in the Newest COVID-19 Hot Spots.* 2020.

2. Patel SY, Mehrotra A, Huskamp HA, Uscher-Pines L, Ganguli I, Barnett ML. Variation in telemedicine use and outpatient care during the COVID-19 pandemic in the United States. *Health Aff (Millwood).* 2021;40(2):349-358. PMID: 33523745

3. Scott SN, Fontana FY, Zuger T, Laimer M, Stettler C. Use and perception of telemedicine in people with type 1 diabetes during the COVID-19 pandemic-results of a global survey. *Endocrinol Diabetes Metab.* 2020;4(1):e00180. PMID: 33532617

4. Haynes SC, Kompala T, Neinstein A, Rosenthal J, Crossen S. Disparities in telemedicine use for subspecialty diabetes care during COVID-19 shelter-in-place orders. *J Diabetes Sci Technol.* 2021;15(5):986-992. PMID: 33719622

5. Ye S, Kronish I, Fleck E, et al. Telemedicine expansion during the COVID-19 pandemic and the potential for technology-driven disparities. *J Gen Intern Med.* 2021;36(1):256-258. PMID: 33105000

6. Pew Research Center. Internet/Broadband Fact Sheet. Accessed September 30, 2022. Available at: https://www.pewresearch.org/internet/fact-sheet/internet-broadband/

7. Nouri S, Khoong EC, Lyles CR, Karliner L. Addressing equity in telemedicine for chronic disease management during the Covid-19 pandemic. *NEJM Catalyst Innovations in Care Delivery.* 2020;1(3)1-13.

8. Crossen SS, Bruggeman BS, Haller MJ, Raymond JK. Challenges and opportunities in using telehealth for diabetes care. *Diabetes Spectr.* 2022;35(1):33-42. PMID: 35308158

9. Tchero H, Kangambega P, Briatte C, Brunet-Houdard S, Retali GR, Rusch E. Clinical effectiveness of telemedicine in diabetes mellitus: a meta-analysis of 42 randomized controlled trials. *Telemed J E Health.* 2019;25(7):569-583. PMID: 30124394

10. Crossen SS, Wagner DV. Narrowing the divide: the role of telehealth in type 1 diabetes care for marginalized communities. *J Diabetes Sci Technol.* 2023 [in press]

11. Sitter KE, Wong DH, Bolton RE, Vimalananda VG. Clinical appropriateness of telehealth: a qualitative study of endocrinologists' perspectives. *J Endocr Soc.* 2022;6(8):bvac089. PMID: 35775013

12. Vimalananda VG, Brito JP, Eiland LA, et al. Appropriate use of telehealth visits in endocrinology: policy perspective of the Endocrine Society. *J Clin Endocrinol Metab.* 2022;107(11):2953-2962. PMID: 36194041

13. Institute of Medicine Committee on Quality of Health Care in America. *Crossing the Quality Chasm: A New Health System for the 21st Century.* The National Academies Press; 2001. Accessed November 29, 2022. Available at: https://www.ncbi.nlm.nih.gov/pubmed/25057539

14. Center for Connected Health Policy. State Telehealth Laws and Reimbursement Policies Report, Fall 2022. Accessed February 4, 2023. Available at: https://www.cchpca.org/resources/state-telehealth-laws-and-reimbursement-policies-report-fall-2022/

15. Interstate Medical Licensure Compact. Accessed February 6, 2023. Available at: https://www.imlcc.org/

What to Do When Patients With Diabetes Have Suboptimal Glycemic Control

Carol H. Wysham, MD. University of Washington, MultiCare Rockwood Clinic, Spokane, WA; Email: chwysham@comcast.net

Educational Objectives

After reviewing this chapter, learners should be able to:

- Identify patient barriers to achievement of good glycemic control.

- Identify and implement changes to the design of their clinic to improve identification and management of patients with suboptimally controlled diabetes.

- Determine when to use technology in assessment and management of diabetes.

Significance of the Clinical Problem

The importance of achievement of good glycemic control for prevention of microvascular complications has been well-demonstrated in patients with type 1 and type 2 diabetes mellitus.[1,2] However, worldwide, most people with diabetes do not achieve glycemic control, especially those who have type 1 diabetes and with increasing duration of diabetes.[3,4] Certain populations with diabetes may have particular challenges to achievement of control: young adults and those with other complex medical issues, limited social support, limited financial resources, and limited proficiency in the language of the country in which they live. There are many explanations for suboptimal management of glycemic control, involving patient-related knowledge and behaviors, provider knowledge and behaviors, and, most importantly, a health care system that is fragmented and is poorly designed to handle the needs of those with chronic illness.[5] The chronic care model has been proposed as a framework around which a system can more effective manage chronic disease.[6] The core elements of the chronic care model include:

1. Delivery system design—coordinated, team-based planned visits to increase efficiency of interactions

2. Self-management support—ensuring patient has knowledge base and support needed to enhance self-care

3. Decision support—evidence-based guidelines

4. Clinical information systems—ability to identify patient-specific, as well as population-based, support to the health care team

5. Community resources—support patients in maintaining a healthy lifestyle

6. Health system—foster a culture based on quality[6]

In a 5-year study, compared with outcomes associated with usual care, patients enrolled in the chronic care model experienced a reduction in cardiovascular disease risk (56.6%), microvascular complications (11.9%), and mortality (66.1%), while substantially reducing costs.[7,8]

Obviously, implementing the full chronic care model requires buy-in from the leadership of involved organizations. However, clinicians can focus on parts of the model that are more in their control:

- Changing how patients with diabetes are scheduled (diabetes-specific visit).

- Delegating to office staff referring for eye examinations, ordering routine laboratory test results, and performing foot examinations.

- Having appropriate experts in technology on the care team.

- Ensuring that there is a system that will promote having all data available before the appointment.

- Working with IT to provide lists of patients with very high hemoglobin A_{1c} values, uncontrolled lipids, high blood pressure, and/or those who have not had an appointment for more than 6 months to target those individuals for more intensive monitoring (ie, remote monitoring)/management (boot camp). This can also be delegated to staff.

- Using diabetes education and care specialists more fully to help assess reasons for suboptimal control and to provide patients with tools needed to help them improve control. We have patients see diabetes care and education specialists before they come for their consultation.

- Using telehealth to complement in-person visits.

- Using diabetes technology to the fullest, which includes encouraging patients to upload their technology data from home. This allows for more remote monitoring, which can be done by the clinic nursing staff or pharmacists.

- Ideally, having a system to track how patients are taking their medications.

- Having ready access to contacts for community health workers, low-cost exercise programs, food banks, patient assistance programs, and mental health professionals.

The National Diabetes Education Program (cdc.gov/diabetes/professional-info/training.html) has pulled together resources to help healthcare teams redesign their practices to improve care of those with diabetes.

Discussion

Globally, diabetes mellitus is threatening to overwhelm health care systems worldwide, due to increased prevalence of diabetes and the increased cost per person. There are an estimated 537 million people with diabetes globally, with expectation to increase by 46% by 2045.[9] Studies have shown that lowering blood glucose, blood pressure, and LDL-cholesterol levels can reduce the risk of long-term complications of diabetes.[10] Despite these data, control of these risk factors remains poor.[11] Total diabetes-related health care expenditure in the United States was estimated to be 237 billion USD in 2017, and globally, expenditure is estimated to be approximately 966 billion USD.[12] The largest expenditures are for hospitalizations and medications for care of diabetes-related complications, which are largely preventable with better risk factor control. These costs do not include lost productivity associated with diabetes, estimated at 90 billion in the United States.[12]

Strategies for Working With Patients With Suboptimally Controlled Diabetes

Fitting into the heath care systems that are currently in place, our goals, as providers of care, are to help patients live fully in the present and in the future by providing care that fits into their lives and helps to prevent future disability and premature mortality by maximizing their risk factor management (*figure 1, following page*).[5] The full American Diabetes Association (ADA) standards of care are available free of charge (https://diabetesjournals.org/care/issue/46/Supplement_1) and are available as an excellent app.

Goals for hemoglobin A_{1c} control should be individualized, but they are generally less than 7.0% (<53 mmol/mol). There have been recent changes in targets for blood pressure and LDL cholesterol in the newest update of the ADA standards of care[5]:

Figure 1. Risk factor management in diabetes mellitus.

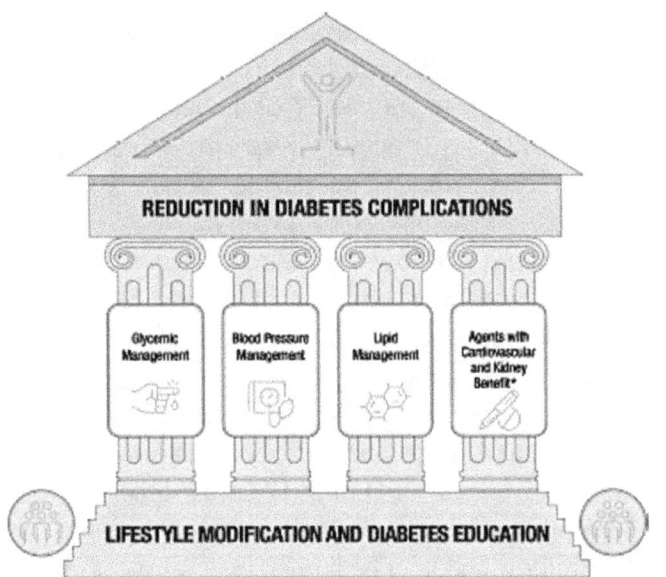

Reprinted from 2023 ADA Standards of Medical Care for Diabetes. *Diabetes Care*, 2023; 46 (Suppl 1): S1-S155. © The American Diabetes Association. (Color—web and EPUB only)

Figure 2. Comprehensive medical evaluation and assessment of comorbidities.

COMPREHENSIVE MEDICAL EVALUATION AND ASSESSMENT OF COMORBIDITIES

BEHAVIORAL FACTORS	• Eating patterns and weight history	✓	✓	✓
	• Assess familiarity with carbohydrate counting (e.g., type 1 diabetes, type 2 diabetes treated with MDI)	✓		✓
	• Physical activity and sleep behaviors	✓	✓	✓
	• Tobacco, alcohol, and substance use	✓		✓
MEDICATIONS AND VACCINATIONS	• Current medication regimen	✓	✓	✓
	• Medication-taking behavior	✓	✓	✓
	• Medication intolerance or side effects	✓	✓	✓
	• Complementary and alternative medicine use	✓	✓	✓
	• Vaccination history and needs	✓		✓
TECHNOLOGY USE	• Assess use of health apps, online education, patient portals, etc.	✓		✓
	• Glucose monitoring (meter/CGM): results and data use	✓	✓	✓
	• Review insulin pump settings and use, connected pen and glucose data	✓	✓	✓
SOCIAL LIFE ASSESSMENT	Social network			
	• Identify existing social supports	✓		✓
	• Identify surrogate decision maker, advanced care plan	✓		✓
	• Identify social determinants of health (e.g., food security, housing stability & homelessness, transportation access, financial security, community safety)	✓		✓

Reprinted from 2023 ADA Standards of Medical Care for Diabetes. *Diabetes Care*, 2023; 46 (Suppl 1): S1-S155. © The American Diabetes Association. (Color—web and EPUB only)

Figure 3. Recommendations for glycemic management.

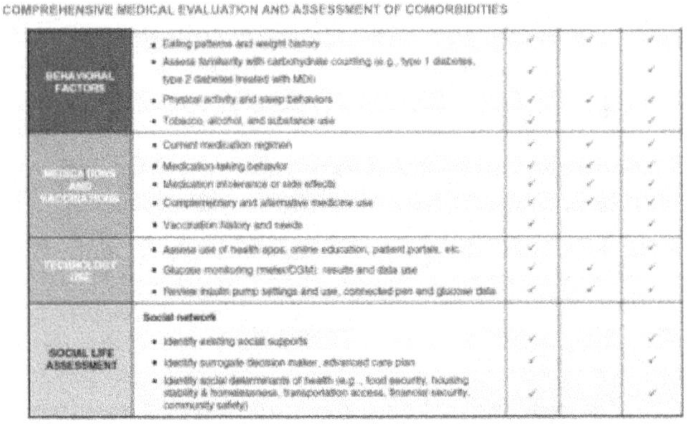

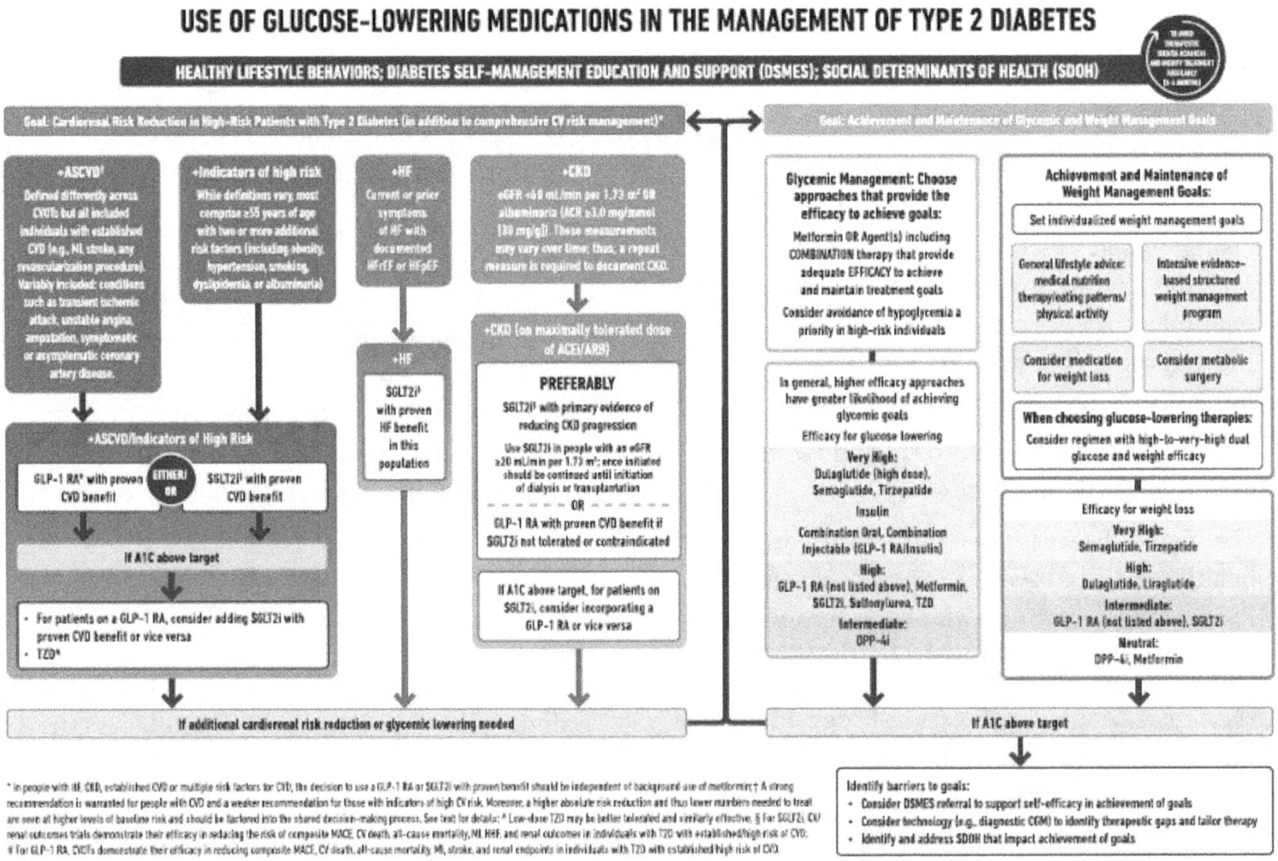

Reprinted from 2023 ADA Standards of Medical Care for Diabetes. *Diabetes Care*, 2023; 46 (Suppl 1): S1-S155. © The American Diabetes Association. (Color—web and EPUB only)

- Blood pressure goal <130/80 mm Hg
- LDL cholesterol <70 mg/dL (<1.81 mmol/L) in patients older than 40 years with 1 additional risk factor or 55 in patients with established cardiovascular disease

In addition to history and physical examination, additional information should be ascertained during the initial visit (*figure 2*).[5] This is often best done by diabetes care and education specialists or office staff before the appointment.

One of the most substantive changes in the ADA standards of care is in the recommendations for glycemic management that stem from the ADA/European Association for the Study of Diabetes report published in 2022 (*figure 3*).[5] These recommendations continue to emphasize the importance of using evidence-based treatments to reduce cardiorenal complications of diabetes; namely, SGLT-2 inhibitors for reducing heart failure and chronic kidney disease progression and GLP-1 receptor agonists for reduction in risk of atherosclerotic cardiovascular disease in patients with known vascular disease and in those with chronic kidney disease. In the absence of these compelling indications, management of weight has been elevated to a much higher level of consideration than in the past. Additionally, the authors recommend choosing the most effective agent to reach weight-loss goals. By choosing a very effective agent that lowers lowering hemoglobin A_{1c} from the beginning, there is likely the potential to maintain more durable control of glycemia and minimize the negative clinical outcomes from therapeutic inertia.[5]

Importantly, each patient must be considered in the context of their own lives and values, and physicians should strive to understand their specific barriers to achieving better metabolic control (*figure 4*).[5] Remembering that management of diabetes is a lifelong process for patients, meeting them where they are, and encouraging even small improvements in lifestyle behaviors (*figure 5*) can make a large difference in their health over time.[5]

When faced with patients who have chronic suboptimal control, I start with the assumption that they want to improve their glycemic control to lead a healthier life. In a survey, 93% of people with diabetes stated that they are willing to do more to manage their diabetes.[13]

I like to start by asking several questions:

1. What does the patient want to live for?
2. What is their schedule for the day?
3. Do they eat out of the house frequently?
4. Who prepares the meals?
5. What activities do they participate in (including housework and gardening)?
6. Is there any reason to doubt the hemoglobin A_{1c} results?
    a. A retrospective study by Dr. Hirsch's group demonstrated discordance between glucose management indicator and hemoglobin A_{1c} value ≥0.5% in 50% of their clinic patients on continuous glucose monitoring. The discordance was ≥1.0% in 225 of their patients.[14]
7. Does the patient have the knowledge and tools to manage their diabetes?
    a. Do we have instructions/educational content in the correct language?
    b. Can they read?
        i. 21% of the US adult population is illiterate
        ii. 54% read below the sixth-grade level
    c. Do they have adequate numeracy skills?
        i. 30% of the US adult population is unable to perform more than simple addition and subtraction
8. Do I have the correct diagnosis, which would alter therapy?
    a. Could the patient have LADA or MODY?

Figure 4. Decision cycle for person-centered glycemic management in type 2 diabetes.

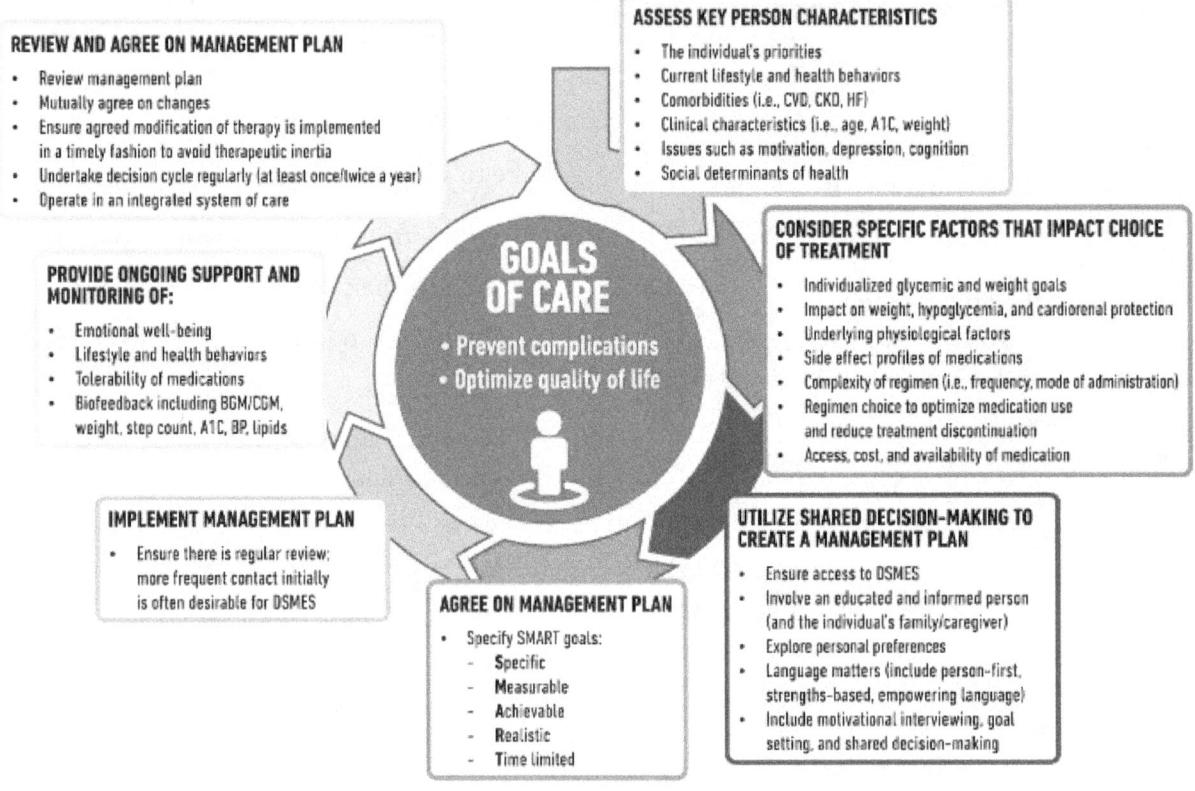

DECISION CYCLE FOR PERSON-CENTERED GLYCEMIC MANAGEMENT IN TYPE 2 DIABETES

REVIEW AND AGREE ON MANAGEMENT PLAN
- Review management plan
- Mutually agree on changes
- Ensure agreed modification of therapy is implemented in a timely fashion to avoid therapeutic inertia
- Undertake decision cycle regularly (at least once/twice a year)
- Operate in an integrated system of care

ASSESS KEY PERSON CHARACTERISTICS
- The individual's priorities
- Current lifestyle and health behaviors
- Comorbidities (i.e., CVD, CKD, HF)
- Clinical characteristics (i.e., age, A1C, weight)
- Issues such as motivation, depression, cognition
- Social determinants of health

PROVIDE ONGOING SUPPORT AND MONITORING OF:
- Emotional well-being
- Lifestyle and health behaviors
- Tolerability of medications
- Biofeedback including BGM/CGM, weight, step count, A1C, BP, lipids

GOALS OF CARE
- Prevent complications
- Optimize quality of life

CONSIDER SPECIFIC FACTORS THAT IMPACT CHOICE OF TREATMENT
- Individualized glycemic and weight goals
- Impact on weight, hypoglycemia, and cardiorenal protection
- Underlying physiological factors
- Side effect profiles of medications
- Complexity of regimen (i.e., frequency, mode of administration)
- Regimen choice to optimize medication use and reduce treatment discontinuation
- Access, cost, and availability of medication

IMPLEMENT MANAGEMENT PLAN
- Ensure there is regular review; more frequent contact initially is often desirable for DSMES

AGREE ON MANAGEMENT PLAN
- Specify SMART goals:
  - Specific
  - Measurable
  - Achievable
  - Realistic
  - Time limited

UTILIZE SHARED DECISION-MAKING TO CREATE A MANAGEMENT PLAN
- Ensure access to DSMES
- Involve an educated and informed person (and the individual's family/caregiver)
- Explore personal preferences
- Language matters (include person-first, strengths-based, empowering language)
- Include motivational interviewing, goal setting, and shared decision-making

Reprinted from 2023 ADA Standards of Medical Care for Diabetes. *Diabetes Care*, 2023; 46 (Suppl 1): S1-S155. © The American Diabetes Association. (Color—web and EPUB only)

9. Do I have the correct glycemic target?

   a. A lower target hemoglobin A_{1c} value should be considered for older patients and those with vascular complications, advanced chronic kidney disease, or geriatric syndromes. *Table 1* shows the recommendations for glycemic targets in elderly patients published by the Endocrine Society, but these targets also pertain to younger individuals with severe vascular/kidney complications.[15]

10. Do I understand the patient's barriers?

    a. Adherence to diet, testing, medications

    b. Persistence with medications

    c. Financial constraints

    d. Access to clinic appointments, contacting the team when needed

    e. Social support

    f. Mental health issues

While attempting to address patients' barriers, we should also be realistic regarding the achievable control due to finances, lack of social support, food insecurity, fear of hypoglycemia, depression, and other mental health issues. The UKPDS and the DCCT both showed very significant improvement in outcomes when hemoglobin A_{1c} was reduced from 10.0% to 8.0%.[1,2]

11. Would the patient benefit from additional technology?

    a. Continuous glucose monitoring

    b. Smart pen

    c. Hybrid closed-loop insulin pump

Figure 5. Importance of 24-hour physical behaviors for type 2 diabetes.

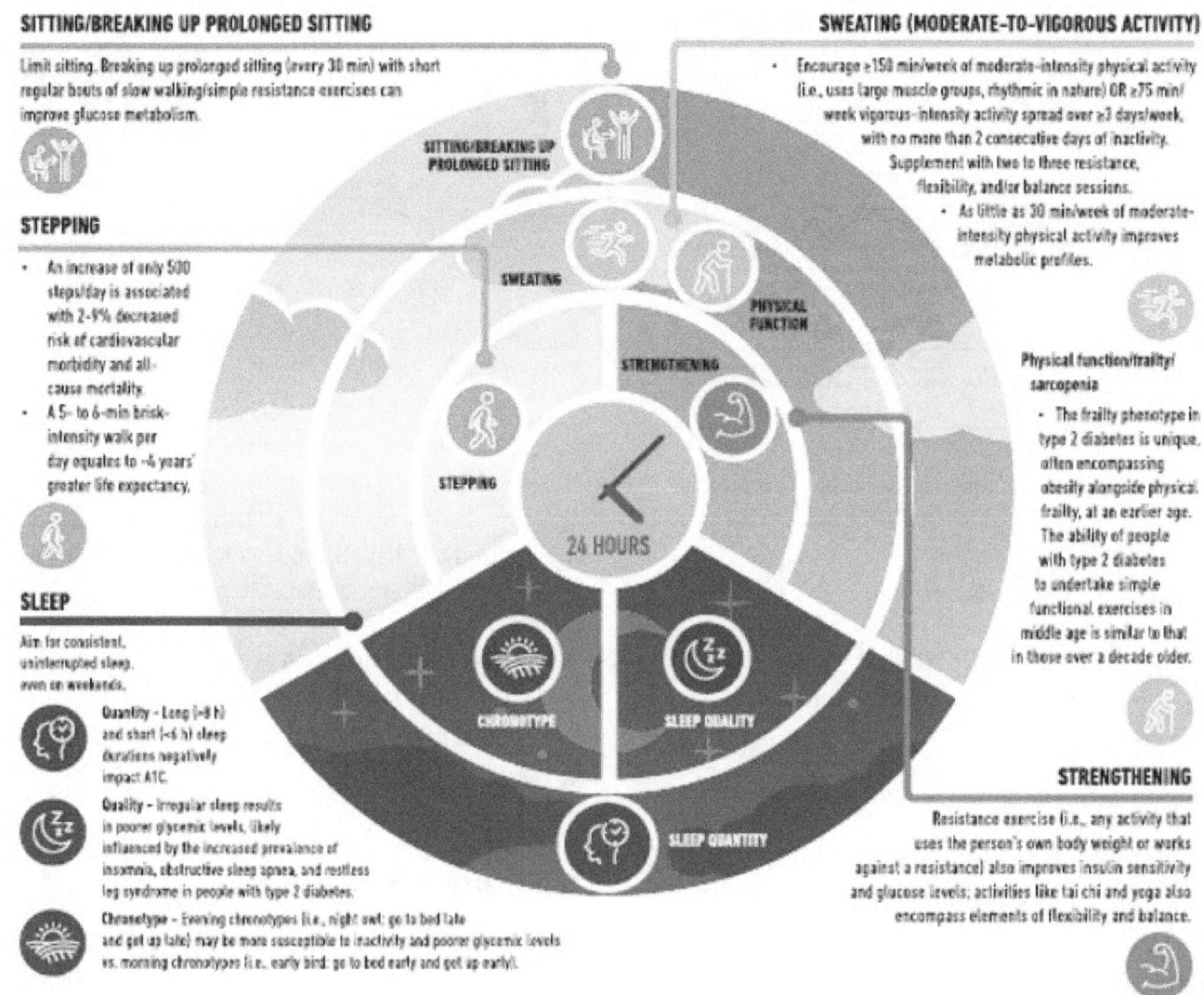

Table 1. Conceptual Framework for Considering Overall Health and Patient Values in Determining Clinical Targets in Adults Aged 65 Years and Older[15]

Overall Health Category		Group 1: Good Health	Group 2: Intermediate Health	Group 3: Poor Health
Patient characteristics		No comorbidities or 1-2 non-diabetes chronic illnesses‡ and No ADL‡ impairments and ≤1 IADL impairment	3 or more non-diabetes chronic illnesses‡ and/or Any one of the following: mild cognitive impairment or early dementia ≥2 IADL impairments	Any one of the following: End-stage medical condition(s)‡‡ Moderate to severe dementia ≥2 ADL impairments Residence in a long-term nursing facility
Reasonable glucose target ranges and HbA1c by group				
Shared decision-making; individualized goal may be lower or higher				
Use of drugs that may cause hypoglycemia (e.g., insulin, sulfonylurea, glinide)	No	Fasting: 80-130 mg/dL Bedtime: 80-160 mg/dL <7.5%	Fasting: 90-150 mg/dL Bedtime: 100-180 mg/dL <8%	Fasting: 100-180 mg/dL Bedtime: 110-200 mg/dL <8.5%‡
	Yes²	Fasting: 90-150 mg/dL Bedtime: 100-180 mg/dL >7.0 and <7.5%	Fasting: 100-150 mg/dL Bedtime: 150-180 mg/dL >7.5 and <8.0%	Fasting: 100-180 mg/dL Bedtime: 150-250 mg/dL >8.0 and <8.5%‡

12. Do I need more information?

    a. Professional continuous glucose monitoring

    b. Personal continuous glucose monitoring

    c. Smart pen

    d. Insulin pump downloads

13. Do I have access to refer the patient to a glycemic management system?

Clinical Case Vignettes

Case 1

A 29-year-old man presents with his mother for evaluation and management of type 1 diabetes. He is developmentally disabled, so she provides most of the history. His treatment regimen consists of glargine insulin, 8 units twice daily; lispro insulin, 4 units with each meal + correction factor of 1 unit per 50 mg/dL over 150 mg/dL. He takes no other medications. His hemoglobin A_{1c} level is 8.8% (73 mmol/mol). His mother seems to remember that he was studied for a genetic problem as a child, when he presented with diabetes around 6 months of age, but she cannot remember the results. They relocated shortly

Figure 6. Risk of complications by hemoglobin A_{1c} level.

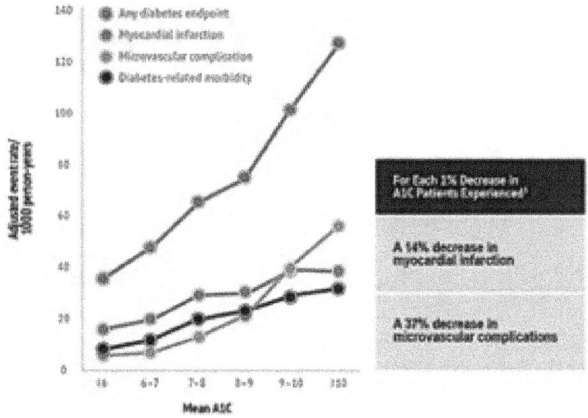

thereafter, and she was under the impression that his diabetes remitted. He was subsequently diagnosed with type 1 diabetes at age 5. He has never been hospitalized for diabetic ketoacidosis. Examination findings and laboratory data are not revealing.

Which of the following is this patient's most likely diagnosis?

A. Typical type 1 diabetes

B. Mitochondrial diabetes

C. Monogenic diabetes

Answer: C) Monogenic diabetes

About 1% to 5% of patients diagnosed with type 1 diabetes have maturity-onset diabetes of the young (MODY) (frequently masquerading as type 1 diabetes).[16] Up to 50% of those with monogenic diabetes may not have a positive family history.

Case 1 (continued)

Which of the following is the best way to proceed?

A. Prescribe a sulfonylurea

B. Recommend genetic testing

C. Ask his mother to find the genetic test results from his youth

Answer: B or C) Recommend genetic testing or ask his mother to find the genetic test results from his youth

The patient's mother found his genetic testing results. He has monogenic diabetes due to a pathogenic variant in the *KCNJ11* gene. This gene is frequently associated with neurocognitive impairment, which may be improved with early introduction of sulfonylurea therapy.[17]

This patient's insulin dosing was cut in half and glimepiride was started, 1 mg once daily. Two days later, his blood glucose control was better. The glimepiride dosage was increased to 2 mg once daily and insulin was stopped. His hemoglobin A_{1c} value 3 months later was 7.1% (54 mmol/mol). Unfortunately, the patient moved shortly thereafter, so long-term follow-up is unavailable. I often refer my patients to the website for monogenic diabetes at the University of Chicago (https://monogenicdiabetes.uchicago.edu). Alternatively, most commercial laboratories have MODY panels.

Case 2

A 67-year-old man presents for evaluation and management of suboptimally controlled type 2 diabetes complicated by obesity and albuminuric stage 3a chronic kidney disease, diagnosed about 10 years ago. His hemoglobin A_{1c} values have ranged between 8.9% and 11.0% (74 and 97 mmol/mol) over the past 2 years. He also has hypertension, hyperlipidemia, and obstructive sleep apnea. He has gained about 15 lb (6.8 kg) over the past year. He has no polyuria, polydipsia, or visual blurring. He does not smoke cigarettes, and he drinks less than 1 serving of alcohol per week.

Current diabetes medications are glargine insulin, 40 units twice daily; aspart insulin, 15 units 3 times daily with meals; and metformin, 1000 mg twice daily. He states he does not miss taking his medication doses or injections. Other medications are ramipril, 10 mg once daily; rosuvastatin, 20 mg daily; and omeprazole, 20 mg once daily. Past medications were glipizide, 20 mg (stopped due to poor control when he started insulin); sitagliptin (lack of efficacy); and pioglitazone (due to fluid retention and weight gain).

On physical examination, he is a healthy appearing man. His BMI is 37 kg/m². His blood pressure is 137/78 mm Hg, and pulse rate is 68 beats/min and regular. He has trace pedal edema, good foot care, with normal pulses, normal sensation to 10-g monofilament, and no deformities. His examination findings are otherwise normal.

Laboratory test results (from 3 months ago):

Hemoglobin A_{1c} = 11.1% (98 mmol/mol)
Glomerular filtration rate = 59 mL/min per 1.73 m²
Albumin-to-creatinine ratio = 120 mg/g creat

Which of the following is the most important element contributing to this patient's suboptimal glycemic control?

A. He is not on enough insulin

B. His lifestyle is not optimal (diet, lack of exercise, poor sleep)

C. He is not taking insulin due to cost

D. He is not taking his medications due to complexity of the regimen

Answer: D) He is not taking his medications due to complexity of the regimen

All of the above are possible; however, patient has excellent insurance. Careful discussion about his schedule, lifestyle, and medication-taking behaviors revealed the following: he is divorced, eats breakfast at home, eats lunch at work and about one-half of his dinners at work. He comes home, watches TV at night, and often awakens at 3 AM in his lounger. He uses continuous positive airway pressure "most of the time." He is very good at taking his medications in the morning, does not take his insulin to work or when he eats out, and often misses his evening dose of basal insulin.

Adherence to medications in patients with chronic disease is often poor. In patients on oral medications, adherence rate (as defined by a medication possession rate of at least 90%) is less than 50% in people taking oral medications, and up to 50% stop taking their medications during 1-year follow-up. Poor medication adherence is linked to suboptimal control, increase in emergency department and hospital visits, and increased mortality. The direct cost of nonadherence to medications for diabetes, hyperlipidemia, and hypertension was about 105.8 billion USD in 2010. Treatment complexity is indirectly associated with adherence rates.[18]

Case 2 (continued)

Which of the following should be the first priority for managing this man's metabolic issues?

A. Glycemic control

B. Weight

C. Lipids

D. Blood pressure

E. Chronic kidney disease

Answer: No correct answer

Obviously, all of the listed answers are important. Some of the above could be accomplished with the addition of a GLP-1 receptor agonist.

Case 2 (continued)

Which of the following is the best suggestion for improving glycemic control?

A. Diabetes education

B. Increasing his basal insulin

C. Adding an SGLT-2 inhibitor

D. Adding a GLP-1 receptor agonist

E. A, C, and D

Answer: E) A, C, and D

Diabetes care and education specialists might be able to help the patient with strategies to improve his adherence.

The first step was to move administration of all of his bedtime medications to the morning. His glargine insulin was switched to 56 units every morning (70% of the total daily dose), and his metformin was changed to metformin XR, 1500 mg every morning. A referral was placed for diabetes education. His C-peptide measurement was 4.7 ng/mL (1.6 nmol/L). Assuming that this was going to confirm that he still had residual insulin secretion, a plan was outlined to add empagliflozin, 10 mg (for his kidneys), and to convert his multiple daily injections to basal + GLP-1 receptor agonist. Semaglutide, 0.25 mg weekly, was started, and his aspart insulin dosage was changed to 8 units 3 times daily. His premeal fingerstick glucose levels stabilized in the range of 130 to 180 mg/dL (7.2-10.0 mmol/L). After 4 weeks, the semaglutide dosage was increased to 0.5 mg weekly and aspart insulin was stopped. His glucose levels remained stable. There was no hypoglycemia. After 4 more weeks, his semaglutide dosage was increased to 1 mg weekly. At a follow-up visit, his hemoglobin A_{1c} value was 7.4% (57 mmol/mol), and he had lost about 8 lb (3.6 kg). He was motivated to continue to work on the dietician's recommendations to choose healthier food at his workplace and to go to a gym before work at least 3 days per week. He declined a continuous glucose monitor and opted for follow-up with his primary care provider.

Case 3

A 62-year-old woman presents for follow-up of type 2 diabetes, which she has had for 16 years. She is 4 years status post Roux-en-Y gastric bypass. Prior to this operation, her glycemic control was variable, but her best hemoglobin A_{1c} values (6.9%-7.3% [52-56 mmol/mol]) were on glargine insulin, 48 units at bedtime + dulaglutide, 1.5 mg weekly. Prior to surgery, she discontinued metformin because of diarrhea. She remained on insulin after surgery. Postoperatively, she has had ongoing issues with nausea, cramping, and intermittent diarrhea.

She maintained good glycemic control on glargine insulin, 10 units daily, with hemoglobin A_{1c} values of 6.6% to 7.1% (49-54 mmol/mol) for 3 years, when her values progressively rose to 8.0% (64 mmol/mol) despite addition of aspart insulin.

She currently takes glargine insulin, 9 units at bedtime + aspart insulin, 1/5 g of carbohydrate + correction factor of 1:50 >150 mg/dL. She monitors her blood glucose with fingerstick glucose every morning and after dinner. She notes her blood glucose values in the morning are

100 to 110 mg/dL (5.6-6.1 mmol/L) and about 150 mg/dL (8.3 mmol/L) after dinner.

Her current BMI is 23.5 kg/m^2.

Laboratory test results:

Hemoglobin A$_{1c}$ = 8.0% (64 mmol/mol)
LDL cholesterol = 67 mg/dL (SI: 1.73 mmol/L)
Glomerular filtration rate = 62 mL/min per 1.73 m^2
Albumin-to-creatinine ratio = 6 mg/g creat
Bariatric labs, normal

She has little insight into why her blood glucose values are so high. She states she eats small meals and takes her insulin with meals.

Which of the following is the most likely explanation for her suboptimal glycemic control?

A. Not taking her aspart insulin before meals

B. Eating high-carbohydrate meals

C. Not counting carbohydrates correctly

D. Her measured hemoglobin A$_{1c}$ may not be accurate

E. All of the above

Answer: E) All of the above

We initiated professional continuous glucose monitoring and arranged for her to follow-up with a dietician. Her continuous glucose monitoring tracing is shown (*figure 7*). Her hemoglobin A$_{1c}$ and glucose management indicator are concordant. The dietician discovered several concerns. She did not really know how to count carbohydrates, she had a very high-carbohydrate diet (fruit smoothies, sweetened coffee drinks, croissants), and she was taking aspart insulin intermittently and generally only after meals.

She was placed on personal continuous glucose monitoring. The MOBILE study showed use of continuous glucose monitoring in insulin-treated participants with type 2 diabetes lowered their hemoglobin A$_{1c}$ by 0.4% over those who use self-monitoring of blood glucose, without an overall change in medications.[19] Continuous glucose monitoring with education targeted at minimizing postprandial glycemic excursions was associated

with a reduction in hemoglobin A$_{1c}$ of 1.5% in non–insulin-treated type 2 diabetes (compared with control group, –0.1%). The continuous glucose monitoring group used less medication, reduced carbohydrate intake, decreased diabetes-related distress, and improved knowledge.[20]

Case 3 (continued)

Despite counseling on low-carbohydrate diet and taking insulin before meals, her control failed to improve.

Which of the following is the best next step?

A. Consider insulin pump

B. Consider GLP-1 receptor agonist

C. Add SGLT-2 inhibitor

D. Enroll her in a glycemic monitoring program

After discussion of the options above, she agreed to try GLP-1 receptor agonist at a low dosage to determine whether she could tolerate it.

Case 4

A 69-year-old woman has a 17-year history of type 1 diabetes. In the preceding 4 years, her median hemoglobin A$_{1c}$ value was 8.4% (68 mmol/mol), with a range of 7.8% to 8.7% (62-72 mmol/mol). She has never had ketoacidosis.

Current regimen:

Basal insulin: detemir 46 units at bedtime.
Carbohydrate coverage: insulin aspart 1/5 g of carbohydrate
Correction: 20
Target: 120 mg/dL (SI: 6.7 mmol/L)

She does not think that she counts carbohydrates well.

She is testing fingerstick glucose 3 to 4 times daily, and her mean glucose value is 202 mg/dL (11.2 mmol/L) (range, 58-220 mg/dL [3.2-12.2 mmol/L]) (*figure 8*).

Hemoglobin A$_{1c}$ = 8.7% (72 mmol/mol)

Figure 7. Patient's CGM tracing (Case 3).

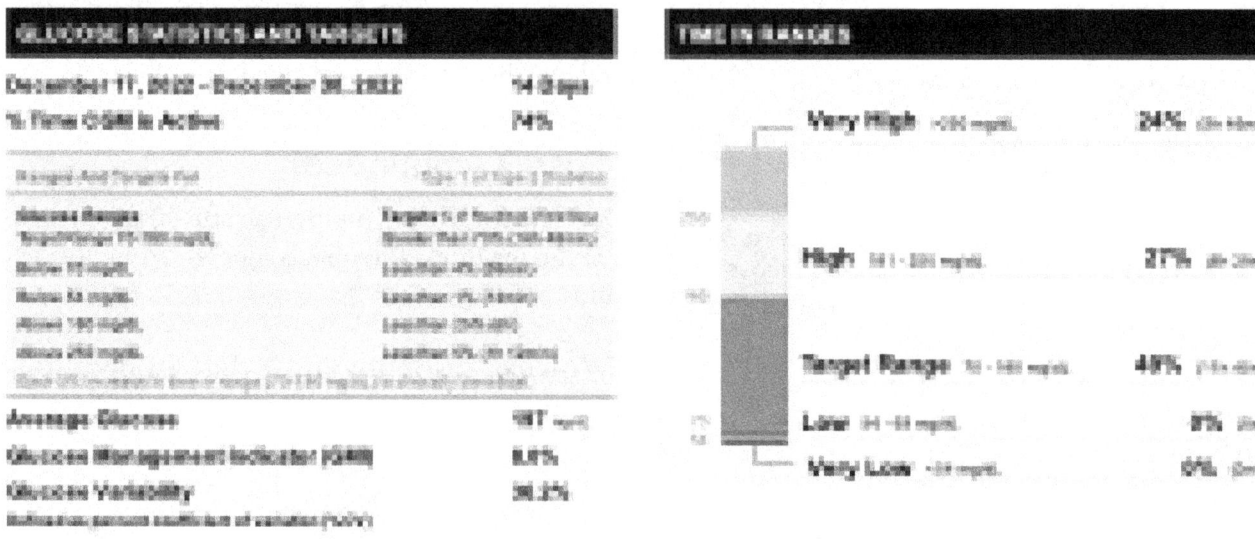

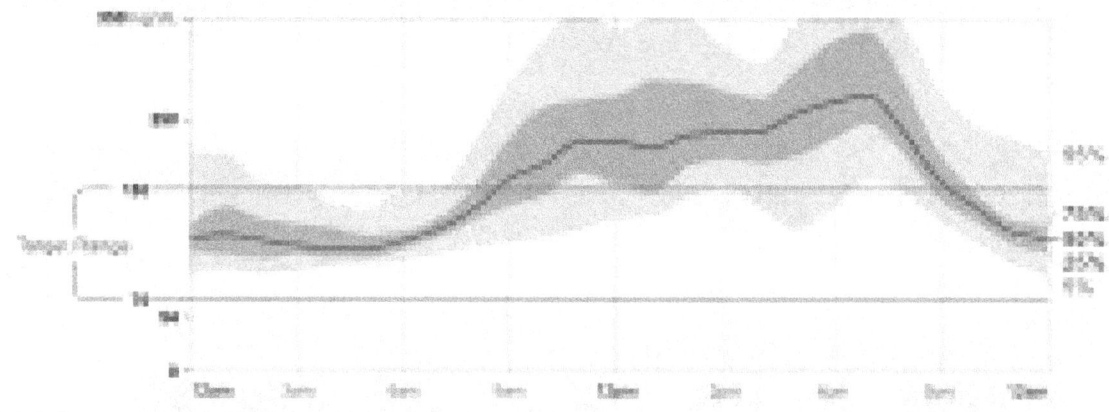

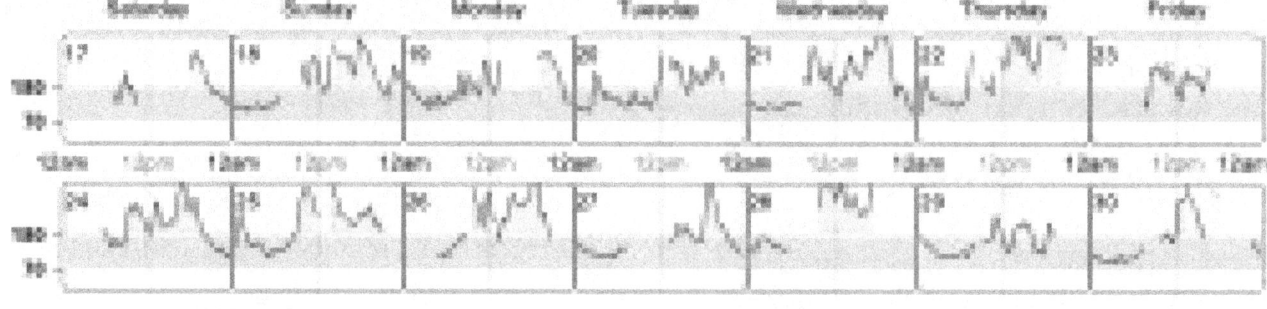

Reprinted from Warshaw H et al. *The Sci of Diab Self Manage & Care*, 2020; 46: 3S-20S. © The Authors. Published by Sage Publications, on behalf of the American Association of Diabetes Educators. (Color—web and EPUB only)

Figure 8. Patient's fingerstick glucose values (Case 4).

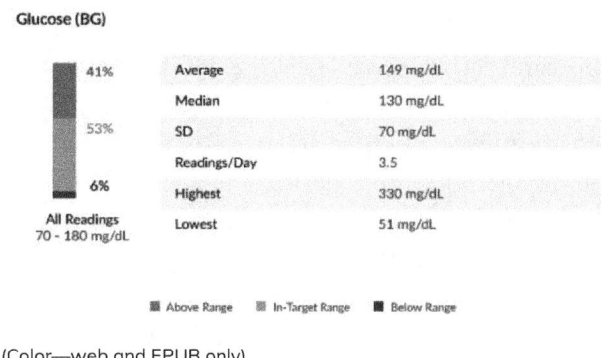

(Color—web and EPUB only)

Which of the following is the best suggestion now?

A. Dietary consultation

B. Personal continuous glucose monitoring

C. C-peptide measurement

D. Insulin pump + continuous glucose monitoring

E. All of the above

Answer: E) All of the above

Many studies have shown improvement in hemoglobin A_{1c} with continuous glucose monitoring in populations with type 1 diabetes.[21] It appears that the improvement in hemoglobin A_{1c} is greater with continuous glucose monitoring than with continuous subcutaneous insulin infusion without a continuous glucose monitor. A retrospective study of patients using continuous subcutaneous insulin infusion or multiple daily injections with and without continuous glucose monitoring showed that patients using multiple daily injections + continuous glucose monitoring had lower hemoglobin A_{1c} than patients using continuous subcutaneous insulin infusion alone (7.7% vs 8.3%, respectively). These results were confirmed in a randomized controlled study.[22]

Case 4 (continued)

The patient declines insulin pump therapy. She does not start the sensor because she is not comfortable with virtual training during the COVID pandemic. The clinic has an available glucose meter to give her (which can perform insulin dose calculations [at the time, smart pens were not available]). Her glycemic control improves significantly. She admits to the dietician that she is very uncomfortable with calculations.

Data from a follow-up visit 3 months later are shown (*figures 9 and 10*).

Figure 9. Patient's blood glucose data (Case 4).

Glucose (BG)

41%	Average	149 mg/dL
	Median	130 mg/dL
53%	SD	70 mg/dL
	Readings/Day	3.5
6%	Highest	330 mg/dL
All Readings 70 - 180 mg/dL	Lowest	51 mg/dL

■ Above Range ■ In-Target Range ■ Below Range

(Color—web and EPUB only)

Figure 10. Patient's blood glucose data (Case 4).

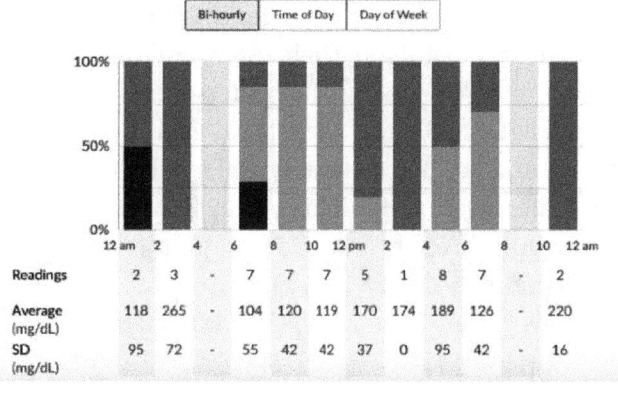

| | Bi-hourly | Time of Day | Day of Week |

	12 am	2	4	6	8	10	12 pm	2	4	6	8	10	12 am
Readings	2	3	-	7	7	7	5	1	8	7	-	2	
Average (mg/dL)	118	265	-	104	120	119	170	174	189	126	-	220	
SD (mg/dL)	95	72	-	55	42	42	37	0	95	42	-	16	

(Color—web and EPUB only)

Her hemoglobin A_{1c} measurement is 7.2% (55 mmol/mol), but with too many low glucose values!

Which of the following is the best suggestion now?

A. Prescribe personal continuous glucose monitoring

B. Change the timing of insulin detemir dosing

C. Recommend insulin pump therapy

D. All of the above

Answer: D) All of the above

I changed her insulin detemir dosing to 10 units in the AM and 30 units in the PM and scheduled her for training in use of a continuous glucose monitor. She declined insulin pump therapy but agreed to start using a smart pen for her aspart doses.

Smart pens, often associated with an app for calculation of insulin doses, can be paired with continuous glucose monitoring data to allow the patient more information about effects of insulin on glucose data and more empowerment for bolusing when glucose is high after meals. Importantly, the reports provide good insight to missed injections, timing of insulin, and whether the patient is overriding the insulin calculator. Galindo and colleagues performed a small study to evaluate impact of smart pen use (with insulin calculations and without continuous glucose monitoring) on changes in hemoglobin A_{1c} in a population of patients with type 2 diabetes on basal insulin ± oral medications. Although the magnitude of change in hemoglobin A_{1c} was relatively small (9.1% to 8.2% compared with 9.3% to 8.4%), the investigators were able to determine that only 53% of the participants were highly adherent (85%+ dosing) and that patients missed an average of 23.6% of their basal insulin doses.[23] It is estimated that 1 missed basal insulin dose per week increases hemoglobin A_{1c} by 0.2% to 0.3%.[24]

A typical report from a smart pen (not from this patient) is shown (*figure 11*).

This patient's data from 3 months later are shown (*figure 12*).

The patient's average glucose value is higher, but her percentage of time spent below target has improved. Her hemoglobin A_{1c} increased to 7.7% (61 mmol/mol). Over the next 2 years, her median hemoglobin A_{1c} was 7.5% (58 mmol/mol), with range of 7.2% to 8.1% (55-65 mmol/mol).

She has an insulin pump but has not yet been fully trained on its use. This patient has true fear of technology, so patience is required.

Case 5

A 76-year-old woman with a 65-year history of type 1 diabetes complicated by coronary artery disease, nonproliferative diabetic retinopathy, and stage 3a chronic kidney disease presents for routine follow-up. She has been on an insulin pump and sensor (not integrated) for many years, without significant improvement in her hemoglobin A_{1c}. Her median hemoglobin A_{1c} value is 10.0% (86 mmol/mol) with a range of 8.9% to 11.5% (74-102 mmol/mol). She admits to missing many boluses, saying she forgets because she is so busy with her grandkids.

She has had multiple visits with diabetes care and education specialists over the years.

Laboratory test results:

Glomerular filtration rate = 55 mL/min per 1.73 m²
Albumin-to-creatinine ratio = 11 mg/g Cr
LDL cholesterol = 43 mg/dL (SI: 1.11 mmol/L)

Baseline sensor tracing is shown (*figure 13*).

What should this patient's hemoglobin A_{1c} be?

A. <7.0% (<53 mmol/mol)

B. <7.5% (<58 mmol/mol)

C. <8.0% (<64 mmol/mol)

D. <8.5% (<69 mmol/mol)

Answer: As low as we can get it, without hypoglycemia

I personally favor less than 8.0% (<64 mmol/mol) for this patient, given her very long history of suboptimal control, with minimal microvascular complications (*see table 1*).

Figure 11. Guide to using the insights by InPen integrated data report (Case 4).

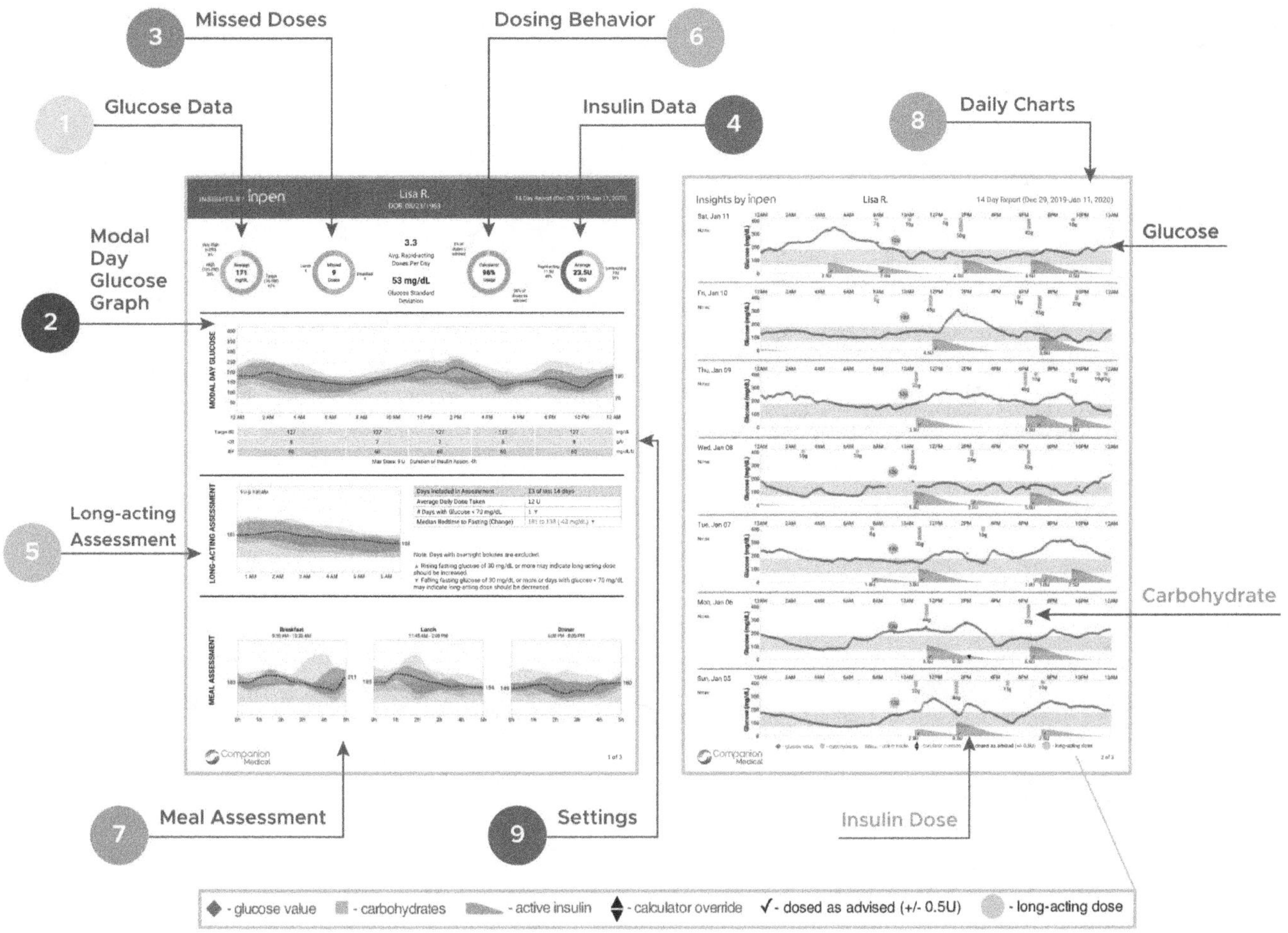

Reprinted from Warshaw H et al. *The Sci of Diab Self Manage & Care.* 2020;46:3S-20S. © The Authors. Published by Sage Publications, on behalf of the American Association of Diabetes Educators. (Color—web and EPUB only)

Case 5 (continued)

Which of the following is the most likely reason for her glycation gap (difference between hemoglobin A_{1c} and glucose management indicator)?

A. Iron deficiency

B. Vitamin C ingestion

C. Chronic alcohol intake

Answer: A) Iron deficiency

This patient had iron deficiency with iron saturation of 6%. No source was found. She did not respond to oral iron. With intravenous iron, her iron levels normalized and glycation gap narrowed. Common reasons for inaccurate hemoglobin A_{1c} values are listed in *table 2.*

Case 5 (continued)

Which of the following is the best next step?

A. Switch her regimen to multiple daily injections because she is not taking her boluses before meals

B. Keep her on insulin pump therapy and enter her into glycemic management program

C. Change to a hybrid closed-loop insulin pump

Answer: C) Change to a hybrid closed-loop insulin pump

Chaudhary et al reported results of a 6-month study using the Medtronic 780G system (hybrid closed-loop) vs multiple daily injections + continuous glucose monitoring in patients with type 1 diabetes and a baseline hemoglobin A_{1c} value of 8.0% or greater (≥64 mmol/mol).

Figure 12. Patient's data from 3 months later (Case 4).

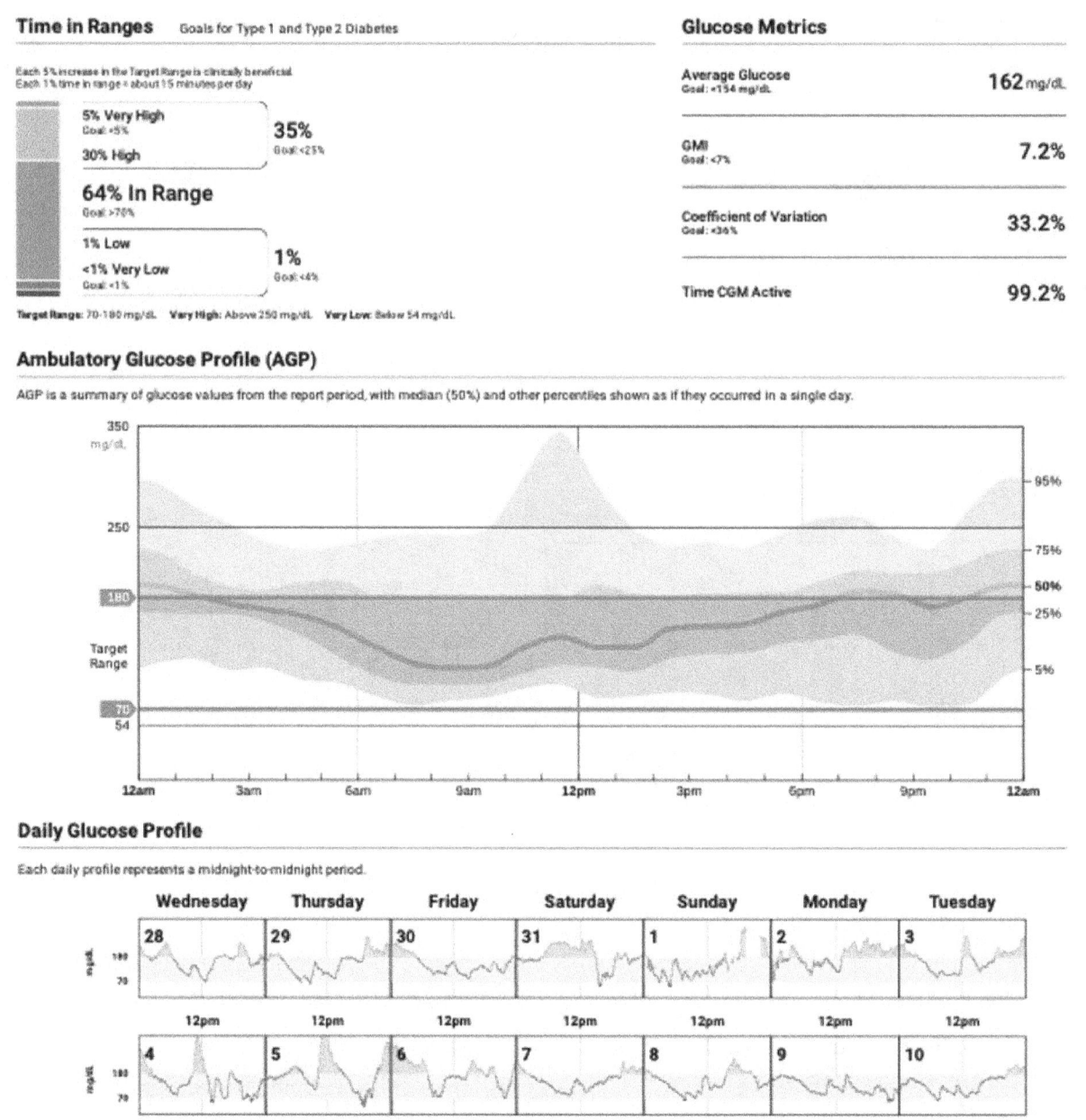

(Color—web and EPUB only)

The mean hemoglobin A_{1c} value was 9.07% (76 mmol/mol) in the hybrid closed-loop group and 9.0% (75 mmol/mol) in the multiple daily injections + continuous glucose monitoring group. The reduction in hemoglobin A_{1c} was −1.54% in the hybrid closed-loop group and –0.3% in the multiple daily injections + continuous glucose monitoring group. There were substantial differences in time in range but no significant change in time spent in the hypoglycemic range

(<70 mg/dL [<3.9 mmol/L]). The investigators suggest that these data and those from other studies support the need to abandon our preconceived notion that these technologies should only be reserved for our "good" patients.[26]

The patient's data from 3 months later are shown (*figure 14*).

This patient would benefit from a glycemic management program. Many of these have been developed, using varied designs. Most programs have

Figure 13. Patient's baseline sensor tracing (Case 5).

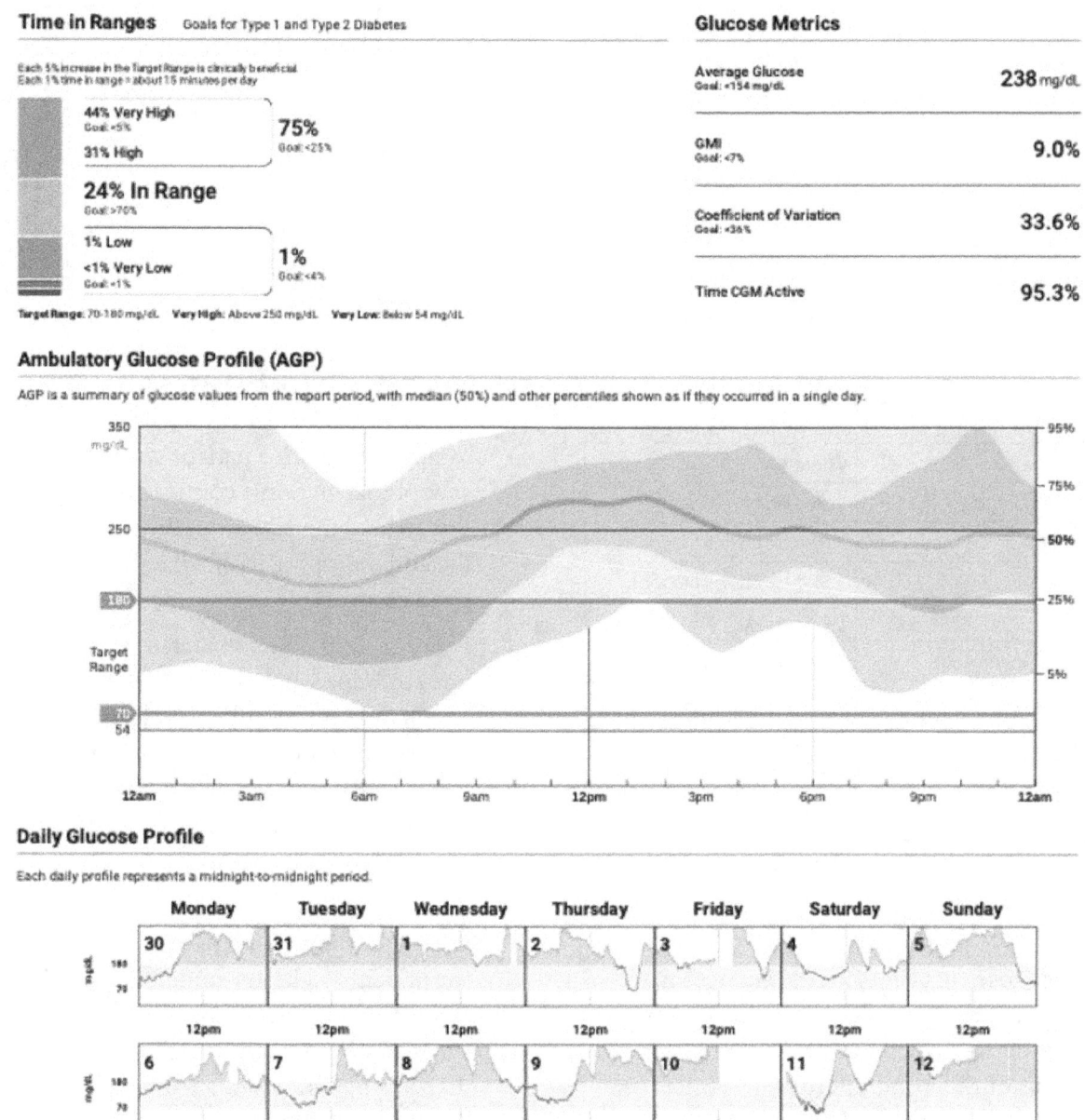

(Color—web and EPUB only)

shown improvement in hemoglobin A_{1c}, averaging around 0.5%, with the magnitude of improvement directly correlating with baseline hemoglobin A_{1c} values. A recent review of the use of virtual care as a method to use for a glycemic management program suggested that the greatest benefit was derived by teleconsultation, followed by telemonitoring. In most programs, the communications are through nurses or pharmacists. Few long-term studies (up to 5 years) have shown ongoing improvement with ongoing intervention.[27]

Another example of a glycemic intervention is Medstar Health's Boot Camp. It is a 12-week intervention targeting patients with uncontrolled diabetes (hemoglobin A_{1c} >9.0% [>75 mmol/mol]). The patient is seen by the diabetes educator for 2 in-person visits for targeted diabetes self-management education and medication adherence strategies. Using a smart meter (which provides real-time blood glucose to the hybrid closed-loop), patients are followed virtually by a diabetes nurse practitioner (via phone, text, or email) who

Table 2. Common Reasons for Inaccurate Hemoglobin A$_{1c}$ (Case 5)

False increase	Comment
Anemia ↓ red blood cell turnover	B$_{12}$, folate, iron deficiency
Asplenia	↑ Red blood cell lifespan
Uremia	Formation of carbamylated hemoglobin
Severe ↑ triglycerides	>1750 mg/dL
Severe ↑ bilirubin	> 20 mg/dL
Chronic alcohol intake	Formation of acetaldehyde-HbA
Chronic salicylate	Mechanism unknown
Lead poisoning	Mechanism unknown
False decrease	**Comment**
Anemia from blood loss	Including hemolysis
Splenomegaly	↓ Red blood cell lifespan
Pregnancy	↓ Red blood cell lifespan
Vitamin E	↓ Glycation
End-stage kidney disease	↓ Red blood cell survival
Variable effects	
Red blood cell transfusion	Generally lower
Hemoglobin variants	
Vitamin C ingestion	Dependent on assay

Adapted from Radin MS. J Gen Intern Med, 2014; 29(2) :388-94. © Society of General Internal Medicine.

monitors glucose real time, makes changes in medications and suggests lifestyle adjustments. They also provide diabetes education and support. In an analysis of this program (using a concurrent matched cohort as controls), hemoglobin A$_{1c}$ was reduced by 3% from baseline in 11.2% of patients compared with 1.4% in the control group. Hospitalizations were reduced in the study group,

with savings estimated at $3086 per person (after cost of the program).[28]

Several commercial programs have been developed and are reporting their results. Some of these results were recently reviewed by Dr. Richard Berganstal at the ATTD meeting (Advanced Technologies and Treatments for Diabetes) in February 2023. *Table 3* provides a high-level summary of his presentation on these programs.[29]

Key Learning Points

- When faced with a patient with chronically suboptimal glycemic control, it is important to understand the patient in the context of their life and their potential barriers to achieving good control.

- Patients should be connected with the tools they need to improve their control—for example, social/financial assistance; referrals to insurance counselors, food banks, social workers, or behavioral health; and changing the medication regimen to meet the patient's lifestyle more appropriately.

- Technology can be used for better understanding of the patient's control or for patients to better understand the impact of food and activity, as well as medication adjustment. Most patients with type 1 diabetes benefit from a hybrid closed-loop insulin pump.

Table 3. Commercial Programs for Glycemic Intervention (Case 5)

Program	Coaching	Virtual consultation	Baseline hemgolobin A$_{1c}$	Hemoglobin A$_{1c}$ change	Glucose management indicator change
UHC Level 2	Yes	Yes	7.7%	−0.8%	...
Welldoc Bluestart	Yes	No*	8.8%	...	−1.1%
Onduo	Yes	Yes	8.9%	−1.6%	...

*Can connect with patient's providers.

Summary of Dr. Richard Berganstal's presentation at ATTD, February 24, 2023, Berlin, Germany.

Figure 14. Patient's data from 3 months later (Case 5).

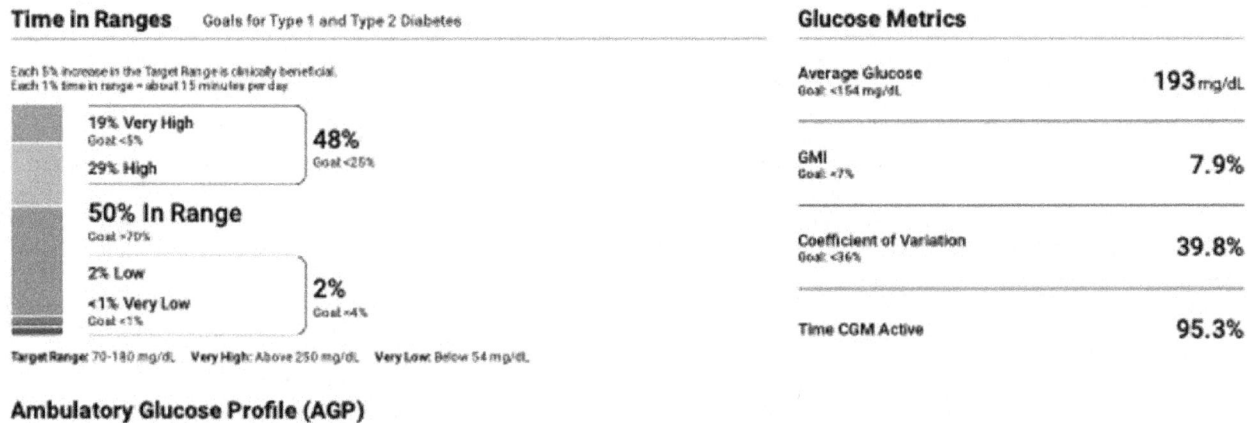

Time in Ranges — Goals for Type 1 and Type 2 Diabetes

Each 5% increase in the Target Range is clinically beneficial.
Each 1% time in range = about 15 minutes per day.

19% Very High — Goal <5%
29% High — **48%** Goal <25%

50% In Range — Goal >70%

2% Low
<1% Very Low — Goal <1% — **2%** Goal <4%

Target Range: 70-180 mg/dL   Very High: Above 250 mg/dL   Very Low: Below 54 mg/dL

Glucose Metrics

Average Glucose — Goal <154 mg/dL	**193** mg/dL
GMI — Goal <7%	**7.9%**
Coefficient of Variation — Goal <36%	**39.8%**
Time CGM Active	**95.3%**

Ambulatory Glucose Profile (AGP)

AGP is a summary of glucose values from the report period, with median (50%) and other percentiles shown as if they occurred in a single day.

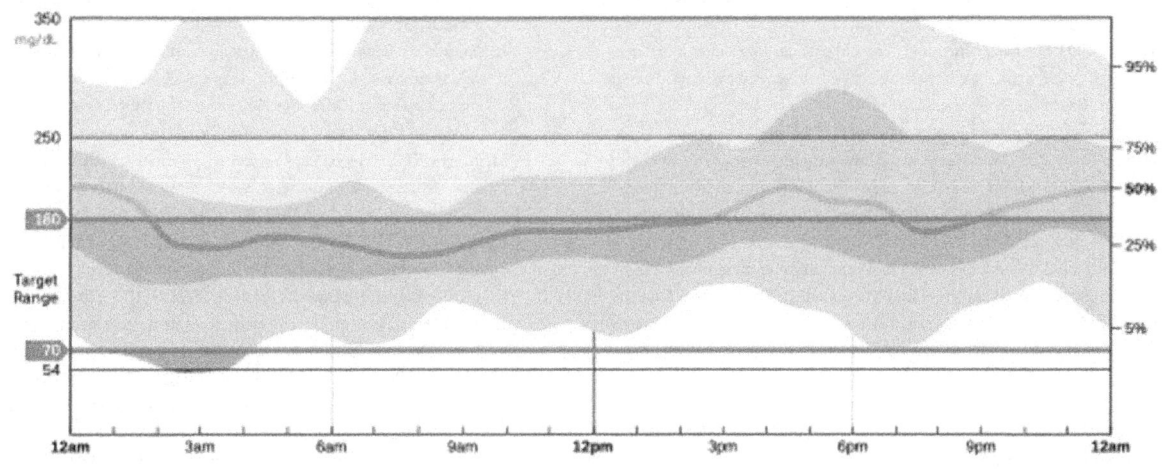

Daily Glucose Profile

Each daily profile represents a midnight-to-midnight period.

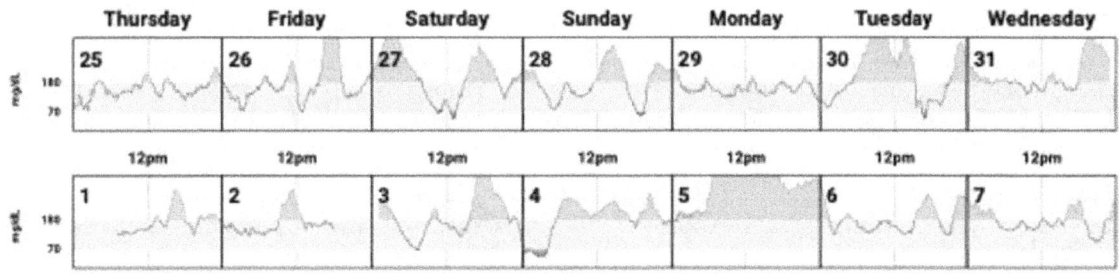

(Color—web and EPUB only)

- Often focusing on other risk factors (blood pressure, cigarette smoking, lipids) is easier and will also have major health impact.

- Finally, remember, the patient who comes into clinic wants to be healthier (or else they would not have made/kept the appointment).

References

1. Stratton IM, Adler AI, Neil HA, et al. Association of glycaemia with macrovascular and microvascular complications of type 2 diabetes (UKPDS 35): prospective observational study. *BMJ.* 2000;321(7258):405-412. PMID: 10938048

2. The Diabetes Control and Complications Trial Research Group, Nathan DM, Genuth S, et al. The effect of intensive treatment of diabetes on the development and progression of long-term complications in insulin-dependent diabetes mellitus. *N Engl J Med.* 1993;329(14):977-986. PMID: 8366922

3. Foster NC, Beck RW, Miller KM, et al. State of type 1 diabetes management and outcomes from the T1D Exchange in 2016-2018. *Diabetes Technol Ther.* 2019;21(2):66-72. PMID: 30657336

4. Valle T, Koivisto V, Reunanen A, Kangas T, Rissanen A. Glycemic control in patients with diabetes in Finland. *Diabetes Care.* 1999;22(4):575-579. PMID: 10189534

5. American Diabetes Association. Standards of medical care in diabetes. *Diabetes Care.* 2023;46(Suppl 1):S1-S155.

6. Stellefson M, Dipnarine K, Stopka C. The chronic care model and diabetes management in US primary care settings: a systematic review. *Prev Chronic Dis.* 2013;10:E26. PMID: 23428085

7. Wan EYF, Fung CSC, Jiao FF, et al. Five-year effectiveness of the multidisciplinary Risk Assessment and Management Programme-Diabetes Mellitus (RAMP-DM) on diabetes-related complications and health care service uses – a population-based and protensity-matched cohort study. *Diabetes Care.* 2018;41(1):49-59. PMID: 29138274

8. Jiao FF, Fung CSC, Wan EYF, et al. Five-year cost-effectiveness of the Multidisciplinary Risk Assessment and Management Programme-Diabetes Mellitus (RAMP-DM). *Diabetes Care.* 2018;41(2):250-257. PMID: 29246949

9. International Diabetes Federation 2022 Diabetes Atlas. http://www.diabetesatlas.org

10. Gaede P, Lund-Anderson H, Parving H-H, Pedersen O. Effect of multifactorial intervention on mortality in type 2 diabetes. *N Engl J Med.* 2008;358(6):580-591. PMID: 18256393

11. Kazemian P, Shebi FM, McCann N, Walensky RP, Wexler DJ. Evaluation of the cascade of diabetes care in the United States, 2005-2016. *JAMA Intern Med.* 2019;179(10):1376-1385. PMID: 31403657 (https://www.cdc.gov/chronicdisease/programs-impact/pop/diabetes)

12. Edelman SV, Wood R, Roberts M, Shubrook JH. Patients with type 2 diabetes are willing to do more to overcome therapeutic inertia: results from a double-blind survey. *Clin Diabetes.* 2020;38(3):222-229. PMID: 32699470

13. Perlman JE, Gooley TA, McNulty B, Meyers J, Hirsch IB. HbA1c and glucose management indicator discordance: a real-world analysis. *Diabetes Technol Ther.* 2021;23(4):253-258.

14. LeRoith D, Biessels GJ, Braithwaite SS, et al. Treatment of diabetes in older adults: an Endocrine Society clinical practice guideline. *J Clin Endocrinol Metab.* 2019;104(5):1520-1574. PMID: 30903688

15. Al-Kandari H, Al-Abdulrazzaq D, Davidsson L, et al. Identification of maturity-onset-diabetes of the young (MODY) mutations in a country where diabetes is endemic. *Sci Rep.* 2021;11(1):16060. PMID: 34373539

16. Bowman P, Day J, Torrens L, et al. Cognitive, neurological, and behavioral features in adults with *KCNJ11* neonatal diabetes. *Diabetes Care.* 2019;42(2):215-224. PMID: 30377186

17. Polonsky WH, Henry RR. Poor medication adherence in type 2 diabetes: recognizing the scope of the problem and its key contributors. *Patient Prefer Adherence.* 2016;10:1299-1307. PMID: 27524885

18. Martens T, Beck RW, Bailey R, et al; MOBILE Study Group. Effect of continuous glucose monitoring on glycemic control in patients with type 2 diabetes treated with basal insulin: a randomized clinical trial. *JAMA.* 2021;325(22):2262-2272. PMID: 34077499

19. Cox DJ, Banton T, Moncrief M, Conaway M, Diamond A, McCall AL. Minimizing glucose excursions (GEM) with continuous glucose monitoring in type 2 diabetes: a randomized clinical trial. *J Endocr Soc.* 2020;4(11):bvaa118. PMID: 33094208

20. Beck RW, Riddlesworth T, Ruedy K, et al; DIAMOND Study Group. Effect of continuous glucose monitoring on glycemic control in adults with type 1 diabetes using insulin injections: the DIAMOND randomized clinical trial. *JAMA.* 2017;317(4):371-378. PMID: 28118453

21. Martin CT, Criego AB, Carlson AL, Bergenstal RM. Advanced technology in the management of diabetes: which comes first-continuous glucose monitor or insulin pump? *Curr Diab Rep.* 2019;19(8):50. PMID: 31250124

22. Galindo RJ, Ramos C, Cardona S, et al. Efficacy of a smart insulin pen cap for the management of patients with uncontrolled type 2 diabetes: a randomized cross-over trial. *J Diabetes Sci Technol.* 2023;17(1):201-207. PMID: 34293955

23. Randløv J, Poulsen JU. How much do forgotten insulin injections matter to hemoglobin A1c in people with diabetes? A simulation study. *J Diabetes Sci Technol.* 2008;2(2):229-235. PMID: 19885347

24. Radin MS. Pitfalls in hemoglobin A_{1c} measurement: when results may be misleading. *J Gen Intern Med.* 2014;29(2):388-394. PMID: 24002631

25. Choudhary P, Kolassa R, Keuthage W, et al; ADAPT Study Group. Advanced hybrid closed loop therapy versus conventional therapy in adults with type 1 diabetes (ADAPT): a randomised controlled study. *Lancet Diab Endocrinol.* 2022;10(10):720-731. PMID: 36058207

26. Chan CB, Popeski N, Hassanabad MF, Sigal RJ, O'Connell P, Sargious P. Use of virtual care for glycemic management in people with types 1 and 2 diabetes and diabetes in regnancy: a rapid review. *Can J Diabetes.* 2021;45(7):677-688. PMID: 34045146

27. Magee MF, Baker KM, Fernandez SJ, et al. Redesigning ambulatory care management for uncontrolled type 2 diabetes: a prospective cohort study of the impact of a Boot Camp model on outcomes. *BMJ Open Diabetes Res Care.* 2019;7(1):e000731. PMID: 31798894

28. Bergenstal R. Presented at the 16th international conference on Advanced Technologies and Treatments for Diabetes, February 24, 2023. Berlin, Germany.

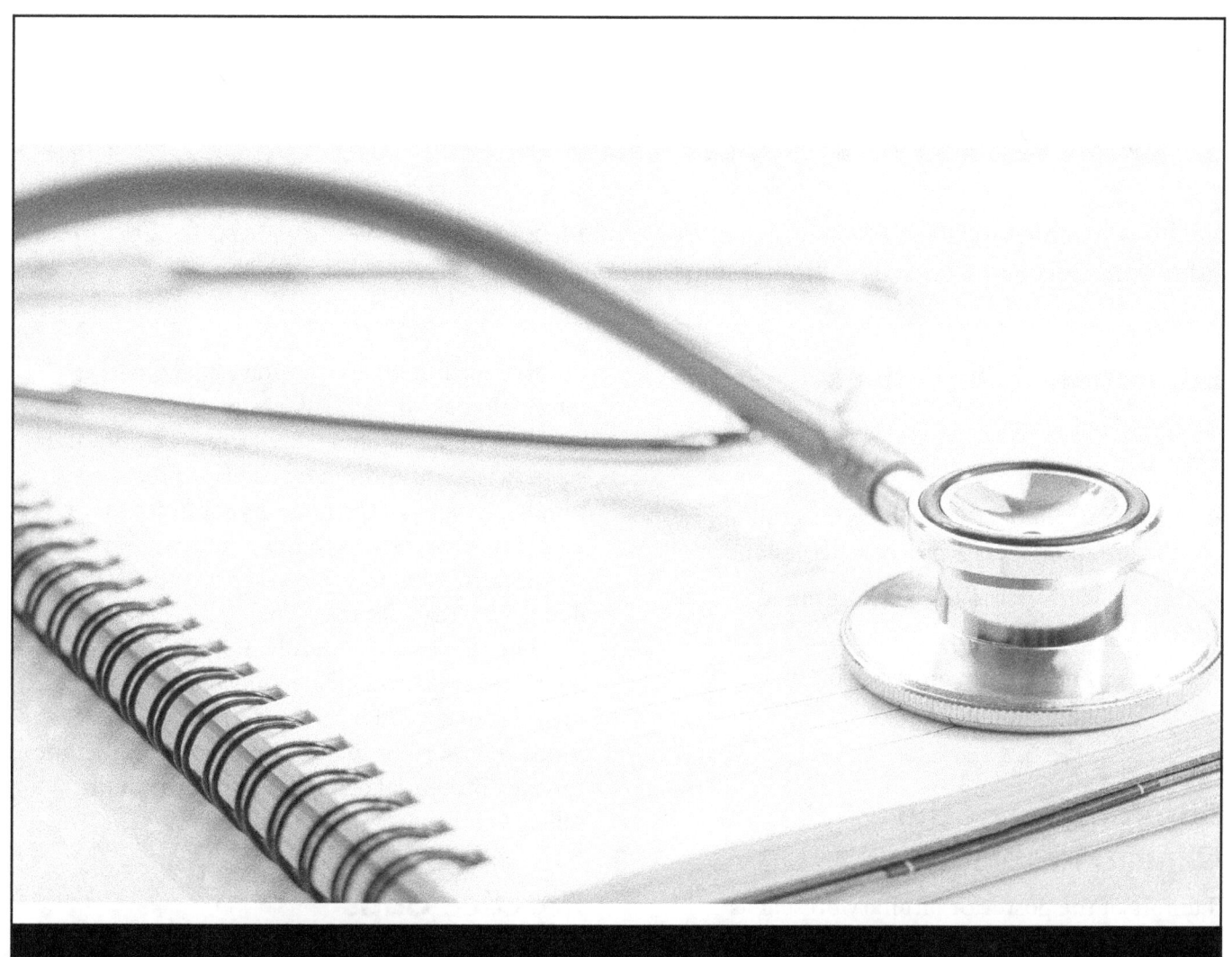

NEUROENDOCRINOLOGY AND PITUITARY

Tumors of the Posterior Pituitary

Michael Buchfelder, MD, PhD. Department of Neurosurgery, University Hospital Erlangen, Erlangen, Germany; Email: michael.buchfelder@uk-erlangen.de

Educational Objectives

After reviewing this chapter, learners should be able to:

- Consider tumors of the posterior pituitary in the differential diagnosis of sellar lesions.

- Describe the pathological background in their classification.

- Treat tumors of the posterior pituitary.

Significance of the Clinical Problem

Tumors of the posterior pituitary present as clinically nonfunctioning, space-occupying lesions of the sellar region. Although the predominant pathology is represented by pituitary adenomas, also referred to as PitNets, there is a wide differential diagnosis, including less common sellar lesions such as craniopharyngiomas and meningiomas. In a large series of sellar lesions, tumors of the posterior pituitary are classified as rare tumors, grouped together with germinomas and metastatic lesions. Recently, all primary posterior pituitary tumors have been subsumed under the term *pituicytoma*,[1] whereas in the past they were known as granular cell tumors, spindle-cell oncocytomas, sellar ependymomas, and pituicytomas. It is pertinent to recognize the new nomenclature to appreciate literature data. Posterior pituitary tumors are usually not recognized as such on the basis of clinical, radiologic, and biochemical features, erroneously defined instead as one of the more frequently occurring pathologies (pituitary adenomas, meningiomas, or papillary craniopharyngiomas). The rate of persistent and recurrent tumors after surgery is high. Although posterior pituitary tumors arise from the neurohypophysis, in contrast to metastases to the pituitary, they do not present with arginine vasopressin (AVP) deficiency (diabetes insipidus).

The lesions are clinically nonfunctioning and are therefore either incidentally discovered or manifest due to their mass effect. However, it is deemed important to take them into consideration for the differential diagnosis of tumors in the sellar region.

Practice Gaps

- Lack of knowledge about posterior pituitary tumors due to their rarity and consequent lack of familiarity among physicians and surgeons leads to failure in recognizing clinical phenotypes, misinterpretation of clinical findings, and delayed diagnosis and management.

- Inconsistency in pathological terminology has hampered the collection of sufficient data to enable assessment of treatment efficacy and prognosis.

Discussion

In the past, primary tumors of the posterior pituitary—the origins of which are nonepithelial cells within the pituitary—were classified as granular-cell tumors, spindle-cell oncocytomas, sellar ependymomas, and pituicytomas. However, taking into account their common genetic and epigenetic characterization, particularly the expression of thyroid transcription factor 1 (TTF-1), the most recent World Health Organization (WHO) classifications from 2017 and 2022 unite them under the term *pituicytoma*, denoting various subtypes.[1]

Pathology

Pituicytomas, granular-cell tumors of the sella, and spindle-cell oncocytomas are a family of rare and typically benign, slowly growing tumors arising from pituicytes within the infundibulum and the posterior pituitary (WHO grade I). These tumors do not represent a clinical and histologic spectrum of a single entity. However, they have morphologic overlap and linked nuclear expression of thyroid TTF-1, which is the keynote feature.[1-3] Pituicytomas have elongated bipolar spindle cells present in sheets and fascicles, and they occasionally adopt a storiform arrangement with perivascular lymphocytes, while granular-cell tumors have sheets and nodules of polygonal cells, small nuclei, abundant periodic acid–Schiff–positive histochemistry, and diastase-resistant granular eosinophilic cytoplasm. Spindle-cell oncocytomas have elongated cells in interlaced fascicles and variable oncocytic features. Spindle-cell oncocytomas exhibit antimitochondrial antibody immunoreactivity, while granular-cell tumors express α1-antitrypsin and CD68 and have intracytoplasmic granules. Focal aggregates of lymphocytes are common. Most cases show low proliferation with rare mitoses. These tumors lack expression of pituitary hormones, transcription factors, and neuroendocrine markers.

Pituicytoma Type

This benign neoplasm is histologically composed of bipolar spindle cells arranged in fascicles or storiform patterns. Cytoplasm is abundant and eosinophilic, but not granular. Histochemistry stain with periodic acid–Schiff is negative. The neoplasm lacks Herring bodies (unlike normal neurohypophysis), as well as Rosenthal fibers and eosinophilic granular bodies (unlike pilocytic astrocytomas). S-100 and vimentin are expressed, although glial fibrillary acidic protein is variable.[3]

Granular-Cell Tumor Type

Microscopically, cells are epithelioid (discrete cell borders) with abundant, coarsely granular eosinophilic cytoplasm (because of accumulation of lysosomes) and are often arranged in sheets or nodules. Periodic acid–Schiff is strongly positive, as well as periodic acid–Schiff with diastase digestion (cells are not glycogen-filled). S-100 is generally positive, and glial fibrillary acidic protein is negative.[3]

Spindle-Cell Oncocytoma Type

Microscopically, these tumors can display quite variable cell shapes, with epithelioid and spindle cells often mixed with eosinophilic to oncocytic cytoplasm and usually arranged in fascicles. In contrast to cytoplasm in granular-cell tumors, cytoplasm is eosinophilic but finely granular because of accumulation of mitochondria. Staining with periodic acid–Schiff is also negative. S-100 is positive, but glial fibrillary acidic protein is negative. Unlike the other diagnostic entities of the neurohypophysis, spindle-cell oncocytomas can recur in up to one-third of cases. Recurrent tumors usually display elevated proliferation indexes and aggressive behavior.[3]

Ependymoma Type

Since the normal pituitary does not contain ependymal cells, the most recent WHO classification has also classified these tumors as pituicytomas of the ependymoma type. The other subtypes are already very rare. However, this subtype is exceedingly rare. Data are sparse in the medical literature.

Epidemiology

Epidemiological data are not available for tumors of the posterior pituitary, which are very rare. Recent systematic reviews of the medical literature reported approximately 270 cases.[4,5] Moreover, most of these tumors reported were single, anecdotal case reports[2,6-10] or small case series.[3,5,11-13] According to the summarized data, posterior pituitary tumors occur most commonly in the middle decades of life with a mean age at onset of 47.7 years (range, 7-83 years). They are exceedingly rare in children, with only 6 cases being reported. There is no difference in incidence rate between males and females (ratio is almost 1:1). The prognosis for these low-grade tumors is generally good with no recurrence following total resection,[11] although the spindle-cell oncocytoma subtype can display more aggressive behavior.

Clinical Presentation

Posterior pituitary tumors are slowly growing lesions, with signs and symptoms usually being secondary to mass effect. Thus, posterior pituitary tumors resemble other slowly expanding, endocrine-inactive tumors of the sellar region, such as pituitary adenomas. Several were incidental radiologic findings, when MRI of the brain was performed for reasons that are unrelated to pituitary disease.[4,5,14] The duration of symptoms prior to diagnosis ranged from a few months to several years. The most common presenting symptoms were visual field defects, followed by hypopituitarism and headache.[4,10,12,14] Commonly encountered endocrine abnormalities were, in decreasing order of frequency, hyperprolactinemia, hypopituitarism, male hypogonadism with low testosterone, and, notably very rarely, AVP deficiency. The clinical presentation mainly depends on tumor size and location. Visual disturbances are commonly caused by compression of the optic chiasma, while headache and hypopituitarism can be induced by compression of the pituitary gland or its surroundings. As for other possible presenting symptoms such as fatigue, dizziness/vertigo, nausea, and vomiting, they are more likely to be the manifestations of hypoglycemia or secondary adrenocortical failure due to hypopituitarism.[4,5,9,14]

Over the last 40 years, 18 consecutive patients with posterior pituitary tumors underwent surgical treatment in our department. Nine patients (4 male, 5 female) were diagnosed with pituicytomas of the granular-cell type, 6 patients (3 males, 3 females) with pituicytomas of the spindle-cell oncocytoma type, and 3 patients (2 males, 1 female) with true pituicytomas. We did not treat pituicytomas of the ependymoma type. Patient age ranged from 26 to 74 years (median, 58 years). The most frequent preoperative symptom in this patient group was visual disturbance.

Radiologic Findings

Most posterior pituitary tumors present as well-defined, solid, contrast-enhancing, intrasellar, parasellar, or suprasellar space-occupying lesions. In contrast to pituitary adenomas and craniopharyngiomas, pituicytomas less frequently exhibit cystic or necrotic portions[13,14] than pituitary adenomas. Whereas the granular-type and "true" pituicytoma type may present as a suprasellar lesion, with the pituitary gland within the normal fossa and the infundibulum clearly visible, the spindle-cell oncocytoma type mostly presents as a complex intrasellar and suprasellar lesion, in which the normal gland cannot be distinguished MRI.[13-15] Only if the solid, enhancing mass is small enough to be clearly identified as arising from the neurohypophysis or infundibulum, and not from the adenohypophysis, can a pituicytoma be considered in the preoperative differential diagnosis.[15] Thus, these tumors are great mimickers.[7]

Biochemical Evaluation

Just like the clinical presentation, the biochemical endocrinological evaluation does not provide a clue to the diagnosis of posterior pituitary tumors. Hormonal testing may reveal all kinds of anterior pituitary function—ranging from unaffected, to partial deficiencies, to total hypopituitarism.[5,9,12-14]

Surgical Treatment

In contrast to operations for pituitary adenomas, the surgical treatment of posterior pituitary tumors is always challenging due to the firmness and high vascularity of the tumors. Moreover, they often display invasive growth into the cavernous sinus, optic apparatus, or the normal pituitary gland.[11,12,14] Their location and extent often necessitates craniotomy, and subtotal or partial tumor resection is the usual outcome. Due to high vascularity, these operations can be associated with significant blood loss. Posterior pituitary tumors can rarely be extracted by curettage. The surgical technique is usually en block resection, which requires extracapsular dissection. As mentioned previously, the histologic subtyping is related to the prognosis.[3,11,12] Data on surgical treatment of sellar ependymoma are hitherto restricted to a few case reports but suggest better outcomes with respect to total resection.[10]

Irradiation

Since some residual tumor usually remains after surgery, irradiation is frequently considered as an adjunct treatment. However, for the relatively small number of patients described in the medical literature, only anecdotal outcomes are reported after conventional fractionated megavoltage irradiation or radiosurgery.[8]

Medical Treatment

Since the *BRAF* V600E pathogenic variant was identified, the use of BRAF inhibitors, such as dabrafenib, has been anecdotally reported with some positive response, but they have not yet been systematically tested.[6]

Clinical Case Vignettes
Case 1

A 68-year-old woman presents with progressive vertigo and gait disturbances over many months. On clinical examination, she has minor visual disturbances. Visual acuity is 0.5 in the right eye and 0.63 in the left eye with considerable restriction of the visual fields. She has no clinical evidence of hormonal excess or hypopituitarism. Laboratory investigation confirms a normal prolactin concentration (2.96 ng/mL [0.13 nmol/L]) and normal pituitary function.

MRI reveals a suprasellar tumor measuring 16 × 16 × 13 mm, which is closely attached to the infundibulum. However, the pituitary, sitting in a normally sized fossa, is virtually unaffected (*see figure 1*).

She undergoes transcranial resection of the tumor via a right frontotemporal craniotomy with dissection and preservation of the infundibulum. She has an uneventful postoperative course, and her visual fields normalize and visual acuity improves. Pituitary function is deemed to be

Figure 1.

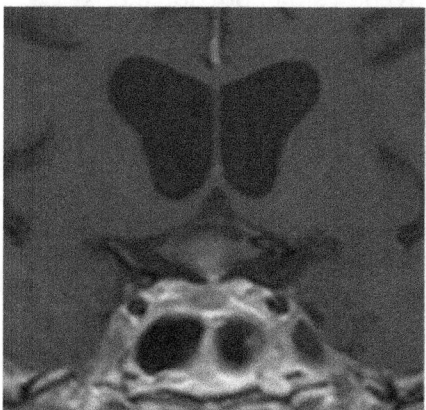
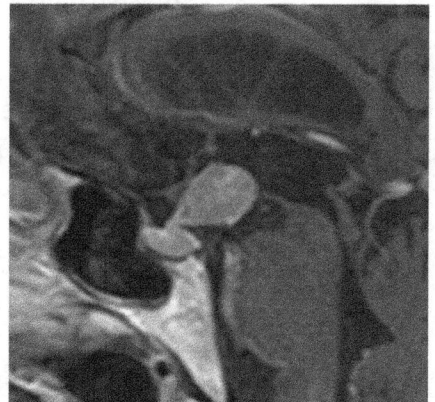
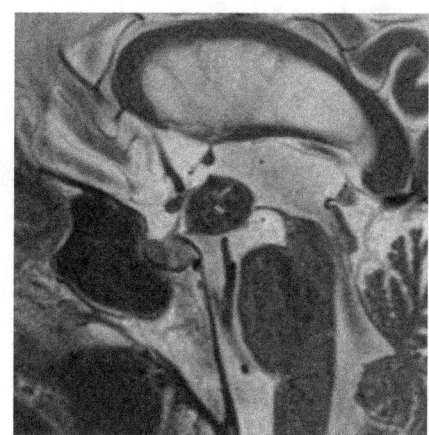

T1-weighted coronal section   **T1-weighted midsagittal section**   **T2-weighted midsagittal section**

preserved on the basis of clinical findings and endocrine testing. She does not develop AVP deficiency. Her most recent follow-up, 1.5 years after surgery, does not reveal any residual lesion. Postoperative pituitary MRI is shown (*see figure 2*).

Figure 2.

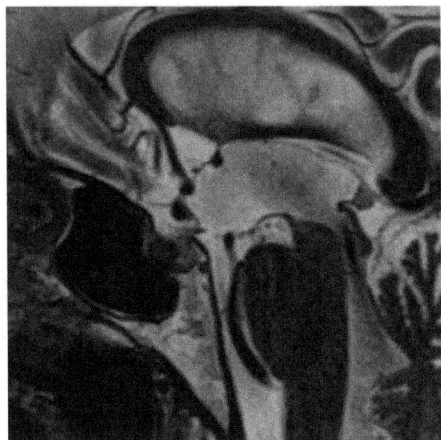

T2-weighted midsagittal section

Histology reveals a granular-type pituicytoma. Hematoxylin-eosin staining shows a relatively well-differentiated tumor with small, round nuclei and finely dispersed chromatin structure (*see figure 3A*). The cytoplasm is periodic acid–Schiff positive. Immunohistochemistry demonstrates weak expression of S-100 as a neuronal marker (*see figure 3B*) and nuclear TTF-1 expression in virtually all tumor cells (*see figure 3C*). Proliferation activity as measured by Ki-67 expression (*see figure 3D*) is low (<3%).

Figure 3.

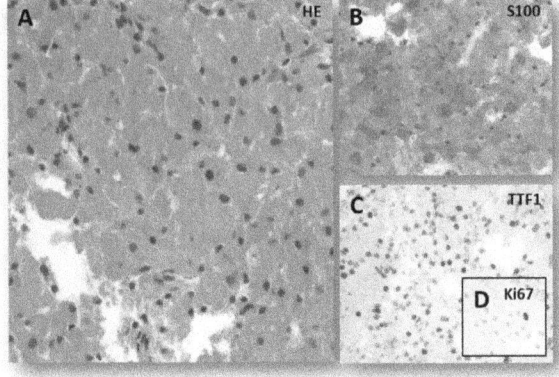

(Color—web and EPUB only)

Case 2

A 63-year-old woman experiences sudden onset of adynamia, fatigue, and vertigo, accompanied by vomiting. She is admitted to the emergency department where severe hyponatremia is diagnosed.

> Sodium = 107 mEq/L (136-142 mEq/L)
>   (SI: 107 mmol/L [136-142 mmol/L])
> Prolactin = 29.9 ng/mL (4-30 ng/mL)
>   (SI: 1.30 nmol/L [0.17-1.30 nmol/L])
> Cortisol, low
> Free T_4, low
> Estradiol, low
> IGF-1, low

This prompts pituitary MRI, which reveals a large intrasellar, suprasellar, and parasellar pituitary tumor (18 × 13 × 13 mm) compromising the optic chiasma. The normal pituitary cannot be differentiated (*see figure 4*).

The patient, however, reports normal visual function. On assessment, visual acuity is normal and visual fields are not restricted. There is no evidence of diabetes insipidus.

She initially undergoes substitution therapy with hydrocortisone and levothyroxine. Sodium concentrations rapidly normalize, and her clinical condition improves dramatically. A nonfunctional pituitary adenoma is suspected. She undergoes transsphenoidal surgery. During the operation, the residual normal pituitary is identified as a thin layer at the bottom of the sella turcica. It is split, and a greyish, fibrous, firm tumor is dissected from the cavernous sinus and arachnoid layer. It is partially removed in small portions. It is extremely vascularized and firmly attached to the cavernous sinus and suprasellar arachnoid. Intraoperative cerebrospinal fluid leakage occurs. However, the postoperative course is uneventful. The patient does well on her substitution treatment and is discharged.

Histology shows fragmented portions of a spindle-cell tumor with moderately chromatin dense nuclei (*see figure 5E*). There are interspersed weakly eosinophilic tumor cells with large cells and round or oval nuclei. Immunostaining reveals strong expression of TTF-1 in the tumor

Figure 4.

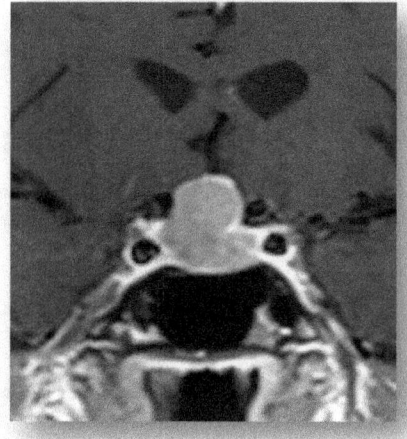

Preoperative pituitary MRI, T1-weighted coronal

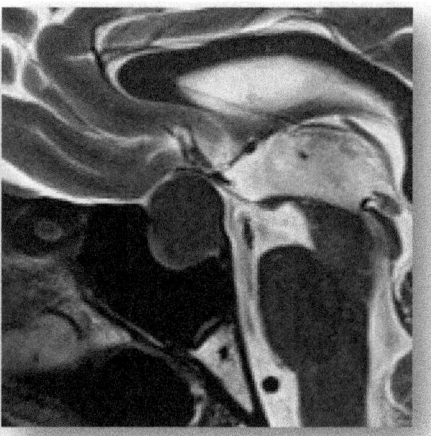

Preoperative pituitary MRI, T2-weighted sagittal

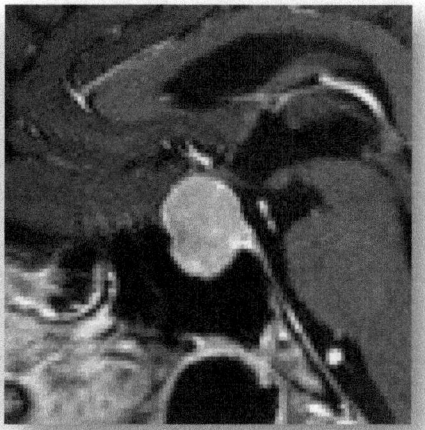

Preoperative pituitary MRI, T1-weighted sagittal

cells (*see figure 5F*). All immunostaining against pituitary hormones is negative. Proliferative activity, as expressed by Ki-67 immunostaining is low (*see figure 5G*). The tumor is thus classified as a pituicytoma of the spindle-cell type due to the TTF-1 expression.

Figure 5.

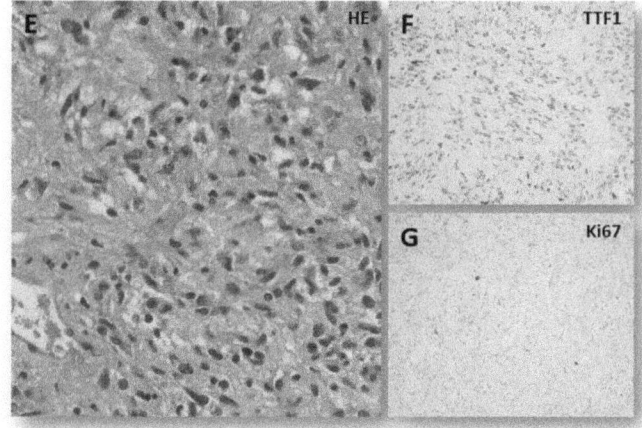

(Color—web and EPUB only)

The delayed routine postoperative MRI after 3 months shows normal postoperative findings with considerable residual tumor. The patient rapidly resumes her full professional activities and maintains her hormonal substitution therapy. There is no evidence of AVP deficiency postoperatively. She attends yearly follow-up appointments and unfortunately experiences progression of her residual lesion. Thus, reoperation or irradiation is being considered. There has been no recovery of anterior pituitary function.

Key Learning Points

- All tumors of the posterior pituitary are called pituicytomas.

- Pituicytomas present as space-occupying intrasellar and extrasellar lesions.

- Diabetes insipidus is not a presenting symptom of pituicytomas.

- Immunohistochemical expression of TTF-1 is the common feature of all 4 subtypes (pituicytoma type, spindle-cell oncocytoma type, granular-cell tumor type, and sellar ependymoma type).

- Although tumors of the posterior pituitary are rare, they should be considered in the differential diagnosis.

References

1. Asa SL, Mete O, Perry A, Osamura RY. Overview of the 2022 WHO classification of pituitary tumors. *Endocrine Pathol.* 2022;33(1):6-26. PMID: 35291028

2. Hong CS, Elsamadicy AA, Fisayo A, et al. Comprehensive genomic characterization of a case of granular cell tumor of the posterior pituitary gland: a case report. *Front Endocrinol.* 2021;12:762095. PMID: 34925233

3. Schmid S, Solomon DA, Perez E, et al. Genetic and epigenetic characterization of posterior pituitary tumors. *Acta Neuropathol.* 2021;142(6):1025-1043.

4. Guerrero-Pérez F, Marengo AP, Vidal N, Iglesias P, Villabona C. Primary tumors of the posterior pituitary: a systematic review. *Rev Endocr Metab Disord.* 2019;20(2):219-238. PMID: 30864049

5. Zhang Y, Teng Y, Zhu H, et al. Granular cell tumor of the neurohypophysis: 3 cases and a systematic literature review of 98 cases. *World Neurosurg.* 2018;118:e621-e630. PMID: 30017767

6. Grenier-Chartrand F, Barrit S, Racu ML, et al. Dabrafenib monotherapy for a recurrent BRAFV600E-mutated TTF-1 positive posterior pituitary tumor. *Acta Neurochir (Wien).* 2022;164(3):737-742. PMID: 35029761

7. Mohan A, Kannoth P, Unni C, Jose BV, Parambil RP, Nandeesh BN. Rare neurohypophyseal tumor presenting as giant pituitary macroadenoma with cavernous sinus invasion – a case report and review of the literature. *Surg Neurol Int.* 2020;11:261-265. PMID: 33024599

8. Oushy S, Graffeo CS, Perry A, Stafford SL, Link MJ, Pollock BE. Single-fraction stereotactic radiosurgery for spindle-cell oncocytoma: preliminary experience and systematic review of the literature. *J Neurooncol.* 2019;144(2):325-332. PMID: 31254265

9. Popovic V, Pekic S, Skender-Gazibara M, Salehi F, Kovacs K. A large sellar granular cell tumor in a 21-year-old woman. *Endocr Pathol.* 2007;18(2):91-94. PMID: 17916999

10. Wang S, Zong W, Li Y, Wang B, Ke C, Guo D. Pituitary ependymoma: a case report and review of the literature. *World Neurosurg.* 2018;110:43-54. PMID: 29102750

11. Ahmed A-K, Dawood HY, Penn DL, Smith TR. Extent of surgical resection and tumor size predicts prognosis in granular cell tumor of the sellar region. *Acta Neurochir (Wien).* 2017;159(11):2209-2216. PMID: 28948361

12. Das L, Vaiphei K, Rai A, et al. Posterior pituitary tumours: patient outcomes and determinants of disease recurrence or persistence. *Endocr Connect.* 2021;10(4):387-400. PMID: 33709954

13. Han F, Gao L, Wang Y, et al. Clinical and imaging features of granular cell tumor of the neurohypophysis: a retrospective analysis. *Medicine (Baltimore).* 2018;97(9):e9745. PMID: 29489677

14. Kandregula S, Shashidhar A, Rao S, et al. Granular cell tumor and spindle cell oncocytoma of the pituitary gland: imaging and intraoperative cytology diagnostic dilemmas and management challenges. *J Neurol Surg A Cent Eur Neurosurg.* 2022;83(5):442-450. PMID: 34911085

15. Shih RY, Schroeder JW, Koeller KK. Primary tumors of the pituitary gland: radiologic-pathologic correlation. *Radiographics.* 2021;41(7):2029-2046. PMID: 34597177

Gastroenteropancreatic Neuroendocrine Neoplasms for Endocrinologists

Wouter W. de Herder, MD, PhD. Erasmus MC and Erasmus MC Cancer Institute, Rotterdam, the Netherlands; Email: w.w.deherder@erasmusmc.nl

Educational Objectives

After reviewing this chapter, learners should be able to:

- Recognize the important role of the endocrinologist in the multidisciplinary team for patients with (functioning) gastroenteropancreatic neuroendocrine neoplasms (NENs).

- Explain the management of hormone-producing gastroenteropancreatic NENs.

- Describe the role of the endocrinologist in the follow-up and surveillance of patients with gastroduodenal NENs in the setting of multiple endocrine neoplasia (MEN) type 1.

Significance of the Clinical Problem

NENs are a diverse group of neoplasms that predominantly arise from the embryonic gut, and they are subdivided into foregut, midgut, and hindgut NENs.[1] General incidence is estimated at 6.98 to 8.8 per 100,000 persons, and it has impressively increased 3.7- to 6.4-fold over the previous 4 decades. Over this period, overall survival has improved for patients with all NEN subtypes.[1-3] Care for patients with gastroenteropancreatic NENs has improved considerably due to better understanding of the underlying key molecular pathways, better classification, advent of PET imaging techniques, and the registration and approval of radionuclide and targeted therapies. Clinicians caring for patients with gastroenteropancreatic NENs should be aware of the heterogeneity of this disease and should be able to provide a tailored diagnostic and therapeutic strategy aimed at controlling hormonal hypersecretion and tumor growth and spread. Because of the rarity of gastroenteropancreatic NENs, affected patients should be discussed in a multidisciplinary team setting with experienced representatives from endocrinology, oncology, gastroenterology, pulmonology, radiology, nuclear medicine, surgery, and pathology. Only through collaboration among these key disciplines can excellent care be delivered.

Practice Gaps

- Patients with gastroenteropancreatic NENs can be seen by different specialists in various hospital settings (eg, endocrinologists, gastroenterologists, oncologists, surgeons). However, a multidisciplinary approach in an expert center is required for optimal patient care.

- Many improvements are needed to achieve a timely and accurate diagnosis.

- Circulating prognostic and predictive markers are generally lacking.

- Knowledge on the biologic processes driving gastroenteropancreatic NENs should be further investigated in preclinical models.

- Histologic diagnosis can be improved through the use of advanced molecular markers.

- Novel nuclear imaging techniques can potentially improve the sensitivity and specificity of functional imaging in NENs.

Discussion

Pathology and Staging

Diagnosis of an NEN is based on its distinctive histologic and immunohistopathologic profile such as expression of the general markers of neuroendocrine differentiation, chromogranin A and synaptophysin. Consequently, histology should be obtained by biopsy or resection in all patients suspected of having an NEN. NEN grading is based on traditional morphologic features, as well as proliferation rate. Proliferation rates are defined by 3 grades (G1, G2, G3) of neuroendocrine tumors (NETs) that use specific numerical ranges of the mitotic count and Ki67 proliferation index and high-grade neuroendocrine carcinomas (NECs). This grading correlates with survival rates.[1,4]

The TNM staging system stages NENs localized to the organ of origin as I or II depending on their size and extent. Tumors with spread to regional nodes are deemed stage III, and those with distant metastases as stage IV. This classification also correlates with survival rates.[1,4]

Genetic (Endocrine) Syndromes

Pancreatic, gastric, duodenal, thymic, and bronchial NENs occur in the spectrum of MEN type 1 (MIM 131100).[5] Pancreatic NENs also occur in persons with von Hippel-Lindau syndrome (MIM 193300). Periampullary somatostatinomas can be diagnosed in patients with neurofibromatosis 1 (MIM 162200). In Pacak-Zhuang syndrome (MIM 603349), pathogenic variants in the *EPAS1* gene lead to the development of somatostatinomas, paragangliomas/pheochromocytomas, and polycythemia. In persons with Mahvash disease (MIM 619290) caused by a pathogenic variant

(P86S) in the glucagon receptor gene (*GCGR*), there is an increased incidence of pancreatic NENs. Insulinomatosis of the pancreas has been documented in patients with *MAFA* pathogenic variants (MIM 147630).[1]

Hormone-Related Symptoms and Syndromes Caused By Gastroenteropancreatic NENs

Carcinoid Syndrome

Carcinoid syndrome is present in about 32% of patients with midgut NETs, and patients with lung carcinoids can also present with this syndrome. The syndrome is rare in persons with metastatic NENs of other primary origins. Carcinoid syndrome is defined by chronic diarrhea and/or flushing in the presence of systemically elevated levels of serotonin or its breakdown product, 5-hydroxyindolacetic acid (5-HIAA). While patients with this syndrome experience long-term survival, their quality of life is often limited due to hormonal symptoms, mesenteric fibrosis, and fibrosis in the heart (endocardium, heart valves—mostly on the right side), known as carcinoid heart disease.[6]

Insulinoma

Insulinomas are pancreatic NENs that can cause severe hypoglycemia through inappropriate secretion of insulin or insulin precursors. The diagnostic Whipple triad consists of (1) symptoms of hypoglycemia, (2) plasma glucose concentration less than 40 mg/dL (<2.2 mmol/L) (guidelines also use 55 mg/dL [3.0 mmol/L] as a cutoff glucose value), and (3) relief of symptoms with the administration of glucose. Approximately 10% of insulinomas are multiple and less than 10% are metastatic at presentation.[7,8]

Gastrinoma

Gastrinomas are NENs that secrete gastrin. Fifty to eighty percent of gastrinomas are localized in the duodenum and 20% to 50% are in the pancreas. Gastric acid hypersecretion can result in severe peptic ulcer disease, which can be resistant to regular treatments, and diarrhea.[9]

VIPoma

VIPomas are NENs that secrete vasoactive intestinal polypeptide (VIP). These tumors can be localized in the pancreas (75%) or in the sympathetic ganglia (25%). Persons with VIPomas experience profuse, large volumes of watery diarrhea that eventually lead to severe electrolyte disturbances. Other symptoms include facial flushing and inhibition of gastric acid secretion.[10]

Glucagonoma

Glucagonomas are pancreatic NENs that secrete glucagon. In most persons with a glucagonoma, there is either new-onset or worsening diabetes mellitus. Glucagon hypersecretion also results in severe weight loss. Furthermore, cheilosis, glossitis, and stomatitis are reported in this setting.[11]

Other Hormonal Syndromes Associated With NENs

Paraneoplastic humoral syndromes in gastroenteropancreatic NENs (mostly pancreatic NENs) are due to ACTH or corticotropin-releasing hormone secretion leading to Cushing syndrome, PTHrP secretion causing hypercalcemia, antidiuretic hormone secretion causing SIADH and hyponatremia, and GHRH excretion causing acromegaly.[12]

Nonfunctioning/Nonsecreting NENs

Given the expanded use of cross-sectional imaging and endoscopic procedures, an increasing number of patients with NENs present without related symptoms, so-called incidentalomas. Also, depending on the location of the nonfunctioning NEN and/or its metastases, symptoms can result from compression, ingrowth, or obstruction of vital structures.[1]

Circulating Markers

Some of the hormones produced by NENs are bioactive and are released in the circulation. Therefore, they are consequently associated with a secretory syndrome (functioning NENs: insulin, gastrin, VIP, glucagon, 5-HIAA). Other markers include chromogranin A, pancreastatin, and the NETest.[1] The NETest is a multianalyte biomarker that gives a single readout through an algorithm. An increased NETest score is a predictor for disease progression and decreased survival.[1]

Imaging Markers

Localization and staging of NENs relies on both morphologic and functional imaging techniques such as CT, MRI, somatostatin receptor imaging using PET, and combinations of these modalities. Endoscopic ultrasonography is a sensitive tool in experienced hands for detecting pancreatic NENs, and it allows for FNA.[1]

Management

Patients with stage 1 to 3 disease might be candidates for curative surgical resection. Surgery for midgut NETs is often palliative; other palliative options include liver-directed therapy.

Hormonal Syndromes

Somatostatin analogues inhibit the secretion of humoral factors by NETs, particularly carcinoid syndrome, VIP, and insulin in malignant metastatic insulinomas. Telotristat ethyl is a serotonin synthesis inhibitor that can alleviate carcinoid syndrome–induced, somatostatin analogue–refractory diarrhea. Prevention of hypoglycemic events is the primary treatment target of insulinoma management. Radical surgical resection of insulinomas for locoregional disease and occasionally distant metastases is recommended if feasible. Frequent meals, if required, and also nightly intake or feeding through a nasogastric or nasoduodenal tube might be needed. Patients with treatment-refractory insulinoma can be managed with parenteral glucose infusion. Drugs used to prevent hypoglycemia include diazoxide, first- and second-generation somatostatin analogues, and glucocorticoids. Second-line antiproliferative treatments such as everolimus and peptide-receptor radionuclide therapy with radiolabeled somatostatin analogues can also alleviate hypoglycemic events. Treatment goals in patients with Zollinger-Ellison syndrome are to prevent pyrosis; reflux; and complications such as ulcers, perforation, and esophageal stricture. Affected patients should be started on high dosages of proton-pump inhibitor therapy. Surgery is the only curative option for duodenal or pancreatic gastrinomas. Somatostatin analogues decrease tumoral gastrin and acid production but neither is registered nor approved for this indication. Treatment of VIPomas should include a combination of high-dosage antidiarrheal agents, as well as somatostatin analogue therapy (octreotide). Patients with glucagonomas can also benefit from treatment with somatostatin analogues, although these drugs are not registered or approved for this indication.

Antineoplastic Treatments in NEN
Somatostatin analogues can have a growth-stabilizing effect in NETs and are generally considered to be first-line systemic therapy for grade 1 and 2 NETs. Somatostatin analogues should not be the primary antiproliferative treatment for fast-growing NENs, massive tumor bulk with local compression of vital structures, or grade 3 disease/NECs.

Peptide-receptor radionuclide therapy with ^{177}Lu-DOTATATE or ^{177}Lu-DOTATOC is an approved second-line treatment in patients with low-grade (grade 1 to 2) gastroenteropancreatic NETs. Second-line targeted therapies in grade 1 to 2 pancreatic NETs include everolimus and sunitinib. Everolimus can also be used as second-line therapy in patients with midgut NETs. Grade 3 pancreatic NETs and NECs can be treated with conventional chemotherapy.[1]

Clinical Case Vignettes

Case 1

A 51-year-old woman is referred for evaluation of suspected NET/carcinoid syndrome. She has hot flashes/flushes during the day and sweats tremendously during the night. She also has diarrhea, mainly after drinking milk, which intensified after she started taking omeprazole, 40 mg daily, for gastroesophageal reflux disease. Laboratory testing documents a chromogranin A concentration of 1288 µg/L (reference range, <94 µg/L).

Which of the following is the best next step?
A. Perform somatostatin receptor imaging (single-photon emission CT/PET) to localize a neuroendocrine tumor
B. Perform upper gastrointestinal endoscopy
C. Recommend no additional investigations
D. Stop omeprazole for at least 1 to 2 weeks and repeat chromogranin A measurement

Answer: D) Stop omeprazole for at least 1 to 2 weeks and repeat chromogranin A measurement

Chromogranin A is the most used circulating general biomarker in NENs. This protein is produced and processed as a component of the neuroendocrine cellular secretory apparatus. The finding of increased chromogranin A is considered to be sensitive and 60% to 90% accurate once a NEN has been identified, but it is an inappropriate first-line diagnostic tool. Measurements are usually nonspecific (10%-35% specificity) since chromogranin A is elevated in other conditions (eg, other neoplasms, cardiac and inflammatory diseases, kidney failure, atrophic gastritis, and in the setting of proton-pump inhibitor or H2-blocker administration). Furthermore, it appears that there is no direct relationship with the levels of circulating chromogranin A and tumoral load, as 30% to 50% of NENs show normal, nonelevated chromogranin A levels. Chromogranin A has a sensitivity of 46% to 100% and specificity of 68% to 90%, respectively, when used to monitor disease progression and response to treatment.[1]

Profound gastric acid inhibition with proton-pump inhibitors can lead to clinically important hypergastrinemia due to hypo/anacidity. Gastrin has a stimulatory effect on the enterochromaffin-like cells of the stomach leading to histamine increase. Generally, not only serum gastrin but also chromogranin A levels increase during potent acid-suppressive therapy. The activation and proliferation of enterochromaffin-like cells resulting in enterochromaffin-like cell hyperplasia can be a source of elevated circulating chromogranin A levels. On cessation of proton-pump inhibitor therapy, normalization of serum chromogranin A and gastrin levels occurs after 1 to 2 weeks.[1,9]

Measurement	While on omeprazole, 40 mg daily	After stopping omeprazole for 2 weeks	While on esomeprazole, 80 mg daily	Reference range
Chromogranin A	1649 µg/L	161 µg/L	1676 µg/L	<94 µg/L
Gastrin	890 ng/L	43 ng/L	470 ng/L	<115 ng/L

In this patient, omeprazole was stopped for 2 weeks, and chromogranin A and gastrin levels were reevaluated (Answer D). Later, esomeprazole was started because of recurrent symptoms of reflux.

Chromogranin A was elevated in the setting of proton-pump inhibitor use. Stopping the proton-pump inhibitor resulted in normalization of chromogranin A. Therefore, no localization studies (Answers A and B) to search for a potential NEN should be performed.

Case 2

A 44-year-old woman is referred for evaluation of hypoglycemic symptoms. For 1.5 years, she has been experiencing episodes of tremors, blurriness, loss of attention, and headaches. There is no excessive perspiration, hunger, or loss of consciousness. She has fewer symptoms when she eats frequent meals. Her weight is 169.8 lb (77 kg); her weight has gradually increased over a period of 3 years (1 to 2 lb/y [0.5 to 0.9 kg/y]). Her primary care provider has documented a very low blood glucose concentration during an episode using a portable glucose sensor.

Additional investigations include a 72-hour fast with the following results:

> After 40 hours; glucose = 23 mg/dL (SI: 1.3 mmol/L), insulin = 3.7 µIU/mL (SI: 25.7 pmol/L) ("hypoglycemic symptoms")
> After 40.5 hours; glucose = 25 mg/dL (SI: 1.4 mmol/L), insulin = 3.0 µIU/mL (SI: 20.8 pmol/L) ("hypoglycemic symptoms")

The fast is stopped and the patient is allowed to eat food. Her hypoglycemic symptoms disappear. Urine toxicology is negative for sulfonylurea or thiazolidinedione (metabolites) derivatives.

Do you agree with the diagnosis of insulinoma in this case? What is the next diagnostic step?

A. Yes; perform CT or MRI of the abdomen

B. Yes; perform [68]Gallium-DOTA-somatostatin analogue PET-CT or PET-MRI

C. No; advise no additional evaluation

D. No; perform a meal test combined with blood glucose measurements

Answer: A) Yes; perform CT or MRI of the abdomen

Endocrine Society guidelines on the biochemical diagnosis of organic hyperinsulinism[8] indicate the following:

- Blood glucose concentration less than 55 mg/dL (<3.0 mmol/L) during symptoms

- Concomitant insulin concentration ≥3.0 µIU/mL (SI: ≥20.8 pmol/L)

- Concomitant C-peptide concentration ≥1.7 ng/mL (SI: ≥0.2 nmol/L)

- Concomitant proinsulin concentration ≥44.1 pg/mL (SI: ≥5 pmol/L)

- Absence of sulfonylurea, thiazolidinedione (metabolites) in the plasma or urine

- β-Hydroxybutyrate ≤0.03 mg/dL (SI: ≤2.7 µmol/L) at end of fast

- Glucose response to 1 mg of glucagon >25 mg/dL (>1.4 mmol/L) at end of fast

Imaging strategies in patients with insulinoma are shown in the *box*.

Imaging	Sensitivity
Transabdominal ultrasonography	9%-65%
3-Phase CT	60%-80%
MRI (T1- and T2-weighted images + fat suppression)	85%-90%
Endoscopic ultrasonography	75%-90%
Arterial calcium stimulation—venous sampling	80%-90%
Angiography	
• Intraoperative localizing techniques	
◦ Palpation	70%
◦ Intraoperative ultrasonography	75%-90%
◦ Palpation + intraoperative ultrasonography	85%-95%
• Nuclear medicine	
◦ Somatostatin receptor scintigraphy SPECT/PET	46%-50%/50%-86%
◦ 18F-DOPA PET	50%
◦ GLP-1 (exendin-4) receptor imaging SPECT/PET	85%-95%

Reprinted from de Herder WW et al. In Feingold KR et al, eds. Endotext. South Dartmouth, MA: MDText.com, Inc. Copyright © 2000 MDText.com, Inc.

According to the guidelines, CT or MRI is considered the first localizing step for an insulinoma. Gallium-68-DOTA-somatostatin analogue PET-CT or PET-MRI is currently not recommended because most localized insulinomas are somatostatin receptor subtype 2 negative. However, most malignant insulinomas and their metastatic spread can be localized using [68]gallium-DOTA-somatostatin analogue PET-CT or PET-MRI. The biochemical investigations are consistent with the biochemical diagnosis of insulinoma, and no additional biochemical testing is required (thus, Answer A is correct).

Case 3

A 44-year-old woman has a positive family history of MEN type 1 and has a pathogenic variant in the *MEN1* gene. She underwent a 3 and one-half gland parathyroidectomy at age 30 years because of multiple gland hyperparathyroidism. Pituitary MRI shows normal findings, and

pituitary function is normal. Serum calcium is within normal limits. Neither chest CT nor mammography shows abnormalities. Laboratory testing documents normal concentrations of blood glucose, gastrin, and serum calcium.

MRI of the abdomen shows a single solid, 1.7-cm, hyperintense lesion in the pancreatic tail and another single solid, 0.9-cm, hyperintense lesion in the pancreatic body. No pathologic lymph nodes are observed, and no other abnormalities are noted. A ^{68}Ga-DOTATATE-PET/CT shows uptake of this radiopharmaceutical agent in both pancreatic lesions. Endoscopic ultrasonography shows 2 hyperechoic lesions in the pancreatic body and tail. Cytologic findings of the largest tail lesion are compatible with a low-grade neuroendocrine tumor (Ki67 index, 1%).

Which of the following is the best next step?

A. First-line peptide-receptor radionuclide therapy with radiolabeled somatostatin analogues or targeted therapy (everolimus/sunitinib)

B. First-line somatostatin analogue therapy

C. Follow-up imaging and watchful waiting

D. Surgical referral for both pancreatic lesions

E. Surgical referral for the largest (tail) pancreatic lesion

Answer: C) Follow-up imaging and watchful waiting

Several studies show that conservative management (Answer C) of patients with MEN type 1 who have a nonfunctioning pancreatic NET 2 cm or smaller is associated with a low risk of disease-specific mortality. The decision to recommend surgery (Answers D and E) to prevent tumor spread should be balanced with operative mortality and morbidity, and patients should be informed about the risk-benefit ratio of conservative vs aggressive management when the nonfunctioning pancreatic NET represents an intermediate risk.[5,13,14]

First-line somatostatin analogue therapy (Answer B) is currently not indicated for these small nonmetastatic lesions, and first-line peptide-receptor radionuclide therapy with radiolabeled somatostatin analogues and targeted therapy (Answer A) are not registered for this specific indication (nonmetastatic pancreatic NEN).

Key Learning Points

- Gastroenteropancreatic NENs can manifest in different ways depending on primary site, size, and hormonal hypersecretion.

- Nonfunctioning pancreatic NENs smaller than 2 cm in patients with MEN type 1 or von Hippel-Lindau disease can be considered for follow-up (watchful waiting).

- Localized insulinomas should preferably be resected.

- Multidisciplinary care in specialized centers is required for the best care of patients with NENs.

- Endocrinologists are essential members of NEN multidisciplinary care teams.

References

1. Hofland J, Kaltsas G, de Herder WW. Advances in the diagnosis and management of well-differentiated neuroendocrine neoplasms. *Endocr Rev.* 2020;41(2):371-403. PMID: 31555796

2. Dasari A, Shen C, Halperin D, et al. Trends in the incidence, prevalence, and survival outcomes in patients with neuroendocrine tumors in the United States. *JAMA Oncol.* 2017;3(10):1335-1342. PMID: 28448665

3. Fraenkel M, Kim M, Faggiano A, de Herder WW, Valk GD, Knowledge NETwork. Incidence of gastroenteropancreatic neuroendocrine tumours: a systematic review of the literature. *Endocr Relat Cancer.* 2014;21(3):R153-R163. PMID: 24322304

4. Rindi G, Mete O, Uccella S, et al. Overview of the 2022 WHO Classification of Neuroendocrine Neoplasms. *Endocr Pathol.* 2022;33(1):115-154. PMID: 35294740

5. Pieterman CRC, van Leeuwaarde RS, van den Broek MFM, et al. Multiple endocrine neoplasia type 1. In: Feingold KR, Anawalt B, Boyce A, et al, eds. Endotext. South Dartmouth, MA: MDText.com, Inc; 2000. PMID: 29465925

6. Grozinsky-Glasberg S, Davar J, et al. European Neuroendocrine Tumor Society (ENETS) 2022 guidance paper for carcinoid syndrome and carcinoid heart disease. *J Neuroendocrinol.* 2022;e13146. PMID: 35613326

7. de Herder WW, Zandee WT, Hofland J. Insulinoma. In: Feingold KR, Anawalt B, Boyce A, et al, eds. Endotext. South Dartmouth, MA: MDText.com, Inc; 2000. PMID: 25905215

8. Cryer PE, Axelrod L, Grossman AB, Heller SR, Montori VM, Seaquist ER, Service FJ; Endocrine Society. Evaluation and management of adult hypoglycemic disorders: an Endocrine Society clinical practice guideline. *J Clin Endocrinol Metab.* 2009;94(3):709-728. PMID: 19088155

9. Jensen RT, Ito T. Gastrinoma. In: Feingold KR, Anawalt B, Boyce A, et al, eds. Endotext. South Dartmouth, MA: MDText.com, Inc; 2000. PMID: 25905301

10. Zandee WT, Hofland J, de Herder WW. Vasoactive intestinal peptide tumor (VIPoma). In: Feingold KR, Anawalt B, Boyce A, et al, eds. Endotext. South Dartmouth, MA: MDText.com, Inc; 2000. PMID: 25905195

11. Zandee WT, Hofland J, de Herder WW. Glucagonoma syndrome. In: Feingold KR, Anawalt B, Boyce A, et al, eds. Endotext. South Dartmouth, MA: MDText.com, Inc; 2000. PMID: 25905270

12. Kaltsas G, Androulakis II, de Herder WW, Grossman AB. Paraneoplastic syndromes secondary to neuroendocrine tumours. *Endocr Relat Cancer.* 2010;17(3):R173-R193. PMID: 20530594

13. van Beek D-J, Pieterman CRC, Wessels FJ, et al. Diagnosing pancreatic neuroendocrine tumors in patients with multiple endocrine neoplasia type 1 in daily practice. *Front Endocrinol (Lausanne).* 2022;13:926491. PMID: 36277719

14. Pieterman CRC, de Laat JM, Twisk JWR, et al. Long-term natural course of small nonfunctional pancreatic neuroendocrine tumors in MEN1-results from the Dutch MEN1 Study Group. *J Clin Endocrinol Metab.* 2017;102(10):3795-3805. PMID: 28938468

Prolactinoma: When Medical Treatment Fails

Niki Karavitaki, MSc, PhD. Institute of Metabolism and Systems Research, School of Medical and Dental Sciences, University of Birmingham and Centre for Endocrinology, Diabetes, and Metabolism, Birmingham, United Kingdom; Email: n.karavitaki@bham.ac.uk

Educational Objectives

After reviewing this chapter, learners should be able to:

- Describe the goals of treatment in patients with prolactinoma.

- Identify alternative management options, as well as their success rates and limitations, when medical treatment with dopamine agonists (DAs) fails due to resistance to these agents.

Significance of the Clinical Problem

Primary goals in the management of patients with prolactinoma are reduction in tumor size, achievement of normal prolactin, and restoration of gonadal function.[1] DAs are currently considered first-line treatment to achieve these targets, with cabergoline being the agent of choice due to its higher efficacy and more optimal tolerability profile.[1,2] A small subset of prolactinomas is resistant to DAs and further management includes various approaches that can be used alone or in combination and tailored to each individual patient. These approaches include switching to another DA, surgical removal of the tumor, and radiotherapy. Cabergoline is effective in most patients whose prolactinomas do not respond to bromocriptine. Surgery can lead to remission of hyperprolactinemia in 71% to 100% of patients with microprolactinomas; however,

recurrence is reported in up to 50% of patients during follow-up. Remission rates are lower in patients with macroprolactinomas, but surgical debulking may lead to improvement of hormonal control on a lower dosage of DA. Risk of postoperative complications and particularly new hypopituitarism are drawbacks of this approach. Radiotherapy, usually offered after surgery, requires many years until biochemical remission is achieved and carries the risk of late toxicities. The value of further medical treatments remains to be assessed.

The criteria defining resistance to DAs are variable throughout the literature. Endocrine Society clinical practice guidelines propose that a failure to achieve normal prolactin concentration on maximally tolerated dosages of DAs and a failure to achieve 50% reduction in tumor size should be regarded as resistance.[1] Nonetheless, there is still discussion on the necessity of both hormonal and tumoral criteria to be fulfilled, as well as on the cutoffs for the dosage, duration of treatment, and degree of prolactinoma shrinkage characterizing resistance. Providing an accurate estimate of the prevalence of primary DA resistance is challenging due heterogeneity among published studies; overall, it has been described in 20% to 30% of patients on bromocriptine and in approximately 10% of those on cabergoline. However, when focusing specifically on cases of macroprolactinoma, these rates decline.[2] The mechanisms implicated in DA resistance are not clearly understood and clinical factors associated with it include male sex, younger age at diagnosis, larger tumor size, and invasiveness.[2] Various options are available for managing patients with prolactinomas who do not respond to DA therapy, which can be used alone or in combination.

Practice Gaps

- Widely accepted criteria defining resistance to DA treatment have not been established.

- Alternatives to DA treatment with robustly proven benefits are not available.

Discussion

In daily clinical practice, lack of achievement of the treatment goals requires confirmation of the patient's adherence to the prescribed DA regimen. Once nonadherence has been excluded, decisions on further steps should also take into account possible clinical benefits achieved with the current DA regimen (eg, restoration of gonadal function, resolution of mass effects [particularly visual disturbances], absence of tumor growth), as well as the patient's wishes and expectations.

When DA treatment fails, various approaches can be used alone or in combination.[3] When there is no concern for tumor mass effect, close surveillance alone may be opted for without normalizing prolactin levels and, when indicated, with gonadal hormone replacement.

Approaches When Medical Treatment Fails

Change to a Different DA

In patients who do not respond to bromocriptine, switching to cabergoline is recommended. Prolactin normalizes in 70% to 85% of these patients, and tumor shrinkage greater than 25% of the pretreatment size is observed in 44% of them.[4,5] Switching to quinagolide cannot be excluded, although a meta-analysis comparing clinical and biochemical outcomes of patients on bromocriptine or quinagolide found no differences.[6] Cabergoline can normalize prolactin and lead to some tumor shrinkage in patients who do not respond to quinagolide,[5,7] suggesting that a switch from quinagolide to cabergoline can be considered. Changing cabergoline to bromocriptine would be anticipated to have a very low success rate; nonetheless, isolated cases of patients with prolactinomas resistant to cabergoline that respond to bromocriptine have been reported.[8]

Surgery

Resection of the prolactinoma is an additional approach in DA-resistant cases. Evaluation of the published outcomes of this strategy is confounded by the inclusion of patients who undergo operation due to DA intolerance or because of patient preference. Taking this into account, achievement of normoprolactinemia after transsphenoidal surgery has been reported in 71% to 100% of patients with microprolactinomas, with subsequent recurrence rates between 0% and 50% (this wide range reflects variable definitions of cure or recurrence, as well as differences in follow-up periods and drop-out rates). Postoperative complications are rare, and development of hypopituitarism has been described in up to 6% of patients.[9] Surgery in patients with macroprolactinomas offers less optimal remission rates and is mainly determined by invasiveness of the tumor.[10] Surgical expertise influences the outcomes.

Radiotherapy

Radiotherapy in the setting of DA-resistant prolactinomas is mainly offered as part of a multimodal treatment approach, usually after surgery. Most contemporary published data describe outcomes of stereotactic radiotherapy techniques; tumor control rates range from 83% to 100% during monitoring periods of 16 to 96 months, whereas biochemical remission requires many years and is reported in 16% to 83% in different series (marginal dose, 15-34 Gy).[11] Monitoring for late radiation-induced toxicities is necessary.[12,13]

Other Management Options

Somatostatin Analogues

Immunochemistry mapping of somatostatin receptors in prolactinoma tissue has revealed expression of all subtypes (particularly subtypes 5 and 2). Although results have not been consistent, small case series and case reports have shown achievement of normal prolactin or tumor shrinkage in a limited number of patients after administration of first- or second-generation long-acting somatostatin analogues. A therapeutic trial in selected cases of DA-resistant, aggressive prolactinomas could be considered as a possible option.[2,14]

Selective Estrogen-Receptor Modulators

Minimal reduction in prolactin levels has been reported following treatment with tamoxifen or raloxifene with no information on the impact on tumor volume. Nonetheless, published data are extremely limited and inconclusive.[2,14]

Metformin

This biguanide reduces lactotroph cells proliferation and promotes their apoptosis both in rat xenografts and in human prolactinoma cell cultures. Despite these promising in vitro findings, the outcomes of metformin administration are conflicting.[2,14,15]

Options for Aggressive/Malignant Prolactinomas

Options for treating aggressive and malignant prolactinomas include temozolomide or other chemotherapeutic agents, immune checkpoint inhibitors, tyrosine kinase inhibitors, inhibitors of mammalian target of rapamycin (mTOR), and peptide radioreceptor therapy.[2,14] Detailed discussion of them is beyond the scope of this chapter.

Clinical Case Vignettes

Case 1

A 32-year-old woman was recently diagnosed with a microprolactinoma (maximum diameter of 5 mm, in proximity to but not invading the left cavernous sinus). She initially presented with a 12-month history of amenorrhea after stopping the oral contraceptive pill, and her monomeric prolactin concentration was 1487 mU/L (109-557 mU/L). Bromocriptine was prescribed with a gradual titration of the dosage to 15 mg daily with minimum reduction of her prolactin to 1214 mU/L after 6 months of treatment. She remains amenorrheic, and she would like to become pregnant in the near future. The patient reports some headaches while on bromocriptine and confirms adherence to this medication regimen. Secondary etiologies for hyperprolactinemia have been excluded.

Which of the following is the best next step?

A. Increase the bromocriptine dosage and wait another 6 months for possible response to the new regimen

B. Stop bromocriptine and offer gonadal hormone replacement with regular monitoring of prolactin

C. Refer the patient for transsphenoidal removal of the microprolactinoma

D. Change bromocriptine to cabergoline and monitor for response

E. Refer the patient for radiotherapy of the microprolactinoma

Answer: D) Change bromocriptine to cabergoline and monitor for response

Most patients whose prolactinomas are resistant to bromocriptine respond to cabergoline (70%-85%) (Answer D), so this would be the most reasonable approach for this patient.

It is unlikely that further increase in the bromocriptine dosage (Answer A) would normalize prolactin, and the patient already reports some possible adverse effects from this medication.

The patient is keen to become pregnant and starting gonadal hormone replacement (Answer B) would not facilitate this.

Transsphenoidal surgery (Answer C) performed by a skilled, experienced surgeon could lead to remission of hyperprolactinemia. However, it carries the risk of hypopituitarism, and it is associated with recurrence of hyperprolactinemia. The patient would like to become pregnant in the near future, so cabergoline is the most appropriate option for her.

Radiotherapy (Answer E) would require many years until it has benefit, and in a number of cases, it fails to lead to biochemical remission. It is usually offered as part of a multimodality approach.

Case 2

A 45-year-old man was recently diagnosed with macroprolactinoma (maximum diameter of 2.3 cm, with suprasellar extension and compression of the optic chiasm and no cavernous sinus invasion). He initially presented with a 6-month history of visual deterioration (which proved to be bitemporal hemianopia), low libido, and erectile dysfunction. His monomeric prolactin concentration was 10,688 mU/L (85-325 mU/L), and he had hypogonadotropic hypogonadism (9:00 AM testosterone, 6 nmol/L [7-27 nmol/L]; FSH, 3.5 IU/L [1.5-12.4 IU/L]; LH, 2.5 IU/L [0.6-12.1 IU/L]). His IGF-1 and thyroid hormones were within the reference range, and he had normal cortisol response on the short cosyntropin-stimulation test. Cabergoline was prescribed with a gradual dose titration up to 3.5 mg per week within 4 weeks. He had no significant adverse effects on DA therapy (only minor gastrointestinal disturbances). Now, during week 8 of treatment, his prolactin concentration is 9882 mU/L, and neuro-ophthalmology review shows no change in bitemporal hemianopia. The patient confirms adherence to his treatment regimen.

Which of the following is the best next step?

A. Increase the dosage of cabergoline and reassess if a change in his management is needed in 3 months

B. Change cabergoline to bromocriptine

C. Refer the patent for radiotherapy

D. Refer the patient for transsphenoidal surgery

E. Add metformin to his regimen

Answer: D) Refer the patient for transsphenoidal surgery

The absence of any improvement of the significant visual disturbances after 8 weeks of cabergoline treatment indicates the DA's lack of tumor effect. This necessitates prompt surgical intervention (Answer D) to release the pressure to the optic chiasm and improve or prevent further visual deterioration.

Increasing the cabergoline dosage (Answer A) would delay the management of the visual disturbances with potential negative sequelae.

Based on the published literature, the chance is slim that bromocriptine (Answer B) would be effective in this case of resistance to cabergoline.

Radiotherapy (Answer C) would not be recommended for a prolactinoma compressing the optic chiasm. This modality could be considered as adjuvant treatment after surgery for a DA-resistant prolactinoma.

Data regarding the addition of metformin (Answer E) in this scenario are conflicting.

Case 3

A 32-year-old man was diagnosed with a macroprolactinoma 18 months ago. At the time of detection, the tumor had maximum diameter of 2.9 cm, showed suprasellar extension without abutting the optic chiasm, and was Knosp 3 on the left and Knosp 1 on the right. He initially presented with a 12-month history of tiredness, low libido, and erectile dysfunction. His monomeric prolactin concentration was 23,000 mU/L (85-325 mU/L), and he had hypogonadotropic hypogonadism (9:00 AM testosterone, 5.2 nmol/L [7-27 nmol/L]; FSH, 0.9 IU/L [1.5-12.4 IU/L]; LH, 1.0 IU/L [0.6-12.1 IU/L]) and secondary hypoadrenalism (cortisol response on short cosyntropin-stimulation test, 270 nmol/L at 30 minutes (>450 nmol/L)). Concentrations of IGF-1 and thyroid hormones were within the reference range. Cabergoline was initiated immediately, and the dosage was gradually increased. In the last 10 months, the dosage has been 7 mg weekly (divided in 3 doses). He states he is adherent to this therapy and has no adverse effects. Eighteen months after starting the DA, his prolactin is now 7000 mU/L and pituitary MRI demonstrates ~25% tumor volume reduction with Knosp 3 on the left. The patient has been on optimal testosterone and glucocorticoid replacement.

Which of the following is the best management approach now?

A. Discuss with the patient the option of surgical debulking of the tumor

B. Increase the dosage of cabergoline to further reduce prolactin levels and tumor size

C. Recommend temozolomide

D. Recommend no management changes

Answer: A) Discuss with the patient the option of surgical debulking of the tumor

This patient's prolactinoma has shown partial response on a relatively high dosage of cabergoline. Given his young age, continuing this dosage in the long-term would be associated with risk of fibrotic valve disease. Surgical debulking of the prolactinoma could improve hormonal control and allow reduction in the cabergoline dosage.[10]

Further increasing of the already high dosage of cabergoline (Answer B) is unlikely to normalize the prolactin.

The patient's prolactinoma has not shown features of aggressive behavior and, hence, temozolomide treatment (Answer C) is not indicated.

Recommending no management changes (Answer E) could be considered given that the patient is on testosterone replacement and his tumor is not threatening his vision. Nonetheless, the high dosage of cabergoline required to achieve only partial response would raise concerns for its long-term safety.

Key Learning Points

- Primary goals in the management of patients with prolactinoma are reduction in tumor size, achievement of normal prolactin, and restoration of gonadal function. These aims are not always achieved in patients treated with DAs (DA resistance), and individualized management approaches are necessary.

- Compared with cabergoline, bromocriptine is associated with higher rates of resistance.

- In patients whose proloactinomas do not respond to bromocriptine, switching to cabergoline is recommended.

- For microprolactinomas, surgery can lead to remission of hyperprolactinemia in 71% to 100% of patients; recurrence has been reported in up to 50%.

- Surgical debulking of a prolactinoma can improve hormonal control, with lower dosages of DA required postoperatively.

- Radiotherapy is mainly offered as part of a multimodal treatment approach, usually after surgery. It leads to high tumor control rates, but it is less successful in normalizing prolactin, which can take a long time to achieve.

References

1. Melmed S, Casanueva FF, Hoffman AR, et al; Endocrine Society. Diagnosis and treatment of hyperprolactinemia: an Endocrine Society clinical practice guideline. *J Clin Endocrinol Metab.* 2011;96(2):273-288. PMID: 21296991

2. Souteiro P, Karavitaki N. Dopamine agonist resistant prolactinomas: any alternative medical treatment? *Pituitary.* 2020;23(1):27-37. PMID: 31522358

3. Vroonen L, Jaffrain-Rea ML, Petrossians P, et al. Prolactinomas resistant to standard doses of cabergoline: a multicenter study of 92 patients. *Eur J Endocrinol.* 2012;167(5):651-662. PMID: 22918301

4. Verhelst J, Abs R, Maiter D, et al. Cabergoline in the treatment of hyperprolactinemia: a study in 455 patients. *J Clin Endocrinol Metab.* 1999;84(7):2518-2522. PMID: 10404830

5. Colao A, Di Sarno A, Sarnacchiaro F, et al. Prolactinomas resistant to standard dopamine agonists respond to chronic cabergoline treatment. *J Clin Endocrinol Metab.* 1997;82(3):876-883. PMID: 9062500

6. Wang AT, Mullan RJ, Lane MA, et al. Treatment of hyperprolactinemia: a systematic review and meta-analysis. *Syst Rev.* 2012;1:33. PMID: 22828169

7. Di Sarno A, Landi ML, Marzullo P, et al. The effect of quinagolide and cabergoline, two selective dopamine receptor type 2 agonists, in the treatment of prolactinomas. *Clin Endocrinol (Oxf)*. 2000;53(1):53-60. PMID: 10931080

8. Iyer P, Molitch ME. Positive prolactin response to bromocriptine in 2 patients with cabergoline-resistant prolactinomas. *Endocr Pract*. 2011;17(3):e55-e58. PMID: 21324816

9. Tampourlou M, Trifanescu R, Paluzzi A, Ahmed SK, Karavitaki N. Therapy of endocrine disease: Surgery in microprolactinomas: effectiveness and risks based on contemporary literature. *Eur J Endocrinol*. 2016;175(3):R89-R96. PMID: 27207245

10. Primeau V, Raftopoulos C, Maiter D. Outcomes of transsphenoidal surgery in prolactinomas: improvement of hormonal control in dopamine agonist-resistant patients. *Eur J Endocrinol*. 2012;166(5):779-786. PMID: 22301915

11. Minniti G, Osti MF, Niyazi M. Target delineation and optimal radiosurgical dose for pituitary tumors. *Radiat Oncol*. 2016;11(1):135. PMID: 27729088

12. Ntali G, Karavitaki N. Efficacy and complications of pituitary irradiation. *Endocrinol Metab Clin North Am*. 2015;44(1):117-126. PMID: 25732648

13. Hamblin R, Vardon A, Akpalu J, et al. Risk of second brain tumour after radiotherapy for pituitary adenoma or craniopharyngioma: a retrospective, multicentre, cohort study of 3679 patients with long-term imaging surveillance. *Lancet Diabetes Endocrinol*. 2022;10(8):581-588. PMID: 35780804

14. Urwyler SA, Karavitaki N. Refractory lactotroph adenomas. *Pituitary*. 2023 [Online ahead of print]. PMID: 36928728

15. Portari LHC, Correa-Silva SR, Abucham J. Prolactin response to metformin in cabergoline-resistant prolactinomas: a pilot study. *Neuroendocrinology*. 2022;112(1):68-73. PMID: 33477154

Management of Challenging Cases of Immune Checkpoint Inhibitor Hypophysitis

Kevin C. J. Yuen, MD. Barrow Pituitary Center, Barrow Neurological Institute, University of Arizona College of Medicine and Creighton School of Medicine, Phoenix, AZ; Email: kevin.yuen@dignityhealth.org

Educational Objectives

After reviewing this chapter, learners should be able to:

- Identify symptoms related to immune checkpoint inhibitor (ICI) hypophysitis and consider pituitary metastasis in the differential diagnosis.

- Identify central adrenal insufficiency (CAI) and diabetes insipidus (now known as arginine vasopressin [AVP] deficiency) in ICI-treated patients.

- Recommend strategies to diagnose and treat challenging endocrinopathies associated with ICI hypophysitis.

Significance of the Clinical Problem

ICI hypophysitis is often unrecognized and can range from isolated to multiple pituitary hormone deficiencies. Severe cases can cause mass effects from pituitary gland enlargement resulting in headaches and visual disturbances, and potentially death from unrecognized adrenal crisis and AVP deficiency.[1] In addition, the pituitary gland is also a target organ for metastatic disease. Fortunately rare, pituitary metastasis only represents 0.4% of all intracranial metastatic tumors and 1% of surgically treated pituitary lesions. Considering the possibility of pituitary metastasis is important in patients with suspected ICI hypophysitis. Furthermore, diagnosing ICI-related CAI and AVP deficiency can also be challenging. With increasing use of ICIs in the oncology space, a better understanding together with a pragmatic diagnostic approach will help clinicians make treatment decisions regarding hormone replacement and whether to maintain, delay, or withdraw ICI treatment. Importantly, patients and clinicians should be counseled not to underestimate or confuse CAI- and AVP deficiency–related symptoms with malignancy-related symptoms and adverse effects from anticancer treatments. Once CAI is diagnosed, physiologic glucocorticoid replacement is recommended, unless adrenal crisis or symptoms of mass effect are present, in which case high-dosage glucocorticoids should be considered. In contrast, AVP deficiency can often be successfully managed with desmopressin.

ICIs have become the mainstay of cancer treatment, but their use is associated with numerous wide-ranging and variable immune-related adverse events affecting the endocrine system.[2] Thyroid and pituitary dysfunction are the 2 most frequent endocrinopathies reported.[3] ICI hypophysitis is also often challenging to detect because the symptoms can be insidious and nonspecific. Fatigue, nausea, vomiting, anorexia, and weight loss may result from CAI, but these symptoms are also common in patients with cancer. Headache is the most common mass effect symptom, whereas visual field defects are more common in non-ICI than ICI hypophysitis because of the relatively milder degree and shorter duration of onset of pituitary enlargement.

In recent years, because of the increasing numbers of patients with cancer who are treated with ICIs, clinicians in a variety of specialties have been called on to manage ICI-mediated endocrinopathies. Hence, all clinicians (eg, endocrinologists, oncologists, primary care providers, and emergency department physicians) should have a high index of clinical suspicion and be well-versed in ICI hypophysitis, so that appropriate treatment decisions can be implemented.

Practice Gaps

- Due to the rarity of ICI hypophysitis and absence of randomized controlled trials, there is no standardized diagnostic workup and treatment algorithm for ICI hypophysitis–related endocrinopathies.

- Patients may already be on high-dosage glucocorticoids as part of their anticancer chemotherapy that directly suppresses their hypothalamic-pituitary-adrenal axis.

- ACTH and cortisol levels are not routinely measured, and cosyntropin-stimulation testing is not sensitive enough to detect acute and mild CAI, resulting in its underdiagnosis.

- Main diagnostic challenges of ICI hypophysitis include nonspecific presenting symptoms, variations in timing of onset, and different ICIs with different mechanisms of action that present with different endocrinopathies.

- Patients may confuse their symptoms with those of their malignancy and anticancer treatments and defer reporting these symptoms.

- Patients are often seen by clinicians who are not sufficiently experienced in diagnosing and treating ICI hypophysitis–related endocrinopathies.

Discussion

ICI hypophysitis is recognized as one of the main adverse effects associated with cancer immunotherapy. Its incidence is higher with CTLA-4 inhibitors (eg, ipilimumab) (0%-17%) than with PD-1 inhibitors (eg, nivolumab and pembrolizumab) (0.5%-2.0%),[4] whereas PD-L1 inhibitors rarely cause hypophysitis.[5,6] The incidence of ICI hypophysitis is also increased when used as combination therapy and with higher CTLA-4 inhibitor dosages, older age, and male sex.[7-9] CAI is frequently reported (20%-75%), followed by gonadal (15%-60%) and TSH (25-58%) deficiencies, and less commonly GH (5%-41%) and prolactin (13%-25%) deficiencies. Multiple pituitary hormone axes (>3 pituitary hormone deficits) can be affected in up to 50% of patients.[10,11] By contrast, hyperprolactinemia and AVP deficiency are relatively rare, affecting only 9% and 1% of patients, respectively.[12,13] Unlike other organs for which the adverse effects can be successfully treated with ICI discontinuation and high-dosage glucocorticoid therapy, damage to pituitary cells—particularly corticotrophs—is often permanent.[11]

In the context of ICI hypophysitis, especially when AVP deficiency is present, it is important to exclude pituitary metastasis. MRI findings and the onset of symptoms may distinguish between these 2 conditions. A recent retrospective study assessed the clinical, biochemical, and radiologic differences in patients with neoplastic and nonneoplastic pituitary stalk pathology. A significantly greater preponderance of AVP deficiency was documented in patients with neoplastic pathology than in those with nonneoplastic pathology. The radiologic features that reached statistical significance were the thickness of the stalk and the heterogeneity of contrast enhancement after administration of the contrast agent.[14] Recently, Fosci et al[15] reported a challenging case of a nivolumab-treated patient with biochemical and radiologic characteristics consistent with the coexistence of hypophysitis and pituitary metastasis, suggesting both pathologies may be responsible in causing AVP deficiency. Another diagnostic challenge is when there are symptoms of polyuria-polydipsia with inappropriate normal or "almost normal" serum osmolality or sodium levels or when primary polydipsia is present. Thus, it is imperative that the diagnosis of AVP deficiency is not missed, as the symptoms of polydipsia and polyuria can often be successfully managed with desmopressin.

When patients present initially with syncope, pyrexia, nausea, and vomiting, these symptoms may not necessarily prompt the patient or the clinician to think about CAI, but rather the underlying cancer burden or the development of a secondary gastrointestinal infection. Also, due to the relatively low incidence of ICI hypophysitis and lack of predictive biomarkers, routine monitoring of pituitary function is not prevalent yet in clinical practice. Furthermore, ICI hypophysitis caused by PD-1 inhibitors usually presents with a normal pituitary gland, whereas CTLA-4 inhibitor–related hypophysitis tends to demonstrate pituitary enlargement on MRI.[16] Glucocorticoid replacement should not be delayed while awaiting pituitary MRI. High-dosage glucocorticoids should be reserved for patients with mass effect symptoms, as there have been some studies that suggest increased mortality following treatment with high dosages.[17] Some studies have implied even if grade 3 to 4 immune-related adverse effects occur, ICI therapy can be continued if there are no tumoral mass effects or it can be temporarily interrupted and resumed when the patient's condition stabilizes.[2] Because CAI tends to persist, when the patient's condition is stabilized on physiological glucocorticoid replacement, periodic monitoring of 8-AM serum cortisol levels is essential to identifying possible hypothalamic-pituitary-adrenal axis recovery. Better survival advantage has been reported for patients with cancer who develop ICI-induced hypophysitis, which may be a silver lining.[18]

Clinical Case Vignettes

Case 1

A 64-year-old woman diagnosed with stage 4 melanoma has been undergoing chemotherapy that includes treatment with ipilimumab and nivolumab. About 6 months before treatment, routine brain MRI was performed as part of surveillance, and the findings were normal. After 3 doses of ipilimumab and nivolumab, she reports increased headaches, dizziness, fatigue, visual blurriness, and excessive thirst and urination. Repeated MRI now demonstrates a 1.3-cm hypoenhancing sellar mass displacing the optic chiasm.

On physical examination, she has dry mouth and dry skin. Her blood pressure is 110/78 mm Hg lying down and 87/65 mm Hg standing. Pulse rate is 88 beats/min. BMI is 23.2 kg/m².

Laboratory test results:

Sodium = 143 mEq/L (136-142 mEq/L) (SI: 143 mmol/L [136-142 mmol/L])
Potassium = 4.5 mEq/L (3.5-5.0 mEq/L) (SI: 4.5 mmol/L [3.5-5.0 mmol/L])
Prolactin = 88 ng/mL (4-30 ng/mL) (SI: 3.83 nmol/L [0.17-1.30 nmol/L])
Plasma glucose = 81 mg/dL (70-99 mg/dL) (SI: 4.9 mmol/L [3.9-5.5 mmol/L])
Free T₄ = 0.7 ng/dL (0.8-1.8 ng/dL) (SI: 9.01 pmol/L [10.30-23.17 pmol/L])
TSH = 0.17 mIU/L (0.5-5.0 mIU/L)
Cortisol = 2.4 µg/dL (6.0-18.4 µg/dL) (SI: 66.2 nmol/L [165.5-507.6 nmol/L])
ACTH = 6 pg/mL (6-50 pg/mL) (SI: 1.3 pmol/L [1.3-11.0 pmol/L])

Which of the following is the most likely diagnosis?

A. Ipilimumab-induced hypophysitis

B. Metastasis

C. Nonfunctioning pituitary macroadenoma

D. Prolactinoma

E. Rathke cleft cyst

Answer: B) Metastasis

The key features of this case—the short history of headaches, rapid growth of the mass, and presence of AVP deficiency—are more likely to suggest pituitary metastasis (Answer B) than ipilimumab-induced hypophysitis (Answer A). In contrast to ipilimumab-induced hypophysitis and pituitary adenomas, metastasis is more likely to also affect posterior pituitary function.[19] In patients with pituitary metastasis, 50% present with AVP deficiency, 25% to 45% with anterior pituitary hormone deficiencies, 30% with visual disturbance, 25% with ophthalmoplegia, and 20% with headache.[20] In cases of pituitary metastasis from melanoma, the clinical presentation is similar to symptoms observed in patients who have pituitary metastasis from other neoplasms. Based on the laboratory results, this patient also has CAI and central hypothyroidism as part of the effects of the metastatic lesion causing anterior hypopituitarism.

Prolactinoma (Answer D) is not likely given the modestly elevated prolactin concentration due to stalk compression from the metastatic disease, short history of tumor appearance on MRI, and presence of AVP deficiency.

Nonfunctioning pituitary macroadenomas (Answer C) are usually slow growing, and given that this patient's brain MRI findings were normal 6 months ago, this tumor type is unlikely. Similarly, Rathke cleft cyst (Answer E) is not likely because of the normal brain MRI 6 months ago. Moreover, nonfunctioning pituitary macroadenomas and Rathke cleft cysts do not tend to cause AVP deficiency.

Hypophysitis is the most frequent and clinically important endocrine-related adverse effect of the CTLA-4 inhibitor ipilimumab (Answer A) that can lead to significant degrees of anterior hypopituitarism, with the overall incidence ranging from 3% to 8%.[3] However, because this patient has a discrete hypoenhancing sellar mass on MRI and a short history of AVP deficiency, ipilimumab-induced hypophysitis is less likely.

Case 2

A 61-year-old woman with metastatic melanoma of the left tibia is schedule to begin treatment with nivolumab. Baseline workup reveals normal electrolytes, hepatic function, and kidney function at the time of treatment initiation and before every session of nivolumab administration. Six months after initiating nivolumab, she develops adrenal insufficiency and hypothyroidism and is treated with hydrocortisone and levothyroxine. Two months later, she presents with polydipsia and polyuria with a urine volume of 4.2 L/24 h.

Laboratory test results:

Sodium = 144 mEq/L (136-142 mEq/L)
(SI: 144 mmol/L [136-142 mmol/L])
Potassium = 4.0 mEq/L (3.5-5.0 mEq/L)
(SI: 4.0 mmol/L [3.5-5.0 mmol/L])
Prolactin = 45 ng/mL (4-30 ng/mL) (SI: 1.96 nmol/L [0.17-1.30 nmol/L])
Glucose = 105 mg/dL (70-99 mg/dL)
(SI: 5.83 mmol/L [3.9-5.5 mmol/L])
Free T$_4$ = 1.0 ng/dL (0.8-1.8 ng/dL)
(SI: 12.87 pmol/L [10.30-23.17 pmol/L])
TSH = 0.98 mIU/L (0.5-5.0 mIU/L)
Cortisol = 1.4 µg/dL (6.0-18.4 µg/dL)
(SI: 38.6 nmol/L [165.5-507.6 nmol/L])
ACTH = 6 pg/mL (6-50 pg/mL) (SI: 1.3 pmol/L [1.3-11.0 pmol/L])
Calcium = 37.6 mg/dL (34.0-40.8 mg/dL)
(SI: 9.4 mmol/L [8.5-10.2 mmol/L])
Urine osmolality = 184 mOsm/kg
(500-800 mOsm/kg) (SI: 184 mmol/kg [500-800 mmol/kg])
Urine specific gravity = 1.003
Plasma osmolality = 310 mOsm/kg
(280295 mOsm/kg) (SI: 310 mmol/kg [280295 mmol/kg])

Pituitary MRI reveals a normal-sized pituitary gland, but the posterior pituitary bright spot is absent in the noncontrast T1 sagittal views.

Which of the following is the most likely diagnosis?

A. Metastasis

B. Nephrogenic diabetes insipidus (AVP resistance)

C. Nivolumab-induced AVP deficiency

D. Psychogenic polydipsia

E. Unmasking of AVP deficiency by hydrocortisone

Answer: C) Nivolumab-induced AVP deficiency

This patient treated with nivolumab for metastatic melanoma presents with a syndrome of polyuria and polydipsia 6 months after starting treatment and 2 months after the diagnosis of anterior hypopituitarism. The diagnosis of nivolumab-induced AVP deficiency (Answer C) is based on biochemical findings that include inappropriately low urine osmolality for serum osmolality and excess urine production. Some of the more common etiologies of AVP resistance are electrolytic disturbances, including hypokalemia and hypercalcemia, and lithium toxicity, which have been excluded in this patient. Metastasis (Answer A) has been excluded based on the findings of a normal pituitary gland on MRI.

ICI hypophysitis tends to be more common in males and typically occurs after 2 to 3 months of immunotherapy. It is more frequently caused by CTLA-4 rather than PD-1 inhibitors.[2] Furthermore, ICIs rarely cause AVP deficiency from an autoimmune process involving the hypothalamo-posterior pituitary region, and dysregulation of the posterior hypothalamic-pituitary axis has been reported in only 14 cases.[21] The pathophysiology of ICI-induced AVP deficiency is unclear and may be linked to multiple pathways, including type 2 and type 4 hypersensitivity reactions, as well as ectopic pituitary CTLA-4 expression.[22] On MRI, AVP deficiency generally manifests as absence of the pituitary bright spot with or without enlargement (2-3 mm) of the pituitary stalk. However, the posterior pituitary bright spot tends to be absent in older individuals.[23] In this patient, the absence of the bright spot favors the diagnosis of AVP deficiency. Another challenge in diagnosing this patient is the relatively normal-sized pituitary on MRI rather than an enlargement of the pituitary gland associated with CTLA-4 inhibitor therapy.[16] This case highlights the need for clinicians to be aware of the potential risk for developing ICI-induced AVP deficiency and the differences in MRI changes with different ICIs. For normoglycemic, normocalcemic, and normokalemic patients presenting with persistent polyuria-polydipsia syndrome during ICI therapy, testing for AVP deficiency with serum and urine specific osmolality, urine specific gravity, and, if required, performing an outpatient water-deprivation test may be necessary to confirm the diagnosis. Treatment for AVP deficiency is similar to that for patients who have not been treated with an ICI (desmopressin).

Based on this patient's history, it is unlikely that she has psychogenic polydipsia (Answer D), nephrogenic diabetes insipidus (AVP resistance) (Answer B), or unmasking of AVP deficiency by hydrocortisone (Answer E), as she presented with polydipsia and polyuria 2 months after commencing hydrocortisone.

Case 3

A 63-year-old man diagnosed with stage 4 bronchial carcinoma undergoes treatment with pembrolizumab. After 6 doses, he presents to the emergency department with frontal headache, dizziness, abdominal pain, diarrhea, nausea, and vomiting. MRI documents global enlargement of the pituitary gland with mild thickening of the pituitary infundibulum.

On physical examination, he has dry mucus membranes and is pyrexial with a temperature of 101.7°F (38.7°C) and blood pressure of 134/86 mm Hg.

Laboratory test results:

Sodium = 125 mEq/L (136-142 mEq/L)
(SI: 125 mmol/L [136-142 mmol/L])
Potassium = 3.4 mEq/L (3.5-5.0 mEq/L)
(SI: 3.4 mmol/L [3.5-5.0 mmol/L])
Creatinine = 1.87 mg/dL (0.74-1.35 mg/dL)
(SI: 165.3 μmol/L [65.4-119.3 μmol/L])
Cortisol (8 AM) 1.2 μg/dL (6.0-18.4 μg/dL)
(SI: 33.1 nmol/L [165.5-507.6 nmol/L])
ACTH (8 AM) = 2.4 pg/mL (6-50 pg/mL)
(SI: 0.5 pmol/L [1.3-11.0 pmol/L])
Prolactin = 48 ng/mL (4-23 ng/mL) (SI: 2.09 nmol/L [0.17-1.00 nmol/L])
Free T_4 = 1.1 ng/dL (0.8-1.8 ng/dL)
(SI: 14.16 pmol/L [10.30-23.17 pmol/L])
TSH = 0.9 mIU/L (0.5-5.0 mIU/L)
Plasma glucose = 65 mg/dL (70-99 mg/dL)
(SI: 3.6 mmol/L [3.9-5.5 mmol/L])
White blood cell count = 4770/μL (4500-11,000/μL)
(SI: 4.77×10^9/L [4.5-11.0×10^9/L])
C-reactive protein = 122.0 mg/L (8.0-10.0 mg/L)
(SI: 1161.9 nmol/L [76.2-95.2 nmol/L])

In addition to fluid resuscitation, which of the following should be used next to treat this patient?

A. Antibiotics

B. Dexamethasone orally, 4 mg every 8 hours

C. Enoxaparin

D. Hydrocortisone intravenously, 100 mg every 8 hours, followed by 200 mg continuous infusion over 24 hours

E. Hydrocortisone orally, 20 mg every 8 hours

Answer: D) Hydrocortisone intravenously, 100 mg every 8 hours, followed by 200 mg continuous infusion over 24 hours

This man treated with pembrolizumab for bronchial carcinoma presents with pyrexia and concurrent symptoms suggestive of a gastrointestinal infection. This is a grade 3 to 4 endocrine immune-related adverse effect associated with PD-1 inhibitor therapy. However, the nonspecific symptoms make the diagnosis of CAI challenging. Patients on ICIs should be reminded that symptoms can evolve over time before the diagnosis becomes evident; therefore, it is important to report these symptoms as they arise. This case illustrates how symptoms can overlap with those of acute illness or underlying malignancy. Unless the clinician has a high degree of suspicion, it would be unlikely to suspect that the patient was developing adrenal crisis and to check morning ACTH and cortisol levels. Treatment with parenteral stress-dose hydrocortisone (Answer D) and rehydration with isotonic saline and subsequent tapering to replacement doses of hydrocortisone is the mainstay of therapy.

Decreasing the dosage of hydrocortisone too rapidly can also result in the re-presentation of pyrexia; a sufficient course of hydrocortisone (4 to 5 days) is required. High-dosage glucocorticoids (prednisolone 1 to 2 mg/kg oral daily) have been proposed for severe immune-related adverse effects in some studies.[2] In this case, parenteral hydrocortisone was administered because of the patient's continued nausea and vomiting. Initiating high-dosage glucocorticoids should be reserved for patients presenting with mass effects (eg, headache and/or visual disturbances) caused by pituitary enlargement,[2] and if the patient does not report any mass effect symptoms, high-dosage glucocorticoids may be withheld. Additionally, if there is concurrent central hypothyroidism, it is important to treat the CAI first before treating with thyroid supplementation to avoid precipitating adrenal crisis.

Administering antibiotics (Answer A) or enoxaparin (Answer C) may be considered, but neither should be administered before glucocorticoids.

Oral hydrocortisone (Answer E) and dexamethasone (Answer B) are not appropriate in the setting of nausea and vomiting.

Given the low likelihood of recovery from CAI,[8,24] it is unknown whether any patient factors (eg, patient age) or treatment strategies (eg, rapid initiation of high-dosage glucocorticoids upon presentation) influence recovery of the axis. In one previous case series, high-dosage glucocorticoids did not alter the outcome of pituitary function recovery.[25] Another possibility is that some patients do not have complete destruction of the corticotrophs (indicated by low, but detectable plasma ACTH) and thus may have a chance of recovery from CAI.[26] Further studies are needed to help understand which factors predict pituitary function recovery.

Key Learning Points

- Although ICIs can cause hypophysitis as part of its immune-related effects profile, the pituitary gland should not be overlooked as a site of metastasis.

- ICI hypophysitis–related CAI can be challenging to diagnose because of nonspecific, insidious symptoms that can mimic acute illness and malignancy; therefore, a high degree of clinical suspicion is indicated.

- Acute symptoms of ICI hypophysitis–related CAI should be treated with physiological glucocorticoids, unless there are symptoms suggestive of mass effects, as high dosages can increase the mortality of these patients.

- Although ICI hypophysitis–related AVP deficiency is very rare and challenging to identify because it can be a complication of anticancer treatments and malignancy itself, once diagnosed, this potentially life-threatening condition can often be successfully managed with desmopressin.

References

1. Arima H, Cheetham T, Christ-Crain M, et al; Working Group for Renaming Diabetes Insipidus. Changing the name of Diabetes Insipidus: a position statement of the Working Group for Renaming Diabetes Insipidus. *J Clin Endocrinol Metab.* 2022;108(1):1-3. PMID: 36355385

2. Brahmer JR, Lacchetti C, Thompson JA. Management of immune-related adverse events in patients treated with immune checkpoint inhibitor therapy: American Society of Clinical Oncology Clinical Practice Guideline summary. *J Oncol Pract.* 2018;14(4):247-249. PMID: 29517954

3. de Filette J, Andreescu CE, Cools F, Bravenboer B, Velkeniers B. A systematic review and meta-analysis of endocrine-related adverse events associated with immune checkpoint inhibitors. *Horm Metab Res.* 2019;51(3):145-156. PMID: 30861560

4. Puzanov I, Diab A, Abdallah K, et al, Society for Immunotherapy of Cancer Toxicity Management Working Group. Managing toxicities associated with immune checkpoint inhibitors: consensus recommendations from the Society for Immunotherapy of Cancer (SITC) Toxicity Management Working Group. *J Immunother Cancer.* 2017;5(1):95. PMID: 29162153

5. Kanie K, Iguchi G, Bando H, et al. Two cases of atezolizumab-induced hypophysitis. *J Endocr Soc.* 2018;2(1):91-95. PMID: 29362727

6. Lupi I, Brancatella A, Cosottini M, et al. Clinical heterogeneity of hypophysitis secondary to PD-1/PD-L1 blockade: insights from four cases. *Endocrinol Diabetes Metab Case Rep.* 2019;19-0102. PMID: 31610523

7. Attia P, Phan GQ, Maker AV, et al. Autoimmunity correlates with tumor regression in patients with metastatic melanoma treated with anti-cytotoxic T-lymphocyte antigen-4. *J Clin Oncol.* 2005;23(25):6043-6053. PMID: 16087944

8. Faje AT, Sullivan R, Lawrence D, et al. Ipilimumab-induced hypophysitis: a detailed longitudinal analysis in a large cohort of patients with metastatic melanoma. *J Clin Endocrinol Metab.* 2014;99(11):4078-4085. PMID: 25078147

9. Maker AV, Yang JC, Sherry RM, et al. Intrapatient dose escalation of anti-CTLA-4 antibody in patients with metastatic melanoma. *J Immunother.* 2006;29(4):455-463. PMID: 16799341

10. Chang LS, Barroso-Sousa R, Tolaney SM, Hodi FS, Kaiser UB, Min L. Endocrine toxicity of cancer immunotherapy targeting immune checkpoints. *Endocr Rev.* 2019;40(1):17-65. PMID: 30184160

11. Kassi E, Angelousi A, Asonitis N, et al. Endocrine-related adverse events associated with immune-checkpoint inhibitors in patients with melanoma. *Cancer Med.* 2019;8(15):6585-6594. PMID: 31518074

12. Albarel F, Gaudy C, Castinetti F, et al. Long-term follow-up of ipilimumab-induced hypophysitis, a common adverse event of the anti-CTLA-4 antibody in melanoma. *Eur J Endocrinol.* 2015;172(2):195-204. PMID: 25416723

13. Deligiorgi MV, Siasos G, Vergadis C, Trafalis DT. Central diabetes insipidus related to anti-programmed cell-death 1 protein active immunotherapy. *Int Immunopharmacol.* 2020;83:106427. PMID: 32244049

14. Sbardella E, Joseph RN, Jafar-Mohammadi B, Isidori AM, Cudlip S, Grossman AB. Pituitary stalk thickening: the role of an innovative MRI imaging analysis which may assist in determining clinical management. *Eur J Endocrinol.* 2016;175(4):255-263. PMID: 27418059

15. Fosci M, Pigliaru F, Salcuni AS, etc. Diabetes insipidus secondary to nivolumab-induced neurohypophysitis and pituitary metastasis. *Endocrinol Diabetes Metab Case Rep.* 2021;2021:20-0123. PMID: 33522491

16. Di Dalmazi G, Ippolito S, Lupi I, Caturegli P. Hypophysitis induced by immune checkpoint inhibitors: a 10-year assessment. *Expert Rev Endocrinol Metab.* 2019;14(6):381-398. PMID: 31842671

17. Faje AT, Lawrence D, Flaherty K, et al. High-dose glucocorticoids for the treatment of ipilimumab-induced hypophysitis is associated with reduced survival in patients with melanoma. *Cancer.* 2018;124(18):3706-3714. PMID: 29975414

18. Kobayashi T, Iwama S, Yasuda Y, et al. Pituitary dysfunction induced by immune checkpoint inhibitors is associated with better overall survival in both malignant melanoma and non-small cell lung carcinoma: a prospective study. *J Immunother Cancer.* 2020;8(2)e000779. PMID: 32606047

19. Javanbakht A, D'Apuzzo M, Badie B, Salehian B. Pituitary metastasis: a rare condition. *Endocr Connect.* 2018;7(10):1049-1057. PMID: 30139817

20. He W, Chen F, Dalm B, Kirby PA, Greenlee JD. Metastatic involvement of the pituitary gland: a systematic review with pooled individual patient data analysis. *Pituitary.* 2015;18(1):159-168. PMID: 24445565

21. Angelousi A, Papalexis P, Karampela A, et al. Diabetes insipidus: a rare endocrine complication of immune check point inhibitors: a case report and literature review. *Exp Ther Med.* 2023;25(1):10. PMID: 36561623

22. Caturegli P, Di Dalmazi G, Lombardi M, et al. Hypophysitis secondary to cytotoxic T-lymphocyte-associated protein 4 blockade: insights into pathogenesis from an autopsy series. *Am J Pathol.* 2016;186(12):3225-3235. PMID: 27750046

23. Bonneville F, Cattin F, Marsot-Dupuch K, Dormont D, Bonneville JF, Chiras J. T1 signal hyperintensity in the sellar region: spectrum of findings. *Radiographics.* 2006;26(1):93-113. PMID: 16418246

24. Downey SG, Klapper JA, Smith FO, et al. Prognostic factors related to clinical response in patients with metastatic melanoma treated by CTL-associated antigen-4 blockade. *Clin Cancer Res.* 2007;13(22 Pt 1):6681-6688. PMID: 17982122

25. Min L, Hodi FS, Giobbie-Hurder A, et al. Systemic high-dose corticosteroid treatment does not improve the outcome of ipilimumab-related hypophysitis: a retrospective cohort study. *Clin Cancer Res.* 2015;21(4):749-755. PMID: 25538262

26. Thapi S, Leiter A, Galsky M, Gallagher EJ. Recovery from secondary adrenal insufficiency in a patient with immune checkpoint inhibitor therapy induced hypophysitis. *J Immunother Cancer.* 2019;7(1):248. PMID: 31511065

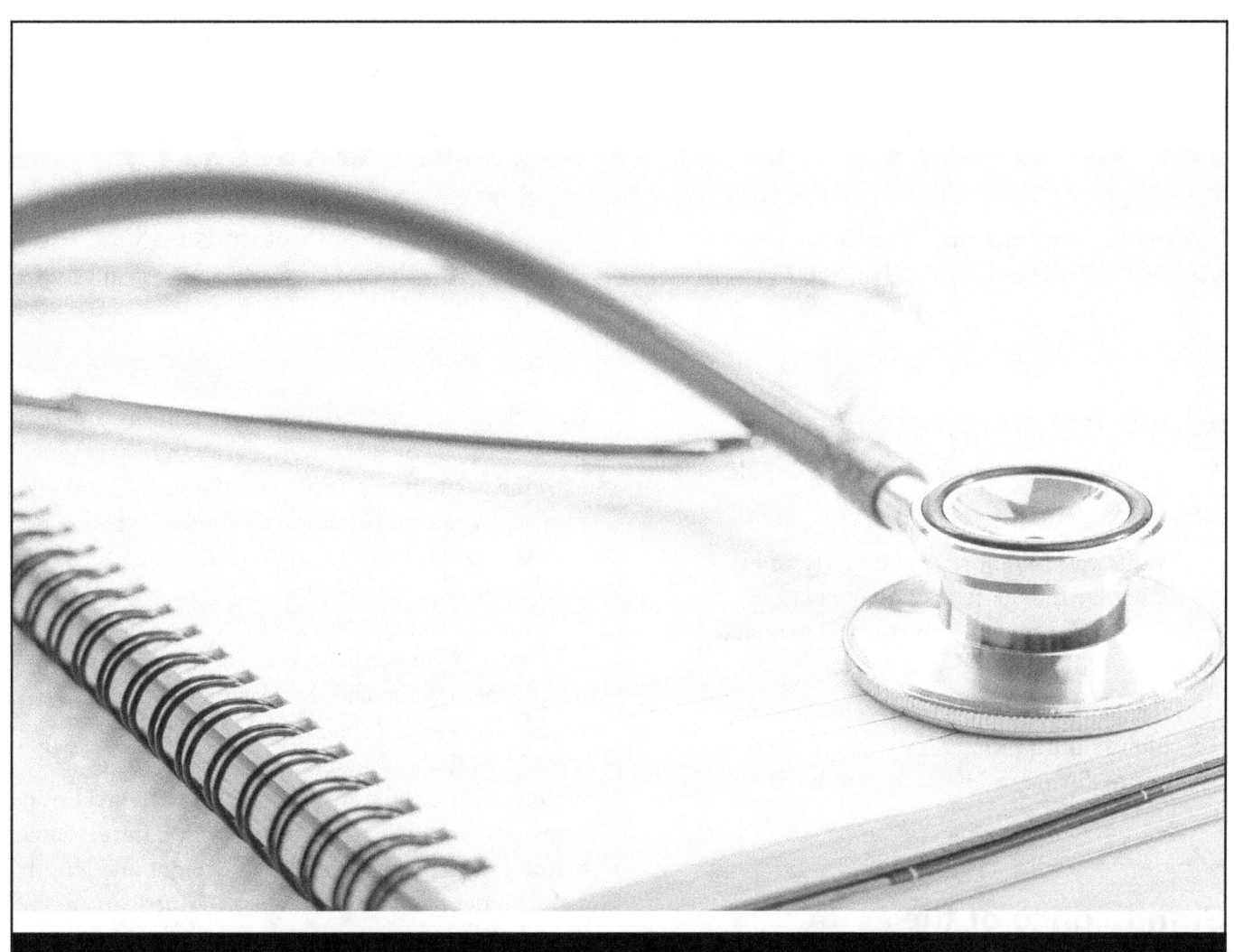

PEDIATRIC
ENDOCRINOLOGY

Growth Hormone Treatment in Children Born Prematurely

Margaret Cristina da Silva Boguszewski, MD, PhD. Department of Pediatrics and the Endocrine Division (SEMPR), Federal University of Parana, Curitiba, Brazil; E-mail: margabogus@uol.com.br

Educational Objectives

After reviewing this chapter, learners should be able to:

- Evaluate a child born prematurely and recognize the possible consequences of gestational age, size at birth, and neonatal comorbidities on postnatal growth.

- Diagnose and discuss treatment for those children born prematurely who have short stature during infancy and childhood.

Significance of the Clinical Problem

Approximately 15 million babies are born with less than 37 completed weeks of gestation across the world every year and are considered preterm. The incidence of preterm birth is increasing worldwide, and more than 1 in 10 babies are born prematurely each year. Survival rates have increased during recent decades with the improvements in neonatal care. With premature birth, babies are deprived of the intense intrauterine growth phase, and postnatal growth failure sometimes occurs. When growth restriction occurs during the early postnatal period with growth rates slower than expected, it is stated that the preterm infant is experiencing extrauterine growth restriction. Some children born prematurely remain short at later ages and in adult life, and the risk of short stature increases if the child is also born small-for-gestational-age (SGA).

Growth failure may be compounded in the presence of intrauterine or extrauterine growth restrictions, extreme prematurity, bronchopulmonary dysplasia, necrotizing enterocolitis, or metabolic bone disease of prematurity. In part due to the heterogeneity of preterm birth and the variability of postnatal outcome, alterations of the GH/IGF-1 axis might also occur. When growth failure occurs and persists during infancy and childhood, children born prematurely might benefit from GH treatment.

Morbidity among preterm infants varies widely. Approximately 80% to 85% of them show catch-up growth after initial growth failure, which is influenced by gestational age, weight and length at birth, neonatal morbidities, and nutritional status. However, substantial growth failure may occur and can be worse if the child was born prematurely and SGA.

Children born prematurely should be followed regularly and evaluated for the effects of prematurity and comorbidities on postnatal growth. In addition to the clinical algorithms for evaluation and diagnosis of short stature, precise characterization of pregnancy and birth condition is required. It is important to document the degree of prematurity, the occurrence of intrauterine growth retardation and small size for gestational age, neonatal comorbidities, and the possibility of extrauterine growth failure due to associated conditions. Together, these characteristics make the evaluation of a preterm infant complex and unique. When growth restriction remains during infancy and childhood, these children might be candidates for GH treatment.

Practice Gaps

- Uncertainty about appropriate growth charts from birth to postnatal life for preterm infants.

- Short children born prematurely might have different associated conditions, including genetic syndromes and/or hormonal deficiencies. All conditions must be carefully evaluated.

- The decision of when to initiate GH treatment is challenging.

Discussion

Gestational age is determined by the length of gestation from the first day of the last menstrual cycle, except for women undergoing assisted reproductive techniques. The term date, or 40 weeks (280 days), is calculated using the information of the last menstrual period. In cases for which this information is unknown or menstrual cycles are irregular, measurements of the embryo or fetus obtained by ultrasonography performed up to 13 weeks and 6 days postconception are accurate to determine or confirm gestational age. In case of assisted reproduction, the expected date of birth is calculated from the day of technical implementation, and in case of in vitro fertilization, from the day of embryo transfer to the uterus. After birth, gestational age can be estimated by physical examination and neurological maturity of the newborn.

Preterm birth usually is subdivided based on gestational age, with extremely preterm occurring at less than 28 weeks of gestational age, very preterm from 28 to 32 weeks, and moderate preterm from 32 to less than 37 completed weeks of gestation. Most babies born prematurely are moderate preterm, and those born between 34 and 36 weeks and 6 days are considered late preterm. When antenatal ultrasonography was not part of the routine for evaluation of GA, babies were considered preterm according to birth weight: extremely low birth weight if weight was less than 1000 g and very low birth weight if weight was less than 1500 g. The disadvantage of this classification is to include in the same group more mature children born SGA and preterm infants born at an appropriate weight for gestational age, with different risk factors for neonatal survival, comorbidities, and growth progression. The more extreme the limit of viability, the more the effects of preterm birth are confounded with those of intrauterine and extrauterine growth restrictions.

The high growth rate observed during fetal life in uncomplicated pregnancies is not repeated in any other stage of life. With preterm birth, infants are deprived of this intense intrauterine growth period. After birth, the intensity of the expected weight loss during the first days of life is associated with gestational age, birth weight, and the time required to achieve full enteral nutrition. After the initial period of weight loss, stabilization of weight is expected with a slight increase in length, followed by the catch-up period. When growth restriction remains during the early postnatal period with growth rates lower than expected, the preterm infant is said to be experiencing extrauterine growth retardation. Persistent growth restriction is more frequent among extremely and very preterm infants and in those with feeding difficulties and comorbidities. After hospital discharge, they are usually shorter and lighter than full-term peers, despite the intense catch-up growth they may have had. In general, growth recovery occurs during the first 2 years of life, when a more stable, healthy condition is expected. In the extreme lower limits of viability (birth weight <500 g or gestational age ≤25 weeks), catch-up growth might occur by 6 years of age or even later. The risk of short stature for the late preterm infants is lower than that of extremely preterm and very preterm infants. The risk of unfavorable growth outcome is higher for preterm infants born at appropriate size for gestational age but with extrauterine growth retardation, for those born prematurely and SGA, for those who still have short stature at 2 years of age, and for those who have rapid weight gain early in childhood.

Adverse exposures during fetal and early postnatal life have been proposed to lead to unfavorable programming effects. In infants born prematurely, the period equivalent to the third trimester of gestation occurs extra utero, with higher risk of alterations in the GH–IGF-1 system. Few and conflicting data are available on GH axis in children who were born prematurely and have short stature during infancy and childhood. The lack of data reflects, in part, the heterogeneity of preterm birth. The same happens with studies on the effects of GH treatment. Few studies are available in which only formerly preterm children are included. Most of the data about growth response to GH treatment in children born prematurely are derived from studies of GH treatment for short stature of different etiologies in which prematurity was not an exclusion criterion. This is especially common in studies involving children born SGA with a high number of infants born prematurely. Apparently, similar response to GH treatment is observed for both preterm and term short children who were born SGA. These studies suggest that when growth failure occurs and persists during infancy and childhood, children born prematurely might benefit from GH treatment.

Clinical Case Vignettes

Case 1

A 1.7-year-old boy, the first child of nonconsanguineous and healthy parents, was born at 31 weeks and 5 days gestation from a twin pregnancy via cesarean delivery after history of fetal distress and single umbilical artery. Birth measurements with respective Z-scores (Intergrowth 21st) were weight, 795 g (–3.88); length, 12.6 in (32 cm) (–3.85); and head circumference, 10.0 in (25.5 cm) (–2.36). Apgar score was 7 at 1 minute after birth but he was transferred to the neonatal intensive care unit because of low birth weight and prematurity. He slowly gained weight and was discharged after 2 months in stable condition with a weight of 2110 g. At 1.7 years of age, his height is now 29.3 in (74.5 cm) (–3.27), weight is 19.0 lb (8.6 kg)

(–2.37) and head circumference is 19.7 in (50 cm) (+1.8) (Z-scores, World Health Organization [WHO] 2016) with consequent relative macrocephaly. No significant additional findings are reported.

Which of the following evaluations (if any) should be performed now?

A. Evaluation of the GH–IGF-1 axis

B. Genetic studies for short stature and small size at birth

C. Reassurance; repeat clinical evaluation in a few months

D. Referral for nutritional counseling to increase caloric intake

E. TSH and free T_4 measurements and celiac screen

Answer: C) Reassurance, repeat clinical evaluation in a few months

This was the first appointment for a 1.7-year-old child born very preterm (<32 weeks of gestation). Approximately 80% of preterm children exhibit growth recovery during the first 2 years of life, with height appropriate for genetic potential between 6 and 12 months of life. After 2 to 3 years of age, height gain usually correlates with parent's height. At 3 years of age, approximately 80% reach normality for head circumference and 70% for weight. The question raised by this case is when to start the investigation for short stature in a child born prematurely and the consideration for genetic studies. The lack of recovery near the second year of life and additional clinical findings would prompt these studies, but at this time, it is reasonable to suggest a clinical reevaluation in a few months (Answer C), as the child has no other clinical or physical findings.

Case 1 (continued)

After approximately 1 year of clinical follow-up, the patient is 2.8 years old (corrected age for gestational age = 2.6 years), and the clinical picture appears unchanged. He presents with moderate speech delay and normal findings on brain MRI.

There are normal findings from a workup for metabolic and gastrointestinal disorders, multiple urine tests, and abdominal ultrasonography. His anthropometric parameters are weight, 22.3 lb (10.1 kg) (–2.58); height, 33.1 in (84 cm) (–2.71); and head circumference, 20.1 in (51 cm) (+1.3) (Z-scores, WHO 2016). Growth velocity is 9.5 cm/y. In addition to relative macrocephaly, physical examination documents low muscle mass. Endocrine laboratory assessment shows normal thyroid and GH function.

Which of the following should be advised at this visit?

A. Due to persistent short stature, discuss GH treatment

B. Recommend genetic studies for short stature and small size at birth

C. Reassure his family that this is a typical scenario for an infant born prematurely and that spontaneous catch-up may occur during the first 10 years of life

D. Reinforce nutritional counseling to increase caloric intake

E. Recommend waiting for the pubertal growth spurt

Answer: A) Due to persistent short stature, discuss GH treatment

Most healthy infants born prematurely have catch-up growth after initial growth failure. However, substantial growth failure may occur and can be worsened if the child was born prematurely and SGA. Previous studies have shown that the incidence of short stature among preterm babies born SGA does not change from 2 to 5 years, reinforcing that catch-up growth in SGA children occurs mainly during the first 2 years of life. Height at 1 year of age and the difference in height between ages 1 and 2 are considered predictors of height at 5 to 6 years of age. Despite normal GH secretion, GH treatment (Answer A) is approved for short children born SGA, including those born preterm. GH therapy can significantly improve growth velocity and adult height.

Case 2

A 4.3-year-old girl is referred because of short stature. She is a child of nonconsanguineous and healthy parents and was born at 34 weeks of gestation via natural delivery after an unremarkable pregnancy. Birth measurements with respective Z-scores (Intergrowth 21st) were weight, 4.2 lb (1.9 kg) (–0.64); length, 16.5 in (42 cm) (–1.40); and head circumference, 12.6 in (32 cm) (0.71). At 4.3 years of age, her height is 37.0 in (94 cm) (–2.45); weight is 28.7 lb (13 kg) (–1.9); and head circumference is 20.9 in (53 cm) (+2.4) (Z-scores, WHO 2016). Target height is at –1 SD. Her medical history is significant for a persistent failure to thrive during the first years of life. Findings on investigation for common pediatric disorders, endocrinological assessment, and karyotype analysis are normal. She starts GH treatment at age 4.6 years with a dosage of 0.03 mg/kg per day. During follow-up, pubarche starts at age 9.6 years and thelarche at 10.9 years. At this age, her height is 53.4 in (136 cm) (–1.12 SD), and bone age is 11 years (Greulich and Pyle method).

Which of the following is the best recommendation for this patient's management?

A. Stop GH treatment and wait for spontaneous pubertal growth spurt

B. Double the GH dosage during puberty

C. Check for adherence to GH therapy and other associated diagnoses

D. Check for adrenal disorders

E. Intensify the monitoring of pubertal progression and skeletal maturation

Answer: E) Intensify the monitoring of pubertal progression and skeletal maturation

Careful monitoring formerly preterm children is recommended during all growth periods, including puberty. They may be shorter than their peers at onset of puberty. Although puberty usually begins at a normal age range and no clear association has been demonstrated between preterm birth and substantially affected pubertal development, it has been suggested that children born prematurely are prone to an earlier onset and faster progression of puberty compared with girls born at appropriate size for gestational age. Therefore, in the case of short stature at onset of puberty or fast progression of puberty compromising growth potential, one of the suggested therapeutic approaches to optimize adult height is to decrease estrogen exposure and slow skeletal maturation while on GH treatment. This effect could be obtained with the combination of GH with the off-label use of GnRH analogues, agents approved for the treatment of central precocious puberty. After a median time of 6 years of GH treatment for boys and 5.3 years for girls, including the 2 years of combined GH and GnRH analogue, GH-treated children born SGA with adult height expectation below −2.5 SDS at onset of puberty have similar adult height compared with those treated with GH only, but with better height expectation at puberty onset. As previously mentioned, prematurity was not an exclusion criterion in the study, and children born moderately preterm were also included. To strengthen the evidence base addressing the question of whether children with short stature associated with preterm birth benefit from pharmacologic interventions, additional studies are needed.

Key Learning Points

- Prematurity might be a reason for growth failure.

- Careful monitoring of children born prematurely is mandatory.

- Short children born prematurely might benefit from GH therapy.

References

1. Hokken-Koelega ACS, van der Steen M, Boguszewski MCS, et al. International consensus guideline on small for gestational age (SGA): etiology and management from infancy to early adulthood. *Endocr Rev.* 2023 [online ahead of print]. PMID: 36635911

2. Boguszewski MCS, Carlsson M, Lindberg A, et al. Near-adult height after growth hormone treatment in children born prematurely-data from KIGS. *J Clin Endocrinol Metab.* 2020;105(7):dgaa203. PMID: 32479603

3. Collett-Solberg PF, Ambler G, Backeljauw PF, et al. Diagnosis, genetics, and therapy of short stature in children: a Growth Hormone Research Society International perspective. *Horm Res Paediatr.* 2019;92(1):1-14. PMID: 31514194

4. Boguszewski MCDS, Cardoso-Demartini AA. Management of endocrine disease: growth and growth hormone therapy in short children born preterm. *Eur J Endocrinol.* 2017;176(3):R111-R122. PMID: 27803030

5. James E, Wood CL, Nair H, Williams TC. Preterm birth and the timing of puberty: a systematic review. *BMC Pediatr.* 2018;18(1):3. PMID: 29310614

6. Wit JM. Should skeletal maturation be manipulated for extra height gain? *Front Endocrinol.* 2021;12:812196. PMID: 34975773

7. van der Steen M, Lem AJ, van der Kaay DCM, Hokken-Koèelega ACS. Puberty and pubertal growth in GH-treated SGA children: effects of 2 years of GnRHa versus no GnRHa. *J Clin Endocrinol Metab.* 2016;101(5):2005-2012. PMID: 26964733

Current Concepts in Delayed Puberty

Yee-Ming Chan, MD, PhD. Division of Endocrinology, Department of Pediatrics, Boston Children's Hospital and Department of Pediatrics, Harvard Medical School, Boston, MA; Email: Yee-Ming.Chan@childrens.harvard.edu

Educational Objectives

After reviewing this chapter, learners should be able to:

- Understand the limitations of the current statistical definition of delayed puberty.

- Evaluate the usefulness and limitations of various tests in evaluating delayed puberty.

- Identify considerations for management of delayed puberty.

Significance of the Clinical Problem

Patients, families, and referring providers can have widely varying reasons for consulting pediatric endocrinology for delayed puberty; determining the specific concerns of all parties helps to guide discussions and decisions about evaluation and management. Constitutional delay is the most common cause of delayed puberty in both girls and boys, but because constitutional delay is a diagnosis of exclusion, other causes of delayed puberty should be ruled out. However, an extensive hunt for a potential underlying cause of delayed puberty is rarely necessary. If delayed puberty is caused by an underlying illness or stressor, the cause can usually be identified on a detailed history and physical examination. While laboratory evaluation should be performed to screen for primary gonadal insufficiency (which produces a pattern of hypergonadotropic hypogonadism), extensive laboratory testing for an occult cause of hypogonadotropic hypogonadism (HH) in an apparently healthy child with delayed puberty is low-yield. Laboratory testing (including genetic testing) is also currently unable to reliably distinguish self-limited constitutional delay from more lasting idiopathic hypogonadotropic hypogonadism (IHH). Individuals with known permanent reproductive endocrine dysfunction should start pubertal induction at an age that is typical for the general population and for the family. For individuals with unexplained delayed puberty, decisions about sex-steroid treatment require an individualized approach that accounts for the concerns of the patient, the goals of care, and the degree of pubertal delay. Whether treatment is pursued or not, patients should be followed to determine if endogenous puberty starts and progresses. Patients should be counseled that the changes of puberty—whether endogenously driven or exogenously induced—are gradual and that it may take years until they feel they have caught up with their peers, and that patience is needed in the meantime.

Concerns about delayed puberty (and associated delays in pubertal growth) are among the most common reasons for consulting a pediatric endocrinology provider, but we have limited knowledge of basic mechanisms by which puberty starts and how the timing of puberty is determined. We also have limited data on outcomes of delayed puberty and the effects of sex-steroid treatment. In the face of ongoing uncertainty about the optimal approach to evaluation and management of delayed puberty, there is currently room for variation in clinical practice.

Practice Gaps

- Lack of understanding of how puberty starts and how pubertal timing is determined.

- Limitations of currently available diagnostic tests.

- Insufficient data on effects of sex-steroid treatment (if any) on long-term outcomes.

Discussion

Defining Delayed Puberty

Because we do not understand the mechanisms that determine when puberty starts, we rely on a statistical definition of delayed puberty. Pubertal timing in the general population exhibits a Gaussian distribution, and delayed puberty is commonly defined as lack of pubertal onset by an age that is 2 standard deviations beyond the population mean (although it is worth noting that the designating 2 standard deviations as a threshold is arbitrary). While most sources define delayed puberty as lack of pubertal onset by age 13 years in girls and 14 years in boys, contemporary data on the timing of puberty suggest that the 2-standard deviation threshold is closer to 12 to 12.5 years for girls and 13.5 years for boys.[1,2] One limitation of using a statistical definition for delayed puberty is that, with the secular trend towards earlier pubertal onset, it is unclear whether the age cutoffs for defining delayed puberty should change and whether doing so would improve or diminish the ability to detect pathological causes of delayed puberty. Indeed, another limitation of the current statistical definition is that it does not distinguish benign variation from pathological causes of delayed puberty.

Also, debating whether a 12-year-7-month-old girl or a 13-year-10-month-old boy meets age criteria for delayed puberty risks overlooking the needs of the patient. It can be helpful to determine early in a visit who is concerned (patient, parents/caregivers, primary care provider) and what the precise concerns are (eg, height, appearance, sports performance, or alternatively, lack of concern because of a strong family history of self-limited delayed puberty).

Causes of Delayed Puberty

Several case series have shown that:

- The most common cause of delayed puberty is constitutional delay, a self-limited delay in pubertal onset, found in ~30% to 50% of girls and ~50% to 75% of boys (*table*).

- The second most common cause of delayed puberty is functional HH, ie, physiologic suppression of the hypothalamic-pituitary-gonadal (HPG) axis by a stressor such as chronic illness/inflammation, undernutrition, or excessive exercise. Functional HH was reported as the cause of delayed puberty in ~20% to 30% of girls and 10% to 35% of boys; however, rates in the general population may be lower, as these case series were from academic medical centers with patients who are more likely to have underlying medical issues.

- The third most common cause of delayed puberty in girls (~15%-25%) is primary ovarian insufficiency (mostly due to Turner syndrome), but primary gonadal insufficiency is less common in boys (~1%-8%).

The remaining causes of delayed puberty are relatively uncommon. These causes include:

- Endocrine conditions such as hyperprolactinemia, hypothyroidism, and Cushing syndrome.

- Pathology broadly affecting the hypothalamus and/or pituitary gland, such as a craniopharyngioma.

- IHH (also called congenital hypogonadotropic hypogonadism, isolated GnRH deficiency, and other names), a pathological deficiency of GnRH production or action. When IHH occurs with anosmia, the combination is called Kallmann syndrome.

Table. Causes of Delayed Puberty Reported in Various Case Series[3]

	Boston 1996-1999 (21)	Copenhagen (16)	Toronto (22)[a]	Helsinki (23)	Boston 2000-2015
Girls	n = 74		n = 20	n = 70	n = 392
Hypergonadotropic hypogonadism	26%		10%[b]	14%	18%
Functional hypogonadotropic hypogonadism	16%		50%	15%	29%
Delayed puberty secondary to another endocrine condition	1%		[b]	0%	8%
Hypogonadotropic hypogonadism because of generalized hypothalamic/pituitary pathology	15%		[b]	1%	3%
Idiopathic hypogonadotropic hypogonadism/ Kallmann syndrome	4%		0%	8%	0.5%
Other syndromes and other causes	8%		10%	6%	9%
Constitutional delay	30%		30%	55%	32%
Boys	n = 158	n = 391	n = 28	n = 174	n = 683
Hypergonadotropic hypogonadism	7%	0.5%	0%[b]	2%	2%
Functional hypogonadotropic hypogonadism	14%	20%	43%	6%	16%
Delayed puberty secondary to another endocrine condition	2%	2%	[b]	0%	5%
Hypogonadotropic hypogonadism due to generalized hypothalamic/pituitary pathology	8%	7%[c]	4%[b]	2%	2%
Idiopathic hypogonadotropic hypogonadism/ Kallmann syndrome	3%		4%	8%	2%
Other syndromes and other causes	4%	0%	0%	0%	4%
Constitutional delay	63%	71%	50%	82%	70%

[a] L. Abitbol and M. Palmert provided additional details through personal communication.

[b] These percentages do not account for 16 girls and boys with previously known hypogonadotropic and hypergonadotropic conditions (eg, Turner syndrome, panhypopituitarism) for whom the specific breakdown of diagnoses was not available.

[c] This reference did not distinguish between these 2 categories of hypogonadotropic hypogonadism. This percentage includes 14 patients with GH deficiency and 13 with hypogonadotropic hypogonadism.

Reprinted from Jonsdottir-Lewis E et al. *J Clin Endocrinol Metab*, 2021; 106(9): e3693-e3703. © The Endocrine Society.

Screening for Occult Causes of Delayed Puberty

Although constitutional delay is the most common cause of delayed puberty, it is a diagnosis of exclusion (as is IHH), and individuals with delayed puberty should be evaluated for other potential causes of pubertal delay. Primary gonadal insufficiency is readily recognizable on laboratory evaluation by a pattern of hypergonadotropic hypogonadism, with elevation of FSH and LH. Most causes of functional HH can be identified through a detailed history and physical examination, including a confidential discussion with the patient about eating patterns and exercise.

Beyond this core evaluation, it is unclear how useful it is to screen an apparently healthy child for occult causes of delayed puberty. One study examined the number of laboratory tests ordered for 64 patients with delayed puberty seen at a single academic center.[4] This analysis revealed wide variation in the number of tests performed, ranging from 3 to 27 tests, with an average of 16 tests performed per patient. In none of the 64 patients did testing identify an issue that was not already suggested by history and physical examination. Anecdotally, I am aware of cases of occult celiac disease and inflammatory bowel disease that were discovered on laboratory evaluation for delayed puberty. My practice for laboratory evaluation is as follows (but I acknowledge that this practice is not evidence-based):

- Measure FSH, LH, and estradiol in girls, testosterone in boys
- Screen for celiac disease
- Assess inflammatory markers (erythrocyte sedimentation rate and/or C-reactive protein)
- Measure TSH and prolactin

It is also unclear which patients require cranial MRI to screen for structural lesions of the hypothalamus and/or pituitary gland. I am not aware of any data on the yield of such screening, but in my experience it is very unlikely to have a pathological finding in a patient with delayed puberty and no other issues. My practice (again, not evidence-based) is to obtain a cranial MRI if:

- There are concerning neurological signs or symptoms
- There is known pituitary pathology outside the HPG axis (although I do not routinely screen for pituitary dysfunction aside from hyperprolactinemia)
- I am beginning to suspect IHH due to increasing age without signs of puberty (~15 years for girls and ~16 years for boys, although I may wait until even later ages if there is a family history of marked constitutional delay).

Distinguishing Constitutional Delay From IHH

In most cases, no underlying cause of delayed puberty is found, and the remaining potential diagnoses are constitutional delay—which is common, self-limited, and does not necessarily require treatment—and IHH—which is rare, usually lifelong, and requires treatment with sex steroids.

Factors that suggest IHH include anosmia, normally timed adrenarche, and in boys, cryptorchidism, micropenis, and low testicular volumes (≤1 mL).[5] Factors that favor constitutional delay include late or absent adrenarche, delayed bone age, childhood growth along a percentile lower than expected for midparental height (although very slow childhood growth of

3 cm/year or less should raise concerns for an underlying stressor), and a family history of constitutional delay. While these factors can be suggestive, none is fully sensitive or specific.

Currently available laboratory studies are also unable to definitively diagnose constitutional delay or IHH, as nicely discussed in reference 6. Tests that have been studied include measurement of LH at baseline or after stimulation with GnRH, baseline inhibin B, and many others. Of these, baseline inhibin B may be the most useful, as very low inhibin B (<30 pg/mL) suggests a diagnosis of IHH[7]; however, not all individuals with IHH have low inhibin B.[8] More recently, small studies have suggested that kisspeptin-stimulated LH[9] and FSH-stimulated inhibin B[10] may have better ability to distinguish constitutional delay from IHH, but larger studies are needed to determine the sensitivity and specificity of these methods.

Genetic testing also has limited prognostic power. While many genes have been associated with IHH, variants in the genes that are more commonly associated with IHH, such as *FGFR1*, exhibit variable penetrance and expressivity: the same genetic variant associated with IHH in one individual may be associated with constitutional delay in a family member.[11] An exception is variants in the *ANOS1* gene, which lies on the X chromosome and is associated with approximately 15% of cases of Kallmann syndrome in males. Variants in *ANOS1* appear to be highly penetrant for both IHH and anosmia. In my practice, I screen for *ANOS1* variants in boys with delayed puberty and anosmia; for other patients, I do not pursue genetic testing.

Whether and When to Treat Delayed Puberty

In general, patients known to have a permanent cause of hypogonadism should have puberty induced within the typical age range for pubertal onset. For individuals with permanent HH, there is no clear marker for when to start pubertal induction. Population averages (~10 years for girls and ~11 years for boys) and family history of pubertal timing can help with the decision when to start pubertal induction.

For those with primary gonadal insufficiency, monitoring gonadotropins can guide when to start treatment. Circulating concentrations of gonadotropins in childhood vary widely across individuals with gonadal insufficiency, with some individuals having gonadotropins in the prepubertal range, others in the pubertal range, and yet others in the hypergonadotropic range.[12,13] Because of this variability, a single finding of elevated gonadotropins does not necessarily signal that it is time to start pubertal induction. My practice is to obtain a baseline measurement of gonadotropins between the ages of 3 and 7 years, and to start monitoring every 6 months starting at age 8 years for girls and 9 years for boys to determine when gonadotropins start to rise above this baseline. However, it may be prudent to wait 6 or even 12 months to start pubertal induction after seeing this initial rise in gonadotropins. Rises in gonadotropins can be detected as early as 1 year prior to the appearance of external signs of puberty,[14] and in individuals with gonadal insufficiency, the loss of negative feedback from gonadal hormones may cause this rise in gonadotropins to be exaggerated.

For individuals with suspected constitutional delay, several studies (mostly of testosterone treatment in boys, and mostly observational, although some have been randomized studies) have shown expected increases in growth and development of secondary sex characteristics with sex-steroid treatment, and some studies also reported improvement in psychosocial outcomes. For long-term outcomes, retrospective analyses of adults who had delayed puberty have not shown any clear effect of sex-steroid treatment on adult height or bone-mineral density.

In the absence of data on long-term outcomes, the primary goal of treatment of constitutional delay with sex steroids is to alleviate psychosocial distress. Some view treatment of constitutional delay with sex steroids as a reasonable method to alleviate psychosocial distress, whereas others feel that such treatment unnecessarily pathologizes and medicalizes normal variation in pubertal timing. Indeed, providers exhibit considerable variation in practice around sex-steroid treatment. Some providers gladly prescribe sex steroids for patients who just meet age criteria for delayed puberty, while others treat only those with marked delay. In general, providers wait longer to induce puberty in girls than in boys and also cite different reasons for treating—primarily bone-mineral density for girls and height and psychosocial considerations for boys.[15] It is unclear whether these differences in practice are clinically justified, and providers should be alert to the possibility of bias in decision-making for girls vs boys with delayed puberty.

In the absence of a clear "right" or "wrong" for whether to treat a patient with presumed constitutional delay with sex steroids, decision-making should be guided by the goals and wishes of the patient. When I discuss sex-steroid treatment with a child with probable constitutional delay, I point out that we currently have no way to predict whether and when puberty will start. Puberty may start soon, or it may not start for several years, or it may never start spontaneously (*figure*),[3] and the patient needs to decide whether it is preferable to avoid potentially starting treatment unnecessarily or to avoid potentially having pubertal development fall even further behind that of one's peers.

Pubertal induction typically starts with low dosages of sex steroids that are gradually increased to adult dosages over a span of 2 to 3 years, and several suggested protocols have been published. It is typically sufficient to monitor growth every 4 months and bone-age x-rays annually. I have not found it clinically useful to monitor serum estradiol or testosterone concentrations.

Unless there is a known permanent cause of delayed puberty, it is important to continue to monitor for signs of pubertal onset, which would generally indicate that treatment is no longer needed. For those receiving estradiol treatment, withdrawal of treatment for 6 to 8 weeks may be needed to assess endogenous activity. For those receiving testosterone treatment, an increase in

The Journal of Clinical Endocrinology & Metabolism, 2021, Vol. 106, No. 9 **e3699**

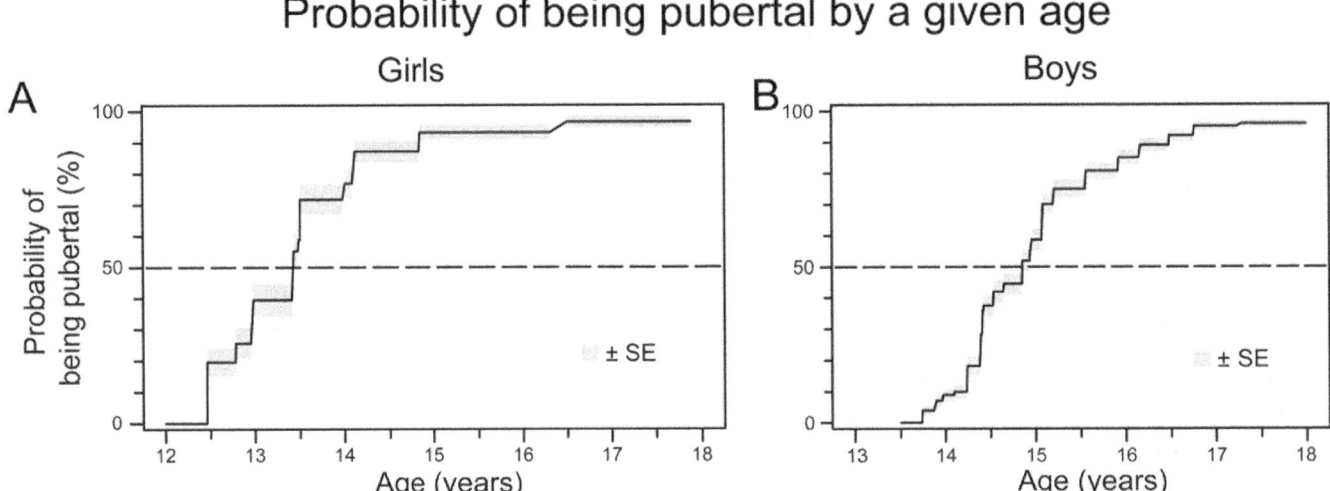

Probability of being pubertal by a given age

Reprinted from Jonsdottir-Lewis E et al. *J Clin Endocrinol Metab*, 2021; 106(9): e3693-e3703. © The Endocrine Society.

testicular volume signals progression into puberty. However, testicular growth may be inhibited by treatment, and periodic laboratory evaluation after withdrawal of treatment may still be needed to detect emerging reproductive endocrine activity.

Some patients are unfamiliar with what to expect with puberty, and counseling that breast tenderness and vaginal discharge are common for estradiol-driven puberty and that erections and nocturnal emissions can occur with testosterone-driven puberty can prevent potentially distressing surprises. For patients who are very eager for the changes of puberty to start, it can be helpful to advise that the changes of puberty are gradual, regardless of whether puberty is endogenously driven or exogenously induced. There may be no obvious effects in the first 3 months of treatment, although growth acceleration can usually be seen by 6 months of treatment. I also advise patients that the effects of sex steroids on body appearance continue well after growth is finished, so it may not be until early adulthood that they that they have fully caught up with their peers, and I counsel them to be patient and reassure them that they will catch up eventually.

Clinical Case Vignettes

Case 1

A 14-year-old girl presents to pediatric endocrine care because of lack of breast development. She is healthy, does not engage in vigorous exercise, and has a normal BMI. She does not have slowing of growth velocity (but also has not had a pubertal growth spurt). Medical history and physical examination findings are unremarkable, and bone age is 12 years. Laboratory test results reveal an LH concentration less than 0.1 mIU/mL.

Which of the following methods is most likely to determine the cause of her delayed puberty?

A. Following over time to determine whether she eventually enters puberty

B. Stimulation testing to assess GH secretion

C. Stimulation testing with GnRH or a GnRH analogue

D. Complete blood cell count, comprehensive metabolic panel, and urinalysis

E. MRI of the brain and pituitary gland

Answer: A) Following over time to determine whether she eventually enters puberty

The most common cause of delayed puberty in girls and boys is constitutional delay, which currently can only be diagnosed retrospectively by observing that a patient enters and progresses through puberty (Answer A). Lack of a pubertal growth spurt is expected in a child with delayed puberty and does not signal GH deficiency. Stimulation testing with GnRH or a GnRH-analogue is neither sensitive nor specific for distinguishing constitutional delay from pathological causes of delayed puberty such as IHH. An extensive laboratory workup in an apparently healthy child is unlikely to identify an occult pathological cause of delayed puberty. Similarly, in the absence of concerning signs or symptoms, cranial MRI is unlikely to reveal a pathological cause.

The patient developed breast buds at 14 years 9 months, achieved menarche at 16 years, and had regular menstrual periods thereafter; thus, a diagnosis of constitutional delay was confirmed.

Case 2

A 13-year-6-month-old boy presents because of concerns about slow growth. He is healthy with no significant medical history, and he reports a normal sense of smell. Family history is notable for IHH associated with a *TACR3* variant in his mother, delayed puberty in his father, and normal pubertal timing in his older brother. Midparental target height is at the 75th percentile, and his childhood growth had been along the 50th percentile. His growth velocity has continued to be fairly constant, but his height is now at the 10th percentile because of lack of a pubertal growth spurt. Physical examination is notable for testicular volumes of 1 mL bilaterally and absence of adrenarchal signs. Bone age is 11 years. Laboratory studies reveal prepubertal gonadotropins and testosterone. Genetic testing shows that he has his mother's *TACR3* variant.

Which of the following is an appropriate conclusion from the patient's evaluation?

A. His declining height percentiles raise concern for GH deficiency

B. He is likely to have an occult illness causing delayed puberty; extensive additional testing is needed to identify a potential underlying cause

C. His general good health, growth along a height percentile lower than that expected for his midparental target height, family history of self-limited delayed puberty, absence of adrenarchal signs, and delayed bone age firmly establish a diagnosis of constitutional delay

D. His testicular volumes of 1 mL and the presence of the *TACR3* variant firmly establish a diagnosis of IHH

E. At this time, it is not possible to determine whether he has constitutional delay or IHH

Answer: E) At this time, it is not possible to determine whether he has constitutional delay or IHH

In the absence of a marked change in growth velocity or a very slow growth velocity (<3 cm/y), the decline in height percentiles commonly seen in individuals with delayed puberty is readily attributable to lack of a pubertal growth spurt. If there are no concerning findings on history or physical examination, the yield of extensive testing for an occult cause of delayed puberty is low. While certain findings may make an eventual diagnosis of constitutional delay or IHH more likely, no single finding or test is definitive, and currently the diagnosis of constitutional delay or IHH can only be made retrospectively, after observing whether a patient eventually enters puberty or not (thus, Answer E is correct).

Case 2 (continued)

The patient does not want to start therapy for delayed puberty and instead prefers to wait for endogenous puberty to start. On follow-up evaluations, testicular volumes and LH remain in the prepubertal range, and at 14 years 9 months the patient begins to consider treatment with testosterone.

Which of the following is the most appropriate counseling and management regarding testosterone treatment?

A. Testosterone treatment is contraindicated because it will cause premature closure of the growth plates

B. Testosterone treatment is contraindicated because constitutional delay is the most likely diagnosis

C. Because constitutional delay is the most likely diagnosis, he can be treated with a 6-month course of testosterone, after which further follow-up is unnecessary

D. Given uncertainty whether he has constitutional delay or IHH, ongoing follow-up is needed to monitor for the emergence of endogenous reproductive endocrine activity

E. Because of the possibility of permanent IHH, he needs to commit to lifelong testosterone treatment

Answer: D) Given ongoing uncertainty whether he has constitutional delay or IHH, ongoing follow-up is needed to monitor for the emergence of endogenous reproductive endocrine activity

Studies of boys with delayed puberty have not shown significant bone-age advancement or compromise of adult height even with dosages of testosterone that would now be considered to be high. Because we currently lack diagnostic tests to distinguish constitutional delay from IHH and because we lack definitive outcome data in individuals treated or not treated with sex steroids for delayed puberty, there is room for practice variation and no "hard rule" for treatment. A discussion of the goals of care and the risks and benefits of treatment can help patients and families decide on the management plan that seems most appropriate to them. Regardless of the decision about sex-steroid treatment, an essential aspect of care is ongoing monitoring to determine whether long-term treatment is needed (Answer D).

With gradually increasing doses of testosterone, the patient achieved robust pubertal growth and reached his midparental target height. Testicular volumes remained 2 mL until age 16 years 9 months, when they were noted to be 3 mL bilaterally. After withdrawal of testosterone treatment, testosterone was 147 ng/dL (5.1 nmol/L). By age 17 years 1 month, testosterone was 466 ng/dL (16.2 nmol/L). He was given a retrospective diagnosis of constitutional delay, and no further testosterone treatment was required.

Key Learning Points

- The current statistical definition for delayed puberty is arbitrary and does not distinguish pathology from normal variation.

- Constitutional delay is the most common cause of delayed puberty, but it is a retrospective diagnosis of exclusion, and current tests cannot reliably distinguish between constitutional delay and IHH.

- Extensive laboratory testing for occult causes of delayed puberty in an apparently healthy individual is low-yield.

- The long-term effects (if any) of constitutional delay are unclear, and the long-term effects of sex-steroid treatment for constitutional delay are similarly unclear.

- Patients with delayed puberty should be monitored for emergence of endogenous reproductive endocrine activity.

References

1. Biro FM, Greenspan LC, Galvez MP, et al. Onset of breast development in a longitudinal cohort. *Pediatrics*. 2013;132(6):1019-1027. PMID: 24190685

2. Herman-Giddens ME, Steffes J, Harris D, et al. Secondary sexual characteristics in boys: data from the Pediatric Research in Office Settings Network. *Pediatrics*. 2012;130(5):e1058-e1068. PMID: 23085608

3. Jonsdottir-Lewis E, Feld A, Ciarlo R, Denhoff E, Feldman HA, Chan YM. Timing of pubertal onset in girls and boys with constitutional delay. *J Clin Endocrinol Metab.* 2021;106(9):e3693-e3703. PMID: 33890108

4. Abitbol L, Zborovski S, Palmert MR. Evaluation of delayed puberty: what diagnostic tests should be performed in the seemingly otherwise well adolescent? *Arch Dis Child.* 2016;101(8):767-771. PMID: 27190100

5. Varimo T, Miettinen PJ, Kansakoski J, Raivio T, Hero M. Congenital hypogonadotropic hypogonadism, functional hypogonadotropism or constitutional delay of growth and puberty? An analysis of a large patient series from a single tertiary center. *Hum Reprod.* 2017;32(1):147-153. PMID: 27927844

6. Harrington J, Palmert MR. Distinguishing self-limited delayed puberty from permanent hypogonadotropic hypogonadism: how and why? *J Clin Endocrinol Metab.* 2021;106(12):e5264-e5266. PMID: 34223894

7. Adan L, Lechevalier P, Couto-Silva AC, et al. Plasma inhibin B and antimullerian hormone concentrations in boys: discriminating between congenital hypogonadotropic hypogonadism and constitutional pubertal delay. *Med Sci Monit.* 2010;16(11):CR511-CR517. PMID: 20980953

8. Pitteloud N, Hayes FJ, Boepple PA, et al. The role of prior pubertal development, biochemical markers of testicular maturation, and genetics in elucidating the phenotypic heterogeneity of idiopathic hypogonadotropic hypogonadism. *J Clin Endocrinol Metab.* 2002;87(1):152-160. PMID: 11788640

9. Chan YM, Lippincott MF, Sales Barroso P, et al. Using kisspeptin to predict pubertal outcomes for youth with pubertal delay. *J Clin Endocrinol Metab.* 2020;105(8):e2717-e2725. PMID: 32232399

10. Chaudhary S, Walia R, Bhansali A, et al. FSH-stimulated inhibin B (FSH-iB): a novel marker for the accurate prediction of pubertal outcome in delayed puberty. *J Clin Endocrinol Metab.* 2021;106(9):e3495-e3505. PMID: 34010394

11. Zhu J, Choa RE, Guo MH, et al. A shared genetic basis for self-limited delayed puberty and idiopathic hypogonadotropic hypogonadism. *J Clin Endocrinol Metab.* 2015;100(4):E646-E654. PMID: 25636053

12. Conte FA, Grumbach MM, Kaplan SL. A diphasic pattern of gonadotropin secretion in patients with the syndrome of gonadal dysgenesis. *J Clin Endocrinol Metab.* 1975;40(4):670-674. PMID: 1127077

13. Grinspon RP, Ropelato MG, Bedecarras P, et al. Gonadotrophin secretion pattern in anorchid boys from birth to pubertal age: pathophysiological aspects and diagnostic usefulness. *Clin Endocrinol (Oxf).* 2012;76(5):698-705. PMID: 22098623

14. Wu FC, Butler GE, Kelnar CJ, Sellar RE. Patterns of pulsatile luteinizing hormone secretion before and during the onset of puberty in boys: a study using an immunoradiometric assay. *J Clin Endocrinol Metab.* 1990;70(3):629-637. PMID: 2407751

15. Zhu J, Feldman HA, Eugster EA, et al. Practice variation in the management of girls and boys with delayed puberty. *Endocr Pract.* 2020;26(3):267-284. PMID: 31859552

Care of Preschool Children With Type 1 Diabetes Mellitus

Linda A. DiMeglio, MD, MPH. Pediatric Endocrinology and Diabetology, Indiana University School of Medicine, Indianapolis, IN. Email: dimeglio@iu.edu

Educational Objectives

After reviewing this chapter, learners should be able to:

- Articulate care considerations unique to very young children with type 1 diabetes mellitus (T1DM).

- Explain successful management strategies for care of youth with T1DM.

- Identify gaps in knowledge regarding care of very young children with T1DM.

Significance of the Clinical Problem

T1DM management in preschool children is challenging. These children depend on others (parents, other family, daycare staff members, babysitters) for all aspects of their care, which includes insulin administration, glucose monitoring, healthy eating, and aspects of physical activity. Because children diagnosed as preschoolers are expected to have a very long diabetes duration, and dysglycemia induces acute and chronic complications, it is important to strive for near-normoglycemia. Also, good treatment habits and lifestyle choices, including family-centered meals, can engrain healthy habits from early childhood that may carry forward throughout life.

The target hemoglobin A_{1c} value for all children with diabetes, including very young children, is less than 7.0% (<53 mmol/mol), which translates to time in the targeted glucose range of 70 to 180 mg/dL (3.9-10 mmol/L) of greater than 70%.[1] To achieve this target, treatment strategies must consider small body sizes; early childhood growth patterns; and evolving stages of cognitive, social, and motor development. Intensive insulin therapy (ideally using pump therapy) should be used with basal insulin and preprandial insulin boluses for food coupled with correction doses as indicated. Fortunately, automated insulin delivery systems are now gradually being approved for this age group. Frequent glucose monitoring is needed; continuous glucose monitoring (CGM) is recommended. When CGM is not available, 7 to 10 blood glucose checks per day with appropriate interpretation and subsequent action are generally required. Diabetes education also must be provided to staff at daycare centers and preschools to promote equal learning and participation for children with T1DM in these settings.

Great demands are placed on families of very young children with diabetes who often have unpredictable behaviors/activity, erratic eating patterns, frequent intercurrent illnesses, and a limited capacity to recognize and articulate symptoms of hypoglycemia or hyperglycemia. Intensive diabetes management requires complex orchestration to manage insulin dosing, diet, physical activity, and glucose values throughout the day and night.[2] Additionally, very high insulin sensitivity can necessitate very small doses of insulin that are often difficult to administer accurately and reproducibly. These complexities can result in high risks both for severe hypoglycemia, resulting in seizure/coma, and for severe hyperglycemia, which itself imparts risk of adverse neurocognitive effects and possible metabolic decompensation.

These youngsters' diabetes management and overall care depends entirely on caregivers. Adult caregivers often experience substantial physical and emotional burdens that can negatively impact the child's diabetes management. Parents of children with diabetes have higher rates of depression than their peers and often report marital strain and feelings of anxiety, guilt, loss of control, and/or isolation. In addition to the emotional effects, there are negative economic and occupational ramifications. As an example, it has been shown that mothers of preschool children often reduce their work hours after a child's diagnosis.

Due in part to the pervasiveness of fear of hypoglycemia rather than concerns for glucose elevations, most youth with T1DM, including very young children, currently experience suboptimal glycemic management.[3] It is now recognized that hyperglycemia is bad for brain development. More time spent in hyperglycemia is associated with slower grey and white matter brain growth.[4] Children with diabetes onset before age 5 years also risk suboptimal cognitive and fine-motor development.

Practice Gaps

- Misunderstanding of differences in the diabetes management of very young children vs older children and teens.

- Caregiver fear of hypoglycemia.

- Few tested effective strategies to optimize use of new technologies to improve care and unrealistic expectations about current devices.

- Care limited by sociodemographic disparities and by lack of educational strategies for primary and secondary caregivers.

Discussion

Historically, young children have underutilized advanced diabetes technologies (continuous subcutaneous insulin infusion, continuous glucose monitoring [CGM], sensor-augmented pump therapy, threshold-suspend pumps, etc). This underuse is shifting, as CGM availability and technologies continue to evolve in ways that make use easier for very young children, including improved insurance coverage, better cloud-based ways to communicate real-time glucose data with caregivers, and approvals for smaller more accurate sensors and automated insulin delivery systems for very young children. Although pump and CGM use is increasing across all race/ethnicity groups and insurance statuses, there remain sharp racial and socioeconomic disparities in new technology use, with lower use in minoritized groups and those of lower socioeconomic status.[5]

Despite modern therapies, care of the youngest children with T1DM remains difficult. Families need to be supported to maintain the health and well-being of the child with diabetes. Parents should be encouraged to adopt a positive, nonjudgmental approach to the needed routines of T1DM management (fingersticks/CGM insertions, meal choices, injections, pump/CGM site changes). Children should also be encouraged to be involved in some of their own diabetes-related management tasks (such as checking blood glucose and making good food choices). It is important that diabetes care teams regularly screen families for social and financial stresses (including food insecurity) and promote optimal health-related quality of life.

Glycemic Targets

Traditional management in young children was targeted to avoid hypoglycemia based on scant data on adverse CNS outcomes related to recurrent seizure/coma. As noted above, there is emerging recognition that hyperglycemia also negatively affects CNS structure and function in young children, creating a need for a paradigm shift. Rather than trying to "err on the high side" with respect to glycemic targets, parents and providers should adopt more balanced approaches aimed at achieving lower glycemic targets while avoiding both frequent hypoglycemia and hyperglycemia.

Both the American Diabetes Association (ADA) and the International Society for Pediatric and Adolescent Diabetes (ISPAD) recommend a target hemoglobin A_{1c} value less than 7.0% (<53 mmol/mol) for all children with T1DM, including the youngest children (*see table*). ISPAD suggests that a target less than 6.5% (<48 mmol/mol) be considered for children using advanced technologies. This target was selected to minimize the time spent in hyperglycemia, the chances of experiencing severe hypoglycemia, and the likelihood of developing hypoglycemia unawareness. Despite caregiver fear of hypoglycemia, many children can reach this target safely, due to the intensive degree of caregiver involvement for children at young ages. In children younger than 6 years, the Diabetes Prospective Follow-up Registry (DPV) reported a mean hemoglobin A_{1c} value of 7.4% (57 mmol/mol) in contrast to the T1DM mean hemoglobin A_{1c} value of 8.2% (66 mmol/mol), which was not accompanied by increased reported severe hypoglycemia, suggesting that this hemoglobin A_{1c} target can be safely achieved in children in this age group.[6] Glucose targets should be clearly stated, agreed on by both the family and the diabetes care team, and tailored to the needs and abilities of the individual child and family.

Table. Recommended Glycemic Targets for Very Young Children

Hemoglobin A_{1c} <7.0% (<53 mmol/mol)		
Glucose targets	**ADA**[7]	**ISPAD**[1,8]
Preprandial	80-130 mg/dL (SI: 5.0-7.2 mmol/L)	70-140 mg/dL (SI: 3.9-7.8 mmol/L)
Peak postprandial	<180 mg/dL (SI: <10.0 mmol/L)	<180 mg/dL (SI: <10.0 mmol/L)
CGM targets		**ISPAD**[8]
		>50% 70-140 mg/dL (SI: 3.9-7.8 mmol/L)
	International consensus guidelines[9]	
	>70%: 70-180 mg/dL (SI: 3.9-10.0 mmol/L)	
	<4%: <70 mg/dL (SI: <3.9 mmol/L)	
	<1%: <54 mg/dL (SI: <3.0 mmol/L)	
	<25%: >180 mg/dL (SI: >10 mmol/L)	
	<5%: >250 mg/dL (SI: >13.9 mmol/L)	
	Glycemic variability (%CV) target ≤36%	

Insulin Therapy

To achieve glycemic targets, intensive insulin therapy must be used. As for older children with T1DM, this involves giving preprandial insulin doses of rapid-acting insulin coupled with basal insulin, and additional corrective doses for hyperglycemia between meals with insulin regimens as close to physiologic insulin secretion as possible. Most very young children need a total daily insulin dose (TDD) of ~0.25 units/kg of insulin immediately after diagnosis. After the remission period, this increases to 0.4 to 0.8 units/kg per day. Insulin-to-carbohydrate ratios can be initially estimated based on a "450" rule (ie, 450/TDD = g of carbohydrates covered by 1 unit of insulin). It is important to note that preschool children generally need proportionally more bolus insulin than older youth, particularly more insulin for ingested carbohydrate at breakfast. Insulin sensitivity can be estimated based on an "1800" rule (eg, 1800/TDD = blood glucose [in mg/dL]) decrease expected with a dose of 1 unit of insulin). Very young children also require greater basal insulin dosing during the evening hours of 9 PM to midnight.[10] Insulin dosing needs to be assessed and adjusted regularly because very young children often experience periods of rapid physical growth.

Insulin pump therapy is the preferred method of insulin delivery; however, multiple daily injections can also be used when insulin pump therapy is not available or feasible. Multiple daily injection therapy for very young children should be administered with syringes/pens with at least one-half unit dosing capacity; use of an injection port can be considered. In some cases, diluted insulin may be needed for precise dosing. Pumps containing diluted insulin should be clearly labeled. Recently, some automated insulin delivery systems have been approved for use for very young children.

Infusion/injection sites should be regularly rotated to reduce the likelihood of lipohypertrophy, scarring, infections, rashes, and dry skin. Skin moisturizers applied to future pump sites (a few days before the site is placed, noting that moisturizers should be avoided 24 hours prior to new pump site/

sensor placement) can help with skin reactions and dryness. Topical hydrocortisone can be used for dryness or irritation after site removal.

Medical Nutrition Therapy

Family-centered meals are beneficial for children with T1DM, as are restrictions that limit "grazing" eating habits and large carbohydrate snacks. To dose insulin appropriately, parents and other caregivers need carbohydrate-counting education. Given the pharmacokinetics of subcutaneous insulin dosing, preprandial insulin dosing is preferable to administering the whole dose during or after a meal or snack.[11] Because breast milk contains approximately 7.4 g of carbohydrate per 100 mL, it is possible to give young infants enough insulin to cover 5 to 7 g of carbohydrate before feeding and enough to cover 15 g if older than 9 months. If the amount of carbohydrate to be consumed is not readily ascertainable, a corrective dose for any hyperglycemia along with a partial food dose for anticipated carbohydrate intake can be given at the start of the meal, with the remainder of the dose delivered at the end of the meal.

Very young children require sufficient nutrition because their brains have a much higher metabolic expenditure than the brains of older children and adults. Young children are at risk of poor growth if they are carbohydrate- or nutrient-restricted. Additionally, data suggest that young children with T1DM are at increased risk of being overweight/obese than older children with T1DM or healthy peers.[12] Parents of children with T1DM often report struggles at mealtimes, including long meal durations and frequent food refusals, even when using insulin pumps. Tailored medical nutrition therapy should be administered by a nutritionist, along with monitoring of growth parameters over time.

Glucose Monitoring

Appropriate diabetes management therapy also requires frequent glucose monitoring. Fingerstick glucose measurements must often be obtained (sometimes 7 to 10 times daily),

using a high-precision glucose meter. Whenever possible, families of young children should use CGM for between-meal values and analysis of glucose trends. Although many young children can test their own blood glucose and begin to interpret the glucose value's meaning, they are not yet able to do this or other diabetes-related tasks completely independently.

Secondary Caregivers

Young children with T1DM often spend significant time with secondary caregivers, often outside their primary home at daycare and at preschools/schools. An atmosphere of trust between the primary caregivers and secondary caregivers is critical. Secondary caregivers must receive adequate diabetes education to ensure both safety and equal participation for the child. Children in school settings should all have a clearly articulated, individualized diabetes management plan in place. Data suggest that optimizing glycemia gives children the best chance at being able to participate fully and to learn.[13]

Engendering Healthy Habits

Early onset of T1DM naturally leads to a potential for a long lifetime exposure to the disease. Longer disease duration increases the likelihood of lifetime disease complications. Therefore, although the data so far are not completely conclusive about the relative contribution of the prepubertal years vs pubertal/postpubertal years to the lifetime development of microvascular complications, it seems logical that establishing good care habits for young children as soon as possible leads to lifelong benefits. Encouraging family habits that promote lifestyles for their children over time that are salutatory and will reduce their risk of subsequent cardiovascular disease is appropriate. These habits include healthy eating and adequate exercise. Many countries recommend at least 60 minutes of moderate to vigorous physical activity for all children. In addition to promoting exercise, parents should be encouraged and given strategies to reduce time spent on sedentary behaviors.

Many of these strategies are primarily drawn from recently published guidelines for care of very young children with diabetes.[8]

Clinical Case Vignettes

Case 1

A 3-year-old boy with T1DM diagnosed at age 9 months presents for a follow-up appointment. He weighs 33 lb (15 kg) and uses an insulin pump.

Which of the following insulin profiles is most likely to be successful in this child?

A. TDD 7 units (basal 4.5 units; bolus 2.5 units)

B. TDD 7 units (corrective dose 1/200 at all meals and snacks)

C. TDD 7 units (insulin-to-carbohydrate ratio 1 unit/15 g at breakfast; 1 unit/40 g at evening meal)

D. TDD 8 units (basal rate 0.3 units/h 12 PM-8 PM; 0.1 unit/h 8 PM-12 AM)

E. TDD 14 units (basal rate 7 units; bolus 7 units)

Answer: C) TDD 7 units (insulin-to-carbohydrate ratio 1 unit/15 g at breakfast; 1 unit/40 g at evening meal)

Most very young children with T1DM require 0.2 to 0.3 units/kg per day of insulin immediately after diagnosis, which then increases to between 0.4 and 0.8 units/kg per day after the remission period.[8] It is typical for them to require more bolus insulin than basal throughout the day, high insulin-to-carbohydrate ratios and corrective doses at breakfast (Answer C), and high basal rates in the later evening hours (8 PM-12 PM).

Case 2

A 5-year-old and her family are managing her T1DM with frequent blood glucose monitoring by fingerstick.

Which of the following is true regarding CGM use for this child?

A. After this child starts CGM, she will be more likely to experience diabetic ketoacidosis

B. CGM uptake for young children is similar, regardless of the child's race and socioeconomic status

C. On average, preschool children who start CGM experience a 15% increase in time in the target range of 70 to 180 mg/dL (3.9-10.0 mmol/L)

D. There is a 20% likelihood that the family will stop using CGM within 1 year

E. Very young children using CGM spend less time in hypoglycemia

Answer: E) Very young children using CGM spend less time in hypoglycemia

CGM use has been shown to decrease time spent in hypoglycemia for very young children with diabetes (Answer E).[14]

Persistence of use is also very high, with more than 90% of children maintaining use out to 52 weeks in the SENCE study (thus, Answer D is incorrect).

CGM use is also associated with decreased glucose variability; however, it has not been associated with increased time in the target range nor improvements in hemoglobin A_{1c} (thus, Answer C is incorrect).

There are no data suggesting that it results in more diabetic ketoacidosis (thus, Answer A is incorrect).

Some data suggest there is lower uptake of CGM for racial minority groups and that there are issues with durable access to technology for children of lower socioeconomic status (thus, Answer B is incorrect).

Case 3

A 4-year-old girl with T1DM diagnosed at age 2 years is a new patient. The mother is pregnant and asks about the risk of diabetes in this soon-to-be born baby (full sibling).

Which of the following is true about the sibling's risk for T1DM?

A. If there are no other affected first-degree family members, the new baby has a 10% lifetime risk of developing T1DM

B. Risk is greater than it would be if her daughter with T1DM had been diagnosed after the age of 7 years

C. Risk is higher if the new baby has an HLA-DQB1*0602 haplotype

D. Risk will be eliminated if she delays feeding the new baby rice cereal until at least 12 months of age

E. There is no way to monitor the child after birth for the possibility of developing the disease until the child has dysglycemia

Answer: B) Risk is greater than it would be if her daughter with T1DM had been diagnosed after the age of 7 years

In general, in the absence of other family history, a sibling of a child with T1DM has a 4% lifetime risk of developing the disease (thus, Answer A is incorrect).

This risk is higher for family members of children diagnosed prior to the age of 7 to 10 years (Answer B).

Risk is lower for those with protective HLA haplotypes such as HLA-DQB1*0602 (thus, Answer C is incorrect).[15]

Although diet may affect risk, there are currently no firm recommendations that will substantively impact future risk (thus, Answer D is incorrect).

It is possible for siblings to be monitored for early signs of development of T1DM by having antibody screening, which can be done starting at the age of 12 months through the Type 1 Diabetes TrialNet research program (https://www.diabetestrialnet.org/) (thus, Answer E is incorrect). General population screening for T1DM is also becoming increasingly available (https://www.jdrf.org/t1d-resources/t1detect/), in part because a therapy (teplizumab) for treating persons with stage 2 diabetes (multiple antibody-positive with dysglycemia but not overt diabetes) is now FDA-approved.

Key Learning Points

- Recent advances in diabetes care including new technological tools (CGM, automated insulin delivery systems) have great potential to enable caregivers and health care providers to provide increasingly effective, tailored therapy, and support for the youngest children with T1DM.

- Both epidemiologic and interventional research must continue to determine how to best serve and care for these children, so that the evidence-based best practices can expand.

References

1. de Bock M, Codner E, Craig ME, et al. ISPAD clinical practice consensus guidelines 2022: glycemic targets and glucose monitoring for children, adolescents, and young people with diabetes. *Pediatr Diabetes.* 2022;23(8):1270-1276. PMID: 36537523

2. ElSayed NA, Aleppo G, Aroda VR, et al. 14. Children and adolescents: standards of care in diabetes-2023. *Diabetes Care.* 2023;46(Suppl 1):S230-S253. PMID: 36507640

3. Foster NC, Beck RW, Miller KM, et al. State of type 1 diabetes management and outcomes from the T1D Exchange in 2016-2018. *Diabetes Technol Ther.* 2019;21(2):66-72. PMID: 30657336

4. Mauras N, Mazaika P, Buckingham B, et al; Diabetes Research in Children Network (DirecNet). Longitudinal assessment of neuroanatomical and cognitive differences in young children with type 1 diabetes: association with hyperglycemia. *Diabetes.* 2015;64(5):1770-1779. PMID: 25488901

5. Willi SM, Miller KM, DiMeglio LA, et al. Racial-ethnic disparities in management and outcomes among children with type 1 diabetes. *Pediatrics.* 2015;135(3):424-434. PMID: 25687140

6. Maahs DM, Hermann JM, DuBose SN, et al; T1D Exchange Clinic Network. Contrasting the clinical care and outcomes of 2,622 children with type 1 diabetes less than 6 years of age in the United States T1D Exchange and German/Austrian DPV registries. *Diabetologia.* 2014;57(8):1578-1585. PMID: 24893863

7. ElSayed NA, Aleppo G, Aroda VR, et al. 6. Glycemic targets: standards of care in diabetes-2023. *Diabetes Care.* 2023;46(Suppl 1):S97-S110. PMID: 36507646

8. Sundberg F, deBeaufort C, Krogvold L, et al. ISPAD clinical practice consensus guidelines 2022: managing diabetes in preschoolers. *Pediatr Diabetes.* 2022;23(8):1496-1511. PMID: 36537520

9. Battelino T, Danne T, Bergenstal RM, et al. Clinical targets for continuous glucose monitoring data interpretation: recommendations from the International Consensus on Time in Range. *Diabetes Care*. 2019;42(8):1593-1603. PMID: 31177185

10. DiMeglio LA, Boyd SR, Pottorff TM, Cleveland JL, Fineberg N, Eugster EA. Preschoolers are not miniature adolescents: a comparison of insulin pump doses in two groups of children with type 1 diabetes mellitus. *J Pediatr Endocrinol Metab*. 2004;17(6):865-870. PMID: 15270404

11. Bell KJ, Smart CE, Steil GM, Brand-Miller JC, King B, Wolpert HA. Impact of fat, protein, and glycemic index on postprandial glucose control in type 1 diabetes: implications for intensive diabetes management in the continuous glucose monitoring era. *Diabetes Care*. 2015;38(6):1008-1015. PMID: 25998293

12. DuBose SN, Hermann JM, Tamborlane WV, et al. Obesity in youth with type 1 diabetes in Germany, Austria, and the United States. *J Pediatr*. 2015;167(3):627-32 e1-e4. PMID: 26164381

13. Cooper MN, McNamara KA, de Klerk NH, Davis EA, Jones TW. School performance in children with type 1 diabetes: a contemporary population-based study. *Pediatr Diabetes*. 2016;17(2):101-111. PMID: 25423904

14. Strategies to Enhance New CGM Use in Early Childhood Study Group. A randomized clinical trial assessing continuous glucose monitoring (CGM) use with standardized education with or without a family behavioral intervention compared with fingerstick blood glucose monitoring in very young children with type 1 diabetes. *Diabetes Care*. 2021;44(2):464-472. PMID: 33334807

15. Insel RA, Dunne JL, Atkinson MA, et al. Staging presymptomatic type 1 diabetes: a scientific statement of JDRF, the Endocrine Society, and the American Diabetes Association. *Diabetes Care*. 2015;38(10):1964-1974. PMID: 26404926

Disorders of Sex Development: Current Concepts and Challenges

David Zangen, MD. Division of Pediatric Endocrinology, Hadassah Medical Center, faculty of Medicine, Hebrew University of Jerusalem, Israel; Email: zangend@hadassah.org.il

Educational Objectives

After reviewing this chapter, learners should be able to:

- Explain the developmental transcriptional cascade in embryonal and pubertal sex development.

- Establish the proper classification of disorders of sex development (DSD).

- Delineate a clinical approach to diagnosis and management of severe cases of DSD.

- Delineate an investigational clinical and molecular genetic approach to unsolved cases of DSD.

Significance of the Clinical Problem

Sex determination of the embryo is established by multiple molecular events that direct the development of germ cells, their migration to the urogenital ridge, and the formation of either a testis or an ovary.[1,2] Aberrations of this process can cause severe clinical outcomes, including major structural genital anomalies, gonadal dysgenesis, problematic gender assignment, and infertility.[3] Development of the mature phenotype of either gender requires normal sex chromosomes ("chromosomal sex"), a normal gonad (testis or ovary; "gonadal sex"), and normal gonadal function (mainly hormone synthesis) and target tissues response ("phenotypic sex"). Pathology of the hormonal pathways leading from gonadal to phenotypic sex has been extensively studied in a variety of DSDs (eg, androgen insensitivity or defects in steroidogenesis). However, the pathogenesis of abnormal gonadal development in chromosomally normal individuals is less understood.

Through analysis of illustrative clinical cases, we will analyze the molecular and clinical diagnostic and management approach and difficulties that characterize these rare but significant and medically challenging conditions.

Practice Gaps

- Ovarian development is not a default when testicular developmental factors are absent.

- The terms *ambiguous genitalia*, *sex reversal*, and *hermaphroditism* are outdated and misleading. XX DSD and XY DSD are the preferred and current nomenclature.

- Early (neonatal or early infantile) genetic diagnosis is essential for major decisions on gender assignment and treatment in DSD.

- Novel genetic etiologies in DSD may have major clinical implications on concomitant extragonadal manifestations, including severe infections or malignant diseases.

Discussion

A major step in elucidating the signaling cascade in testicular development occurred in the early 1990s with the finding of the *SRY* gene as the gonadal determining factor towards a testis. XY individuals lacking *SRY* develop phenotypically as females, and XX individuals carrying the *SRY* gene on the tip of their X chromosome are born phenotypically as males with male gonads (a testis) in their scrotum. This finding enabled intensive studies that have successfully elucidated several downstream transcription factors that are necessary and which determine testicular development such as SOX-9 and SF-1. As such, in the last decade of the 20th and the first decade of the 21st century, ovarian development was considered to occur as a default pathway when *SRY* is lacking.

The clinical entity of females with ovarian dysgenesis and normal karyotype (46,XX) (MIM #233300),[2] namely with XX DSD, is a rare, genetically heterogeneous disorder that is characterized by underdeveloped, dysfunctional ovaries (streak ovaries), with subsequent lack of spontaneous pubertal development, primary amenorrhea, uterine hypoplasia, and hypergonadotropic hypogonadism (clinically similar to the XO DSD—Turner syndrome but without its classic extragonadal manifestations). In the last 15 years, XX DSDs with ovarian dysgenesis have been shown to be caused by autosomal recessive pathogenic variants in the genes encoding the FSH receptor, WNT4,[4] r-spondin,[5] PSMC3IP,[6] MCM9,[7] MCM8,[8] STAG3,[9] SYCE1,[10] and NUP107.[15] These and other studies indicate that ovarian development

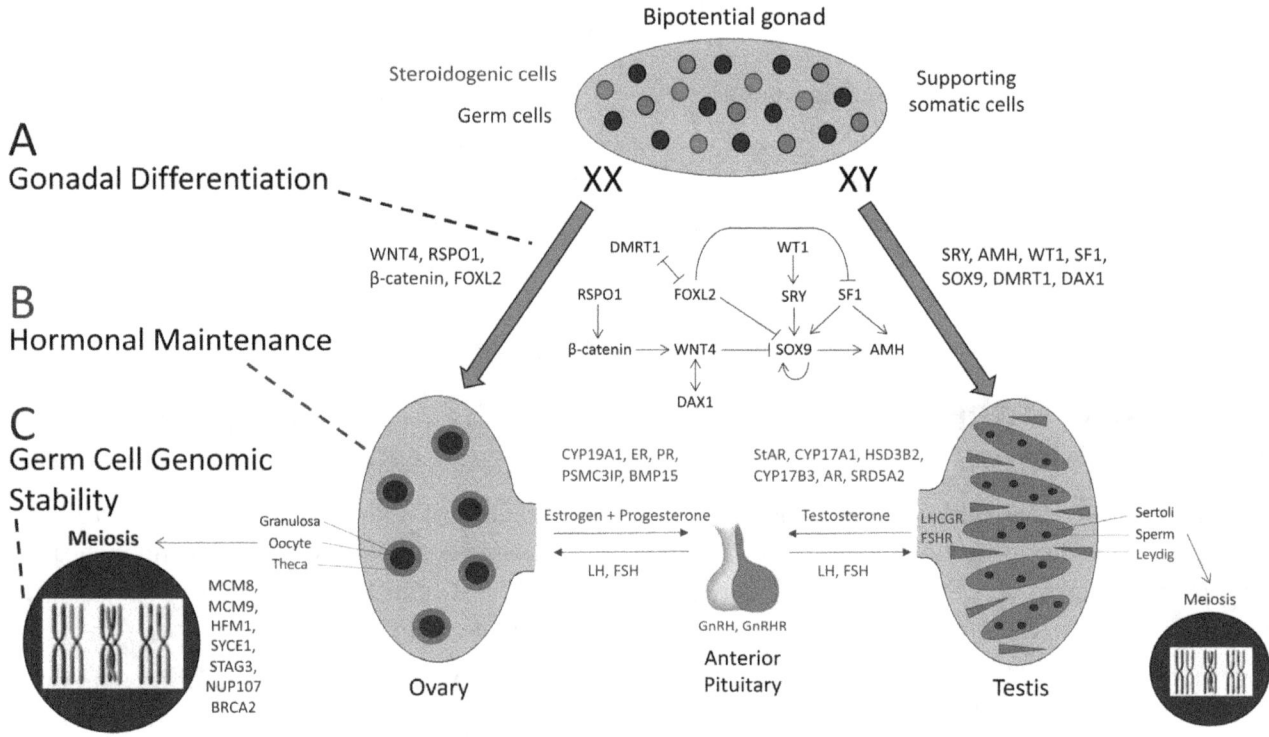

Schematic illustration of gonadal development and the genes involved in its 3-subgroup process. Bipotential gonad is composed of cells that will develop into supporting somatic cells (blue), steroidogenic cells (green), or germ cells (red). **A.** In blue: primary gonadal differentiation and development, from the bipotential gonad, into either ovaries or testis. The genes involved in these processes are primarily transcription factor genes. In an XY gonad, these genes are SRY, AMH, WT1, SF1, SOX9, DMRT1, and DAX1. In an XX gonad, these genes are WNT4, RSPO1, β-catenin, and FOXL2. The male and female transcription factor genes interact and regulate each other, thus determining gonadal development. **B.** In green: subsequent hormonal signaling from both the anterior pituitary/hypothalamus (LH, FSH, and GnRH and their receptors) and from the gonad itself—testosterone in the testis (eg, STAR, CYP17A1, and HSD3B2 genes) and estrogen in the ovary (eg, CYP19A1, ER, PR, PSMC3IP, and BMP15 genes) are crucial for gonadal development and maintenance. **C.** In red: germ-cell meiosis. Genes involved in homologous recombination and DNA damage repair are involved in both oocyte and sperm meiosis, but they are essential for survival in the female ovary, thus characterizing a new subgroup of genes important for ovarian development. (Color—web and EPUB only)

is an active process that involves both signaling pathways, opposing testis signaling pathways, and cross-talk between somatic and germ cells (*see figure*). Thus, ovarian development is not a passive process unfolding in the absence of *SRY*, the testis-determining gene on the Y chromosome. Nevertheless, delineation of the downstream signaling cascades orchestrating ovarian development remains rudimentary, and the identification of new genes underlying XX ovarian dysgenesis has remained challenging because of the genetic heterogeneity in XX gonadal dysgenesis, as well as the small number of families with multiple affected individuals. Thus, there is a compelling need to identify additional players involved in sex determination, which will provide new tools to dissect the molecular regulation of ovarian development.[16,17]

An important change has been recently made in the classification of the conditions associated with maldevelopment of the gonads and genital phenotype of males and females. The terms *ambiguous genitalia*, *hermaphroditism*, *pseudohermaphroditism*, *sex reversal*, and *gonadal dysgenesis* have been renamed to XY DSD and XX DSD (with its milder and much more common phenotype being premature ovarian insufficiency).

Clinical Case Vignettes

Case 1

A 9-month-old otherwise healthy baby girl born to consanguineous Palestinian parents from the Gaza Strip comes for consultation regarding gender assignment. Physical examination findings are unremarkable. The baby has normal-appearing female external genitalia, but a gonad is palpated in both labia.

Which of the following is a true or clinically relevant statement at this stage?

A. LH, FSH, and testosterone measurements will be informative and help in making the diagnosis

B. The place of birth is relevant for the handling and clinical treatment of such a case

C. Removal of the testis in early childhood is indicated given the increased risk for malignancy

D. Urine biochemical analysis is not a practical diagnostic tool in this case

E. A quick genetic diagnosis will not influence the treatment, as the external phenotype is female and the patient is already growing up as a female

Laboratory testing revealed low LH, FSH, and testosterone; a relatively low 17-hydroxyprogesterone value; and a 46,XY karyotype. On ultrasonography, the observed gonads were consistent with testes, and no uterus or ovaries were identified.

As previously noted, one would try to make the diagnosis through the 3 major sexual developmental stages as follows: (1) karyotype analysis indicates a "normal" XY **chromosomal sex**; (2) labial palpation of gonads and ultrasonography indicate "normal" male **gonadal sex** (with further evidence of an absent uterus, indicating functionality of anti-mullerian hormone secreted by the Sertoli cells). The phenotypic sex is female, making the general diagnosis of **XY-DSD**.

When the pathophysiology of XY DSD is in the stage of phenotypic sex, the clinical investigation should assess for a defect in steroidogenesis (mainly androgen synthesis) or androgen insensitivity. The well-being and growth of this 9-month-old baby indicate that there is no severe deficiency of either glucocorticoids or mineralocorticoids, so there is probably no major StAR, side-chain cleavage enzyme, or 3β-hydroxysteroid dehydrogenase pathogenic variant. Normal blood pressure, serum electrolyte values, and ACTH concentration, which are indicated in the assessment, confirmed that the pathology is only in androgen synthesis or beyond.

The fact that the gonads were within the labia and not in the inguinal canals hints towards the presence of testosterone and a responsive androgen receptor in utero. The descent of the testis to the scrotum is known to be influenced initially by the insulinlike 3

(INSL3) protein, but the final descent is probably dependent on testosterone action. There are 2 ways to biochemically distinguish between 17β-hydroxysteroid dehydrogenase (17HSDB3) deficiency and 5α-reductase deficiency. The first is the long hCG test in which the testosterone-to-androstenedione ratio is low in patients with 17HSDB3 deficiency. The second is the urine metabolome assay (after 6 months of age) in which a low ratio between α- and β-reduced steroid metabolites establishes the diagnosis of 5α-reductase dysfunction. Both tests have normal results in the setting of androgen insensitivity (or possibly a slightly high testosterone value in the hCG test).

Currently, the gold standard of proper diagnosis that will importantly influence prognosis and early gender assignment is whole-exome next-generation sequencing conducted in the neonatal period or early infancy. In this case, genetic testing and the urine metabolome assay indicated that this patient has 5α-reductase deficiency with a Y91H homozygous pathogenic variant in the *SRD5A2* gene.

The clinical neonatal presentation with a completely female genital phenotype at birth in 5α-reductase deficiency dysfunction is relatively rare. Only 7% of individuals with 5α-reductase deficiency have completely female external genitalia. Most have either clitoromegaly or hypospadias and micropenis at birth.[11] A similar neonatal phenotype is found in individuals with *17HSDB3* pathogenic variants.[12] In contrast to the clinical course of androgen insensitivity, the clinical course at puberty in both 5α-reductase deficiency and 17HSDB3 dysfunction involves virilization, and more than 60% of affected individuals choose to change their original female gender to male.[13]

Gender identity formulates during the first few years of life and is considered to be fully achieved by 5 years of age. Gender orientation is a different element of the identity, and it classically formulates much later, during puberty.

The possibility of identifying an exact genetic diagnosis and therefore predicting the clinical course of the disease in each patient s has led to a major change in the attitude towards gender assignment in individuals with 5α-reductase deficiency or 17HSDBS deficiency. Knowing that 100% of affected persons will go through virilization, and more than 60% of such patients will go through the devastating change in gender identity during puberty may allow for a more comprehensive decision regarding the gender assignment in the neonatal/infantile period by the parents and the multidisciplinary team. Furthermore, one should assume that the reported unwillingness to change gender identity in the remaining 30% of cases may be due to the complexity of such a decision when gender identity has been completely formed at 5 years of age. Assigning a male gender before 1 year of age may mitigate this complexity.

Another consideration regarding virilization during puberty in persons with XY DSD who have no internal female organs is the major effect of the values, the culture, and the social impact of the chosen gender assignment on the patient and his/her family. In the currently described case, according to the patient's parents and local community leaders, raising the patient with a female gender identity would have caused her to have a miserable life, being de-facto imprisoned in her household as a girl with no personal independence and with significant damage to the whole family social status within the community. The patient's parents decided, against most of the multidisciplinary team recommendations (especially the urologists), to try for an optimal anatomical solution for rearing the patient as a male despite completely female external genitalia. The use of topical/local dihydrotestosterone cream for a short period of 2 months resulted in growth of a penis- or clitoris-like structure. The demonstrates that even in such severe cases (practically aphalia), such therapy may enable the first and then second reconstructive operations when the urethra is placed within the penile structure.

Case 2

A 13.3-year-old girl from a consanguineous family presents to the emergency department with abdominal pain. Physical examination reveals abdominal wall sensitivity with no rigidity or peritoneal signs. Pubertal development is Tanner stage 1 for breasts and stage 2 for pubic hair. She has normal-appearing female external genitalia. She had pneumococcal sepsis at 9 months of age and periorbital cellulitis and bacteremia at 20 months of age. In the last 6 months, she was evaluated for short stature.

On abdominal ultrasonography, fecal impaction is identified in the colon, and the spleen is not visible.

Which of the following is a true or clinically relevant statement at this stage?

A. In this 13.3-year-old patient, an intensive workup (LH-releasing hormone test, etc) for evaluation of delayed puberty is not indicated

B. The finding of asplenia is irrelevant to her general clinical presentation

C. Her expected karyotype will be 46,XY

D. Finding gonads in the inguinal canal in such a patient indicates a high probability of normal transcriptional signaling towards gonadal development

E. Assuming there is pathologic pubertal development, a monogenetic etiology may not explain the full clinical phenotype

Blood smear revealed target cells and Howell-Joley bodies indicative of clinical asplenia. Confirmatory CT revealed asplenia but also 2 gonads consistent with testes in the inguinal canals. Reaching the inguinal canal probably indicates normal action of INSL3, but testosterone levels were most likely low or undetected.

Given a normal predicted chromosomal sex (karyotype pending...) and gonadal sex (testes appearance), steroidogenesis was evaluated. As expected, mineralocorticoids and glucocorticoids were normal. Androgens and estradiol were undetectable. LH and FSH values were high. Karyotype returned as 46,XY. *SRY* gene was

identified on PCR testing. The diagnosis was XY DSD with gonadal failure.

At this point, medicine and molecular science meet. The clinical observation of asplenia in a patient with XY DSD is so rare that a unifying genetic etiology was considered. The parental consanguinity prompted the search for homozygous pathogenic variants causing the rare phenotype. An intensive PubMed search did not find an association between the 2 findings (asplenia and severe XY DSD). However, a search in articles describing the detailed phenotype of mice with knockout of genes known in 2012 to cause XY DSD found that *SF1* knockout mice had a severe reduction in their spleen size. In such a case, whole-exome sequencing was not necessary; only the *SF1* gene was sequenced in the patient and family members. A homozygous *SF1/NR5A1* pathogenic variant was identified. The variant (1) segregated well in the family, (2) was conserved through evolution, (3) was expected to cause dysfunction by genetic prediction tools and programs, (4) was located in an important gene domain, and (5) was not prevalent (less then 1%) in a matched cohort from the same ethnic background. These findings make it highly probable that the homozygous variant is indeed responsible for the rare phenotype observed.

SF-1 is a nuclear receptor that is involved in early stages of both testicular and ovarian development but also is a transcription factor for steroidogenic genes such as 17,20-lyase and also for genes such as *AMH* and *INSL3*. Pathogenic variants in *SF1* cause a variety of XY DSD, from minimal hypospadias to severe sex reversal DSD and, in rare homozygous cases, also adrenal insufficiency. A search was performed to learn about the genes that are required for spleen development. TLX-1/Hox-11 that has been shown to control the genesis of the spleen was found to have 3 SF-1 binding elements in its gene promoter. The Arg103Gly pathogenic variant in the asplenic patient had indeed a 70% reduction of SF-1 binding to the TLX-1 promoter, thereby causing lower TLX-1 protein expression and asplenia.[14]

The Arg103Gly pathogenic variant also causes decreased binding and transactivation of the 17,20-lyase promoter, resulting in the decreased androgen synthesis and the resulting XY DSD.

Elucidating the role of SF-1 in both gonadal differentiation and spleen development led to the identification of 10 other families in the region, one of which had lost a 2.5-year-old daughter due to pneumonia, which is now explained by asplenia that was not recognized clinically in a timely manner.

This association based on a single case has therefore a significant and possibly life-saving clinical implications in persons with *SF1* pathogenic variants causing DSD where pneumococcal vaccination and preventive therapy are indicated. Alternatively, when younger patients are identified with asplenia, there should be awareness of the possible coexistence of a DSD.

Case 3

Two sisters of Ethiopian Jewish ancestry born to nonconsanguineous parents presented sequentially with primary amenorrhea at 14.5 years of age. The older sister had acute myelogenous leukemia at age 5 years, which resolved completely following relatively mild medical treatment with no alkylating agents.

Physical examination revealed normal cognition, absence of spontaneous pubertal development (Tanner stage 1), mild microcephaly, several café-au-lait macules, and vitiligo.

Results of general laboratory tests were normal, but LH and FSH concentrations were high, indicating hypergonadotropic hypogonadism. The ovaries were not detected on ultrasonography. Both sisters had a 46,XX karyotype (thus, making the diagnosis of XX DSD).

A faulty DNA repair gene was suspected as the cause of the microcephaly, café-au-lait spots, but also of the ovarian dysgenesis and the primary amenorrhea. Chromosomal breakage was assessed using an assay that relied on the alkylating agent mitomycin C. Both sisters demonstrated a significantly higher rate of both spontaneous and mitomycin-induced number of breaks. The high number of candidate genes involved in DNA repair justified whole-exome sequencing to identify the genetic cause of the ovarian dysgenesis. Both affected sisters were compound heterozygotes for 2 *BRCA2* pathogenic variants that cause a decrease in *BRCA2* transcription and subsequently the protein. *BRCA2* is a major DNA repair gene, and the small amount of the protein in these patients is not able to recruit the RAD 51 protein to DNA breakage sites.

Fetal ovarian development depends on an appropriate chromosomal sex having 2 copies of the X chromosome. Gonadal sex as an ovary depends on the relatively newly characterized WNT, r-spondin, β-catenin, and ovarian developmental transcriptional cascade. Proper hormone secretion and action (maintenance factors (eg, LH, FSH, LHR, FSHR, aromatase, etc) give rise to normal phenotypic sex. These stages in ovarian development resemble the testicular developmental cascade, but in the case of the ovary, there is another major group of genes that are crucial for meiosis and normal fetal oocyte formation in utero. DNA repair genes are required for proper homologous recombination that is an integral part of meiosis in the developing fetal ovary. When repair is not done, homologous recombination and meiosis fail and oocytes do not survive. With no oocytes, there is no ovary. This phenomenon was exemplified in the drosophila *BRCA2* knockout model.[18] Drosophila lacking the dmBRCA2 had severely underdeveloped ovaries, no eggs, and no progeny, mimicking in a way the human *BRCA2* dysfunction model.[19]

Interestingly, the mother who carried 1 of the pathogenic variants was diagnosed with ovarian cancer due to a surveillance performed based on the *BRCA2* pathogenic variants identified in her daughters.

Each year, more DNA repair genes and other genes that are required for proper meiosis are identified as genetic etiologies of ovarian dysgenesis and XX DSD. *MCM8*, *MCM9*, *PSMC3IP*, *STAG3*, and *SYCE1* are just a few examples. In patients with primary amenorrhea who have an XX karyotype, clinician should look for clinical findings such as microcephaly, café-au-lait spots, or vitiligo, which might suggest dysfunction in DNA repair genes. Furthermore, chromosomal breakage assays should probably be advocated, and if positive, routine cancer surveillance should be recommended for these patients and their at-risk family members.

Key Learning Points

- The new nomenclature of XY DSD and XX DSD reflects the concepts of no default in development but rather a set of master positive transcriptional regulators for each type of gonad, which suppresses the positive set of the alternative gonad (namely, SRY, SOX9, and SF-1 for the testis and WNT-4, r-spondin 1, and β-catenin for the ovary).

- The availability of relatively simple and cheap whole-exome sequencing enables not only early diagnosis but also more comprehensive and optimal decisions regarding gender assignment in the neonatal and infantile age prior to formation of gender identity.

- Studying the molecular basis for the associations of DSD and clinical features that are supposedly unrelated (eg, recurrent bacterial infections or signs of dysfunctional DNA repair) in single patients may be clinically significant in the diagnosis and treatment of patients with DSD and their family members.

References

1. MacLaughlin DT, Donahoe PK. Sex determination and differentiation. *N Engl J Med.* 2004;350(4):367-378. PMID: 14736929

2. Park SY, Jameson JL. Minireview: transcriptional regulation of gonadal development and differentiation. *Endocrinology.* 2005;146(3):1035-1042. PMID: 15604204

3. Sultan C, Paris F, Jeandel C, Lumbroso S, Galifer RB, Picaud J-C. Ambiguous genitalia in the newborn: diagnosis, etiology and sex assignment. *Endocr Dev.* 2004;7:23-38. PMID: 15052995

4. Biason-Lauber A, Konrad D, Navratil F, Schoenle EJ. A WNT4 mutation associated with Mullerian-duct regression and virilization in a 46,XX woman. *N Engl J Med.* 2004;351(8):792-798. PMID: 15317892

5. Kamata T, Katsube K, Michikawa M, Yamada M, Takada S, Mizusawa H. R-spondin, a novel gene with thrombospondin type 1 domain, was expressed in the dorsal neural tube and affected in Wnts mutants. *Biochim Biophys Acta.* 2004;1676(1):51-62. PMID: 14732490

6. Zangen D, Kaufman Y, Zeligson S, et al. XX ovarian dysgenesis is caused by a PSMC3IP/HOP2 mutation that abolishes coactivation of estrogen-driven transcription. *Am J Hum Genet.* 2011;89(4):572–579. PMID: 21963259

7. Wood-Trageser MA, Gurbuz F, Yatsenko SA, et al. MCM9 mutations are associated with ovarian failure, short stature, and chromosomal instability. *Am J Hum Genet.* 2014;95(6):754-762. PMID: 25480036

8. Tenenbaum-Rakover Y, Weinberg-Shukron A, Renbaum P, et al. Minichromosome maintenance complex component 8 (MCM8) gene mutations result in primary gonadal failure. *J Med Genet.* 2015;52(6):391-399. PMID: 25873734

9. Le Quesne Stabej P, Williams HJ, James C, et al; GOSgene. STAG3 truncating variant as the cause of primary ovarian insufficiency. *Eur J Hum Genet.* 2016;24(1):135-138. PMID: 26059840

10. de Vries L, Behar DM, Smirin-Yosef P, Lagovsky I, Tzur S, Basel-Vanagaite L. Exome sequencing reveals SYCE1 mutation associated with autosomal recessive primary ovarian insufficiency. *J Clin Endocrinol Metab.* 2014;99(10):E2129-E2132. PMID: 25062452

11. Maimoun L, Philibert P, Cammas B, et al. Phenotypical, biological, and molecular heterogeneity of 5α-reductase deficiency: an extensive international experience of 55 patients. *J Clin Endocrinol Metab.* 96(2):296-307. PMID: 21147889

12. Levy-Khademi F, Zeligson S, Lavi E, et al. The novel founder homozygous V225M mutation in the HSD17B3 gene causes aberrant splicing and XY-DSD. *Endocrine.* 2020;69(3):650-654. PMID: 32372306

13. Batista RL, Inácio M, Arnhold IJP, et al. Psychosexual aspects, effects of prenatal androgen exposure, and gender change in 46,XY disorders of sex development. *J Clin Endocrinol Metab.* 2019;104(4):1160-1170. PMID: 30388241

14. Zangen D, Kaufman Y, Banne E, et al. Testicular differentiation factor SF-1 is required for human spleen development. *J Clin Invest.* 2014;124(5):2071-2075. PMID: 24905461

15. Weinberg-Shukron A, Renbaum P, Kalifa R, et al. A mutation in the nucleoporin-107 gene causes XX gonadal dysgenesis. *J Clin Invest.* 2015;125(11):4295-4304. PMID: 26485283

16. Online Mendelian Inheritance in Man, OMIM. McKusick-Nathans Institute of Genetic Medicine, Johns Hopkins University (Baltimore, MD), 2008. Available at: http://wwwncbinlmnihgov/omim/

17. Cederroth CR, Pitetti JL, Papaioannou MD, Nef S. Genetic programs that regulate testicular and ovarian development. *Mol Cell Endocrinol.* 2008;265-266:3-9. PMID: 17208359

18. Ashburner M, Bergman CM. Drosophila melanogaster: a case study of a model genomic sequence and its consequences. *Genome Res.* 2005;15(12):1661-1667. PMID: 16339363

19. Weinberg-Shukron A, Rachmiel M, Renbaum P, et al. Essential role of BRCA2 in ovarian development. *N Engl J Med.* 2018;379(11):1042-1049. PMID: 30207912

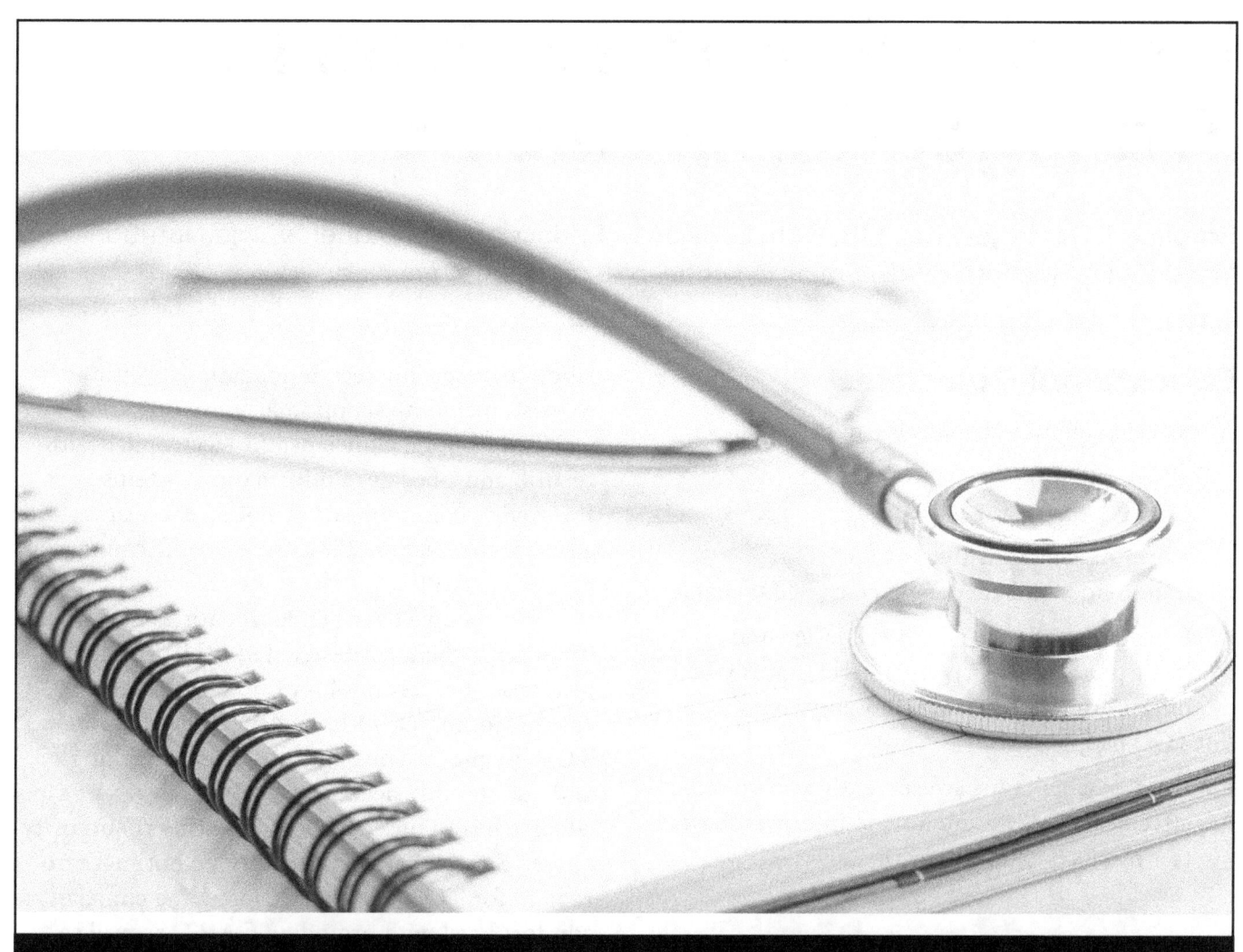

REPRODUCTIVE ENDOCRINOLOGY

Use of Laboratory Tests in Transgender Medicine

Caroline J. Davidge-Pitts, MB, BCh. Division of Endocrinology, Diabetes, and Nutrition, Mayo Clinic, Rochester, MN; Email: Davidge-pitts.caroline@mayo.edu

Educational Objectives

After reviewing this chapter, learners should be able to:

- Describe the basic principles of gender-affirming hormone therapy (GAHT) in transgender and gender-diverse (TGD) people.

- Explain the importance of sex designated at birth, gender identity, and GAHT status when interpreting sex-specific laboratory tests in TGD people.

- Identify which tests are currently known to be affected by GAHT and how to interpret these test results in clinical practice.

Significance of the Clinical Problem

GAHT can be life-saving treatment for many TGD people. GAHT typically includes estradiol and an antiandrogen in transgender women and testosterone in transgender men.[1] Nonbinary people may or may not use GAHT, or they may require lower dosages. GAHT leads to changes in physiological processes that can influence sex-specific laboratory testing. Although there is a lack of data from large populations, an increasing number of studies have been published to address the importance of correct interpretation of laboratory testing in TGD people.[2-6] Unfortunately, many barriers to developing laboratory-specific recommendations continue to exist, including suboptimal communication strategies among clinicians, the electronic health record, and laboratory information systems.[7] Improving communication among these areas will advance the quality of inclusive and affirming care to TGD patients.

TGD people have gender identities that differ from their sex designated at birth. The *table* describes terminology often used in this space.[8] Compared with the general population, TGD people face multiple obstacles in seeking and maintaining health care, with high rates of adverse health outcomes in the setting of minority stress.[9] Several barriers to receiving optimal care remain for TGD individuals, including clinician comfort level with providing GAHT, as well as with correct interpretation of standard laboratory test results in response to GAHT and surgical care. Using the correct reference interval is not only affirming to the patient but also important to prevent overdiagnosis or underdiagnosis of medical conditions. Establishing the natural history of changes in laboratory results in the TGD population on GAHT can help clinicians understand what laboratory tests do change, when to anticipate these changes, and how to interpret these changes when making clinical decisions. Unfortunately, there continue to be significant gaps in optimal interpretation of laboratory test results in the TGD community. Additionally, in the era of the electronic medical record, further barriers to affirming care can exist due to system design issues in laboratory information systems.

Table. Selected Terminology in the Care of TGD Individuals

Term	Definition
Terms representing independent aspects of one's identity (ie, not the same things)	
Gender identity	The innate and internal sense of gender that is not visible to other people
Sex designated at birth	Also hear "sex assigned at birth," "assigned female at birth," "assigned male at birth"
Gender expression	The external manifestations of a person's gender; may or may not conform to the socially defined behaviors and external characteristics that are historically referred to as masculine or feminine (eg, clothing, haircut, jewelry, social interactions, speech patterns)
Sexual orientation	Term that characterizes pattern of romantic or sexual attraction to other people, independent of gender identity
Terms used when discussing gender identity	
Gender incongruence	When a person's gender identity or gender expression differs from that person's sex recorded at birth or what is typically associated with the designated sex recorded at birth; not everyone with gender incongruence has gender dysphoria or seeks treatment
Gender dysphoria	The distress and unease associated with gender incongruence; the phrase "gender identity disorder" is no longer used, particularly after the 2013 American Psychiatric Association's DSM-5 replaced it with "gender dysphoria"
Transgender	An adjective that encompasses people whose gender identity or gender expression differs from their sex recorded at birth; independent of the decision whether to use GAHT or undergo gender-affirming surgery, and inclusive of gender nonbinary people; the terms "transgendered" and "transgenders" should not be used Examples: A person who was assigned female at birth but whose gender identity or gender expression is (more) male/masculine may identify as a transgender man, transgender male, transmasculine, or something else A person who was assigned male at birth but whose gender identity or gender expression is (more) female/feminine may identify as a transgender woman, a transgender female, transfeminine, or something else
Gender nonbinary	May represent people who identify and present themselves as both or alternatively male and female, as neither male nor female, or with a gender identity outside the male/female binary; may include genderqueer, gender-fluid, pan-gender, polygender
Cisgender	An adjective for people whose gender identity and gender expression align with their sex recorded at birth (ie, not transgender)

Reprinted from Iwamoto SJ et al. *Ther Adv Endocrinol Metab*, 2019; 10: January-December. © 2019 The Authors.

Practice Gaps

- Lack of transgender-specific reference intervals for sex-specific laboratory tests based on large population data.

- Uncertain timing of sex-specific laboratory test changes in response to GAHT.

- Low clinician comfort level in interpreting laboratory test results in TGD individuals, often due to lack of training or experience.

- Lack of knowledge of hormone-sensitive screening test results that should prompt a clinical action (eg, PSA for prostate cancer screening).

- Laboratory testing intervals in nonbinary individuals on low-dosage GAHT.

- Barriers to adequate communication among laboratory systems and the electronic medical record.

Discussion

GAHT raises the sex steroid that is congruent with the person's gender identity and decreases the endogenous sex steroid through negative feedback on the hypothalamic-pituitary-gonadal axis. The goal of GAHT is to induce physical changes that align with a person's gender identity, thereby alleviating the distress associated with gender dysphoria/gender incongruence.[1] Studies show that gender-affirming medical and surgical interventions help to alleviate gender dysphoria and lead to improved well-being.[10,11] Not all TGD people pursue medical therapy. For those who do, GAHT[1] for transgender women typically involves estradiol in combination with an antiandrogen (such as spironolactone) to decrease testosterone production and block its action at the androgen receptor. In transgender men, testosterone therapy exerts masculinizing effects through the androgen receptor, while causing a decrease in endogenous estrogen production. People who identify as nonbinary can proceed with medical therapy that depends on their embodiment goals. This might include full-dosage GAHT, low-dosage GAHT, or no GAHT at all.

An ideal laboratory result is one that has an established reference interval specific to the TGD patient population. There are multiple barriers to establishing reliable reference intervals, including lack of large population data. Currently, sex-specific analytes are assigned to "male" and/or "female" reference intervals, with the onus on the health care clinician to appropriately interpret the result depending on the clinical situation.

Laboratory tests results in TGD people might be influenced by many factors. GAHT can have a direct effect on certain organs such as the kidney or bone marrow, leading to changes in physiological processes. Laboratory tests might also be influenced by the route of administration of the prescribed hormone (oral, sublingual, intramuscular, subcutaneous) with resultant differences in pharmacokinetic action. In the past, appropriate interpretation of test results in TGD was guided by retrospective or observational studies; however more recently, prospective studies[2-6] have provided much needed data on multiple analyte reference intervals in the TGD population.

Measurement of Kidney Function

Serum creatinine levels and estimated glomerular filtration rate (eGFR) are important tools in diagnosing and monitoring kidney disease. Furthermore, accurate assessment of kidney function can be important in several clinical situations, for example, correct dosing of medications and correct identification of kidney transplant candidates. In our recent study,[12] we found that creatinine values in transgender men on testosterone increased as early as 3 months after starting GAHT with a new baseline stabilizing by 6 months. The average increase in creatinine at 6 months was 0.21 mg/dL (18.5 µmol/L) ($P = .02$). In transgender women, creatinine values were found to be significantly decreased by –0.03 mg/dL (2.6 µmol/L) at 3 months ($P = .04$) and –0.1 mg/dL (8.8 µmol/L) at 6 months ($P < .01$). Current eGFR equations make it challenging to interpret and care for the kidney health of TGD people. It has therefore been suggested that use of cystatin C–based equations or more direct GFR determinations might be more appropriate in TGD people. Cystatin C, however, has not yet been studied in the transgender population.

Hematology

GAHT leads to changes in hemoglobin/hematocrit and red blood cell count in TGD people due to an effect on erythropoiesis. Testosterone therapy leads to higher hemoglobin/hematocrit levels than those in cisgender women, whereas transgender women on estradiol have lower hemoglobin/hematocrit levels than cisgender men.[5] Therefore, the reference interval for the affirmed gender should be used in interpretations of complete blood cell counts in TGD people on stable hormone therapy.

Metabolic Tests

GAHT leads to changes in weight and metabolic risk factors in TGD people. Per Endocrine Society guidelines,[1] weight, blood pressure, and lipids should be measured at regular intervals while a patient is on GAHT. In transgender men who have been on GAHT for 1 year, LDL cholesterol increases from baseline and HDL cholesterol decreases.[13] In transgender women, variable data exist describing no change or an increase in HDL-cholesterol levels.[13,14] A meta-analysis reported that estradiol therapy was associated with an increase in triglycerides without significant change in total cholesterol or other lipoprotein fractions.[13] The impact of lipid changes on overall health and long-term risk in the TGD population is unknown, especially in the absence of reliable risk calculators. Nevertheless, awareness of potential changes in lipids following GAHT could aid appropriate interpretation and subsequent clinical decision-making.

Liver Function Tests

Liver function analytes, including alkaline phosphatase, alanine transaminase, aspartate transferase, and gamma-glutamyl transferase, increase in transgender men on testosterone therapy compared with levels cisgender women.[4] The degree of elevation might increase the concentration above the upper normal limit in the female range but remain normal in the male range. In transgender women, a minimal effect or a slight decrease in liver enzymes can be expected. A change in liver mass might be a potential explanation for changes in liver function tests, but this has not been studied in the TGD population.

Cardiology

A cross-sectional prospective study of healthy transgender individuals prescribed testosterone or estradiol for 12 months or more revealed that differences in concentration of high-sensitivity cardiac troponin and N-terminal pro–brain natriuretic peptide between transgender men and transgender women were similar to differences observed between cisgender men and cisgender women.[3] Therefore, sex hormone status may be a stronger driver of the differences between men and women for biomarkers of cardiac disease. Consequently, for TGD people on stable hormone therapy, the affirmed gender can be used for deciding which reference intervals to use.

Prolactin

Prolactin is a hormone that is responsive to estrogen, and increased exposure to exogenous estrogen could potentially lead to a rise in prolactin levels. This is important to consider in transgender women on GAHT[2] who might have an upward trend of their prolactin above the male range but still within the female range. Use of the male range in this situation may lead to an inaccurate diagnosis of hyperprolactinemia and subsequent unnecessary testing. In transgender men on testosterone, it is recommended to use the prolactin reference interval for cisgender women.[6]

Additional Considerations and Unknowns

Additional considerations include how to correctly interpret laboratory tests in nonbinary people on low-dosage hormone therapy. Nonbinary people might not have hormone levels within the binary female or male range, which can pose a challenge for determining the most appropriate reference interval to use with sex-specific laboratory tests. Like many areas of medical decision-making in transgender health, reporting of both male and female reference intervals might be helpful in such situations. However, laboratories might be challenged in correctly identifying when to report both intervals using only information provided in the electronic medical record.

Another area of concern and consideration is submission of tests that in the past have mostly been associated with a specific sex, such as pregnancy and Papanicolaou tests. If these tests are ordered and/or performed in someone who has a male identification marker in the electronic medical record, they could be mistakenly cancelled or discarded. This again highlights the importance of adequate communication between the electronic medical record and laboratory systems. In addition, use of the organ inventory, a tool in the electronic medical record that documents the presence or absence of a person's organs, could be helpful in reducing the reliance on sex and gender markers in the medical record alone.

Clinical Case Vignettes

Case 1

A 25-year-old transgender woman comes to clinic after recent evaluation in the emergency department for abdominal pain. She is a longstanding patient and has been on GAHT with estradiol and spironolactone for the last 5 years without interruption. Her sex steroid levels have consistently been at goal within the female range for at least 2 years. Blood tests were performed in the emergency department, and she was found to have hemoglobin and hematocrit values slightly below the laboratory's lower limit of normal. It was recommended in the emergency department that she follow-up with her primary care provider for evaluation.

Which of the following is the best recommendation?

A. Find out whether the male or female reference range for hemoglobin and hematocrit was used in the emergency department's laboratory

B. Reassure her that this is an expected finding with hormone therapy and no follow-up is needed

C. Reduce her estradiol dosage to allow the testosterone to increase and thus stimulate erythropoiesis

D. Refer her to hematology to investigate the cause of low hemoglobin and hematocrit

E. Repeat an urgent complete blood cell count and perform a peripheral smear after today's visit

Answer: A) Find out whether the male or female reference range for hemoglobin and hematocrit was used in the emergency department's laboratory

Although this patient has been on GAHT for 5 years, she might not have officially changed her legal sex. Many laboratory systems use legal sex when deciding which laboratory reference intervals to report. In this vignette, it is important to ask which laboratory interval was used in the interpretation of her hemoglobin and hematocrit (Answer A). If the male interval is used, it is not uncommon to see the hemoglobin and hematocrit values fall below the lower reference interval limit due to reduction in erythropoiesis. However, if her value was below the female reference range, then further evaluation is warranted. Based on this information, reassuring her that this is an expected finding with hormone therapy and no follow-up is needed (Answer B) is incorrect.

Additional testing and referrals would not be needed until establishment of the correct reference range, so referring to hematology to investigate the cause of low hemoglobin and hematocrit (Answer D) or repeating an urgent complete blood cell count and performing a peripheral smear after today's visit (Answer E) is incorrect.

Reducing her estradiol dosage to allow the testosterone to increase and thus erythropoiesis to ensue (Answer C) is incorrect because her sex steroids concentrations are at goal.

Case 2

A 40-year-old transgender man is referred from his primary care physician for elevated creatinine. He initiated GAHT 2 years ago for gender dysphoria/incongruence. He is otherwise generally healthy, although he does report an increase in weight and blood pressure since starting GAHT. He does not take any medications other than the testosterone prescribed. He is a nonsmoker.

On physical examination, his blood pressure is 140/85 mm Hg, pulse rate is 75 beats/min, and BMI is 32 kg/m². Examination findings are otherwise unremarkable.

On review of his laboratory tests, it is apparent that he has had an increase in creatinine over the last year compared with his prehormone baseline value 2 years ago. He has no dysuria or hematuria.

Baseline creatinine = 0.8 mg/dL (SI: 70.7 μmol/L)
1 year = 1.0 mg/dL (SI: 88.4 μmol/L)
2 years = 1.5 mg/dL (SI: 132.6 μmol/L)

Which of the following is the best next step in management?

A. Ask him to reduce his dietary protein

B. No referrals needed, plan to improve his blood pressure and recheck creatinine in 6 months through primary care

C. Reassure him that the elevation in creatinine is related to testosterone therapy and the creatinine level should plateau soon

D. Refer for kidney biopsy

E. Refer him to nephrology for evaluation of unexpected elevation in creatinine

Answer: E) Refer him to nephrology for evaluation of unexpected elevation in creatinine

GAHT with testosterone increases muscle mass and decreases fat mass. GAHT may also have a direct impact on kidney function through effects on nephrosclerosis and tubular atrophy and by acting on cortical and medullary volumes. Our study at Mayo Clinic[12] revealed that creatinine values in transgender men on testosterone had already increased 3 months after starting GAHT with a new baseline stabilizing by 6 months. The average increase in creatinine at 6 months was 0.21 mg/dL (18.5 μmol/L) (*P* = .02). Based on this information, his creatinine has increased more than would be expected with testosterone alone and therefore requires evaluation (thus, Answer E is correct and Answer C is incorrect).

Although lifestyle changes and blood pressure improvement (Answers A and B) could potentially prevent worsening of kidney function in certain diseases, the diagnosis is still unknown.

Kidney biopsy (Answer D) would not be indicated until evaluation by nephrology.

Case 3

A 60-year-old transgender woman presents to clinic for yearly follow-up. She initiated GAHT 12 years ago and completed vaginoplasty 5 years ago. She is doing generally well and has no concerns today. On review of systems, she has started to notice more nocturia over the last year. Her only medications are an estradiol patch, 0.1 mg/24 h, and rosuvastatin for dyslipidemia.

Her vital signs and physical examination findings are normal.

Laboratory testing shows estradiol and testosterone concentrations within the female range. She recently had a visit with her primary care provider who was uncertain whether PSA should be measured.

Which of the following is the best recommendation?

A. Measure PSA, using the standard reference range to guide care

B. Measure PSA, using a different reference range to guide care

C. Measure PSA, but counsel her that we do not have a specific reference range to guide care in transgender women on GAHT

D. Recommend not measuring PSA because of her advanced age

E. Recommend not measuring PSA because she completed vaginoplasty and therefore no longer has a prostate

Answer: C) Measure PSA, but counsel her that we do not have a specific reference range to guide care in transgender women on GAHT

During vaginoplasty, the prostate is not removed, and therefore recommendations for prostate cancer screening follow cisgender guidelines (thus, Answer E is incorrect).[1] Based on her age, she will qualify for prostate cancer screening if she wishes (thus, Answer D is incorrect).

In the setting of long-term GAHT and gonadectomy, this patient has testosterone concentrations in the female range. Considering that the prostate is androgen-sensitive, one would anticipate that PSA levels would drop with GAHT. The PSA value that should prompt an investigation for prostate cancer in this setting is unknown (thus, Answers A and B are incorrect). Some experts consider a concentration greater than 1.0 ng/mL (>1.0 µg/L) to be an indication for referral,[15] but clear-cut data are lacking. Thus, the best option is to measure PSA, but counsel her that we do not have a specific reference range to guide care in transgender women on GAHT (Answer C). Prostate cancer incidence is believed to be lower in transgender women than in cisgender men.[16]

Key Learning Points

- Multiple barriers to optimal care exist for TGD people; optimal care includes reliable and clinically meaningful interpretation of laboratory test results.

- Many laboratory tests have sex-specific reference intervals. It is important to apply the most appropriate reference interval when interpreting test results in TGD individuals on stable hormone therapy.

- Incorrect interpretation of sex-specific laboratory tests in this population might lead to overdiagnosis or underdiagnosis of medical conditions.

- More data are needed to better define specific reference intervals in TGD people.

- Better communication strategies are needed among clinicians, the electronic medical record, and laboratory information systems to optimize reporting and interpretation of laboratory tests.

References

1. Hembree WC, Cohen-Kettenis PT, Gooren L, et al. Endocrine treatment of gender-dysphoric/gender-incongruent persons: an Endocrine Society clinical practice guideline. *J Clin Endocrinol Metab.* 2017;102(11):3869-3903. PMID: 28945902

2. Greene DN, Schmidt RL, Winston McPherson G, et al. Reproductive endocrinology reference intervals for transgender women on stable hormone therapy. *J Appl Lab Med.* 2021;6(1):15-26. PMID: 32674116.

3. Greene DN, Schmidt RL, Christenson RH, et al. Distribution of high-sensitivity cardiac troponin and N-terminal pro-brain natriuretic peptide in healthy transgender people. *JAMA Cardiol.* 2022;7(11):1170-1174. PMID: 36197689

4. Humble RM, Greene DN, Schmidt RL, et al. Reference intervals for clinical chemistry analytes for transgender men and women on stable hormone therapy. *J Appl Lab Med.* 2022;7(5):1131-1144. PMID: 35584132

5. Greene DN, McPherson GW, Rongitsch J, et al. Hematology reference intervals for transgender adults on stable hormone therapy. *Clin Chim Acta.* 2019;492:84-90. PMID: 30771301

6. Greene DN, Schmidt RL, Winston-McPherson G, et al. Reproductive endocrinology reference intervals for transgender men on stable hormone therapy. *J Appl Lab Med.* 2021;6(1):41-50. PMID: 33241847

7. Goldstein Z, Corneil TA, Greene DN. When gender identity doesn't equal sex recorded at birth: the role of the laboratory in providing effective healthcare to the transgender community. *Clin Chem.* 2017;63(8):1342-1352. PMID: 28679645

8. Iwamoto SJ, Defreyne J, Rothman MS, et al. Health considerations for transgender women and remaining unknowns: a narrative review. *Ther Adv Endocrinol Metab.* 2019;10:2042018819871166.

9. Valentine SE, Shipherd JC. A systematic review of social stress and mental health among transgender and gender non-conforming people in the United States. *Clin Psychol Rev.* 2018;66:24-38. PMID: 29627104

10. Nguyen HB, Chavez AM, Lipner E, et al. Gender-affirming hormone use in transgender individuals: impact on behavioral health and cognition. *Curr Psychiatry Rep.* 2018;20(12):110. PMID: 30306351

11. Wernick JA, Busa S, Matouk K, Nicholson J, Janssen A. A systematic review of the psychological benefits of gender-affirming surgery. *Urol Clin North Am.* 2019;46(4):475-486. PMID: 31582022

12. Maheshwari A, Dines V, Saul D, Nippoldt T, Kattah A, Davidge-Pitts C. The effect of gender-affirming hormone therapy on serum creatinine in transgender individuals. *Endocr Pract.* 2022;28(1):52-57. PMID: 3447418

13. Maraka S, Singh Ospina N, Rodriguez-Gutierrez R, et al. Sex steroids and cardiovascular outcomes in transgender individuals: a systematic review and meta-analysis. *J Clin Endocrinol Metab.* 2017;102(11):3914-3923. PMID: 28945852

14. Streed CG Jr, Beach LB, Caceres BA, et al; American Heart Association Council on Peripheral Vascular Disease; Council on Arteriosclerosis, Thrombosis and Vascular Biology; Council on Cardiovascular and Stroke Nursing; Council on Cardiovascular Radiology and Intervention; Council on Hypertension; and Stroke Council. Assessing and addressing cardiovascular health in people who are transgender and gender diverse: a scientific statement from the American Heart Association. *Circulation.* 2021;144(6):e136-e148. PMID: 34235936

15. UCSF Transgender Care, Department of Family and Community Medicine, University of California San Francisco. Guidelines for the primary and gender-affirming care of transgender and gender nonbinary people. 2nd ed. Deutsch MB, ed. June 2016. Available at transcare.ucsf.edu/guidelines. Accessed January 2023.

16. de Nie I, de Blok CJM, van der Sluis TM, et al. Prostate cancer incidence under androgen deprivation: nationwide cohort study in trans women receiving hormone treatment. *J Clin Endocrinol Metab.* 2020;105(9):e3293-e3299. PMID: 32594155

Managing the Nonreproductive Comorbidities of Polycystic Ovary Syndrome

Andrea Dunaif, MD. Hilda and J. Lester Gabrilove Division of Endocrinology, Diabetes, and Bone Disease, Icahn School of Medicine and Mount Sinai Health System, New York, NY; Email: andrea.dunaif@mssm.edu

Educational Objectives

After reviewing this chapter, learners should be able to:

- Describe the nonreproductive comorbidities of polycystic ovary syndrome (PCOS).

- Critically assess the diagnostic criteria for PCOS.

- Review management of nonreproductive comorbidities of PCOS.

Significance of the Clinical Problem

Women who fulfill the National Institutes of Health (NIH) diagnostic criteria for PCOS of hyperandrogenism and ovulatory dysfunction, which is usually manifested by chronic oligomenorrhea, are at the greatest risk for nonreproductive comorbidities.[1] Obesity substantially exacerbates this risk.[1] There is no need to assess ovarian morphology for the diagnosis of PCOS in women with hyperandrogenism and ovulatory dysfunction,[2] a recommendation endorsed by the International Evidence-Based Guideline for the Assessment and Management of Polycystic Ovary Syndrome.[3] The magnitude of the risk for nonreproductive comorbidities is controversial in women with ovulatory menstrual cycles and hyperandrogenism, who would be classified as having non-NIH

Rotterdam PCOS, if they have polycystic ovarian morphology (PCOM). However, the assessment of ovarian morphology is not needed to manage hyperandrogenic symptoms such as hirsutism in ovulatory women with hyperandrogenism.[4] Further, there is no evidence that the presence or absence of PCOM affects metabolic risk in ovulatory women with hyperandrogenism. There is also no difference in metabolic risk in women with NIH PCOS based on the presence or absence of PCOM.

Most studies of therapy for nonreproductive comorbidities of PCOS are constrained by small sample size, short duration, and lack of randomized clinical trial design. Further, reproductive features rather than nonreproductive comorbidities are frequently the primary study endpoints; therefore, studies are often not adequately powered to assess nonreproductive outcomes. Consequently, therapeutic decisions for nonreproductive comorbidities are frequently extrapolated from conditions other than PCOS. There are minimal data on the optimal therapies for these comorbidities in the setting of PCOS. Lifestyle modification, metformin, and GLP-1 receptor agonists are effective for the management of nonreproductive comorbidities in PCOS. Despite concerns about their potential adverse effects on insulin sensitivity, in practice, hormonal contraceptives do not appear to decompensate glucose tolerance, although this question has not been directly investigated in appropriately designed trials.

PCOS is a heterogeneous disorder that affects up to 20% of premenopausal women worldwide, depending on the diagnostic criteria applied. It is the leading cause of hirsutism, oligomenorrhea, and anovulatory infertility.[4,5] PCOS is now recognized as a major metabolic disorder due to its frequent association with insulin resistance.[1] Affected women have a ~4-fold increased risk for type 2 diabetes mellitus (T2DM), as well as increased risk for other disorders that are associated with insulin resistance, such as metabolic syndrome and nonalcoholic fatty liver disease (NAFLD).[1] Further, T2DM in women with PCOS has a significantly younger age of onset than it does in reproductively normal women. Thus, women with PCOS and T2DM often have a more prolonged exposure to the deleterious effects of dysglycemia. There is an increased prevalence of obesity in PCOS that exacerbates both the metabolic and reproductive morbidities of the syndrome.[1] PCOS is also associated with anxiety, depression, and reduced quality of life.[6]

There have been no large longitudinal studies of women with PCOS that have followed women through the seventh and eighth decades of life when cardiovascular events become prevalent in women.[7] Therefore, it remains unknown whether PCOS actually increases the risk for such events. However, there is mounting evidence from prospective cohort studies using irregular menses as a proxy for PCOS that this finding is associated with increased risk for cardiovascular disease,[7,8] cancer (including nongynecologic malignancies),[9] and premature mortality.[10] These observations strongly suggest that PCOS—at least NIH PCOS (hyperandrogenism + ovulatory dysfunction)—has substantial adverse long-term health outcomes. Adolescent and adult women with PCOS have major reproductive, metabolic, and psychiatric morbidities.[1,6] The US health care–related economic burden of PCOS was $8 billion in 2020 alone. Despite PCOS's high prevalence and major morbidities, affected women remain remarkably underserved. Diagnosis is frequently delayed and physicians are often poorly informed about PCOS.[11]

Practice Gaps

- Paucity of high-quality evidence to support practice guidelines.

- Lack of knowledge among endocrinologists and primary care providers of the appropriate diagnostic evaluation for PCOS and its nonreproductive comorbidities.

- Lack of high-quality randomized clinical trials of optimal therapies for the management of nonreproductive comorbidities when they occur in women with PCOS.

Discussion

Diagnostic Criteria

Given the lack of information on the cause(s) of PCOS, its diagnosis has been based on the phenotypic features of the syndrome, as with the diagnosis of many medical disorders. There are 3 internationally recognized sets of PCOS diagnostic criteria: NIH, Rotterdam, and Androgen Excess Society. Despite their designation as consensus criteria, all are based on expert opinion rather than on a formal consensus process.[2,12] The original NIH diagnostic criteria require the presence of hyperandrogenism and ovulatory dysfunction. The Rotterdam criteria added PCOM and require the presence of at least 2 of the 3 key reproductive traits resulting in 3 phenotypes: hyperandrogenism and ovulatory dysfunction ± PCOM (also known as NIH PCOS), as well as 2 additional non-NIH Rotterdam phenotypes: hyperandrogenism and PCOM, and ovulatory dysfunction and PCOM. The Androgen Excess Society criteria require the presence of hyperandrogenism, reducing the number of phenotypes to 2: hyperandrogenism and ovulatory dysfunction ± PCOM, and hyperandrogenism and PCOM. All of the criteria require the exclusion of other disorders that present similarly to PCOS, for example, nonclassic adrenal 21-hydroxylase deficiency, hyperprolactinemia, abnormal thyroid function, Cushing syndrome, and androgen-secreting neoplasms. Fortunately, serious conditions such as Cushing syndrome and androgen-secreting neoplasms are quite rare in women presenting with features of PCOS.[2,13]

The prevalence of PCOS differs according to the diagnostic criteria applied. The prevalence of the NIH PCOS phenotype of hyperandrogenism and ovulatory dysfunction ± PCOM is 5% to 8% in premenopausal women. The Rotterdam criteria added 2 additional non-NIH phenotypes: (1) hyperandrogenism and PCOM and (2) ovulatory dysfunction and PCOM, resulting in prevalence rates of 8% to 20%. These prevalence estimates are remarkably consistent across racial and ethnic groups. Metabolic risk is greatest in NIH PCOS compared with risk in non-NIH Rotterdam PCOS phenotypes.[1] The diagnostic criteria for PCOS in adolescents have been modified to reflect the fact that menstrual cycles are typically anovulatory in the early postmenarchal transition and that polycystic ovaries are a common finding in adolescents. According to these guidelines,[14] the diagnosis of PCOS cannot be made until 2 years after menarche, and PCOM cannot be used as a diagnostic criterion until 8 years after menarche. Thus, the NIH criteria are used for the diagnosis of PCOS in adolescents. Women with PCOS see, on average, 4 physicians prior to diagnosis.[11] The difficulty in physician diagnosis of PCOS implies that diagnostic criteria are poorly disseminated, difficult to use, and/or poorly understood. Surveys suggest that endocrinologists use the NIH diagnostic criteria more frequently than the Rotterdam diagnostic criteria.

There are evidence-based guidelines for the diagnosis and management of PCOS, such as those published in 2013 by the Endocrine Society[5] and the 2018 International Evidence-Based Guideline.[3] However, the quality of the evidence upon which these guidelines are based is predominantly low due to a paucity of randomized clinical trials. Of the 34 recommendations in the Endocrine Society Clinical Practice Guideline,[5] the evidence supporting 24 of these was rated as low or very low. There were almost 175 recommendations in the International Guideline,[3] of which only 31 were ranked as evidence-based, the rest were

clinical consensus recommendations or clinical practice points. There is agreement that the presence or absence of PCOM does not have any implications regarding the nonreproductive comorbidities of PCOS.[5] Further, there is no evidence to support the addition of assessment of PCOM to the diagnosis of NIH PCOS.[3] Indeed, the International Evidence-Based Guidelines[3] state that ovarian ultrasonography is not needed for the diagnosis of PCOS in women with hyperandrogenism and ovulatory dysfunction (ie, NIH PCOS). Similarly, the recently updated Endocrine Society Guideline on Hirsutism[4] states that demonstrating PCOM to diagnose ovulatory PCOS is unlikely to affect management of hirsutism.

Nonreproductive Comorbidities of PCOS

The main nonreproductive comorbidities of PCOS are obesity, impaired glucose tolerance or prediabetes, T2DM, and metabolic syndrome characterized by increased triglycerides and waist circumference with low HDL cholesterol. Affected women also have an increased risk for sleep disordered breathing, NAFLD, and elevated blood pressure. The insulin resistance that is a common feature of the syndrome[1] has an important role in the pathogenesis of these comorbidities. It is the result of a distinctive postbinding defect in insulin-receptor signaling. Pancreatic β-cell dysfunction contributes to dysglycemia. These abnormalities of insulin secretion and action are independent of but greatly exacerbated by obesity. Elevated androgens contribute to nonreproductive comorbidities by direct actions on adipose tissue distribution and function, hepatic steatosis, lipid metabolism, and, possibly, glucose homeostasis. Androgens may also have a role in sleep disordered breathing.

Numerous studies demonstrate that the NIH criteria define the phenotype with the most severe insulin resistance and associated metabolic risk.[1] Many studies have indicated that ovulatory women with hyperandrogenism have normal insulin sensitivity, whereas others have suggested that they have mild insulin resistance.[1] There have been no studies that have specifically assessed whether there is increased risk for T2DM or other nonreproductive comorbidities in ovulatory women with hyperandrogenism. However, there is an association between elevated androgens and cardiometabolic risk in epidemiologic studies of premenopausal and postmenopausal women, as well as in women who are otherwise reproductively normal.

Genomic Insights into PCOS

PCOS and its associated traits are a highly heritable, suggesting a genetic contribution to their pathogenesis. More than 20 genetic susceptibility loci have been reproducibly mapped for PCOS in genome-wide association studies in European and in Han Chinese case-control cohorts, many of which are shared among these ethnic groups.[12] Biologic pathways implicated include gonadotropin secretion and action, androgen biosynthesis, and metabolic homeostasis. However, a recent meta-analysis found that the genetic architecture was generally similar when NIH PCOS, non-NIH Rotterdam PCOS, and PCOS by self-report cohorts were compared. In other words, the current PCOS diagnostic criteria do not identify genetically distinct subsets of affected women. In contrast, using unsupervised hierarchical clustering of PCOS quantitative phenotypic traits, we have identified discrete and reproducible subtypes.[15] We designated these subtypes as "reproductive," characterized by higher LH and SHBG levels with relatively low BMI and insulin levels, and "metabolic," characterized by increased glucose, and insulin levels with lower SHBG and LH levels. In genome-wide association studies, these subtypes were associated with novel genome-wide significant loci suggesting that they had distinct genetic architectures. These findings suggest that clustering algorithms capture biologically relevant subtypes of PCOS and provide a data-driven approach to PCOS diagnosis.

The major susceptibility loci for PCOS differ from those for T2DM and obesity, although genetically determined BMI and glycemic traits are causally related to PCOS and these disorders share genetic architecture.[12] Nevertheless, it appears that T2DM and obesity in PCOS differs genetically from T2DM and obesity in the general population. Analogous to our recent findings of PCOS subtypes, clustering has identified subtypes of T2DM and obesity. Further, there appear to be subtype-specific optimal therapies for T2DM and obesity. Taken together, these findings suggest that the optimal therapies for PCOS-related T2DM and obesity may differ from those therapies in the absence of PCOS. There have been no randomized clinical trials that have investigated which therapies are superior for nonreproductive comorbidities in women with PCOS compared with unaffected women.

Clinical Case Vignettes
Case 1

A 25-year-old woman presents for the evaluation of oligomenorrhea and inability to lose weight. She experienced menarche at age 14 years and subsequently had 2 to 3 menstrual bleeds annually. She has a few terminal hairs on her chin that she removes with waxing every 2 weeks. She began to gain weight around the time of menarche and her weight increased by 50 lb (22.7 kg) during her first year of college. She attends 3 aerobics classes per week and follows a "Mediterranean" diet. Nevertheless, she reports that she is unable to lose weight. She was evaluated by her gynecologist for these problems several years ago who performed ovarian ultrasonography and started her on metformin, which she did not tolerate. Her family history is noteworthy for T2DM in her father.

On physical examination, her blood pressure is 130/85 mm Hg and pulse rate is 82 beats/min. Her BMI is 37.8 kg/m², and she has a normal habitus. There is no increased terminal hair growth. She has moderate acanthosis nigricans with skin tags on her neck and in her axillae. Her examination findings are otherwise normal.

Laboratory test results:

> Urine pregnancy test, negative
> Testosterone = 56 ng/dL (<58 ng/dL)
> (SI: 1.93 nmol/L [<2.01 nmol/L])
> SHBG = 40.1 nmol/L (24.6-122.0 nmol/L)
> Bioavailable testosterone = 21 ng/dL (<16 ng/dL)
> (SI: 0.73 nmol/L [<0.56 nmol/L])
> DHEA-S = 350 µg/dL (<263 µg/dL) (SI: 9.49 µmol/L
> [<7.13 µmol/L])
> 17-Hydroxyprogesterone (8 AM) = 175 ng/dL
> (<200 ng/dL) (SI: 5.30 nmol/L [<6.06 nmol/L])
> Prolactin = 20 ng/mL (<25 ng/mL) (SI: 0.87 nmol/L
> [<1.09 nmol/L])
> TSH = 2.0 mIU/L (0.4-4.5 mIU/L)
> FSH = 3.0 mIU/L (<40 mIU/L)
> Hemoglobin A_{1c} = 5.4% (<5.6%) (35.5 mmol/mol
> [<37.3 mmol/mol])

Which of the following additional tests/measurements would best determine her diagnosis?

A. Androstenedione measurement

B. Ovarian ultrasonography

C. LH measurement

D. 11-Ketotestosterone measurement

E. None

Answer: E) None

The diagnosis of PCOS can be made by NIH, Rotterdam, and Androgen Excess Society criteria by the presence of hyperandrogenism—clinical (ie, hirsutism) and biochemical (elevated total and bioavailable testosterone and DHEA-S levels)—as well as chronic anovulation indicated by oligomenorrhea. This patient has elevated circulating bioavailable testosterone and DHEA-S levels. She does not have clinical signs of androgen excess. However, patients frequently remove terminal hairs, so asking the patient to indicate the distribution and density of terminal hair growth using an image of a Ferriman-Gallwey chart can be helpful. Other disorders have been excluded with normal TSH, prolactin, and 17-hydroxyprogesterone levels.

There is no need to do additional androgen testing (eg, androstenedione [Answer A]).

Ovarian ultrasonography (Answer B) is not needed for the diagnosis.

In the United States, these studies are often not interpreted according to Rotterdam criteria for PCOM. Although increased LH relative to FSH levels is a common feature of PCOS, LH levels (Answer C) are not part of any diagnostic criteria for PCOS. FSH levels can be measured to assess whether there is evidence for premature ovarian insufficiency, which is in the differential diagnosis for oligomenorrhea.

11-Oxyandrogens are a recently appreciated major pool of androgens derived primarily from the adrenals that are elevated in PCOS, as well as in other disorders of androgen excess. 11-Ketotestosterone (Answer D) is a bioactive 11-oxyandrogen with a potency similar to that of testosterone. However, it is not a validated androgen measurement for the diagnosis of PCOS.

Case 1 (continued)

Additional laboratory testing is performed:

> Fasting glucose = 85 mg/dL (<100 mg/dL)
> (SI: 4.72 mmol/L [<5.55 mmol/L])
> Glucose (2-h post 75-g oral glucose challenge) =
> 180 mg/dL (<140 mg/dL) (SI: 9.99 mmol/L
> [<7.77 mmol/L])
> Total cholesterol = 210 mg/dL (<200 mg/dL)
> (SI: 5.44 mmol/L [<5.18 mmol/L])
> LDL cholesterol = 110 mg/dL (<100 mg/dL)
> (SI: 2.85 mmol/L [<2.59 mmol/L])
> HDL cholesterol = 40 mg/dL (≥50 mg/dL)
> (SI: 1.04 mmol/L [≥1.30 mmol/L])
> Triglycerides = 180 mg/dL (<150 mg/dL)
> (SI: 2.03 mmol/L [<1.70 mmol/L])

Which of the following pharmacologic therapies should be recommended?

A. Combined oral contraceptive pill

B. Metformin

C. Liraglutide or semaglutide

D. Spironolactone

E. Pioglitazone

Answer: C) Liraglutide or semaglutide

As little as a 5% reduction of body weight can result in improvements in testosterone levels and resumption of ovulatory menses in women with PCOS. Small studies indicate the GLP-1 receptor agonists (liraglutide and semaglutide [Answer C]) are effective for weight loss in the setting of PCOS. Antiobesity medications should always be combined with lifestyle modification. The patient has impaired glucose tolerance and fulfills criteria for metabolic syndrome. There are no studies of diabetes prevention in women with PCOS. However, the Diabetes Prevention Program (DPP), which studied individuals with prediabetes, demonstrated that a 5% to 10% reduction of body weight with an intensive lifestyle intervention produced the greatest decrease in risk of progression to T2DM (58%). It also significantly reduced the prevalence of metabolic syndrome in individuals with prediabetes. Metformin (Answer B) reduced the incidence of T2DM (31%) and metabolic syndrome in the DPP. Meta-analyses indicate that metformin improves menstrual frequency and slightly decreases fasting glucose, LDL-cholesterol levels, and systolic blood pressure in women with PCOS. Metformin may result in weight loss of approximately 4.4 lb (2 kg). However, the patient did not tolerate metformin in the past. GLP-1 receptor agonists are much more effective than metformin for weight loss.

The patient has relative contraindications to combined oral contraceptive pills (Answer A), as she has obesity, impaired glucose tolerance, and elevated triglyceride levels.

She does not have clinically significant hirsutism, so there is no indication for the antiandrogen spironolactone (Answer D).

Pioglitazone (Answer E) is a possibility, but there are concerns about using thiazolidinediones in reproductive-aged women because of weight gain, potential effects on bone density, and safety during pregnancy.

The patient will need intermittent progestin-induced withdrawal bleeding for endometrial protection. However, it is likely that she will resume ovulatory menses with as little as ~5% weight loss. Progestin-only contraceptives would also provide endometrial protection.

Case 2

A 33-year-old woman presents for evaluation of hirsutism and acne. She has had irregular menses since menarche at age 14 years with cycle lengths of 3 to 6 months. She had severe acne as an adolescent and had a course of oral isotretinoin at that time. She began to note increasing terminal hair growth on her chin and sideburn area during college. She has also had recurrent acne lesions. Her dermatologist prescribed spironolactone, 50 mg once daily orally. She has never had hormonal testing, but her gynecologist ordered ovarian ultrasonography. She is of Italian ancestry. A maternal cousin has hirsutism and was recently diagnosed with PCOS. Her father has dyslipidemia and pancreatitis. He has no history of coronary artery disease.

On physical examination, her blood pressure is 115/70 mm Hg, pulse rate is 84 beats/min, BMI is 26.6 kg/m², and waist circumference is 39.4 in (100 cm). She has a normal habitus.

There is increased terminal hair in the sideburn, chin, and presacral areas, with a Ferriman-Gallwey score of 16. There is no acanthosis nigricans. The rest of the examination findings are normal.

Laboratory test results:

> Testosterone = 72 ng/dL (<58 ng/dL)
>   (SI: 2.50 nmol/L [<2.01 nmol/L])
> SHBG = 71.3 nmol/L (24.6-122.0 nmol/L)
> Bioavailable testosterone = 18 ng/dL (<16 ng/dL)
>   (SI: 0.62 nmol/L [<0.56 nmol/L])
> DHEA-S = 500 µg/dL (<263 µg/dL)
>   (SI: 13.55 µmol/L [<7.13 µmol/L])
> 17-Hydroxyprogesterone (8 AM) = 175 ng/dL
>   (<200 ng/dL) (SI: 5.30 nmol/L [<6.06 nmol/L])
> Prolactin = 20 ng/mL (<25 ng/mL) (SI: 0.87 nmol/L
>   [<1.09 nmol/L])
> TSH = 2.0 mIU/L (0.4-4.5 mIU/L)

What additional testing should be performed to determine her diagnosis?

A. Androstenedione measurement

B. Ovarian ultrasonography

C. LH measurement

D. Adrenal CT

E. None

Answer: E) None

The diagnosis of PCOS can be made by NIH, Rotterdam, and Androgen Excess Society criteria by the presence of hyperandrogenism—clinical (ie, hirsutism) and biochemical (elevated total and bioavailable testosterone and DHEA-S levels) —as well as chronic anovulation indicated by oligomenorrhea. This patient meets the criteria (thus, Answer E is correct).

There is no need for measurement of additional androgens (Answer A) or ovarian ultrasonography (Answer B) to confirm the diagnosis of PCOS. LH levels (Answer C) are frequently increased in women with PCOS, but they are not part of any current diagnostic criteria.

Although the patient's DHEA-S level is elevated, it is not above the threshold (600-700 µg/dL [16.26-18.97 µmol/L]) at which adrenal CT (Answer D) would be indicated to exclude an adrenal neoplasm.

Case 2 (continued)

Additional test results:

Hemoglobin A$_{1c}$ = 5.2% (≤5.6%) (33.3 mmol/mol [≤37.3 mmol/mol])

Total cholesterol = 180 mg/dL (<200 mg/dL) (SI: 4.66 mmol/L [<5.18 mmol/L])

LDL cholesterol = 90 mg/dL (<100 mg/dL) (SI: 2.33 mmol/L [<2.59 mmol/L])

HDL cholesterol = 40 mg/dL (≥50 mg/dL) (SI: 1.04 mmol/L [≥1.30 mmol/L])

Triglycerides = 150 mg/dL (<150 mg/dL) (SI: 1.70 mmol/L [<1.70 mmol/L])

Which of the following therapies should be recommended?

A. Combined oral contraceptive pill and spironolactone, 100 mg twice daily

B. Progestin intrauterine device

C. Metformin

D. Liraglutide or semaglutide

E. Dexamethasone

Answer: A) Combined oral contraceptive pill and spironolactone, 100 mg twice daily

A combined oral contraceptive pill alone or in combination with an antiandrogen (Answer A) would be appropriate first-line therapy for androgenic symptoms. If symptoms are severe, it is reasonable to begin with the combination of a combined oral contraceptive pill and antiandrogen. In the United States, the antiandrogen of choice is spironolactone, although there are no FDA-approved antiandrogens for the treatment of hirsutism, acne, or alopecia in women. It is preferred to ensure adequate contraception during antiandrogen treatment, usually with combined oral contraceptive pills, since antiandrogens cross the placenta and interfere with the virilization of a male fetus. There are also additive beneficial effects of combined oral contraceptive pills and antiandrogens.

Progestin-only contraceptives (Answer B) are an option to provide contraception when using spironolactone in women who have contraindications to combined oral contraceptive pills.

Metformin (Answer C) is less effective than combined oral contraceptive pills for the treatment of hirsutism.

The patient is below the BMI thresholds (≥27 kg/m^2 with 1 BMI-related complication or ≥30 kg/m^2) for GLP-1 receptor agonist therapy (Answer D).

Dexamethasone (Answer E) is not recommended for the treatment of hirsutism because it is less effective than combined oral contraceptive pills and antiandrogens, even in patients with nonclassic 21-hydroxylase deficiency. It also has an unfavorable adverse effect profile.

Case 2 (continued)

The patient returns for follow-up after 6 months. She reports that her acne has improved and that her facial terminal hair has become finer and lighter, and she has to remove it less frequently. However, her primary care physician noted that her triglyceride levels were elevated at the time of her annual physical exam.

Additional test results:

> Total cholesterol = 180 mg/dL (<200 mg/dL)
> (SI: 4.66 mmol/L [<5.18 mmol/L])
> LDL cholesterol, cannot be calculated
> HDL cholesterol = 40 mg/dL (≥50 mg/L)
> (SI: 1.04 mmol/L [≥1.30 mmol/L])
> Triglycerides = 600 mg/dL (<150 mg/dL)
> (SI: 6.78 mmol/L [<1.70 mmol/L])

Should her therapy be modified?

A. No, there is no contraindication to continuing combined oral contraceptive pills and spironolactone

B. Yes, metformin should be added

C. Yes, combined oral contraceptive pills should be discontinued

D. Yes, combined oral contraceptive pills should be discontinued and she should be started on progestin-only contraception

E. Yes, atorvastatin should be added

Answer: D) Yes, combined oral contraceptive pills should be discontinued and she should be started on progestin-only contraception

Estrogen-containing combined oral contraceptive pills can cause increases in circulating triglyceride levels. The patient's value of 600 mg/dL (6.78 mmol/L) is of concern, particularly with a family history of pancreatitis, so it is prudent to switch to progestin-only contraception (Answer D), such as a progestin intrauterine device.

She requires adequate contraception given the potential adverse effects of spironolactone on a male fetus (thus, Answer C is incorrect).

There is no indication for the addition of metformin (Answer B) or atorvastatin (Answer E).

Case 3

A 17-year-old girl had menarche at age 14 years. She was evaluated with abdominal ultrasonography at age 15 years after an episode of right-sided pelvic pain. She was informed that she had polycystic ovaries and was prescribed a combined oral contraceptive pill. She does not recall her menstrual pattern prior to combined oral contraceptive pills or whether any hormonal testing was performed. She has not had menses since her combined oral contraceptive pill was stopped 6 weeks ago because she developed migraines with aura. Her major concern is weight gain.

On physical examination, her blood pressure is 110/70 mm Hg, pulse rate is 82 beats/min, and BMI is 28.3 kg/m² (93rd percentile for age and sex). Body habitus is normal. There is no increased terminal hair growth or acne, and the remaining exam findings are normal.

Laboratory test results:

> Total testosterone = 40 ng/dL (<58 mg/dL)
> (SI: 1.39 nmol/L [<2.01 nmol/L])
> SHBG = 130 nmol/L (24.6-122.0 nmol/L)
> Bioavailable testosterone = 6 ng/dL (<16 ng/dL)
> (SI: 0.21 nmol/L [<0.56 nmol/L])
> DHEA-S = 200 μg/dL (<263 μg/dL) (SI: 5.42 μmol/L
> [<7.13 μmol/L])
> 17-Hydroxyprogesterone (8 AM) = 175 ng/dL
> (<200 ng/dL) (SI: 5.30 nmol/L [<6.06 nmol/L])
> Prolactin = 20 ng/mL (<25 ng/mL) (SI: 0.87 nmol/L
> [<1.09 nmol/L])
> TSH = 2.0 mIU/L (0.4-4.5 mIU/L)

What additional testing should be performed now to determine her diagnosis?

A. None, hormonal testing should be repeated at least 3 months after combined oral contraceptive pills have been stopped

B. Ovarian ultrasonography

C. LH measurement

D. Progesterone measurement

E. Pelvic MRI

Answer: A) None, hormonal testing should be repeated at least 3 months after combined oral contraceptive pills have been stopped

The effects of estrogen-containing combined oral contraceptive pills to increase hepatic production of SHBG can take at least 3 months to reverse. Accordingly, endogenous hormone production cannot be accurately assessed prior to adequate wash-out (Answer A).

It is possible that a progesterone level (Answer D) would indicate recent ovulation before menses occurred. However, it would be appropriate to wait until menses resume to assess ovulation.

In adolescents within 8 years of menarche, ovarian ultrasonography (Answer B) is not part of the diagnostic criteria for PCOS because of the high prevalence of PCOM in girls in this age range.

Pelvic MRI (Answer E) has not been shown to be superior to ovarian ultrasonography for detecting PCOM.

Case 3 (continued)

Additional testing 4 months after combined oral contraceptive pills have been stopped:

Testosterone = 54 ng/dL (<58 ng/dL)
(SI: 1.87 nmol/L [<2.01 nmol/L])
SHBG = 40.0 nmol/L (24.6-122.0 nmol/L)
Bioavailable testosterone = 20 ng/dL (<16 ng/dL)
(SI: 0.69 nmol/L [<0.56 nmol/L])
DHEA-S = 200 µg/dL (<263 µg/dL) (SI: 5.42 µmol/L
[<7.13 µmol/L])
Fasting glucose = 85 mg/dL (<100 mg/dL)
(SI: 4.72 mmol/L [<5.55 mmol/L])
Glucose (2-h post 75-g oral glucose challenge) =
180 mg/dL (<140 mg/dL) (SI: 9.99 mmol/L
[<7.77 mmol/L])
Total cholesterol = 180 mg/dL (<200 mg/dL)
(SI: 4.66 mmol/L [<5.18 mmol/L])
LDL cholesterol = 90 mg/dL (<100 mg/dL)
(SI: 2.33 mmol/L [<2.59 mmol/L])
HDL cholesterol = 40 mg/dL (≥50 mg/dL)
(SI: 1.04 mmol/L [≥1.30 mmol/L])
Triglycerides = 150 mg/dL (<150 mg/dL)
(SI: 1.70 mmol/L [<1.70 mmol/L])

AST = 76 U/L (<40 U/L) (SI: 1.27 µkat/L
[<0.67 µkat/L])
ALT = 88 U/L (<32 U/L) (SI: 1.47 µkat/L
[<0.53 µkat/L])

Her menses have not resumed.

Which of the following therapies would be appropriate?

A. Spironolactone

B. Metformin

C. Liraglutide or semaglutide

D. Dexamethasone

E. Etonogestrel/ethinyl estradiol vaginal ring

Answer: B) Metformin

Metformin (Answer B) is an appropriate therapy because it results in resumption of regular menstrual cycles in approximately 40% of women with PCOS after 6 months of treatment. Metformin is frequently associated with modest weight loss, and it may also reverse her impaired glucose tolerance. The elevated AST and ALT suggest the presence of NAFLD. Metformin treatment is also associated with decreases in hepatic steatosis in women with PCOS.

This patient does not have symptoms of androgen excess, so there is no indication for spironolactone (Answer A).

Liraglutide and semaglutide (Answer C) are FDA-approved for adolescents aged 12 to 17 years with a BMI in the 95th percentile or greater for age and sex; the patient is not at this BMI threshold. There is no indication for treatment with dexamethasone (Answer D), and it may worsen glucose tolerance.

Estrogen-containing contraceptives (Answer E) are contraindicated because the patient has migraines with aura.

Key Learning Points

- Women with NIH PCOS, ovulatory dysfunction, and hyperandrogenism are at greatest risk for nonreproductive comorbidities.

- Ultrasonography assessment of ovarian morphology is not needed for the diagnosis of NIH PCOS.

- Therapies for nonreproductive comorbidities are not well-studied in women with PCOS but appear to have similar efficacy to that seen in the general population with these comorbidities.

References

1. Diamanti-Kandarakis E, Dunaif A. Insulin resistance and the polycystic ovary syndrome revisited: an update on mechanisms and implications. *Endocr Rev.* 2012;33(6):981-1030. PMID: 23065822

2. Chang S, Dunaif A. Diagnosis of polycystic ovary syndrome: which criteria to use and when? *Endocrinol Metab Clin North Am.* 2021;50(1):11-23. PMID: 33518179

3. Teede HJ, Misso ML, Costello MF, et al; International PCOS Network. Recommendations from the international evidence-based guideline for the assessment and management of polycystic ovary syndrome. *Clin Endocrinol (Oxf).* 2018;89(3):251-268. PMID: 30024653

4. Martin KA, Anderson RR, Chang RJ, et al. Evaluation and treatment of hirsutism in premenopausal women: an Endocrine Society clinical practice guideline. *J Clin Endocrinol Metab.* 2018;103(4):1233-1257. PMID: 29522147

5. Legro RS, Arslanian SA, Ehrmann DA, et al, Endocrine Society. Diagnosis and treatment of polycystic ovary syndrome: an Endocrine Society clinical practice guideline. *J Clin Endocrinol Metab.* 2013;98(12):4565-4592. PMID: 24151290

6. Dokras A, Stener-Victorin E, Yildiz BO, et al. Androgen excess- Polycystic Ovary Syndrome Society: position statement on depression, anxiety, quality of life, and eating disorders in polycystic ovary syndrome. *Fertil Steril.* 2018;109(5):888-899. PMID: 29778388

7. Guan C, Zahid S, Minhas AS, Ouyang P, Vaught A, Baker VL, Michos ED. Polycystic ovary syndrome: a "risk-enhancing" factor for cardiovascular disease. *Fertil Steril.* 2022;117(5):924-935. PMID: 35512976

8. Solomon CG, Hu FB, Dunaif A, et al. Menstrual cycle irregularity and risk for future cardiovascular disease. *J Clin Endocrinol Metab.* 2002;87(5):2013-2017. PMID: 11994334

9. Wang S, Wang Y-X, Sandoval-Insausti H,et al. Menstrual cycle characteristics and incident cancer: a prospective cohort study. *Hum Reprod.* 2022;37(2):341-351. PMID: 34893843

10. Wang Y-X, Arvizu M, Rich-Edwards JW, et al. Menstrual cycle regularity and length across the reproductive lifespan and risk of premature mortality: prospective cohort study. *BMJ.* 2020;371:m3464. PMID: 32998909

11. Gibson-Helm M, Teede H, Dunaif A, Dokras A. Delayed diagnosis and a lack of information associated with dissatisfaction in women with polycystic ovary syndrome. *J Clin Endocrinol Metab.* 2017;102(2):604-612. PMID: 27906550

12. Dapas M, Dunaif A. Deconstructing a syndrome: genomic insights into PCOS causal mechanisms and classification. *Endocr Rev.* 2022;43(6):927-965. PMID: 35026001

13. Azziz R, Carmina E, Dewailly D, et al; Androgen Excess Society. Positions statement: criteria for defining polycystic ovary syndrome as a predominantly hyperandrogenic syndrome: an Androgen Excess Society guideline. *J Clin Endocrinol Metab.* 2006;91(11):4237-4245. PMID: 16940456

14. Pena AS, Witchel SF, Hoeger KM, et al. Adolescent polycystic ovary syndrome according to the international evidence-based guideline. *BMC Med.* 2020;18(1):72. PMID: 32204714

15. Dapas M, Lin FTJ, Nadkarni GN, et al. Distinct subtypes of polycystic ovary syndrome with novel genetic associations: an unsupervised, phenotypic clustering analysis. *PLoS Med.* 2020;17(6):e1003132. PMID: 32574161

Testosterone Replacement Therapy: Navigating the Pharmacologic Landscape

Frances J. Hayes, MB BCh BAO. Reproductive Endocrine Unit, Massachusetts General Hospital, Boston, MA; Email: fhayes@mgh.harvard.edu

Educational Objectives

After reviewing this chapter, learners should be able to:

- Describe the different testosterone formulations available to treat hypogonadism in men.

- Explain the pros and cons of the different agents and thus identify the best fit for an individual patient.

Significance of the Clinical Problem

For patients who meet criteria for hypogonadism and have no contraindications to testosterone replacement, a variety of treatment options are available to restore testosterone levels to the normal range. The past 2 decades have seen a surge in use of testosterone replacement for treatment of male hypogonadism.[1] There has also been a substantial increase in the number of formulations approved by the US FDA to treat hypogonadal patients. Available options now include the traditional intramuscular injections of testosterone esters (enanthate and cypionate); gels of different concentrations (1%, 1.62%, 2%); patches; oral; and depot formulations of testosterone undecanoate; nasal testosterone; and pellets (*table*).[2] It is therefore imperative for endocrinologists to be familiar with the various treatment modalities, so that they can optimally manage these patients. The decision about which formulation to prescribe can be influenced by several factors, including patient and physician preference, pharmacokinetics of the formulation, ease of use, cost, insurance coverage, and adverse effect profile. Adverse effects of testosterone can be formulation-specific or a class effect. If a patient has derived benefit from testosterone replacement but is experiencing a formulation-specific adverse effect, an alternative preparation should be prescribed.

Practice Gaps

- Several clinical practice recommendations have been published to guide physicians on the optimal management of men with androgen deficiency.[2-4] However, evidence suggests that adherence to these guidelines is poor and that substantial gaps in knowledge remain.[5,6]

Discussion

Given the multitude of FDA-approved testosterone formulations that are now available, it can be challenging for physicians who have not specialized in this area to become familiar with all of these options and make a well-informed choice.

The starting dose of treatment is guided by the pubertal status of the patient. In patients with a congenital cause of hypogonadism such as Kallmann syndrome, the goal of treatment is to induce puberty at a tempo similar to that which occurs physiologically. In this situation, testosterone replacement is started at very low dosages such as 25 to 50 mg of a testosterone ester every 3 to 4 weeks and gradually titrated upwards to doses that are sufficient to induce secondary sexual characteristics and growth without unduly advancing epiphyseal maturation and compromising final height. By contrast, a full adult replacement dose can be initiated in men with adult-onset hypogonadism where the goal is to correct symptoms of hypogonadism and restore normal sexual function, body composition, and bone health by returning testosterone levels to the middle of the reference range for healthy, eugonadal men of similar age. This goal is most commonly achieved by replacing testosterone using one of the FDA-approved formulations available (*table*). Factors that influence the type of testosterone prescribed include patient and physician preference, pharmacokinetics of the

formulation, ease of use, cost, insurance coverage, and adverse effect profile.

Testosterone esters, including enanthate and cypionate, have been used for the treatment of male hypogonadism for more than 7 decades. They have the advantage of being the least expensive of the testosterone replacement modalities, and they predictably restore testosterone levels to the normal range. However, they have unfavorable pharmacokinetics characterized by significant fluctuation in serum testosterone between peak and trough values. The esters are typically injected at 2-week intervals with levels reaching peak concentrations 24 to 48 hours after the injection followed by a gradual decline to the low-normal range before the next injection is due. When the interval between injections is extended to every 3 weeks, peak concentrations tend to be

Table. Testosterone Formulations Approved to Treat Hypogonadism

Formulation	Typical dosage	Advantages	Disadvantages
Testosterone enanthate and cypionate	150-200 mg intramuscularly every 2 weeks or 75-100 mg weekly	Low cost if self-administered; flexible dosing options	Discomfort of intramuscular injection; peaks and troughs may cause fluctuation in symptoms; more likely to cause erythrocytosis
Testosterone undecanoate in oil	750 mg at start, at 4 weeks, and then every 10 weeks	Long duration of action	Large injection volume; small risk of pulmonary oil microembolism
Testosterone transdermal 1%, 1.62%, and 2%) gels	50-100 mg of 1% gel 40.5-81 mg of 1.62% gel 40-70 mg of 2% gel	Ease of use Good skin tolerance Flexibility of dosing	Potential to transfer to female partner or child; testosterone levels may vary from one application to the next; rarely skin irritation
Testosterone axillary solution	60-120 mg applied daily in axillae using applicator	Good skin tolerance Flexibility of dosing	Potential to transfer to female partner or child; testosterone levels may vary from one application to the next; rarely skin irritation in a small percentage of men
Testosterone transdermal patch	4-6 mg applied daily to nonpressure areas	Easy to apply No risk of transference	Skin irritation at application site is common
Testosterone pellets	Pellets containing 600-1200 mg testosterone implanted subcutaneously in buttocks or abdomen	Long duration of action	Requires surgical incision for insertion; pellets may extrude spontaneously, risk of infection and hematoma
Testosterone nasal gel	11 mg 3 times daily	Rapid absorption Avoidance of first-pass metabolism	Multiple daily dosing; local nasal side effects; not suitable for men with nasal disorders
Testosterone undecanoate capsule	Taken by mouth twice daily; dosage varies with formulation	Oral administration Avoidance of first-pass metabolism	Increase in blood pressure

Reprinted from Bhasin et al. *J Clin Endocrinol Metab*, 2010; 95(6):2536–2559. © The Endocrine Society.

supraphysiologic and testosterone levels may fall to the hypogonadal range by the time the next injection is administered. Such wide excursions in serum testosterone concentrations can, in turn, cause undesirable swings in mood, libido, and energy levels. Given the pharmacokinetics of testosterone esters, they also tend to increase hematocrit more than transdermal testosterone preparations, especially when high dosages are given at less frequent intervals.

A longer-acting depot formulation of another testosterone ester called testosterone undecanoate was approved in Europe in 2003 and in the United States in 2014. In Europe and Australia, this product consists of a 4-mL injection containing 1000 mg of testosterone undecanoate dissolved in castor oil and can be self-administered every 12 weeks after a loading dose. The formulation approved for use in the United States differs in a few respects. First, it contains a lower dose of 750 mg in 3 mL and is administered every 10 weeks. Second, the US FDA has stipulated that the injection be administered in an office or hospital setting by a registered health care provider and that the patient be monitored for 30 minutes because of the potential risk of pulmonary oil microembolism and anaphylaxis, although both are rare with an incidence of 1.5 cases per 10,000 and 0.4 cases per 10,000 injections, respectively.

The development of transdermal testosterone delivery systems in the 1990s represented a significant advance in the treatment of male hypogonadism because they are easier to use and thus have greater patient acceptability. The first preparation to be approved was a scrotal patch, which resulted in stable testosterone levels over a 24-hour period. However, in some hypogonadal men the surface area of the scrotum was not large enough to accommodate this large patch; it was quickly replaced by nonscrotal patches and is no longer available. These second-generation nonscrotal transdermal patches can be applied to the back, abdomen, thighs, and upper arms. They are currently available in doses of 2 and 4 mg. However, many patients experience skin irritation from these patches due to the permeation

enhancers added to facilitate absorption of testosterone. In about 10% of patients, these skin reactions are sufficiently severe to warrant discontinuation of therapy.

In 2000, a 1% transdermal testosterone gel became available in 25- and 50-mg packets, which could be applied to the upper arms and shoulders and resulted in steady state testosterone concentrations over a 24-hour period. The incidence of skin irritation with the transdermal gel is low. Since then, several other brand name and generic gel formulations have been approved. The preparations differ in their concentrations (1%, 1.62%, and 2%), packaging (packets, tubes, multidose pump dispensers), and cost. A risk of all transdermal testosterone gels is the potential for transference during intimate contact, which could result in virilization of a female partner or precocious puberty in a child. However, when appropriate precautions (ie, washing hands after application and covering the application site with clothing) are followed, the incidence of secondary exposure with gels is rare, estimated at 8 cases per 1.8 million prescriptions.

A formulation containing subcutaneous pellets of testosterone was approved by the US FDA in 2008. Under local anesthesia, a trocar is used to insert 3 to 6 pellets into the subdermal fat of the abdomen, buttocks, or thigh, which provide physiologic levels of testosterone for a period of 3 to 6 months. While this preparation has the advantage of a long duration of action, there is a risk of extrusion and infection, as well as the need for a minor surgical procedure.

A nasal testosterone preparation is also approved for the treatment of hypogonadism in men. For physiological testosterone levels to be achieved, the gel must be sprayed into the nostrils 3 times per day using a metered dose pump applicator. Local adverse effects, including rhinorrhea, nose bleeds, and sinusitis, can occur, and it is therefore not a suitable option for men with allergies or sinusitis.

In recent years, the US FDA has approved several oral formulations of testosterone undecanoate in capsule form. These agents, which are lipophilic, are absorbed through the lymphatic system. As a result, they are not subject to first-pass metabolism by the liver and do not cause hepatoxicity unlike prior oral preparations comprising methyltestosterone. Labeling information for these products includes a boxed warning about possible increases in blood pressure and cardiovascular events. These preparations should be taken with food and require twice-daily administration. Depending on the formulation (*table*), different dose strengths and dosing options are available.

Clinical Case Vignettes

Case 1

A 72-year-old man returns for follow-up of hypogonadism 3 months after starting replacement with injections of testosterone enanthate, 200 mg every 2 weeks. His libido has improved on this regimen, but he continues to feel tired and sometimes takes an afternoon nap. Physical examination findings are notable only for a BMI of 36 kg/m². Pretreatment, he had 2 morning testosterone values in the hypogonadal range (180 and 210 ng/dL [6.2 and 7.3 nmol/L]) and a hematocrit measurement of 50% (0.50). On treatment, a trough testosterone level drawn right before an injection is due is 315 ng/dL (10.9 nmol/L), and his hematocrit is now 54% (0.54).

Which of the following is the best next step in this patient's management?

A. Switch from testosterone enanthate to cypionate at the current dosage

B. Increase the testosterone dosage to 250 mg every 2 weeks

C. Continue his current testosterone regimen but arrange for him to have monthly phlebotomy

D. Schedule a sleep study

Answer: D) Schedule a sleep study

The pharmacokinetics of testosterone cypionate and enanthate are similar. Hence, switching esters (Answer A) will not improve the patient's symptoms. Increasing the testosterone dosage

(Answer B) is not appropriate for 2 reasons. First, the patient's testosterone concentration is already in the desired range for a trough level, namely at the lower end of the normal range. Second, a higher dose would cause a further increase in an already elevated hematocrit. The baseline hematocrit of 50% for this hypogonadal patient is high. In fact, a baseline hematocrit greater than 48% (and greater than 50% for men living at higher altitudes) is a relative contraindication to testosterone therapy because these men are more likely to develop a hematocrit level greater than 54% when treated with testosterone. Occasionally, phlebotomy (Answer C) may be necessary for testosterone therapy to be continued in a hypogonadal patient, but it is important to exclude other causes of erythrocytosis such as sleep apnea, chronic obstructive pulmonary disease, or polycythemia rubra vera before doing so.

The Endocrine Society clinical practice guidelines recommend that the underlying cause of erythrocytosis be investigated before androgen therapy is prescribed. Given the patient's obesity and history of daytime somnolence, the possibility of obstructive sleep apnea should be considered, and a sleep study should be scheduled (Answer D). In most patients in whom a diagnosis of obstructive sleep apnea is confirmed, initiation of continuous positive airway pressure will normalize, or at least lower, the hematocrit level. While not given as an answer option in this vignette, switching the patient's formulation from an intramuscular to transdermal testosterone preparation is also likely to be of benefit, as the latter is less likely to cause high peak levels that stimulate red cell production.

Case 2

A 65-year-old man wishes to discuss treatment for newly diagnosed hypogonadism. When informed of various options, he is not keen on the idea of having to apply a testosterone gel or patch daily and expresses a preference for injections. He has read about the long-acting depot formulation of testosterone undecanoate and asks about potential adverse effects.

Which of the following is a potential adverse effect that this patient might experience as a result of treatment with testosterone undecanoate injections?

A. Significant fluctuations in energy levels and mood

B. Skin irritation

C. Cough and shortness of breath following the injection

D. Jaundice

E. Flulike illness

Answer C) Cough and shortness of breath following the injection

The long-acting intramuscular formulation of testosterone undecanoate has the advantage of having a superior pharmacokinetic profile compared with other injectable formulations such as enanthate and cypionate, and it has the ability to maintain testosterone levels more consistently in the normal range over a 10-week period. The absence of marked swings in serum testosterone levels means that fluctuations in energy and mood (Answer A) are not typical adverse effects.

Skin irritation (Answer B) can occur in as many as 50% of patients whose hypogonadism is treated with a testosterone patch, but this adverse effect is not seen with intramuscular testosterone undecanoate.

Pulmonary oil microembolism is an acute reaction to injection of an oil-based compound and has been reported as an adverse event related to testosterone preparations formulated in oil. Symptoms of pulmonary oil microembolism include the urge to cough, shortness of breath (Answer C), throat tightening, chest pain, dizziness, and syncope. These symptoms have been reported with all testosterone injections but are more common with testosterone undecanoate (1.5 cases/10,000 injections) because of the larger injection volume of 3 mL.

When ingested orally, testosterone is broken down by the liver and has the potential to cause liver damage, including cholestatic jaundice, peliosis hepatis, and hepatomas.

However, testosterone formulations administered intramuscularly bypass the liver, so jaundice (Answer D) is incorrect.

Flulike symptoms (Answer E) have not been reported with testosterone undecanoate injections.

Case 3

A 35-year-old man presents for evaluation of decreased libido and erectile dysfunction. He has been working long hours and is under a lot of stress. He and his wife would like to start a family in the next 6 months.

On physical examination, his BMI is 35 kg/m², he is well virilized, and testicular volume is 25 mL bilaterally.

Results of hormone workup:

> Total testosterone (8 AM) = 275 ng/dL
> (SI: 9.5 nmol/L) and 290 ng/dL (SI: 10.1 nmol/L)
> (280-1000 ng/dL [SI: 9.7-34.7 nmol/L])
> LH = 2.5 IU/L
> FSH = 3.2 IU/L
> Prolactin = 10 ng/mL (SI: 0.43 nmol/L)

Which of the following medications is most appropriate for this patient at this juncture?

A. A testosterone gel

B. A phosphodiesterase inhibitor

C. Injections of hCG alone

D. Injections of hCG plus recombinant FSH

Answer B) A phosphodiesterase inhibitor

This patient has total testosterone levels at or just below the lower end of normal but given his increased BMI, he is likely to have low SHBG levels, which would account for the lower total testosterone level. There is no evidence that he has any organic disease affecting the hypothalamus, pituitary, or testes. Testosterone therapy (Answer A) is incorrect, and for patients desiring fertility, testosterone is particularly unhelpful given the likelihood that it will suppress endogenous FSH secretion and spermatogenesis. Studies from male contraceptive trials show that approximately two-thirds of men have recovery of spermatogenesis within 6 months of discontinuing testosterone therapy.[7] However, both the time course and extent of recovery of spermatogenesis after treatment cessation are variable. Although the doses of testosterone used in male contraceptive regimens are considerably higher than those used to treat hypogonadism, it is nonetheless prudent to counsel patients with plans to start a family about implications for fertility.

This patient's main symptom is sexual dysfunction in the setting of significant stress. Therefore, a trial of a phosphodiesterase inhibitor (Answer B) is the most appropriate next step in that it is likely to alleviate his symptoms without compromising fertility, which will become especially important when he and his wife are actively trying to conceive and trying to time intercourse to ovulation.

Patients with significant hypogonadotropic hypogonadism can be offered gonadotropin therapy, which would stimulate both testosterone secretion and spermatogenesis.[8] However, given that this patient has borderline testosterone levels, it is quite possible that intratesticular testosterone concentrations are preserved and that sperm production may not be suppressed. Thus, initiating treatment with hCG (Answer C) would not be appropriate without first doing a semen analysis. The combination of hCG and FSH (Answer D) is only indicated for patients with congenital hypogonadotropic hypogonadism and prepubertal testes, which does not apply to this patient.

Key Learning Points

- In the absence of a contraindication, testosterone replacement can be initiated with one of the formulations listed in the *table*, with the choice depending on patient and physician preference, adverse effect profile, cost, and insurance coverage.

- In patients with congenital causes of hypogonadism, testosterone replacement should be started at very low dosages and gradually titrated upwards to dosages that are sufficient to induce secondary sexual characteristics and growth without unduly advancing bone age and compromising final height.

- For hypogonadal patients desiring fertility in the near future, testosterone therapy is not the optimal choice given the likelihood that it will suppress endogenous FSH secretion and spermatogenesis.

- Adverse effects of testosterone can be formulation-specific or a class effect. If a patient has derived benefit from testosterone replacement but is experiencing a formulation-specific adverse effect, an alternative preparation should be prescribed.

REFERENCES

1. Layton JB, Li D, Meier CR, et al. Testosterone lab testing and initiation in the United Kingdom and the United States, 2000 to 2011. *J Clin Endocrinol Metab.* 2014;99(3):835-842. PMID: 24423353

2. Bhasin S, Brito JP, Cunningham GR, et al. Testosterone therapy in men with hypogonadism: an Endocrine Society clinical practice guideline. *J Clin Endocrinol Metab.* 2018;103:1715-1744. PMID: 29562364

3. Wang C, Nieschlag E, Swerdloff R, et al. Investigation, treatment and monitoring of late-onset hypogonadism in males: ISA, ISSAM, EAU, EAA and ASA recommendations. *Eur J Endocrinol.* 2008;159:507-514. PMID: 18955511

4. Mulhall JP, Trost LW, Brannigan RE, et al. Evaluation and management of testosterone deficiency: AUA guideline. *J Urol.* 2018;200;423-432. PMID: 29601923

5. Grossmann M, Anawalt BD, Wu FCW. Clinical practice patterns in the assessment and management of low testosterone in men: an international survey of endocrinologists. *Clin Endocrinol (Oxf).* 2015;82(2):234-241. PMID: 25154540

6. Malik RD, Wang CE, Lapin B, Lakeman JC, Helfand BT. Characteristics of men undergoing testosterone replacement therapy and adherence to follow-up recommendations in metropolitan, multicenter healthcare system. *Urology.* 2015;85(6):1382-1388. PMID: 25862121

7. Liu PY, Swerdloff RS, Christenson PD, Handelsman DJ, Wang C; Hormonal Male Contraception Summit Group. Rate, extent, and modifiers of spermatogenic recovery after hormonal male contraception: an integrated analysis. *Lancet.* 2006;367:1412-1420. PMID: 16650651

8. King T, Hayes FJ. Long-term outcome of idiopathic hypogonadotropic hypogonadism. *Curr Opin Endocrinol Diabetes Obes.* 2012;19(3):204-210. PMID: 22499222

Management of Functional Hypogonadism in Men

Michael S. Irwig, MD. Beth Israel Deaconess Medical Center and Harvard Medical School, Boston, MA; Email: mirwig@bidmc.harvard.edu

Educational Objectives

After reviewing this chapter, learners should be able to:

- Distinguish between organic and functional causes of male hypogonadism.

- Recognize the effects of obesity on SHBG and testosterone.

- Employ strategies to manage functional hypogonadism in men.

Significance of the Clinical Problem

Functional hypogonadism is relatively common among adult men and refers to low testosterone levels with no recognizable structural pathology in the hypothalamic-pituitary-gonadal axis. Etiologies of functional hypogonadism include obesity, chronic illnesses (ie, diabetes mellitus), opioid use, excessive exercise, and inadequate sleep.

The management of men with functional hypogonadism is often uncertain and usually depends on the etiology and degree of testosterone suppression. Most causes are potentially reversible such as obesity, opioid use, excessive exercise, and inadequate sleep. Addressing the underlying cause is recommended when feasible and may result in the normalization of endogenous testosterone levels without the risks and costs associated with testosterone therapy.

Over the past decade in the United States and elsewhere, there has been an explosion in the number of men having testosterone tests, requests for testosterone therapy, and testosterone prescriptions. In the United States, there is a growing problem of inappropriate and off-label prescribing of testosterone through direct-to-consumer online platforms and some for-profit specialty clinics promoting men's health and antiaging treatments.[1,2] Much of this prescribing is not done by physicians but by nurse practitioners, physician assistants, and nonmedically licensed individuals.[2]

Practice Gaps

- Lack of a proper understanding of the testosterone reference range and its limitations.

- The management of functional hypogonadism in men is often uncertain.

Discussion

Endocrinologists are increasingly referred men with low or borderline-low testosterone levels, which are most often due to functional hypogonadism. Functional hypogonadism is a diagnosis of exclusion that refers to low testosterone levels in the setting of no recognizable structural pathology in the hypothalamic-pituitary-gonadal axis (see table).[3] A similar term is "late-onset hypogonadism," but this term historically has focused more on the age-related decline in testosterone. In contrast, organic causes of hypogonadism include structural pathology such as Kallmann syndrome, Klinefelter syndrome, and hypopituitarism. Functional hypogonadism is relatively common among adult men, with rates as high as 12%.

Table. Organic Hypogonadism vs Functional Hypogonadism in Middle-Aged and Older Men

	Organic hypogonadism	Functional hypogonadism
Condition	Proven hypothalamic-pituitary-thyroid axis pathology (structural, destructive, or congenital disease)	No recognizable structural intrinsic hypothalamic-pituitary-thyroid axis pathology. No specific pathologic etiologies of functional hypogonadism (diagnosis of exclusion)
Reversibility	Established disease state, organic and generally irreversible hypothalamic-pituitary-thyroid pathology	Hypothalamic-pituitary-thyroid axis suppression is functional and may be reversible
Symptoms/signs	Specific: eunuchoidism. More specific/objective: low libido, small testes, loss of male hair, gynecomastia	Less specific: erectile dysfunction, low energy and mood
Testosterone levels	Unequivocally, consistently, and severely low	Borderline-low, fluctuating around the lower limit of assay range, occasionally severely low
Gonadotropin levels	Elevated (primary hypogonadism) or low/inappropriately normal (secondary hypogonadism)	Usually in the normal range, occasionally low (secondary hypogonadism)
Association of low testosterone with symptoms	Causal	Uncertain, symptoms may be predominantly or partially due to comorbid illness
Testosterone therapy	Replacement	Replacement?
Benefits of therapy	Marked symptomatic and somatic response (except fertility)	Symptomatic and somatic response less well established
Risks of therapy	Considered low relative to benefits	Unknown

Reprinted from Grossmann M & Matsumoto AM. *J Clin Endocrinol Metab*, 2017; 102(3): 1067-1075. © by The Endocrine Society.

Clinicians and patients are commonly confronted with misconceptions and misinformation regarding testosterone levels and testosterone therapy. For example, younger men may believe that normal testosterone levels for them need to be in the upper one-third or upper half of the reference range. Another common misconception is that androgen deficiency is the most common etiology underlying many nonspecific symptoms such as low energy, depressed mood, and erectile dysfunction. Many men also mistakenly believe that initiating testosterone therapy will suddenly ameliorate all of their common nonspecific symptoms.

Few signs and symptoms of male hypogonadism are very specific (*see box*).[4] Low energy is a highly prevalent symptom associated with a myriad of medical and psychiatric conditions from sleep apnea to depression. Of the sexual symptoms, low libido is a bit more specific than erectile dysfunction for androgen deficiency. Erectile dysfunction is primarily a function of aging due to atherosclerosis and changes to the vasculature. It is also associated with many chronic diseases such as diabetes mellitus, hyperlipidemia, hypertension, and kidney disease. Erectile dysfunction may also represent an adverse medication effect of an antihypertensive, diuretic, antidepressant, antipsychotic, anticonvulsant, barbiturate, benzodiazepine, anticholinergic or antispasmodic.

A lack of a proper understanding of the testosterone reference range represents another major barrier to optimal practice. Some clinicians overly fixate on whether a given value is outside of the reference range without adequate attention to whether the abnormal test result is actually clinically significant. The reference range for testosterone is based on healthy adult men aged 19 to 39 years who do not have obesity. The cutpoints for low and high testosterone values are simply arbitrary statistical percentiles that are not based on clinical signs or symptoms. For example, the harmonized reference range for total testosterone in adult men has been calculated as 264 to 916 ng/dL (9.2-31.8 nmol/L).[5] Although

Box. Symptoms and Signs Suggestive of Testosterone Deficiency in Men

Specific symptoms and signs

- Incomplete or delayed sexual development
- Loss of body hair (axillary and pubic)
- Very small testes (<6 mL)

Suggestive symptoms and signs

- Reduced sexual desire (libido) and activity
- Decrease spontaneous erections, erectile dysfunction
- Breast discomfort, gynecomastia
- Eunuchoidal body proportions
- Inability to father children, low sperm count
- Height loss, low-trauma fracture, low bone mineral density
- Hot flushes, sweats

Nonspecific symptoms and signs associated with testosterone deficiency

- Decreased energy, motivation, initiative, and self-confidence
- Feeling sad or blue, depressed mood, persistent low-grade depressive disorder
- Poor concentration and memory
- Sleep disturbance, increased sleepiness
- Mild unexplained anemia (normochromic, normocytic)
- Reduced muscle bulk and strength
- Increased body fat, body mass index

Reprinted from Bhasin S et al. J Clin Endocrinol Metab, 2018; 103(5): 1715-1744. © The Endocrine Society; Adapted from Bhasin S. Andrology, 2018; 6(1): 151–157. © American Society of Andrology and European Academy of Andrology.

testosterone concentrations often decline with age, the reference range does not adjust for age. The Massachusetts Male Aging Study calculated the lower limit of the reference range for men based on decade of life.[6] For men in their 40s, the value was 251 ng/dL (8.7 nmol/L). For men in their 70s, it was 156 ng/dL (5.4 nmol/L).

Men with overweight and obesity have lower mean levels of total testosterone (*see figure 1*).[7] According to the European Male Aging Study, as compared with men who have a normal BMI, men with overweight have a mean total testosterone concentration that is 66 ng/dL (2.3 nmol/L) lower.[8] For men with obesity, it is 147 ng/dL (5.1 nmol/L) lower. This difference in testosterone concentration according to BMI is largely explained by lower mean levels of SHBG.[7] Obesity is also associated with increased

conversion of testosterone to estrogen in adipose tissue. Estrogen causes potent negative feedback at the level of the hypothalamus and pituitary to lower testosterone production.

Figure 1. Relationships among age, BMI, and hormones

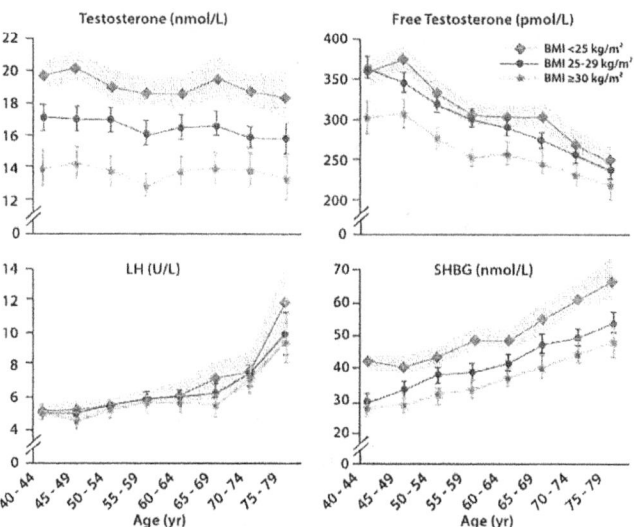

The cohort was stratified according to BMI into 3 groups: nonobese (BMI <25 kg/m²), overweight (BMI ≥25 to <30 kg/m²), and obese (BMI ≥30 kg/m²). Mean (95% CI in shaded area and vertical lines) total and free testosterone and SHBG were significantly lower in the overweight and obese groups at all ages, compared with patients who did not have obesity. The total testosterone and SHBG age trends in the 3 BMI categories were similar (indicating no interaction between BMI and age); the free testosterone age trend in the obesity group was less steep than in the other 2 groups (indicating an interaction between BMI and age). Mean LH was not significantly different among the 3 groups at the median age of 60 years. LH was higher in the patients older than 70 years without obesity compared with levels in the patients with overweight or obesity, due to a negative BMI-age interaction. Reprinted from Wu FC et al. J Clin Endocrinol Metab, 2008; 93(7): 2737-45. © The Endocrine Society.

When managing men with borderline testosterone levels and sexual symptoms, the main clinical question is whether the symptoms are a result of androgen deficiency. To help address this question, the European Male Aging Study assessed the association between sexual symptoms and serum concentrations of total testosterone. This study found that the probability for erectile dysfunction increased when the total testosterone concentration was less than 245 ng/dL (<8.5 nmol/L) and that the frequency of sexual thoughts declined when the total testosterone concentration was less than 230 ng/dL (<8.0 nmol/L).[9] Another study was a randomized controlled trial that rendered 177 healthy older men hypogonadal with the GnRH agonist goserelin. Men were subsequently randomly assigned to different doses of a testosterone or placebo gel. This study found that changes in sexual desire and erectile function were only statistically significant in the group of men whose mean total testosterone concentration was less than 100 ng/dL (<3.5 nmol/L).[10]

To distinguish between organic and functional causes of male hypogonadism, clinicians should always begin by taking a careful history to elicit established medical diagnoses, as well as potential causes that have yet to be diagnosed. On physical examination, attention should be paid to the testicular exam, which may identify testicular (primary) causes of hypogonadism such as Klinefelter syndrome. A careful reconciliation of medications should be performed because many medications have sexual adverse effects.

Functional hypogonadism is often associated with borderline-low testosterone levels, in contrast to the severely and unequivocally low levels seen in many organic causes (*see box*). Whereas there is often a clear causal relationship between low testosterone and a particular sign and symptom with organic causes, the relationship for functional hypogonadism is often uncertain. Another uncertainty is the benefit-to-risk ratio of testosterone therapy in men with borderline-low levels.

Treatment of men with borderline-low testosterone levels may or may not involve testosterone, as many causes of functional hypogonadism are reversible. For example, when a man tapers off opioids, his testosterone levels may recover or normalize. Likewise, when a man with obesity loses weight, his endogenous testosterone levels may rise (*see figure 2*).[3,11] There is no consensus on what testosterone concentration should be used to guide testosterone therapy. In a consensus statement on late-onset hypogonadism from 2008, it was stated that

testosterone therapy is not indicated for men with total testosterone levels greater than 350 ng/dL (>12.1 nmol/L) and that beneficial effects are usually seen when the concentration is less than 230 ng/dL (<8.0 nmol/L).[12] This consensus statement illustrated that there is uncertainty whether to recommend or prescribe testosterone to men with total testosterone levels between 230 and 350 ng/dL (8.0-12.1 nmol/L), which is a large proportion of men referred to endocrinology clinics for functional hypogonadism.

Figure 2. Effect of weight loss on testosterone levels

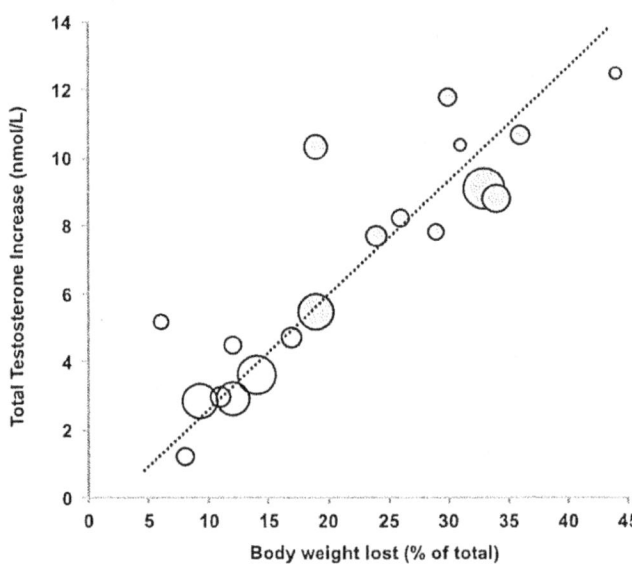

Each datum point refers to an individual study, and the size of the datum point is proportional to the size of the study, ranging from 10 to 293 men. Open circles represent studies where weight loss was achieved by diet and exercise and filled circles represent studies where weight loss was achieved by bariatric surgery. Reprinted from Grossmann M & Matsumoto AM. *J Clin Endocrinol Metab*, 2017; 102(3): 1067-1075. © The Endocrine Society.

To help clinicians manage men with functional hypogonadism, a 2020 clinical practice guideline was developed by the European Academy of Andrology that was endorsed by the European Society of Endocrinology.[13] It contains 33 recommendations in which the level of evidence was graded.

Clinical Case Vignettes

Case 1

A 47-year-old man presents to discuss restarting testosterone therapy for low testosterone. The patient went through normal puberty and fathered a biological child with no difficulty. In his 20s, he used 2 cycles of anabolic steroids over 2 summers. He states that weightlifting has been a very important activity for him. Three years ago, he got into opioids (oxycodone and heroin), which he used for approximately 1 year. For the past 2 years, he has been on methadone and is hoping to taper off over the next few months. He has lost 60 lb (27.2 kg) over the past year through diet and exercise.

One year ago, the patient presented to another physician with concerns of low energy and low libido. He had a low total testosterone concentration (115 ng/dL [4.0 nmol/L]) with a normal SHBG concentration 3.4 μg/mL (30 nmol/L). He was prescribed intramuscular testosterone, which he took for approximately 6 months. He estimates that his libido was an 8 out of 10 while on testosterone. He has been off testosterone for about 6 months and currently reports fatigue, a lower libido (4 out of 10), and erectile dysfunction.

Apart from the opioid use and history of anabolic steroid use, there are no other causes of primary or secondary hypogonadism. His medical history is also relevant for alcohol use disorder complicated by an episode of acute pancreatitis, hypertension, and asthma. Medications are methadone, 45 mg daily; amlodipine; and salbutamol as needed. He does not have a regular sexual partner. He quit drinking alcohol 2 months ago. He does not smoke cigarettes but vapes. He exercises 3 days per week.

On physical examination, his blood pressure is 141/93 mm Hg, and pulse rate is 90 beats/min. His height is 71 in (180.3 cm), and weight is 204 lb (92.5 kg) (BMI = 28.4 kg/m^2). He is muscular and has normal genitalia with 12 mL testes bilaterally.

Laboratory test results:

> 8-AM total testosterone = 250 and
> 233 ng/dL (280-800 ng/dL) (SI: 8.7 and
> 8.1 nmol/L [9.7- 27.8 nmol/L])
> LH, normal
> FSH, normal
> Hematocrit = 46% (41%-51%) (SI: 0.46 [0.41-0.51])

The patient requests to restart testosterone therapy given his symptoms and because he is an avid weightlifter.

In this man with opioid-induced hypogonadism, will testosterone therapy clinically improve his libido?

A. No

B. Yes

C. Possibly

Answer: C) Possibly

Two randomized controlled trials provide helpful information that can be used to counsel patients with opioid-induced hypogonadism. The first was a trial of 84 men aged 18 to 64 years who were taking at least 20 mg of hydrocodone daily (or morphine equivalent dose) for 4 or more weeks for chronic noncancer-related pain.[14] The patients had at least 1 morning total testosterone value less than 350 ng/dL (<12.1 nmol/L). They were randomly assigned to a 1% topical testosterone gel or placebo gel for 3 months with a target total testosterone concentration between 500 and 1000 ng/dL (17.4-34.7 nmol/L). According to the International Index of Erectile Function, there was a statistically significant increase in sexual desire with a treatment difference of 1 on a scale of 0 to 10. It is unclear how much of a clinically meaningful benefit this would have in any given patient.

The second randomized controlled trial enrolled 41 men who were taking at least 50 mg daily of morphine (or equivalent dose) for 3 or more months for chronic noncancer-related pain.[15] The patients had at least 2 morning total testosterone values less than 346 ng/dL (<12.0 nmol/L). They were randomly assigned to intramuscular testosterone undecanoate, 1000 mg, or placebo for 6 months. According to a validated Danish questionnaire, the men in the testosterone-treated group were having more sexual intercourse as evidenced by the days since coitus which was 18 days in the testosterone-treated group and 365 days in the placebo group.

Case 1 (continued)

In this man with opioid-induced hypogonadism, will testosterone therapy clinically improve his erectile dysfunction?

A. No

B. Yes

C. Possibly

Answer: C) Possibly

Two randomized controlled trials provide inconsistent results. The first study was a trial of 84 men aged 18 to 64 years who were taking at least 20 mg hydrocodone daily (or morphine equivalent dose) for 4 or more weeks for chronic noncancer-related pain.[14] They all had at least 1 morning total testosterone value less than 350 ng/dL (<12.1 nmol/L). They were randomly assigned to a 1% topical testosterone gel or placebo gel for 3 months with a target total testosterone concentration between 500 and 1000 ng/dL (17.4-34.7 nmol/L). According to the International Index of Erectile Function, there was no difference between the groups.

The second randomized controlled trial enrolled 41 men who were taking at least 50 mg daily of morphine (or equivalent dose) for 3 or more months for chronic noncancer-related pain.[15] They all had at least 2 morning total testosterone values less than 346 ng/dL (<12.0 nmol/L). They were randomly assigned to intramuscular testosterone undecanoate, 1000 mg, or placebo for 6 months. According to a validated Danish questionnaire, the prevalence of erectile dysfunction was 25% in those receiving testosterone treatment vs 63% in those receiving placebo.

Case 2

A 30-year-old man is referred by his nurse practitioner for consultation regarding management of the following symptoms over the past 3 to 4 years: decreased libido, nervousness, fatigue, cold intolerance, confusion, and insomnia. The patient underwent normal puberty and has not attempted to father children. He has no known causes of primary or secondary hypogonadism. His medical history is notable for hyperlipidemia. He takes various supplements and vitamins.

On physical examination, his blood pressure is 148/77 mm Hg and BMI is 27 kg/m². Examination findings are unremarkable, and testicular volume is normal.

Laboratory test results (sample drawn at 11 AM):

Total testosterone = 351 ng/dL (348-1197 ng/dL) (SI: 12.2 nmol/L [12.1-41.5 nmol/L])
Free testosterone = 65 pg/mL (52-280 pg/mL) (SI: 2.3 nmol/L [1.8-9.7 nmol/L])
Estradiol = 34.6 pg/mL (7.6-42.6 pg/mL) (SI: 127.0 pmol/L [27.9-156.4 pmol/L])
LH = 5.1 mIU/mL (1.7-8.6 mIU/mL) (SI: 5.1 IU/L [1.7-8.6 IU/L])
FSH = 7.0 mIU/mL (1.5-12.4 mIU/mL) (SI: 7.0 IU/L [1.5-12.4 IU/L])
TSH = 2.8 mIU/L (0.5-5.0 mIU/L)

Which of the following is the best next step?

A. Administer the Patient Health Questionnaire 9 (PHQ-9)

B. Do nothing

C. Offer a 3-month trial of testosterone

D. Recheck an 8-AM testosterone panel and measure SHBG

Answer: A) Administer the Patient Health Questionnaire 9 (PHQ-9)

This patient's hormonal test results are within their respective reference ranges. Rechecking an 8-AM testosterone panel and measuring SHBG (Answer D) may actually complicate the situation. If the repeated testosterone value comes back slightly low, the patient may assume that androgen deficiency is the cause of his signs and symptoms and insist on treatment. When there is a discrepancy (one measurement is normal and the other is low), the normal testosterone value usually trumps the low value. We interpret the difference as normal variability due to LH pulses. A discrepancy between the total and free testosterone from the same sample may indicate a high or low SHBG, but this was not the case for this patient. His BMI is 27 kg/m², which could be associated with a lower SHBG (*see figure 1*).

A trial of testosterone (Answer C) should not be offered based on only 1 borderline testosterone value but could be considered with at least 2 consistently low concentrations. It is quite possible that a repeat testosterone measurement would be very robust.

While reassuring the patient that his hormone levels are all within the reference range is correct, doing nothing (Answer B) would miss the opportunity to uncover depression, which is a very common diagnosis among men presenting with borderline-low testosterone levels. In a study of 200 men referred to an endocrinology clinic for evaluation of borderline-low testosterone values (200-350 ng/dL [6.9-12.1 nmol/L]), 56% had either known depression, a PHQ-9 score of 10 or higher, or were taking an antidepressant.[16] The patient in this vignette turned out to have suicidal ideation and severe depression with a score of 24 on the PHQ-9. Administering the PHQ-9 (Answer A) is therefore correct.

Case 3

A 44-year-old man is referred by his primary care physician for multiple low testosterone values. The patient underwent normal puberty. He has fathered 2 biological children with no difficulty and his wife would like a third child. Over the past 5 years he has noticed a progressive decline in his energy, libido, and erectile function. He also has gained 50 lb (22.7 kg) over this period. He tried sildenafil, which helped with his erectile function but caused headaches. He then switched to tadalafil as needed, which he uses on a regular basis.

Apart from obesity, he has no other causes of primary or secondary hypogonadism. His medical history is notable for prediabetes, hypertension, anxiety, and depression. His medications are hydrochlorothiazide, metoprolol, sertraline, and venlafaxine. He drinks 4 to 5 alcoholic beverages per week and does not smoke cigarettes. Exercise is minimal.

On physical examination, his blood pressure is 143/86 mm Hg and pulse rate is 72 beats/min. His BMI is 31.0 kg/m². Examination findings, including those on genital exam, are normal.

Laboratory test results:

> 8-AM total testosterone = 218 ng/dL (264-916 ng/dL) (SI: 7.6 nmol/L [9.2-31.8 nmol/L])
> Repeat 8-AM total testosterone = 235 ng/dL (264-916 ng/dL) (SI: 8.2 nmol/L [9.2-31.8 nmol/L])
> LH, normal
> FSH, normal
> SHBG = 2.2 µg/mL (1.1-5.6 µg/mL) (SI: 20 nmol/L [10-50 nmol/L])

Which of the following is the best next step?

A. Measure 8-AM total testosterone and calculated free testosterone

B. Measure prolactin and perform pituitary-directed MRI

C. Offer a 3-month trial of clomiphene or hCG

D. Offer a 3-month trial of testosterone

E. None of the above

Answer: E) None of the above

Measuring 8-AM total testosterone and calculated free testosterone (Answer A) would be low yield, as the vignette already provides 2 low total testosterone values and an SHBG value.

Measuring prolactin and performing pituitary-directed MRI (Answer B) would be incorrect, as pituitary MRI is recommended for patients for a total testosterone concentration less than 150 ng/dL (<5.2 nmol/L).

According to some guidelines on male hypogonadism, multiple low testosterone values in combination with signs and symptoms would be an indication to offer therapy (Answers C or D) to increase testosterone levels. However, the potential health benefits of testosterone, clomiphene, or hCG are uncertain for this patient. In a man who desires fertility in the near future, offering testosterone (Answer D) is not a good option because it could impair sperm production. Long-term efficacy and safety data are lacking for men such as this patient who are treated with clomiphene or hCG (Answer C).

Lifestyle changes offer this patient the best chance to improve his overall health. In particular, he could benefit from exercise. Men with higher fitness levels have lower mortality rates than men with lower fitness levels. Exercise and weight loss would also improve his hypertension and reduce the risk of the prediabetes progressing to diabetes.

Key Learning Points

- Functional hypogonadism is often reversible if the underlying issue is addressed.

- Most of the symptoms attributed to hypogonadism are nonspecific.

- For men with sexual symptoms, review potential adverse medication effects.

- Most patients must be educated about the normal variability of testosterone levels and factors that are associated with lower testosterone concentrations.

- Many men referred for borderline-low testosterone concentrations have either overweight/obesity and/or depression.

References

1. Irwig MS, Fleseriu M, Jonklaas J, et al. Off-label use and misuse of testosterone, growth hormone, thyroid hormone, and adrenal supplements: risk and costs of a growing problem. *Endocr Pract.* 2020;26(3):340-353. PMID: 32163313

2. Dubin JM, Jesse E, Fantus RJ, et al. Guideline-discordant care among direct-to-consumer testosterone therapy platforms. *JAMA Intern Med.* 2022;182(12):1321-1323. PMID: 36469030

3. Grossmann M, Matsumoto AM. A perspective on middle-aged and older men with functional hypogonadism: focus on holistic management. *J Clin Endocrinol Metab.* 2017;102(3):1067-1075. PMID: 28359097

4. Bhasin S, Brito JP, Cunningham GR, et al. Testosterone therapy in men with hypogonadism: an Endocrine Society clinical practice guideline. *J Clin Endocrinol Metab.* 2018;103(5):1715-1744. PMID: 29562364

5. Travison TG, Vesper HW, Orwoll E, et al. Harmonized reference ranges for circulating testosterone levels in men of four cohort studies in the United States and Europe. *J Clin Endocrinol Metab.* 2017;102(4):1161-1173. PMID: 28324103

6. Mohr BA, Guay AT, O'Donnell AB, McKinlay JB. Normal, bound and nonbound testosterone levels in normally ageing men: results from the Massachusetts Male Ageing Study. *Clin Endocrinol (Oxf).* 2005;62(1):64-73. PMID: 15638872

7. Wu FC, Tajar A, Pye SR, et al; European Male Aging Study Group. Hypothalamic-pituitary-testicular axis disruptions in older men are differentially linked to age and modifiable risk factors: the European Male Aging Study. *J Clin Endocrinol Metab.* 2008;93(7):2737-2745. PMID: 18270261

8. Tajar A, Forti G, O'Neill TW, et al; EMAS Group. Characteristics of secondary, primary, and compensated hypogonadism in aging men: evidence from the European Male Ageing Study. *J Clin Endocrinol Metab.* 2010;95(4):1810-1818. PMID: 20173018

9. Wu FC, Tajar A, Beynon JM, et al; EMAS Group. Identification of late-onset hypogonadism in middle-aged and elderly men. *N Engl J Med.* 2010;363(2):123-135. PMID: 20554979

10. Finkelstein JS, Lee H, Burnett-Bowie S-AM, et al. Dose-response relationships between gonadal steroids and bone, body composition, and sexual function in aging men. *J Clin Endocrinol Metab.* 2020;105(8):2779-2788. PMID: 32480409

11. Corona G, Rastrelli G, Monami M, et al. Body weight loss reverts obesity-associated hypogonadotropic hypogonadism: a systematic review and meta-analysis. *Eur J Endocrinol.* 2013;168(6):829-843. PMID: 23482592

12. Wang C, Nieschlag E, Swerdloff R, et al. Investigation, treatment and monitoring of late-onset hypogonadism in males: ISA, ISSAM, EAU, EAA and ASA recommendations. *Eur J Endocrinol.* 2008;159(5):507-514. PMID: 18955511

13. Corona G, Goulis DG, Huhtaniemi I, et al. European Academy of Andrology (EAA) guidelines on investigation, treatment and monitoring of functional hypogonadism in males: endorsing organization: European Society of Endocrinology. *Andrology.* 2020;8(5):970-987. PMID: 32026626

14. Basaria S, Travison TG, Alford D, et al. Effects of testosterone replacement in men with opioid-induced androgen deficiency: a randomized controlled trial. *Pain.* 2015;156(2):280-288. PMID: 25599449

15. Glintborg D, Vaegter HB, Christensen LL, et al. Testosterone replacement therapy of opioid-induced male hypogonadism improved body composition but not pain perception: a double-blind, randomized, and placebo-controlled trial. *Eur J Endocrinol.* 2020;182(6):539-548. PMID: 32213659

16. Westley CJ, Amdur RL, Irwig MS. High rates of depression and depressive symptoms among men referred for borderline testosterone levels. *J Sex Med.* 2015;12(8):1753-1760. PMID: 26129722

Approach to Nonbinary Adolescents and Young Adults

Karine Khatchadourian, MD, MSc. Department of Pediatrics, University of Ottawa, Ottawa, Ontario, Canada; Email: kkhatchadourian@cheo.on.ca

Daniel L. Metzger, MD. Department of Pediatrics, University of British Columbia, Vancouver, British Columbia, Canada; Email: dmetzger@cw.bc.ca

Educational Objectives

After reviewing this chapter, learners should be able to:

- Describe current estimated prevalence rates of trans and nonbinary people.

- Explain clinical challenges in the endocrine management of nonbinary adolescents and young adults.

- Review current treatment options for nonbinary adolescents based on the young person's pubertal status and goals.

Significance of the Clinical Problem

Over the last decade, the number of people identifying as nonbinary has grown exponentially, along with referrals to gender clinics worldwide. Nonbinary is used as an umbrella term referring to individuals who experience their gender as outside of the gender binary categories of male or female.[1] Often individuals use "they/them" pronouns; these people can use numerous terms to describe themselves (eg, nonbinary and gender fluid), and they identify to various degrees with binary-associated genders (eg, nonbinary man/woman).

Recent North American data suggest that 0.8% to 1.5% of youth aged 15 to 24 years identify as transgender or gender-nonconforming. Of these, roughly one-third identify as nonbinary.

Canada is the first country to provide census data on transgender and nonbinary people.[2] Of the nearly 30.5 million people in Canada 15 years of age and older living in private households in 2021, 100,815 self-identified as transgender (59,460) or nonbinary (41,355), accounting for 0.33% of the population in this age group. Based on results of a Canadian study[3] administered across the country to 923 transgender youth 14 to 25 years of age, 41% identified as nonbinary individuals; of these, 82% were assigned female sex at birth. Those identifying as nonbinary report poorer mental health outcomes and higher rates of self-harm in the past year, compared with those who identified as transgender men or transgender women. Other studies are also noting more psychological problems in youth who identify as nonbinary. It is hypothesized that nonbinary individuals' poorer mental-health outcomes are explained by a paucity of information and resources and a lack of nonbinary models.[4-6]

A 2022 report from the Williams Institute in the United States identified that among US adults older than 17 years, 0.5% identify as trans/gender-nonconforming (38.5% transgender women, 35.9% transgender men, 25.6% gender-nonconforming).[7] The percentage of youth identifying as trans/gender-nonconforming was 1.4% in those 13 to 17 years of age and 1.3% in those 18 to 24 years of age.

The US Census Household Pulse Survey is administered to Americans 18 years of age and older. Data from 2021 show that for those respondents assigned female sex at birth, 0.6%

identify as trans, 0.3% identify as male, and 1.7% identify as neither cis nor trans.[8] For those respondents assigned male sex at birth, 0.6% identify as trans, 0.4% identify as female, and 0.7% identify as neither cis nor trans.

In a new and evolving field, ethical issues can arise when providing care to nonbinary adolescents and young adults. The basic ethical principle of what is in the best interest for the patient should remain at the forefront of any clinical decision-making. Using published ethical decision-making frameworks can be helpful when faced with clinical challenges. The medical risks of using medication off-label with current knowledge gaps should be weighed against the benefits of initiating treatment for the well-being and safety of the patient.

Practice Gaps

- There are very few peer-reviewed publications discussing the optimal medical care of people identifying as nonbinary who do not wish to follow a conventional binary gender-affirming hormone regimen. To our knowledge, there are no controlled trials of any nonstandard hormone regimens designed specifically for nonbinary people. Alternative medical therapies for nonbinary people (including "microdosing" and the off-label use of medications known to alter hormone synthesis and tissue-level action) have been proposed in the literature, and these are likely already being used in some clinical settings.

- Long-term safety and efficacy data are completely lacking for these therapies. In considering treating nonbinary youth who have not fully completed either a testosterone- or estrogen-directed pubertal pathway, one must consider the added theoretical risks of long-term effects of these alternative therapies, particularly in terms of bone-mineral accretion, neuropsychiatric development, and cardiovascular and metabolic risks.

Discussion

Our first case highlights the challenges of initiating treatment with a GnRH analogue for a gender nonbinary adolescent who wants to remain on therapy until they have hysterectomy and salpingo-oophorectomy as an adult.

Many nonbinary people desiring some hormone therapy use "microdosing," that is, the use of subphysiologic doses of testosterone and/or estradiol to achieve partial masculinization or feminization. Clinicians may be faced with a nonbinary individual who presents at Tanner stage 2 who desires long-term pubertal suppression. This causes an ethical dilemma where one can argue that long-term or lifelong pubertal suppression is not possible because of negative health effects. To demonstrate the potential harm this may cause on the bones, one must look at the remains of historical figures. The famous castrato Gaspare Pacchierotti of the 18th century had evidence of vertebral fractures and a decrease in cortical bone density in long bones, along with other fascinating findings.[9]

Our second case highlights the inherent difficulty in helping youth achieve their nonbinary embodiment goals with the use of hormones that act in a fairly binary manner.

A number of medical therapies have been suggested in the literature[10,11] for the treatment of nonbinary people (see table). These include progestins, selective estrogen receptor modulators (SERMs), 5α-reductase and aromatase inhibitors, and nonsteroidal androgen-receptor blockers. The list contains medications familiar to most endocrinologists, in that they primarily affect either the synthesis or the end-organ actions of sex hormones. Many of these medications are licensed for use in other medical conditions, but their use in otherwise healthy nonbinary people must be considered off-label at this time. Many of these medications have significant adverse effects, and many have no licensed indication in the pediatric age group.

Table. Proposed Novel Uses of Hormones and End-Effect–Modulating Medications for Nonbinary People.

Drug class/action	Examples	Proposed general use	Proposed use in AMAB	Proposed use in AFAB	Adverse effects
Progestins: • Inhibition of GnRH–LH/FSH–gonadal axis • Stimulates P receptors • Complex/variable bone effects	• Micronized progesterone • Medroxyprogesterone acetate • Cyproterone • Norethindrone • Progestin-containing intrauterine devices • Etonogestrel implant	• *Pubertal suppression • ? Partial bone protection in those on GnRHa (norethindrone can ↓ bone mineral density loss in postmenopausal cis women)	• *Androgen suppression • *↑ breast growth • *↑ libido when T is suppressed • *Cardiovascular protection • *Mood effects • Incomplete lowering of T without use of GnRHa	• *Menstrual suppression (without the need for T) • *Contraception	• Many possible, depending on actual medication • Incomplete menstrual cessation, contraception • Effects on bones still a matter of debate • Some have androgenic profiles, some thrombogenic risks • Cyproterone: meningioma
Selective estrogen receptor modulators (SERMs): • Mixed agonist and antagonist action on ERα and β with variable tissue specificities • Some SERMs ↑ LH, FSH and T levels 2° ↓ feedback	• Tamoxifen • Raloxifene • Ospemiphene • Bazedoxifene		• Allow for E_2-like bone protection with minimal effects on breast • Produce some E_2-like changes in fat and skin		Mostly known from cis women being treated for breast cancer: • Hair loss, nausea, mood changes • Menopausal symptoms • Risk of thromboembolic events (DVT ↑54%, pulmonary embolism ↑91%) • Risk of type 2 diabetes ↑31% and ↑ triglycerides w/ hepatic steatosis • ↑ T levels may produce undesired effects
5α-reductase inhibitors: • ↓ conversion of T to DHT in skin, hair • Can ↑ T levels and thus E_2 levels	• Finasteride • Dutasteride	• ↓ androgen-dependent hair loss	• For those taking E_2 but wanting to preserve erectile function, could allow for use of some T, but lessen effect on skin/hair	• For those taking T but wanting to minimize androgen-dependent hair growth	Mostly known from cis men taking a 5αRI for prostatic hyperplasia, balding: • ↑ T and E_2 levels might be counter-productive • ? Can promote the growth of high-grade prostate cancer in some people • May be associated with rates of depression and low mood • ↓ libido, ↑ sexual dysfunction

Drug class/action	Examples	Proposed general use	Proposed use in AMAB	Proposed use in AFAB	Adverse effects
Aromatase inhibitors: • Block conversion of T → E_2 and androstenedione → E_1 • ↑ T levels in cis boys	• Anastrozole • Letrozole		• ↓ breast growth in those taking spironolactone	• ↑ Final height • ↓ feminizing effects of endogenous E_2 • ↓ feminizing effects of T in obesity	Mostly known from cis women being treated for breast cancer: • Hot flashes • ↓ bone accretion
Nonsteroidal androgen-receptor blockers • ↓ androgen action • ↑ T and E_2	• Flutamide • Bicalutamide		• ↓ masculinization but preserve bone density		• Hepatotoxicity, can be fulminant

*Currently being used for this indication in binary people (although evidence may be weak or nonexistent for some indications). Abbreviations: T, testosterone; E_2, 17β-estradiol; AMAB, assigned male sex at birth; AFAB, assigned female sex at birth. Reprinted from Cocchetti C et al. *J Clin Med*, 2020; 9(6): 1609. © by the authors. Published by MDPI, Basel, Switzerland; Xu JY et al. *Front Endocrinol*, 2021; 12:701364. © by the authors. Published by Frontier Media S.A.

Since many of these therapies affect sex hormone levels and/or action and secondarily bone mineral accretion and maintenance, one needs to consider that they could have long-lasting effects on bone health and osteoporosis and fracture risk. In postmenopausal women, a daily estrogen dose of 0.5 mg orally or 25 mcg transdermally is sufficient to prevent osteoporosis. In elderly men, an estradiol concentration 16 pg/mL or greater (≥60 pmol/L) is thought to prevent fracture risk. These values could be used to guide the use of alternative therapies in nonbinary adults who have achieved peak bone mass.

However, the use of these therapies in youth who have not achieved peak bone mass (thought to happen in the early to mid-20s) could have serious consequences for long-term bone health. The serum levels of sex hormones required to achieve peak bone mass are unknown, but it is recognized that even partially hypogonadal cisgender young adults have decreased bone mineral density.[12]

In addition to bone health, many of these therapies have known risks (eg, increased incidence of thrombosis with the use of selective estrogen receptor modulators) and likely unknown cardiovascular and metabolic effects.[10,11]

One last area of concern is how these therapies may alter the neurocognitive effects of sex hormones in the pubertal brain. The effects that puberty blockers have on neurocognitive development in trans youth is currently an area of active research, but essentially nothing is known about the effects of these novel alternative therapies.

In addition to hormone-based medical therapies, some nonbinary people would theoretically benefit from the use of medications that can enhance (minoxidil) or suppress (eflornithine) androgen-dependent hair growth. Some people benefit from the use of laser or electrolysis for unwanted hair removal. Lastly, many nonbinary people seek a wide variety of gender-affirming surgeries to achieve their embodiment goals.[11]

Clinical Case Vignettes
Case 1

A 14-year-old youth assigned female at birth uses "they/them" pronouns. After being assessed by a trans-competent mental health specialist and diagnosed with gender dysphoria, the youth is referred to endocrinology. The patient knew they were different from a young age. They cut their hair short in grade 1. They knew from grade 5 they were nonbinary, and they came out to their friends and at school between grades 6 and 7. They are now in grade 8. They have been consistent with identity for the last year. They came out to their parents 1 year before assessment. For this patient, menarche was "the worst thing in the world." They have had menses for 2 years now and gender dysphoria is rated as 9/10. They say, "I hate being in my body." Gender issues affect their mood a lot, and they often get anxious. They had a suicide attempt 3 months ago with an overdose of medication, and they continue to self-harm and have ongoing passive suicidal ideation. Bone age is 16 years, and BMI is at the 75th percentile. Their embodiment goal is to stop periods with puberty blockers. They are not interested in gender-affirming hormones in the future, nor in bottom surgery; they are interested in top surgery, hysterectomy, and salpingo-oophorectomy.

Which of the following is the best next step for this individual?

A. Discussing all options of menstrual suppression including a GnRH analogue, combined estrogen-progestin medications, oral progestins, depot and subdermal progestin, and intrauterine devices; then coming to a decision based on individual/ family's treatment preference

B. Encouraging oral progestins, continuous combined hormonal contraceptive, or medroxyprogesterone depot to suppress menses, as the patient is postpubertal with no future goals of testosterone treatment

C. Recommending not starting treatment yet because they have not experienced gender incongruence long enough

D. Starting a GnRH analogue, as this is the best option for menstrual suppression now

Answer: A) Discussing all options of menstrual suppression including a GnRH analogue, combined estrogen-progestin medications, oral progestins, depot and subdermal progestin, and intrauterine devices, then coming to a decision based on individual/family's treatment preference

If this patient had not completed puberty (was in Tanner stages 2 to 4), starting a GnRH analogue (Answer D) would have been the best option.

Recent WPATH guidelines recommend providers consider menstrual suppression agents for adolescents experiencing gender incongruence who may not desire testosterone therapy, who desire but have not yet begun testosterone therapy, or in conjunction with testosterone therapy for breakthrough bleeding.[1] The use of a GnRH analogue can still be considered given an individual's goals; however, we would recommend this is used for short-term treatment (roughly 1 to 2 years).

Recommending against treatment (Answer C) is incorrect, as this individual's experience of gender incongruence can be considered marked and sustained.

One could argue that the patient is postpubertal and that starting a treatment other than a GnRH analogue (Answer B) would prevent the future conversation of having to stop the GnRH analogue at some point. If the patient were older than 15 to 16 years, we would lean more towards recommending methods of menstrual suppression other than a GnRH analogue.

After discussing various methods of pubertal/ menstrual suppression (Answer A), the patient was started on a GnRH analogue.

The patient, who is now 16 years and 9 months, has been on the blocker for more than 2 years and still does not desire gender-affirming hormones in the future. They get extremely anxious and panicky when other menstrual-suppression options are discussed, as they know there will not be a guarantee that other medications will stop menses completely.[13-16] They want a hysterectomy/ salpingo-oophorectomy as soon as this is possible (must be 18 years old where they live).

On review of bone density, the lumbar-spine bone mineral density has dropped from −0.5 to −2.2 SD, and the lumbar spine bone mineral content has dropped from 44.19 to 41.68 g. The thoracic lumbar spine x-ray shows mild diffuse osteopenia and slight decreased height of the lower thoracic vertebrae.

At this point, the clinician strongly recommends discontinuing the GnRH analogue, given the threat to bone health. Other options of menstrual suppression are discussed with the patient.[13-16] However, they want to continue the GnRH analogue for a few more years.

What would happen if they remained on a GnRH analogue as long as they desired? One could consider initiating a bone-protective medication (such as a bisphosphonate) to optimize bone accrual for a few years, until the GnRH analogue is discontinued at the time of gonadectomy. Adding another off-label medication is not without risks, but this can be an ethically justifiable option.

The ethical issues surrounding the long-term use of unopposed puberty blockers in trans youth have been the subject of a number of publications that offer frameworks for ethical decision-making, balancing the youth's right to autonomy vs their short- and long-term physical and mental well-being.[17,18]

If the patient continues to desire oophorectomy when they reach an age at which they would be eligible, they would need counseling about the issue of prolonged hypogonadism. The minimal dose or duration of treatment with testosterone or estradiol to achieve peak bone mineral density is unknown.

Case 2

A 12-year-old patient was assigned male sex at birth. They have never clearly seemed to identify with or show preference for playing with boys or girls. They keep to themself, like to read and draw, but are not particularly active. They do OK socially in the presence of siblings and parents. They have kept their hair long in a ponytail since grade 1 and wear clothes that are not particularly gendered. They started expressing concern in grades 4 and 5 that they were going to "get hairy and grow a big penis." With puberty, the patient has become more anxious about body changes. When asked about pronouns, the patient says, "I don't know, just call me 'K'." They have had several sessions with a trans-competent mental health specialist and is diagnosed with mild, but clearly worsening, gender dysphoria. At this time, they have no clear embodiment goals, no clear binary or transfeminine identification. A diagnosis of neurodiversity is raised, but no significant learning problems are identified. After this assessment, the patient is offered a GnRH analogue at mid-Tanner stage 2, which will allow more time to map out their gender journey, and this relieves their agitation.

Now, 2 years later, at age 14 years, the diagnosis of autism spectrum disorder has been confirmed, and the patient has been participating in counseling. They have decided they identify as nonbinary and use "he/they" pronouns. They have met other nonbinary kids and found similarities with some of them, but also some differences. The patient says the closest term heard to describe themself is "demiboy." He also thinks he is asexual. His embodiment goals now are to appear "a bit masculinized, not like a little boy, not like a man": a deeper voice, but no body hair/beard and no breasts; they are not interested in "sexual stuff."

Which of the following is the best treatment plan for this patient now?

A. Add finasteride once they start developing facial hair

B. Continue the GnRH analogue but add back low-dosage testosterone

C. Discontinue the GnRH analogue and allow full male puberty to start

D. Discontinue the GnRH analogue because it has been 2 years, and hold off on other hormones until they have a clearer idea of what they want

E. Wait to discontinue the GnRH analogue, and hold off on other hormones until they have a clearer idea of what they want

Answer: B) Continue the GnRH analogue but add back low-dosage testosterone

The patient has developed relative clear, age-appropriate embodiment goals (thus, Answers D and E are incorrect). In most cases, use of a GnRH analogue for more than 2 years is avoided without the addition of a sex hormone. Continuing the GnRH analogue but adding back low-dosage testosterone (Answer B) allows the clinician to control the amount of masculinization that occurs and allows the patient to decide the pace of dosage changes.

Discontinuing the GnRH analogue and allowing full male puberty to start (Answer C) is incorrect in that this patient is seeking partial masculinization.

There are no studies in youth (or adults) for the off-label use of a 5α-reductase inhibitor (Answer A) to prevent beard growth.

Key Learning Points

- Recent North American data suggest that 0.8% to 1.5% of youth aged 15 to 24 years identify as transgender or gender-nonconforming. Of these, roughly one-third identify as nonbinary.

- Providing care to nonbinary youth is a new paradigm for pediatric and adult endocrinologists who want to help their patients achieve their often nonbinary embodiment goals with relative binary-acting hormones.

- Ethical issues arise when patients and providers have to balance the use of treatment options that are potentially unsafe or off-label with the patient's long-term physical and mental health safety and well-being.

- Novel treatment regimens for nonbinary people—with as yet no studies to justify their routine use—are being proposed to help modify or enhance current hormone replacement regimens for binary trans people. Extreme caution must be used with these medications, especially in nonbinary youth those who have not achieved peak bone mass.

- We have lots to learn about how best to help nonbinary people!

References

1. Coleman E, Radix AE, Bouman WP, et al. Standards of care for the health of transgender and gender diverse people, version 8. *Int J Transgend.* 2022;23(Supp 1):S1-S259. PMID: 36238954

2. Statistics Canada. (2022). Census of population Canada. https://www150.statcan.gc.ca/n1/daily-quotidien/220427/dq220427b-eng.htm. Accessed 25 February 2023.

3. Veale JF, Watson RJ, Peter T, Saewyc EM. Mental health disparities among Canadian transgender youth. *J Adolesc Health.* 2017;60(1):44-49. PMID: 28007056

4. Fiani CN, Han HJ. Navigating identity: experiences of binary and non-binary transgender and gender non-conforming (TGNC) adults. *Int J Transgend.* 2019;20(2-3):181-194. PMID: 32999605

5. Jones BA, Pierre Bouman W, Haycraft E, Arcelus J. Mental health and quality of life in non-binary transgender adults: a case control study. *Int J Transgend.* 2019;20(2-3):251-262. PMID: 32999611

6. Nicholas L. Queer ethics and fostering positive mindsets toward non-binary gender, genderqueer, and gender ambiguity. *Int J Transgend.* 2019;20(2-3):169-180. PMID: 32999604

7. Herman JL, Flores AR, O'Neill KK. How many adults and youth identify as transgender in the United States? The Williams Institute, UCLA School of Law, 2022.

8. United States Census Bureau (2021). Sexual orientation and gender identity in the Household Pulse Survey. https://www.census.gov/library/visualizations/interactive/sexual-orientation-and-gender-identity.html. Accessed 25 February 2023.

9. Zanatta A, Zampieri F, Scattolin G, Bonati MR. Occupational markers and pathology of the castrato singer Gaspare Pacchierotti (1740–1821). *Sci Rep.* 2016;6:28463. PMID: 27350433

10. Cocchetti C, Ristori J, Romani A, Maggi M, Fisher AD. Hormonal treatment strategies tailored to non-binary transgender individuals. *J Clin Med.* 2020;9(6):1609. PMID: 32466485

11. Xu JY, O'Connell MA, Notini L, Cheung AS, Zwickl S, Pang KC. Selective estrogen receptor modulators: a potential option for non-binary gender-affirming hormonal care? *Front Endocrinol.* 2021;12:701364. PMID: 34226826

12. Laitinen E-M, Hero M, Vaaralahti K, Tommiska J, Raivio T. Bone mineral density, body composition and bone turnover in patients with congenital hypogonadotropic hypogonadism. *Int J Androl.* 2012;35(4):534-540. PMID: 22248317

13. Carswell JM, Roberts SA. Induction and maintenance of amenorrhea in transmasculine and nonbinary adolescents. *Transgend Health.* 2017;2(1):195-201. PMID: 29142910

14. Gomez AM, Do L, Ratliff GA, Crego PI, Hastings J. Contraceptive beliefs, needs, and care experiences among transgender and nonbinary young adults. *J Adolesc Health.* 2020;67(4):597-602. PMID: 32527572

15. Kanj RV, Conard LAE, Corathers SD, Trotman GE. Hormonal contraceptive choices in a clinic-based series of transgender adolescents and young adults. *Int J Transgend.* 2019;20(4):413-420. PMID: 32999626

16. Pradhan S, Gomez-Lobo V. Hormonal contraceptives, intrauterine devices, gonadotropin-releasing hormone analogues and testosterone: menstrual suppression in special adolescent populations. *J Pediatr Adolesc Gynecol.* 2019;32(5S):S23-S29. PMID: 30980941

17. Notini L, et al. "No one stays just on blockers forever": clinicians' divergent views and practices regarding puberty suppression for nonbinary young people. *J Adolesc Health.* 2021;68(6):1189-1196. PMID: 33121900

18. Pang KC, Notini L, McDougall R, et al. Long-term puberty suppression for a nonbinary teenager. *Pediatrics.* 2020;145(2):e20191606. PMID: 31974217

Fertility Preservation Considerations for Gender-Diverse Adolescents and Young Adults

Leena Nahata, MD. Department of Pediatrics, The Ohio State University College of Medicine, Center for Biobehavioral Health, The Abigail Wexner Research Institute, Division of Endocrinology, Nationwide Children's Hospital, Columbus, OH; Email: leena.nahata@ nationwidechildrens.org

Educational Objectives

After reviewing this chapter, learners should be able to:

- Describe research on fertility perspectives in transgender and gender-diverse (TGD) populations.

- Identify potential fertility-related risks of gender-affirming interventions.

- Characterize fertility preservation (FP) options for gender-diverse adolescents and young adults.

Significance of the Clinical Problem

Research shows a wide spectrum of fertility-related perspectives in TGD populations. Studies in TGD adults demonstrate that many desire genetically related children, yet they frequently face barriers to accessing reproductive health care.[1] Studies in TGD adolescents highlight more varied perspectives, with some adolescents endorsing a desire for genetically related children in the future, and others reporting disinterest in genetic parenthood.[2] Most TGD adolescents acknowledge their fertility-related perspectives may evolve over time.[2] In this context, it is essential to provide counseling about potential impacts of medical and surgical gender-affirming interventions on reproductive capacity.[3] Puberty blockers inhibit gamete maturation and suppress the hypothalamic-pituitary-gonadal axis but do not appear to have permanent effects on fertility.[3] Studies on exogenous testosterone effects are mixed, with some studies showing negative effects on reproductive function and others showing pregnancies (planned and unplanned) during or after testosterone treatment.[4] Estrogen appears to impair spermatogenesis.[5] Prospective, longitudinal studies have not been conducted to examine long-term effects of these hormonal interventions on fertility. Gender-affirming surgeries involving the reproductive organs have obvious and often permanent effects on reproductive capacity.[3] Given these risks, FP options should be discussed before initiating each of these interventions and on an ongoing basis thereafter.[3] Sperm cryopreservation is an established, effective, and typically noninvasive FP option for pubertal birth-assigned males.[6] Oocyte and embryo cryopreservation are also established FP options, but they are more intensive, invasive, and expensive.[6] Gonadal tissue cryopreservation should be offered to TGD adults undergoing gonadectomy.[3]

Reproduction is a basic human right, and infertility is known to result in negative psychosocial outcomes.[7] Research in populations experiencing fertility impairment due to effects of their medical conditions or treatments (such as chemotherapy) shows psychological distress and regret about missed opportunities for FP.[7,8] Thus, guidelines have been published by organizations such as the American Society for Reproductive Medicine, highlighting the need for timely and comprehensive fertility counseling.[6]

An expanding body of literature has focused on fertility perspectives and practices in TGD populations, with the following key findings: (1) many TGD adults desire genetically related children, and efforts are needed to increase access to inclusive reproductive health care[1]; (2) while fertility-related attitudes vary widely among TGD adolescents and their caregivers, families endorse wanting more information about FP options[2,9]; (3) gender-affirming therapies appear to have variable effects on reproductive capacity, ranging from transient effects to increasingly permanent effects—larger, prospective, longitudinal studies are needed to better understand these effects[3]; (4) reproductive health counseling practices in TGD populations remain inconsistent[9]; (5) providers report gaps in knowledge and training regarding this topic, in addition to structural barriers (eg, high out-of-pocket costs of FP techniques, limited access to reproductive specialists).[10,11]

Practice Gaps

- Fertility-related risks of gender-affirming interventions are not fully understood, and many providers report inadequate knowledge and training on this topic.

- Reproductive health counseling remains inconsistent in TGD adolescent and young adult populations.

- Structural barriers are commonly reported, including high cost of FP and lack of access to reproductive specialists.

Discussion

Fertility-Related Perspectives in TGD Populations

Infertility is known to cause psychosocial distress.[7] Most fertility-related research has been conducted in oncology, showing cancer survivors and their families regret having missed opportunities for fertility preservation.[8] Organizations such as the American Society for Reproductive Medicine have thus recommended comprehensive counseling, including a discussion about potential fertility-related risks and fertility preservation options, prior to gonadotoxic therapy.[6] While research has been more limited in TGD populations, studies show many TGD adults desire genetically related children.[1] Published cases of transgender individuals experiencing pregnancy and/or receiving assisted reproductive technologies have demonstrated a wide spectrum of experiences and highlighted areas where more inclusive systems are needed.[12]

Fertility-related attitudes are more variable in the TGD adolescent population. Studies show low FP rates, particularly in the United States, with many transgender adolescents stating they do not want genetically related children and/or do not wish to be parents at all.[2] Other reasons for declining FP include cost, urgency to start treatment, and dysphoria associated with FP procedures.[2] Notably, a number of these adolescents acknowledge their fertility-related perspectives and parenthood goals may change over time, and both adolescents and their caregivers report a desire for information about FP.[2] According to the *World Professional Association for Transgender Care Standards of Care, Version 8*, reproductive health counseling should be provided to all individuals and families prior to gender-affirming medical and surgical treatments that may negatively impact fertility.[3] These discussions should address fertility-related risks, FP options, and the need for contraception, and should continue on an ongoing basis.[3]

Fertility-Related Risks

Given the lack of prospective, longitudinal studies, it remains unclear whether and the extent to which various gender-affirming treatments may impact fertility. Further, it is important to distinguish fertility (using one's own gametes to conceive a child) from capacity to carry a pregnancy. Puberty blockers, or GnRH analogues, prevent gamete maturation and suppress the hypothalamic-pituitary-gonadal axis, but they do not appear to have permanent effects on fertility.[3] Specifically, puberty progresses and/or there is resumption of menses/spermatogenesis after discontinuation of puberty blockers. The most permanent effects on reproductive function are caused by gender-affirming surgeries.[3] Studies suggest the effects of gender-affirming hormones (eg, exogenous testosterone and estrogen) may be partially reversible,[3] as summarized below, although it is difficult to predict the degree of effects on a given individual.

Studies examining the effects of exogenous testosterone on reproductive function have shown conflicting results, with some showing polycystic ovarian morphology and uterine changes and others suggesting these effects are transient and/or do not affect clinical fertility outcomes.[4] Conclusions have been difficult to draw given potentially confounding effects of other hormonal interventions, limitations of study design (observational and of limited duration), and high rates of polycystic ovary syndrome at baseline in this population.[4] Notably, several pregnancies (planned and unplanned) have been reported during and after exogenous testosterone therapy, and therefore it should not be considered an effective contraception method.[4]

Antiandrogens and estrogens have been shown to impair spermatogenesis and result in diminished testicular volumes; findings have been mixed regarding how long this effect may last (a few months to several years) if treatment is discontinued.[5] Again, conclusions are limited by a lack of longitudinal, prospective studies, and studies have shown a higher proportion of sperm abnormalities at baseline in transgender women compared with sperm abnormalities in cisgender men (potentially in part due to behavioral factors).[13]

Fertility Preservation Options

Established FP options, or those with proven efficacy, include cryopreservation of sperm, oocytes, and embryos (if there is a partner or identified donor). These options should be offered to postpubertal individuals, after which a spectrum of assisted reproductive technologies may be used to conceive a child.[6] Sperm cryopreservation has been used for decades with samples remaining viable for many years.[6] Semen samples are most often produced via masturbation, and sperm may be found in individuals whose sexual development is Tanner stage 2 to 3 or higher.[6] If an individual is unable or unwilling to produce a sample using this method (eg, due to sexual inexperience or dysphoria), more invasive methods could be offered by a urologist.[3] These alternative options include testicular sperm extraction and electroejaculation, and they carry more risks given that they are more invasive and use some type of anesthesia.[3] Oocyte retrieval is costly, invasive, and intensive, typically requiring a hormonal stimulation protocol followed by transvaginal monitoring and retrieval of oocytes.[6]

Evidence-based FP options are limited for prepubertal patients, as cryopreservation of gonadal tissue is less established.[6] Testicular tissue cryopreservation, via testicular biopsy, is the only FP option available for prepubertal or early pubertal boys; this procedure has been performed in several hundred boys (eg, prior to chemotherapy) with a live birth reported in a primate but not yet in humans, and is thus still considered experimental.[6] More than 130 live births have been reported from cryopreserved ovarian tissue, but most of these have been from postpubertal cisgender women, and all occurred after tissue was retransplanted.[6] Less is known about the efficacy of this technique in prepubertal individuals, and reported live birth rates are lower than those reported using oocytes.[6,14] Given that gonadotoxic effects of testosterone remain unclear and that ovarian tissue cryopreservation in prepubertal children often requires removal of an entire ovary, which may negatively impact future fertility, this option should primarily be offered to adults who are pursuing oophorectomy.[3]

Fertility-Related Practice Gaps and Barriers

Despite published guidelines recommending timely and comprehensive reproductive health counseling,[3] studies show inconsistent practice patterns.[9] Clinicians report inadequate knowledge about this topic and a desire for more training.[10,11] Structural barriers are also frequently noted, including high costs of FP techniques and assisted reproductive technologies (often with limited insurance coverage), lack of access to reproductive specialists, and systems that are not inclusive of TGD populations.[10,11] Further, ethical dilemmas may arise, particularly in the context of reproductive health care for adolescents where shared decision-making involves the patient, caregiver(s), and clinician(s).[15] Interdisciplinary teams are essential to delivering high-quality, equitable health care, with both medical and mental health clinicians who are (1) trained to work with TGD populations, (2) well-versed on this topic, and (3) able to help families navigate complexities such as discordance between adolescent and parent fertility-related perspectives and/or dysphoria associated with FP.[3,15]

Clinical Case Vignettes

Case 1

A 15-year-old transgender female presents with her parents to endocrinology clinic for estrogen therapy. She was referred by a behavioral health colleague. Based on physical examination, sexual development is Tanner stage 4. She has not received any gender-affirming interventions in the past.

Her parents state that they are supportive of her identity but are concerned about the potential adverse effects of estrogen, including on her future fertility. She states she does not like children and does not care about her fertility. Her parents acknowledge her perspective, with the caveat that her attitude about parenthood may change in the future.

Which of the following is the best recommendation in this situation?

A. Provide information about sperm cryopreservation and encourage her and her parents to discuss this option as a family, after which you all can meet again

B. Provide information about testicular tissue cryopreservation and encourage her and her parents to discuss this option as a family, after which you all can meet again

C. Reassure her and her family that estrogen has no known negative effects on fertility, so there is no need to consider FP

D. Suggest starting a GnRH analogue instead of estrogen and then consider FP in 6 months

E. Tell her that she should complete FP given that she is a minor and her parents are responsible for all medical decisions

Answer: A) Provide information about sperm cryopreservation and encourage her and her parents to discuss this option as a family, after which you all can meet again

Studies show estrogen therapy may impair spermatogenesis (thus, Answer C is incorrect), so pretreatment FP is recommended. At Tanner stage 4, sperm cryopreservation (Answer A) would be the appropriate option.

Testicular tissue cryopreservation (Answer B) is the only fertility preservation option available for prepubertal or early pubertal boys and is experimental.

GnRH analogue therapy (Answer D) would suppress the hypothalamic-pituitary-gonadal access and make it more difficult to cryopreserve sperm in 6 months.

While this patient's ability to plan for her future may be limited based on her developmental stage, it is also important to respect her autonomy and encourage family communication (thus, Answer E is incorrect).

Case 2

A 14-year-old nonbinary individual born with female anatomy has been treated with a GnRH analogue starting at age 12 years (Tanner stage 4). At their clinic visit today, the discussion involves stopping the GnRH analogue and starting testosterone treatment.

Which of the following is the best advice?

A. Testosterone is known to cause infertility; oocyte cryopreservation is recommended, and contraception is unnecessary, regardless of sexual activity

B. Testosterone is known to cause infertility; ovarian tissue cryopreservation is recommended, and contraception is unnecessary, regardless of sexual activity

C. Testosterone might impair fertility, and the patient can consider oocyte cryopreservation prior to starting testosterone; another form of contraception should still be used to prevent unplanned pregnancy if they have sexual intercourse with a sperm-producing partner

D. The patient is a minor, so oocyte cryopreservation should not be discussed

E. There is no need to discuss fertility preservation before testosterone therapy, as the patient's history of GnRH analogue treatment has likely resulted in permanent infertility

Answer: C) Testosterone might impair fertility, and the patient can consider oocyte cryopreservation prior to starting testosterone; another form of contraception should still be used to prevent unplanned pregnancy if they have sexual intercourse with a sperm-producing partner

Studies regarding fertility effects of testosterone have shown mixed results, so oocyte cryopreservation should be offered to postpubertal females (rather than ovarian tissue cryopreservation), but contraception is still essential to prevent unplanned pregnancy (thus, Answers A and B are incorrect).

GnRH analogue therapy is not known to cause permanent infertility (thus, Answer E is incorrect).

Finally, while fertility perspectives are variable and many TGD adolescents decline FP, guidelines state FP should be routinely offered prior to gender-affirming interventions (thus, Answer D is incorrect).

Case 2 (continued)

Shortly after that visit, the patient stops the GnRH analogue, starts testosterone, and decides not to proceed with FP. Four years later, the patient is 18 years old and seeking a total abdominal hysterectomy with bilateral salpingo-oophorectomy.

Which of the following is the best advice?

A. FP options should be discussed prior to surgery, including oocyte cryopreservation and ovarian tissue cryopreservation

B. FP would not be useful since the patient is planning to have a hysterectomy

C. Oocyte cryopreservation would not possible since the patient has been treated with testosterone; the only viable option is ovarian tissue cryopreservation

D. The patient declined FP in the past, so it would be best not to address this issue again

E. The patient should proceed with the surgery right now as planned; fertility can be addressed in the future

Answer: A) FP options should be discussed prior to surgery, including oocyte cryopreservation and ovarian tissue cryopreservation

According to the recently published *World Professional Association for Transgender Care Standards of Care, Version 8*, FP should be offered prior to any gender-affirming medical or surgical intervention that could negatively impact fertility (thus, Answer A is correct and Answer E is incorrect).

Discussions should occur on an ongoing basis, as perspectives on family building may evolve over time (thus, Answer D is incorrect), and clinicians should distinguish between fertility (having a genetically related child) vs pregnancy (thus, Answer B is incorrect).

Finally, several publications have described pregnancies (planned and unplanned) and successful oocyte cryopreservation in individuals who have received testosterone therapy (thus, Answer C is incorrect).

Case 3

A 21-year-old transgender female presenting to endocrinology to discuss gender-affirming treatments. She has been undergoing a social transition over the past year. During the discussion about estrogen therapy and potential effects on fertility, she becomes tearful. She states that she has always wanted to have genetically related children but is not sure if she will be comfortable masturbating to produce the sample. Plus, she is wondering if it would be weird to be a mother yet have a child with her sperm.

Which of the following is the best way to guide this patient?

A. Since masturbation is the only way a semen sample can be collected for cryopreservation, the patient will have to decide how she would like to proceed

B. Tell her that she is not a good candidate for estrogen therapy

C. Encourage her to talk about these concerns with her therapist and offer to refer her to a urologist to discuss alternative sperm retrieval options, after which she can return to clinic and proceed with estrogen therapy

D. Prescribe estrogen and advise her that adoption would be her best option for parenthood

E. Tell her that she can start estrogen therapy and then decide in 6 to 12 months if she wants to bank sperm

Answer: C) Encourage her to talk about these concerns with her therapist and offer to refer her to a urologist to discuss alternative sperm retrieval options, after which she can return to clinic and proceed with estrogen therapy

This patient's concerns are understandable and have been reported by TGD populations. These concerns should be addressed appropriately to avoid future regret, and they do not make her ineligible for gender-affirming hormones (thus, Answers B and D are incorrect). She should be encouraged to talk about her concerns with her therapist and she could be referred to a urologist to discuss alternative sperm retrieval options (Answer C).

Further, although self-stimulation is the first-line option, alternative methods such as electroejaculation or testicular sperm extraction could be considered (thus, Answer A is incorrect).

Finally, based on the current body of evidence, we cannot conclude that spermatogenesis would be intact after 6 to 12 months of estrogen therapy (thus, Answer E is incorrect).

Key Learning Points

- Gender-affirming hormonal interventions and surgeries may impact reproductive capacity to varying degrees, and sometimes irreversibly.

- To mitigate psychosocial distress and prevent regret, reproductive health counseling (including fertility-related risks, FP options, and need for contraception) should routinely occur before initiating these gender-affirming therapies and should continue on an ongoing basis.

- Sperm, oocyte, and embryo cryopreservation are the first-line FP options for TGD adolescent and young adult populations; gonadal tissue cryopreservation is the only available option for prepubertal children and should be offered to TGD adults in the context of gonadectomy.

- Patient, provider, and structural barriers must be addressed to facilitate shared decision-making about FP and improve access to high-quality, equitable care for TGD populations.

- Prospective, longitudinal research is needed to clarify fertility impacts of gender-affirming treatments and to examine reproductive health outcomes in this population.

References

1. Defreyne J, Van Schuylenbergh J, Motmans J, Tilleman KL, T'Sjoen GGR. Parental desire and fertility preservation in assigned female at birth transgender people living in Belgium. *Fertil Steril.* 2020;113(1):149-157.e2. PMID: 31727413

2. Nahata L, Chen D, Quinn GP, et al. Reproductive attitudes and behaviors among transgender/nonbinary adolescents. *J Adolesc Health.* 2020;66(3):372-374. PMID: 32029201

3. Coleman E, Radix AE, Bouman WP, et al. Standards of care for the health of transgender and gender diverse people, version 8. *Int J Transgend Health.* 2022;23(Suppl 1):S1-S259. PMID: 36238954

4. Moravek MB, Kinnear HM, George J, et al. Impact of exogenous testosterone on reproduction in transgender men. *Endocrinology.* 2020;161(3):bqaa014. PMID: 32105330

5. Jindarak S, Nilprapha K, Atikankul T, et al. Spermatogenesis abnormalities following hormonal therapy in transwomen. *Biomed Res Int.* 2018;2018:7919481. PMID: 29808166

6. Practice Committee of the American Society for Reproductive Medicine. Fertility preservation in patients undergoing gonadotoxic therapy or gonadectomy: a committee opinion. *Fertil Steril.* 2019;112(6):1022-1033. PMID: 31843073

7. Ellis SJ, Wakefield CE, McLoone JK, Robertson EG, Cohn RJ. Fertility concerns among child and adolescent cancer survivors and their parents: a qualitative analysis. *J Psychosoc Oncol.* 2016;34(5):347-362. PMID: 27269305

8. Stein DM, Victorson DE, Choy JT, et al. Fertility preservation preferences and perspectives among adult male survivors of pediatric cancer and their parents. *J Adolesc Young Adult Oncol.* 2014;3(2):75-82.

9. Chen D, Matson M, Macapagal K, et al. Attitudes toward fertility and reproductive health among transgender and gender-nonconforming adolescents. *J Adolesc Health.* 2018;63(1):62-68. PMID: 29503031

10. Tishelman AC, Sutter ME, Chen D, et al. Health care provider perceptions of fertility preservation barriers and challenges with transgender patients and families: qualitative responses to an international survey. *J Assisted Reprod Genet.* 201936(3):579-588. PMID: 30604136

11. Chen D, Kolbuck VD, Sutter ME, Tishelman AC, Quinn GP, Nahata L. Knowledge, practice behaviors, and perceived barriers to fertility care among providers of transgender healthcare. *J Adolesc Health.* 2019;64(2):226-234. PMID: 30661518

12. Hoffkling A, Obedin-Maliver J, Sevelius J. From erasure to opportunity: a qualitative study of the experiences of transgender men around pregnancy and recommendations for providers. *BMC Pregnancy Childbirth.* 2017;17(Suppl 2):332. PMID: 29143629

13. de Nie I, Meissner A, Kostelijk EH, et al. Impaired semen quality in trans women: prevalence and determinants. *Hum Reprod.* 2020;35(7):1529-1536. PMID: 326132241

14. Fraison E, Huberlant S, Labrune E, et al. Live birth rate after female fertility preservation for cancer or haematopoietic stem cell transplantation: a systematic review and meta-analysis of the three main techniques; embryo, oocyte and ovarian tissue cryopreservation. *Hum Reprod.* 2023;38(3):489-502. PMID: 36421038

15. Nahata L, Campo-Engelstein LT, Tishelman A, Quinn GP, Lantos JD. Fertility preservation for a transgender teenager. *Pediatrics.* 2018;142(3):e20173142

Exogenous estrogens are associated with increased risk of venous thromboembolism (VTE) in a dose-dependent fashion.[8] Ethinyl estradiol is associated with a higher VTE risk than other estrogen products. It is not clear to what degree risk may also be related to route of administration, duration of hormone therapy, product choice (other than avoiding ethinyl estradiol), or other factors.

Although the VTE risk related to exogenous estrogens has resulted in surgeons asking transfeminine patients to suspend hormone therapy in the perioperative period, the only data to date found that hormone therapy during the perioperative period did not alter VTE risk in transfeminine people in a tertiary care setting with an aggressive VTE prophylaxis program.[9]

Data to date do not include rigorous evidence supporting a benefit of progestogen therapy for transgender women, including for breast growth. The only data for progestogens documents harm.[5] When added to conjugated equine estrogen therapy in older cisgender women, medroxyprogesterone is associated with greater risk for heart disease and breast cancer. Progestogens are associated with increased VTE risk when added to estrogen regimens (eg, in oral contraceptives for younger cisgender women). When paired with estrogens for transgender women, the progestogen cyproterone acetate is associated with elevated prolactin, decreased HDL cholesterol, and rare meningiomas—none of which are seen when estrogens are paired with GnRH agonists or spironolactone.

Adult Masculinizing GAHT

The typical masculinizing GAHT regimen consists of testosterone therapy (*box 2*) to achieve typical male levels of circulating testosterone (300-1000 ng/dL [10.4-34.7 nmol/L]). The most common routes of administration are weekly injections and daily transdermal gels. Patches, longer-acting injections, implanted pellets, and buccal patches may also be available.

Box 2. Masculinizing GAHT Regimens

Testosterone

Parenteral

- Testosterone esters (cypionate or enanthate), 50-100 mg intramuscularly/subcutaneously
  - weekly (some give larger doses every 2 weeks)
- Testosterone undecanoate, 1000 mg every 12 weeks

Transdermal

- Testosterone gel, 60-120 mg daily
- Testosterone patch, 2-8 mg daily

Oral

- Testosterone undecanoate, 160-240 mg daily

Adapted from Safer JD & Tangpricha V. N Engl J Med, 2019; 381(25): 2451-2460. © Massachusetts Medical Society.

While there have been observations connecting exogenous testosterone to increased blood pressure and LDL-cholesterol levels and decreased HDL-cholesterol levels, no significant differences in cardiac mortality outcomes are observed when studies of transgender men are pooled and compared with outcomes in the general population.[10,11]

There have not been observations of increased rates of malignancy associated with masculinizing GAHT.

Clinical Case Vignettes
Case 1

A 22-year-old transgender woman who had feminizing GAHT prescribed by her primary care provider comes to the endocrinology clinic because her testosterone concentration is reportedly above the typical target. She would like guidance regarding what to do next.

The patient has no relevant medical or mental health history. She became aware of her female gender identity in high school, but on reflection, her feminine gender identity goes back as far as she can remember. She decided to start gender-affirming medical treatment in college and started GAHT 2 years ago.

Her physical examination findings are normal and include modest breast development.

The patient's GAHT regimen consists of oral estradiol, 6 mg daily, and oral bicalutamide, 50 mg daily. She takes no other medications.

Laboratory test results:

> Total testosterone = 95 ng/dL (SI: 3.3 nmol/L)
> Estradiol = 250 pg/mL (SI: 917.8 pmol/L)

Which of the following would be the most reasonable change to her medication regimen?

A. Add ethinyl estradiol

B. Add micronized progesterone

C. Increase 17β-estradiol

D. Replace with conjugated equine estrogens

Answer: C) Increase 17β-estradiol

17β-Estradiol (Answer C) is the preferred estrogen for GAHT relative to the other options offered. The literature reports a notable decrease in observed VTE when the estrogen of choice changes from ethinyl estradiol to 17β-estradiol. There are modest data for increased VTE risk with conjugated equine estrogens that are not observed with 17β-estradiol. Data with micronized progesterone are few, but other progestogens have been associated with increased VTE risk, increased coronary artery disease risk, and increased breast cancer risk in some populations, at least when used for long periods. Although the guidelines include a target estradiol range of 100 to 200 pg/mL (367.1-734.2 pmol/L), it is not clear how that should be nuanced relative to the goal to suppress testosterone below 50 ng/dL (<1.7 nmol/L). Total testosterone measured by liquid chromatography–tandem mass spectrometry is the most reliable assay.

Case 1 (continued)

Which of the following medications should replace bicalutamide?

A. Finasteride

B. Increased estrogen dosing

C. Micronized progesterone

D. Spironolactone

Answer: D) Spironolactone

Although rare, the concern with bicalutamide is fulminant hepatitis resulting in death. There is no warning and no way to monitor. Per the guidelines, spironolactone (Answer D) is the preferred agent. Finasteride (Answer A) has only been demonstrated to have efficacy when used to decrease conversion of typically male levels of testosterone to dihydrotestosterone. Benefit to people with lower circulating levels of testosterone (cis women) has not been established. Conservative options include replacing bicalutamide with a GnRH agonist. It remains to be established if even a slightly higher estrogen dose would be safer than bicalutamide.

Case 2

A 35-year-old transgender woman who has been taking GAHT for 13 years has a plan for vaginoplasty with an experienced surgeon. The surgeon is aware that exogenous estrogens may be associated with increased risk of VTE. The patient has no relevant medical or mental health history. She became aware of her female gender identity in childhood, and she decided to start gender-affirming medical treatment in college.

The patient's gender-affirming hormone medication regimen consists of oral estradiol, 4 mg daily, and oral spironolactone, 200 mg daily. She takes no other medication.

Findings on physical examination are normal and include significant breast development.

Laboratory test results:

> Total testosterone = 25 ng/dL (SI: 0.87 nmol/L)
> Estradiol = 110 pg/mL (SI: 403.8 pmol/L)

The surgery team reaches out to Endocrinology for guidance regarding the recommended strategy for VTE prophylaxis for this patient.

Which of following approaches would best minimize this patient's VTE risk in the perioperative period?

A. Begin short-term anticoagulation therapy

B. Change oral regimen to a topical regimen

C. Hold estradiol

D. Recommend early ambulation after surgery

Answer: D) Recommend early ambulation after surgery

Three studies have documented no increased VTE risk in aging transgender women who use transdermal estrogen products. While there are no comparative studies, the data to date suggest that transdermal products can be safe in that setting.

However, the only data collected to date show no increase of VTE risk for TGD people who maintain their hormone regimens while undergoing surgery (including those taking estrogens and having vaginoplasty), at least in the setting of an intense VTE prophylaxis regimen in a tertiary care setting that includes early ambulation (Answer D). It is not clear that there is a harm on which to improve with either a change in the estrogen treatment regimen (Answers B or C) or with an anticoagulation approach (Answer A) not otherwise indicated.

Case 3

A 24-year-old transgender person presents to an endocrinology clinic for advice regarding low-dosage testosterone. The patient was recorded as female on the original birth certificate and now uses they/them pronouns. The patient has no relevant medical history. They have never had GAHT or surgery. They are interested in an androgynous appearance but want to avoid facial hair or voice deepening.

Physical examination findings are normal.

Laboratory test results:

Total testosterone = 35 ng/dL (SI: 1.2 nmol/L)

Which of the following is the best recommendation for this patient?

A. Begin testosterone at a low-dosage and stop if there are unwanted changes

B. Begin testosterone only if willing to accept masculinizing changes

C. Combine testosterone with estrogens to achieve the patient's goals

D. Explain that testosterone is not indicated

Answer: B) Begin testosterone only if willing to accept masculinizing changes

Some TGD people may be interested in low-dosage regimens. As long as hypogonadism is avoided, there are no data to suggest concern for regimens across the spectrum from typical male to typical female. However, it is not reliably possible to titrate to specific physical endpoints or to choose the tissues that will respond to exogenous hormone therapy. Therefore, hormone therapy only makes sense if the patient recognizes that they (or some of their tissues) may be more sensitive or less sensitive than they might prefer. Testosterone can be prescribed in low dosages, but the patient should be comfortable with some facial hair, some lowering of the voice, and even some misgendering with "he" pronouns (Answer B). Although this patient uses "they" pronouns and wants a low-dosage hormone regimen, those are not necessarily connected and the goals need to be asked independently of the pronouns. Some people using "they" pronouns may want binary hormone regimens and some people using binary pronouns (he or she) may want low-dosage regimens.

Case 4

A 27-year-old transgender man presents to an endocrinology clinic for counsel regarding reproductive organs. He has no relevant medical history. He has been treated with testosterone since age 18 years and had chest masculinization surgery at that time. The patient's GAHT regimen consists of subcutaneous testosterone cypionate, 80 mg self-administered by the patient weekly.

The patient is in a relationship with a 35-year-old cisgender female partner. They have discussed having children, which has prompted this clinic visit.

Physical examination findings are normal. There is no significant breast tissue. Examination of external genitalia demonstrates clitoromegaly consistent with the history of testosterone treatment.

Laboratory test result (48 hours after testosterone injection):

Total testosterone = 655 ng/dL (SI: 22.7 nmol/L)

Which of the following is the best advice for the patient now?

A. Add a progestogen to the GAHT regimen to preserve ovarian reserve

B. Decrease testosterone dosage to determine if menses can be induced

C. Retain ovaries to preserve fertility options during potential childbearing years

D. Undergo hysterectomy and bilateral oophorectomy now to mitigate future cancer risk

Answer: C) Retain ovaries to preserve fertility options during potential childbearing years

Fertility preservation for transmasculine people may include oocyte cryopreservation or retaining ovaries through potential childbearing years. The patient has no history of oocyte cryopreservation. It may be that the couple will use the cis partner's oocytes and uterus along with donor sperm. That would be easiest. However, stimulated oocyte retrieval from the patient's ovaries could be an option. The best recommendation is to retain the ovaries to preserve fertility options during potential childbearing years (Answer C). There are no data for increased ovarian cancer risk in transgender men relative to cisgender women. In any case, oophorectomy to address that concern could happen when the patient is older than he is now.

Case 5

A 19-year-old transgender woman is hospitalized after a suicidal gesture. The patient and the inpatient team determine that she will likely remain in the hospital for 10 days. The inpatient team wants to simplify the medical regimen as much as possible. She has no significant medical history. She has a history of depression treated with bupropion. This is her first-ever mental health hospitalization.

The patient reports that she became aware of her female gender identity in childhood and began taking GnRH agonist therapy when puberty began. She started GAHT at age 17 years and has been on a stable regimen for 12 months. The patient's GAHT consists of oral estradiol, 4 mg daily, and oral spironolactone, 200 mg daily. She also takes lamotrigine.

Physical examination findings are normal and include significant breast development.

Laboratory test results:

Total testosterone = 35 ng/dL (SI: 1.2 nmol/L)
Estradiol = 125 pg/mL (SI: 458.9 pmol/L)

The inpatient psychiatry team discontinues estradiol and spironolactone on admission and reaches out to Endocrinology for guidance regarding recommended strategy.

Which of the following is the best recommendation?

A. Continue GAHT as prescribed outpatient

B. Cut GAHT dosing in half

C. Increase 17β-estradiol dosage

D. Suspend GAHT

Answer: A) Continue GAHT as prescribed outpatient

The primary message from this case is to avoid the introduction of variables when the mental health situation is unstable. While recommendations often point out the wisdom of delaying GAHT until any relevant medical and mental health morbidity is appropriately addressed, the opposite may also be true. That is, someone on a stable

GAHT regimen is likely to do better if that is left in place (Answer A) while other concerns are addressed, such as mental health instability.[5]

Key Learning Points

- 17β-Estradiol is the preferred estrogen for GAHT.

- Progestogens have been associated with increased VTE risk, increased coronary artery disease risk, and increased breast cancer risk in some populations, at least when used for long periods.

- Fertility preservation is a major consideration prior to any gender-affirming medical intervention, including treatment to delay puberty.

- Gender labels and hormone treatment desires are not necessarily connected; goals need to be inquired about independently of pronouns.

- A patient on a stable GAHT regimen is likely to do better if that is left in place while other concerns, such as mental health instability, are addressed.

References

1. Hembree WC, Cohen-Kettenis PT, Gooren L, et al. Endocrine treatment of gender-dysphoric/gender-incongruent persons: an Endocrine Society clinical practice guideline. *J Clin Endocrinol Metab.* 2017;102(11):3869-3903. PMID: 28945902

2. Flores AR, Herman JL, Gates GJ, Brown TNT. How many adults identify as transgender in the United States? https://williamsinstitute.law.ucla.edu/publications/trans-adults-united-states/. Accessed March 10, 2021.

3. Safer JD. Research gaps in medical treatment of transgender/nonbinary people. *J Clin Invest.* 2021;131(4):e142029. PMID: 33586675

4. Fernández Rodríguez M, Menéndez Granda M, Villaverde González A. Gender incongruence is no longer a mental disorder. *J Ment Health Clin Psychol.* 2018;2:6-8

5. Coleman E, Radix AE, Bouman WP, et al. Standards of care for the health of transgender and gender diverse people, version 8. *Int J Transgend Health.* 2022;23(Supp 1):S1-S259. PMID: 36238954

6. Safer JD, Tangpricha V. Care of transgender persons. *N Engl J Med.* 2019;381(25):2451-2460. PMID: 31851801

7. Tebbens M, Heijboer AC, T'Sjoen G, Bisschop PH, den Heijer M. The role of estrone in feminizing hormone treatment. *J Clin Endocrinol Metab.* 2022;107(2):e458-e466. PMID: 34632510

8. Vinogradova Y, Coupland C, Hippisley-Cox J. Use of hormone replacement therapy and risk of venous thromboembolism: nested case-control studies using the QResearch and CPRD databases. *BMJ.* 2019;364:k4810. PMID: 30626577

9. Kozato A, Fox GWC, Yong PC, et al. No venous thromboembolism increase among transgender female patients remaining on estrogen for gender-affirming surgery. *J Clin Endocrinol Metab.* 2021;106(4):1586-1590. PMID: 33417686

10. T'Sjoen G, Arcelus J, Gooren L, Klink DT, Tangpricha V. Endocrinology of transgender medicine. *Endocr Rev.* 2019;40:97-117. PMID: 30307546

11. Slack DJ, Safer JD. Cardiovascular health maintenance in aging individuals: the implications for transgender men and women on hormone therapy. *Endocr Pract.* 2021;27(1):63-70. PMID: 33475503

Long-Term Outcomes After Gender-Affirming Surgeries

Brielle Weinstein, MD. Department of Surgery, Rush University Medical Center, Chicago, IL; Email: Brielle_Weinstein@rush.edu

Rebecca B. Schechter, MD. Highland Park, IL; Email: Rebeccabschechter@gmail.com

Loren S. Schechter, MD. Department of Surgery, Rush University Medical Center, Chicago, IL; Email: Loren_Schechter@rush.edu

Educational Objectives

After reviewing this chapter, learners should be able to:

- Identify the surgical options available to help gender-diverse individuals.

- Explain the preoperative and postoperative care of individuals undergoing gender-affirming surgery.

- Describe significant outcome measures used to evaluate individuals undergoing gender-affirming surgery.

Significance of the Clinical Problem

Gender incongruence refers to an individual whose gender identity is different from their sex assigned at birth. Gender dysphoria describes the distress and/or impairment resulting from gender incongruence. Some people with gender dysphoria seek medical and/or surgical interventions with goals to align their body (ie, anatomy and secondary sex characteristics) with their gender identity. Using guidelines developed by the World Professional Association for Transgender Health (WPATH) referred to as the *Standards of Care Version 8 (SOC8)* and the Endocrine Society, health care providers can provide personalized and medically necessary care for individuals with gender incongruence/dysphoria. Optimal care requires a multidisciplinary approach involving primary care professionals, mental/behavioral health professionals, endocrinologists, surgeons, and other health professionals (ie, pelvic floor physical therapists, social workers, advanced practice providers, etc).

Gender-affirming surgeries are designed to align physical and anatomic characteristics with a person's gender identity. Transfeminine surgeries include augmentation mammaplasty, vaginoplasty, facial feminization, and body-contouring procedures. Transmasculine surgeries include top surgery (gender-affirming mastectomy), metoidioplasty (lengthening of the hormonally hypertrophied clitoris), phalloplasty, and body contouring. Surgical complication rates are commensurate with those in other complex reconstructive procedures. In appropriately selected individuals, gender-affirming surgery alleviates or ameliorates gender dysphoria, improves mental health outcomes, reduces negative health outcomes, and improves body self-image. "Regret" is a complex and often mischaracterized condition. Nevertheless, "regret" remains uncommon. Levels of evidence to support surgical interventions are consistent with those in many other areas of plastic surgery.

The number of individuals who identify as transgender or gender diverse (TGD) and who seek medical care continues to increase.[1] While awareness of TGD rights has improved in recent years, the TGD population remains vulnerable and frequently stigmatized. TGD people throughout the world experience discrimination, prejudice, and violence resulting in marginalization, poor health, and, in some cases, death. The overarching objective of gender-affirming care is to help TGD people optimize their physical health and psychological well-being to achieve lasting comfort and fulfillment.[1] In addition to providing individualized, patient-centered care, health care professionals should facilitate access to safe and effective care.

Practice Gaps

- Misinformation/misinterpretation of the nature of care and evidence supporting it.

- Lack of access due to limited providers with expertise in gender-affirming care.

Discussion

Multidisciplinary Care With Guidance From WPATH and the Endocrine Society

Gender-affirming surgery is delivered within a complex health care system and requires collaboration among health care professionals. While not all members of the team may practice within the same institution (or city, state, country), these individuals should communicate (often in writing) their findings and recommendations. Experts in different disciplines can bolster each other's understanding of a patient's request(s) and strengthen the shared decision-making process. Primary care and mental/behavioral health professionals should be willing to participate in the aftercare of surgical patients. This includes social and emotional support, as well as assistance with medical and/or surgical follow-up.

Both WPATH and the Endocrine Society provide health care professionals with guidelines to evaluate and care for TGD individuals.[1,2] WPATH's *SOC8*, released in 2022, based its

recommendations on evaluation of published literature, background evidence, and consensus expert opinion. These guidelines are intended to be flexible, providing health care professionals a framework within which to care for TGD individuals. Recommendations incorporate the need for attention to benefits and harms, values, and preferences.

The surgeon often meets TGD individuals after they have established longitudinal relationships with mental/behavioral health and medical experts. The surgeon gains insight into the needs and expectations of an individual from the individual themselves, as well as from other treating health care providers. These longitudinal relationships help patients explore and solidify which procedures, if any, will benefit their mental and physical health. To provide "informed consent," patients need to understand not only the technical aspects and risks of surgery but also how surgery will affect other aspects of their lives (family, professional, intimate relationships, etc). Understanding and optimizing the psychosocial and medical conditions of individuals undergoing gender-affirming surgical interventions supports high-quality care, helps manage patient expectations, and allows the field to advance.

Transfeminine Surgery

Transwomen may request vaginoplasty, augmentation mammaplasty, facial feminization, and body-contouring procedures to meet their individual goals. Often, vaginoplasty and breast augmentation can be performed concurrently, at one surgical setting.

Vaginoplasty
Penile inversion vaginoplasty is the most commonly performed vaginoplasty technique. However, individuals treated with GnRH analogues before completing puberty may not have sufficient penile length, and alternative procedures (ie, intestinal vaginoplasty, peritoneal vaginoplasty, additional skin grafts) may be required.[3] Pertinent preoperative discussions include existing genitourinary function, sexual

goals, fertility, hair removal, and nicotine use. Surgeons may recommend cessation of hormones preoperatively for a potential risk of increased venous thromboembolic events,[4] although this is debated.

Most complications following vaginoplasty are minor and self-limited (wound healing disruptions).[5] Rates of serious complications, such as rectal or genitourinary injury and/or reoperation for wound complications, following vaginoplasty are low and comparable to complications of other genitourinary reconstruction surgeries.[6-9] Risk factors, such as advanced age, BMI, diabetes, and cigarette smoking history, may be associated with complications.[10,11] In addition, nonadherence with postoperative protocols (dilation and activity restrictions) has been associated with surgical complications.[9] With this in mind, preoperative strategies (surgical "prehabilitation") to understand possible barriers to aftercare (caregiver support, safe housing, food security, transportation, etc) help ensure adherence.

The *SOC8* provides references of 8 prospective, 15 retrospective, and 3 cross-sectional studies that evaluate vaginoplasty.[1] As a whole, these studies have concluded that gender-affirming vaginoplasty improves quality of life, decreases gender dysphoria, and improves body image. Rates of regret are low (0%-8%).

Augmentation Mammaplasty
Breast augmentation is often requested with vaginoplasty or as an independent procedure. Preoperative breast cancer screening should be considered based on patient age, personal/family history, physical examination, and duration of hormone use.[1] Imaging guidelines are published by the American College of Radiology.[12] Feminizing hormones contribute to breast growth and feminization of the chest/torso. While *SOC8* does not require hormone use prior to breast augmentation, estrogen can aid in breast development, skin expansion, and subsequent implant placement. Augmentation mammaplasty has been shown to consistently improve body

image satisfaction and general satisfaction with a trend toward improved depression and anxiety scores.[13-15] Historically, insurance providers considered breast augmentation a "cosmetic" procedure. As noted in the *SOC7*, these procedures can have a radical and permanent effect on quality of life.[16] *SOC8* considers breast augmentation to be medically necessary when performed on the basis of gender incongruence/gender dysphoria and recommends insurance coverage.[1]

Facial Feminization
Facial feminization surgery is a constellation of reconstructive procedures aimed to modify "masculine" characteristics of the face to create a more feminine appearance. This may involve hairline lowering, brow lift, frontal sinus recession, rhinoplasty, genioplasty, mandibular angle contouring, and chondrolaryngoplasty, among others. As detailed in *SOC8*, reported patient satisfaction levels range between 72% and 100% following facial feminization procedures.[1] Additionally, one international, prospective study demonstrated that facial procedures improved mid-term and long-term quality of life.[17] *SOC8* also consider these procedures to be medically necessary when performed on the basis of gender incongruence/gender dysphoria and recommends insurance coverage.[1]

Transmasculine Surgery

Transmasculine surgeries may include mastectomy, genital surgery (metoidioplasty/phalloplasty, hysterectomy/oophorectomy, colpectomy/colpocleisis), facial, and body-contouring procedures. Chest surgery is the most commonly performed procedure. Many of these procedures are performed in a staged manner. Others (ie, mastectomy and hysterectomy) may be combined in a single surgical setting.

Chest Surgery
The goals of chest surgery include contouring of the chest by removal of breast tissue and excess skin, reduction and repositioning of the nipple-areola complex, release of the inframammary

crease, liposuction of the chest (when necessary), and, when possible, minimization of chest scars and preservation of nipple sensitivity. Preoperative mammography should be considered in individuals with risk factors for breast cancer, such as age, personal or family history of breast cancer, and physical examination findings.[12] Choice of surgical technique depends on breast volume, breast ptosis, and skin elasticity. Small breasts with elastic skin envelopes may be amenable to periareolar incisions, whereas larger breasts with loss of skin elasticity (manifested by striae and breast ptosis) may require the traditional "double-incision" approach. Complications are generally self-limited (ie, healing disruptions), but also include hematoma, seroma, infection, and loss of nipple graft(s).[18-20] Hematoma is the most commonly reported reason for reoperation in the acute postoperative period.[19] Revision requested for aesthetic concerns may be surgeon- and technique-dependent. In the senior author's practice, revisions occur in less than 5%, while rates in the literature vary between 9.0% and 40.4%.[18-20] Rates of revision may also vary with body habitus (ie, obesity).

Studies referenced in *SOC8* assessed improvement in quality of life following chest surgery. These studies included preoperative and postoperative surveys.[1] Significant improvements in breast satisfaction, psychosocial well-being, sexual satisfaction, and physical well-being are reported.[1] Almost all participants reported improved body image, higher quality of life, and improved self-esteem.

Metoidioplasty/Phalloplasty

Masculinizing genital surgery is a complex procedure that may involve construction of a phallus, often a urethra, and may include removal of the vaginal canal (and/or uterus and ovaries). Surgical goals include an aesthetic phallus and scrotum, standing micturition, and the ability to engage in penetrative intercourse. Procedures include metoidioplasty (lengthening of the hormonally hypertrophied clitoris), urethral lengthening, pedicle or free tissue transfer,

monsplasty (removal of skin and subcutaneous fat in the lower abdominal region), and penile and/ or scrotal implants. A shared decision-making process with the use of decisional aids helps meet patients' individual goals while balancing risks of the procedure(s). Various staging regimens are used for phalloplasty. The rationale for staging the procedures is to reduce the frequency and magnitude/impact of complications and to isolate urinary and healing-related complications. While the radial forearm flap is the most commonly used phalloplasty technique, anterior lateral thigh, lower abdomen (superficial circumflex iliac perforator flaps (suprapubic flaps), and back (musculocutaneous latissimus dorsi) are also options. Urethral reconstruction, placement of penile and testicular implants, scrotoplasty, and other procedures may be performed at different stages.

Complications following phalloplasty can be classified as urinary-, flap- (ie, healing), or prosthetic-related. In a systematic review and meta-analysis, urinary complications included a urinary fistula rate of 34.1% and urinary stricture rate of 25.4%.[21] Total flap loss is uncommon (3%), but partial flap loss is more common (11%).[21] Despite challenges, patients report long-term satisfaction[22] and improved quality of life.[23] A reported 75% to 100% of study participants were able to void while standing, 77% to 95% of participants reported satisfaction with their sexual function, and no participants reported regret.[1]

Surgery in Adolescents

While the number of adolescents identifying as gender diverse continues to increase, there is no unifying reason to explain how young persons come to understand their gender needs. Multidisciplinary teams working with adolescents and their families should explore all aspects of development when collectively determining whether an intervention meets a person's needs. Discussion with the adolescent and their parents/caregivers includes, but is not limited to reproductive options (including breastfeeding), sexual function, regret and/or evolution of gender identity (including gender fluidity), and family/social support. Transgender youth are a vulnerable group at risk for life-threatening behaviors.[24] Decisions as to whether to perform surgical interventions and the timing of surgical interventions require considerable discussion. Surgery on adolescents requires a multidisciplinary approach with professionals from behavioral/mental health, primary care, and surgery. While surgery on adolescents is uncommon, it may be considered in select people on an individual, case-by-case basis.

In carefully selected adolescents who exhibit sustained and severe distress following breast development, chest surgery may be considered. Compared with transmasculine youth who did not undergo top surgery, adolescents and young adults with gender dysphoria who underwent top surgery have shown significant improvement in gender dysphoria, gender congruence, and body image satisfaction.[25,26] Complication rates were low,[25,26] and self-reported regret was near zero.[25] Genital surgery, although rare in adolescents, may be performed in highly select people on a case-by-case basis. Again, and importantly, input from the multidisciplinary team is essential, and discussions include, but are not limited to reproductive options, sexual function, regret and/or evolution of gender identity (including gender fluidity), and family/social support.

Clinical Case Vignettes

Case 1

A 42-year-old transgender woman (she/her) presents for gender-affirming vaginoplasty. She has taken estrogen for more than 10 years. Her goals include a vagina capable of receptive intercourse. She is not interested in fertility preservation. She has no family history of breast cancer.

In counseling the patient on the surgical process of penile inversion vaginoplasty, which of the following structures is used to form the clitoris?

A. Glans penis

B. Penile shaft skin

C. Scrotal skin

D. Skin graft

E. Urethra

Answer: A) Glans penis

A portion of the glans penis (Answer A) is maintained on the dorsal penile nerves and vessels to form the clitoris in gender-affirming vaginoplasty. In penile inversion technique, the scrotal skin is used as a skin graft to line the vaginal canal, the penile shaft skin is used to form the introitus and labia minora, the urethra is used to form the new urethral meatus and labia minora.

Case 2

A 28-year-old transgender man (he/him) presents for evaluation for masculinizing chest surgery. He has been taking testosterone for 6 years and has been binding his chest during that time. He reports no family history of breast or ovarian cancer. He is contemplating whether he wants to maintain his nipple areolar complex following surgery. He ultimately decides to forego surgical reconstruction of the nipple-areola complex and opts for reconstruction with tattoo.

On physical examination, the patient has large, pendulous breasts with grade 3 ptosis and loss of skin elasticity with striae present. No palpable masses, lymphadenopathy, skin retraction, nipple retraction, or discharge are noted.

Which of the following techniques will best allow the surgeon to meet the patient's goals (flat contour of the chest) and remove excess skin and breast tissue?

A. Double incision mastectomy with nipple areolar graft

B. Double incision mastectomy without nipple areolar graft

C. Liposuction

D. Periareolar/keyhole mastectomy

E. Wise-pattern breast reduction

Answer: B) Double incision mastectomy without nipple areolar graft

Multiple incision patterns can be used for gender-affirming mastectomy. Patient-specific goals, anatomy, and risks are considered in a shared decision-making process to determine the best option for each patient. Based on his physical examination, a double-incision technique will be required to remove skin and glandular tissue. The nipple-areola complex will not be replaced, as he opted for nipple-areola tattoo (thus, Answer B is correct and Answer A is incorrect).

Liposuction (Answer C) may be used as an adjunct to contour the periphery of the chest.

The periareolar approach (Answer D) does not allow for sufficient skin resection, and skin redundancy can be anticipated following surgery.

A Wise-pattern breast reduction (Answer E) is most commonly used in cisgender women as a treatment for breast hypertrophy and symptomatic macromastia. Its utility in masculinizing chest surgery is limited.

Case 3

A 38-year-old transgender man (he/him) presents for masculinizing bottom surgery. His goals include standing micturition, closure of the vaginal canal, and penetrative intercourse. He has taken testosterone for more than years. He has not had a hysterectomy or oophorectomy. He is not interested in fertility preservation.

Which of the following procedures will help this patient meet his current goal?

A. Hysterectomy alone

B. Metoidioplasty with urethral lengthening

C. Monsplasty

D. Radial forearm phalloplasty with urethral lengthening, hysterectomy, colpectomy with colpocleisis, and placement of penile prosthesis

E. Testicular implants

Answer: D) Radial forearm phalloplasty with urethral lengthening, hysterectomy, colpectomy with colpocleisis, and placement of penile prosthesis

Phalloplasty with urethral lengthening, hysterectomy (+/- oophorectomy), colpectomy with colpocleisis, and staged placement of a penile prosthesis (Answer D) are required to accomplish this patient's goals. If colpectomy and colpocleisis are requested, a hysterectomy must be performed (to prevent uterine secretion). While these procedures may be performed in a staged fashion, this constellation will be required to provide: (1) a phallus capable of standing micturition and penetrative intercourse and (2) closure of the vaginal canal with masculinization of the perineum.

Metoidioplasty (release of the clitoris) with urethroplasty (Answer B) will allow for standing micturition. However, penetrative intercourse is not possible following metoidioplasty.

If colpectomy/colpocleisis (removal of the vaginal lining with closure of the vaginal canal) is requested, a hysterectomy is required (Answer A) because once the vaginal canal is closed, there is no path for egress of uterine secretions. This necessitates a hysterectomy.

Monsplasty (Answer C) is used to resect the skin and fatty tissue overlying the pubis. This is typically performed to masculinize the pubic region and allow additional exposure of the phallus.

Testicular implants (Answer E) are performed as the last stage of masculinizing genital surgery. The implants fill the scrotal sac. Most often, testicular implants are not performed concurrent with urethral reconstruction due to risks of implant infection and extrusion.

Key Learning Points

- In appropriately selected individuals, gender-affirming surgery can alleviate gender dysphoria and improve quality of life.

- Optimal care for TGD individuals requires a multidisciplinary team with frequent communication.

- Regret following gender-affirming surgery is uncommon.

References

1. Coleman E, Radix AE, Bouman WP, et al. Standards of care for the health of transgender and gender diverse people, version 8. *Int J Transgend Health.* 2022;23(Suppl 1):S1-S259. PMID: 36238954

2. Hembree WC, Cohen-Kettenis PT, Gooren L, et al. Endocrine treatment of gender-dysphoric/gender-incongruent persons: an Endocrine Society clinical practice guideline. *J Clin Endocrinol Metab.* 2017;102(11):3869-3903. PMID: 28945902

3. van de Grift TC, van Gelder ZJ, Mullender MG, Steensma TD, de Vries ALC, Bouman MB. Timing of puberty suppression and soptions for transgender youth. *Pediatrics.* 2020;146(5):e20193653. PMID: 33106340

4. Kozato A, Fox GWC, Yong PC, et al. No venous thromboembolism increase among transgender female patients remaining on estrogen for gender-affirming surgery. *J Clin Endocrinol Metab.* 2021;106(4):e1586-e1590. PMID: 33417686

5. Weinstein B, Schechter L. Wound healing complications in gender-affirming surgery. *Neurourol Urodyn.* [Online ahead of print]

6. Pan S, Honig SC, Gender-affirming surgery: current concepts. *Curr Urol Rep.* 2018;19(8):62. PMID: 29881906

7. Gaither TW, Awad MA, Osterberg EC, et al. Postoperative complications following primary penile inversion vaginoplasty among 330 male-to-female transgender patients. *J Urol.* 2018;199(3):760-765. PMID: 29032297

8. Ferrando CA. Adverse events associated with gender affirming vaginoplasty surgery. *Am J Obstet Gynecol.* 2020;223(2):267.e1-267.e6. PMID: 32446999

9. Levy JA, Edwards DC, Cutruzzula-Dreher P, et al. Male-to-female gender reassignment surgery: an institutional analysis of outcomes, short-term complications, and risk factors for 240 patients undergoing penile-inversion vaginoplasty. *Urology.* 2019;131:228-233. PMID: 31207304

10. Buncamper ME, van der Sluis WB, van der Pas RSD, et al. Surgical outcome after penile inversion vaginoplasty: a retrospective study of 475 transgender women. *Plast Reconstr Surg.* 2016;138(5):999-1007. PMID: 27782992

11. Massie JP, Morrison SD, Van Maasdam J, Satterwhite T. Predictors of patient satisfaction and postoperative complications in penile inversion vaginoplasty. *Plast Reconstr Surg.* 2018;141(6):911e-921e. PMID: 29794711

12. Expert Panel on Breast Imaging, Brown A, Lourenco AP, et al. ACR Appropriateness Criteria transgender breast cancer screening. *J Am Coll Radiol.* 2021;18(11S):S502-S515. PMID: 34794604

13. Weigert R, Frison E, Sessiecq Q, Al Mutairi K, Casoli V. Patient satisfaction with breasts and psychosocial, sexual, and physical well-being after breast augmentation in male-to-female transsexuals. *Plast Reconstr Surg.* 2013;132(6):1421-1429. PMID: 24281571

14. Zavlin D, Schaff J, Lelle J-D, et al. Male-to-female sex reassignment surgery using the combined vaginoplasty technique: satisfaction of transgender patients with aesthetic, functional, and sexual outcomes. *Aesthetic Plast Surg.* 2018;42(1):178-187. PMID: 29101439

15. Fakin RM, Zimmermann S, Kaye K, Lunger L, Weinforth G, Giovanoli P. Long-term outcomes in breast augmentation in trans-women: a 20-year experience. *Aesthet Surg J.* 2019;39(4):381-390. PMID: 29901707

16. Coleman E. Standards of care for the health of transsexual, transgender, and gender-nonconforming people, version 7. *International Journal of Transgenderism.* 2012;13(4):165-232.

17. Morrison SD, Capitan-Canadas F, Sanchez-Garcia A, et al. Prospective quality-of-life outcomes after facial feminization surgery: an international multicenter study. *Plast Reconstr Surg.* 2020;145(6):1499-1509. PMID: 32459779

18. Monstrey S, Selvaggi G, Ceulemans P, et al. Chest-wall contouring surgery in female-to-male transsexuals: a new algorithm. *Plast Reconstr Surg.* 2008;121(3):849-859. PMID: 18317134

19. Kaariainen M, Salonen K, Helminen M, Karhunen-Enckell U. Chest-wall contouring surgery in female-to-male transgender patients: a one-center retrospective analysis of applied surgical techniques and results. *Scand J Surg.* 2017;106(1):74-79. PMID: 27107053

20. Cregten-Escobar P, Bram Bouman M, Buncamper ME, Mullender MG. Subcutaneous mastectomy in female-to-male transsexuals: a retrospective cohort-analysis of 202 patients. *J Sex Med.* 2012;9(12):3148-3153. PMID: 23035854

21. Wang AMQ, Tsang V, Mankowski P, Demsey D, Kavanagh A, Genoway K. Outcomes following gender affirming phalloplasty: a systematic review and meta-analysis. *Sex Med Rev.* 2022;10(4):499-512. PMID: 36031521

22. Papadopulos NA, Ehrenberger B, Zavlin D, et al. Quality of life and satisfaction in transgender men after phalloplasty in a retrospective study. *Ann Plast Surg.* 2021;87(1):91-97. PMID: 33661220

23. Oles N, Darrach H, Landford W, et al. Gender affirming surgery: a comprehensive, systematic review of all peer-reviewed literature and methods of assessing patient-centered outcomes (part 2: genital reconstruction). *Ann Surg.* 2022;275(1):e67-e74. PMID: 34914663

24. Rosenthal SM, Challenges in the care of transgender and gender-diverse youth: an endocrinologist's view. *Nat Rev Endocrinol.* 2021;17(10):581-591. PMID: 34376826

25. Olson-Kennedy J, Warus J, Okonta V, Belzer M, Clark LF. Chest reconstruction and chest dysphoria in transmasculine minors and young adults: comparisons of nonsurgical and postsurgical cohorts. *JAMA Pediatr.* 2018;172(5):431-436. PMID: 29507933

26. Ascha M, Sasson DC, Sood R, et al. Top surgery and chest dysphoria among transmasculine and nonbinary adolescents and young adults. *JAMA Pediatr.* 2022;176(11):1115-1122. PMID: 36156703

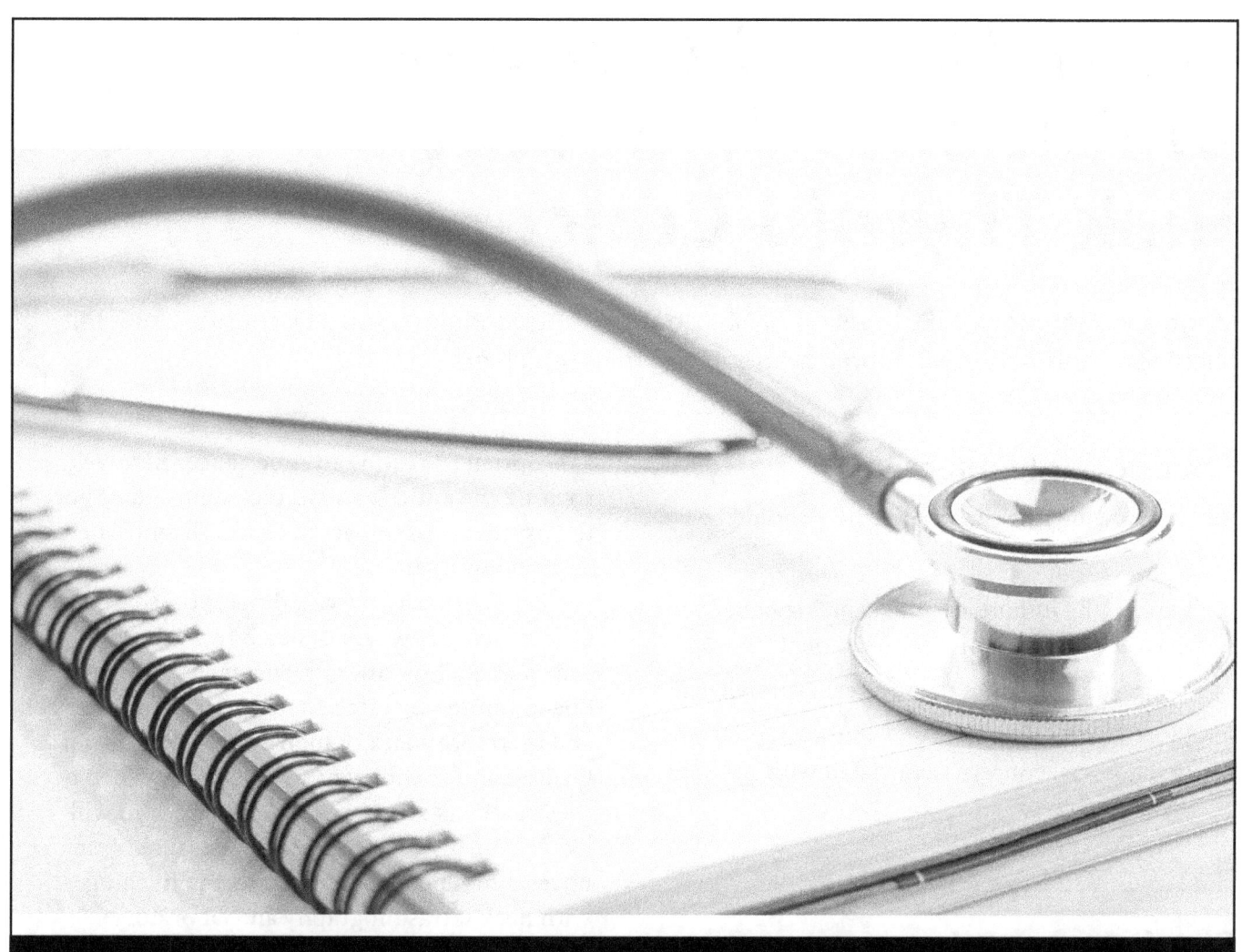

THYROID

Long-Term Management of Patients With Low-Risk Thyroid Cancer

Megan R. Haymart, MD. Division of Metabolism, Endocrinology, and Diabetes, University of Michigan, Ann Arbor, MI; Email: meganhay@med.umich.edu

Educational Objectives

After reviewing this chapter, learners should be able to:

- Explain the importance of balancing benefits-risks and tailoring care to the patient.

- Define de-escalation of long-term surveillance.

- Illustrate the importance of addressing the psychosocial concerns associated with being a cancer survivor.

Signficance of the Clinical Problem

Thyroid cancer is a common endocrine malignancy, and most patients with thyroid cancer are diagnosed with low-risk differentiated thyroid cancer. Neck ultrasonography (including evaluation of the lateral neck) and unstimulated serum thyroglobulin and thyroglobulin antibody measurement are mainstays in long-term thyroid cancer surveillance. Although in recent years, clinicians have begun to tailor treatment to disease severity, uncertainty remains regarding optimal, tailored, long-term surveillance, especially in the setting of less intensive treatment. Surveillance strategy should be tailored to the patient, the disease, and the treatment. In the setting of prior treatment with total thyroidectomy, there are patients at low risk in whom de-escalating ultrasonography surveillance may be appropriate. Treating thyroid cancer involves treating the entire patient, including addressing the psychosocial impact of cancer diagnosis and management.

Patients with low-risk differentiated thyroid cancer have a low risk of death from thyroid cancer and a low risk of recurrence. However, due to limited research funding for thyroid cancer and therefore a lack of high-quality data, it can be difficult for clinicians to determine which of these patients at low risk are the few who will likely have disease progression. Because of this uncertainty, many patients undergo imaging with neck ultrasonography and laboratory evaluation with thyroglobulin for many years, sometimes lifelong monitoring. The goal of this continued surveillance is to detect recurrence, but the risks include false-positive findings, patient worry and distress, and, in some instances, additional unwarranted treatments with risks of complications and adverse effects.

In recent years, there has been a transition towards less-intensive surgical and medical treatment for some patients with low-risk thyroid cancer. This includes use of lobectomy instead of total thyroidectomy and less use of radioactive iodine and suppressive doses of thyroid hormone replacement. Although this is a shift towards tailored care, it does complicate long-term surveillance strategies. Limited data are available on how to follow-up patients long-term when they have had conventional treatment with total thyroidectomy and radioactive iodine, and even fewer data are available about optimal surveillance when they have had less-intensive treatment.

Per the National Cancer Institute of the National Institutes of Health, an individual is considered a cancer survivor from the time of cancer diagnosis through life. Since the median age at the time of thyroid cancer diagnosis is 51 years, since thyroid cancer is the most common cancer in individuals aged 16 to 33 years, and since the likelihood of survival is high for most patients, time spent as a cancer survivor can be many, many years. Being diagnosed with any cancer, including thyroid cancer, can lead to cancer-related worry, distress, and in some instances, worse quality of life. Young adults are especially vulnerable to cancer-related worry. Optimal management of the psychosocial concerns of a thyroid cancer survivor can be complex, especially given system-level constraints such as clinic time restrictions and limited clinician availability.

Practice Gaps

- Uncertainty of how to tailor the use of neck ultrasonography, and subsequent downstream management, to the patient.

- Determining when to de-escalate the long-term surveillance strategy for thyroid cancer survivors and assessing what de-escalation of surveillance involves.

- Guiding how to best support the psychosocial concerns of thyroid cancer survivors.

Discussion

Defining Optimal Long-Term Surveillance

Optimal long-term surveillance should be determined based on patient factors (eg, life expectancy), tumor characteristics (eg, tumor size, lymph node metastases, etc), and type of treatment (eg, total thyroidectomy with radioactive iodine therapy, total thyroidectomy without radioiodine, and lobectomy). The primary reason for long-term surveillance is to detect recurrence. The key components of long-term surveillance for low-risk thyroid cancer are neck ultrasonography (including lateral neck) and measurement of serum thyroglobulin with thyroglobulin antibodies.

Laboratory Evaluation

Measuring TSH at the same time as thyroglobulin is useful because thyroglobulin can rise in parallel to higher TSH. Ideally, a comparison of thyroglobulin trends will be in the setting of similar TSH values. In addition, about 20% of patients have positive thyroglobulin antibodies and, in this setting, thyroglobulin is not as useful, but antibodies can be used as a surrogate marker. A rise in thyroglobulin antibodies can sometimes suggest cancer recurrence.

Imaging

Neck ultrasonography, which should include evaluation of the lateral neck, is the primary imaging modality for low-risk differentiated thyroid cancer, especially for papillary thyroid cancer. Most papillary thyroid cancer recurrences occur in neck lymph nodes. The role of thyroglobulin measurement is less clear in the setting of residual thyroid tissue (eg, after lobectomy), and therefore, in this scenario, neck ultrasonography alone is the method of long-term surveillance.

De-escalation of Surveillance

"De-escalation" is defined as reducing the intensity of something. For many patients at low risk, neck ultrasonography is performed every year or every other year during the initial years after diagnosis. However, at some point, if there has been no recurrence and if (in the instance of a patient who had total thyroidectomy) thyroglobulin remains undetectable and there are no positive thyroglobulin antibodies, it is reasonable to decrease the frequency of or to eliminate the use of neck ultrasonography. Because thyroglobulin is a reliable assay in individuals who do not have antibodies or residual thyroid lobes, after a period of ultrasonography surveillance, patients can be followed with laboratory testing, with neck ultrasonography added only if thyroglobulin levels rise. However, whether de-escalation can occur after 5 years of surveillance with ultrasonography vs after 10 years is debated. In addition, the role of de-escalation for patients who had lobectomy or have positive antibodies is unknown.

Addressing the Psychosocial Concerns of Cancer Survivors

Several studies have found that thyroid cancer survivors, including those with low-risk disease, can experience worse quality of life, distress, and cancer-related worry. One study found that self-reported quality of life in thyroid cancer survivors is similar to or worse than the quality of life of survivors of other cancer types. Patients who are diagnosed at a younger age, with comorbidities, with preexisting depression, who overestimate mortality risk, who have a fear of recurrence, and who have adverse effects or complications from prior thyroid cancer treatments are more likely to report worse quality of life. The cancer-related worry, distress, and worsening of quality of life can persist many years after diagnosis. Clinicians should be aware that a cancer diagnosis, including a thyroid cancer diagnosis, affects patients' psychosocial well-being. Clinicians should be prepared to offer online and in-hospital resources when appropriate.

Clinical Case Vignettes

Case 1

A 40-year-old woman with a history of a 2.3-cm classic variant of papillary thyroid cancer treated with total thyroidectomy 3 years ago has no history of lymph node involvement. Total thyroidectomy was followed by treatment with 30 mCi of radioactive iodine.

Neck ultrasonography in clinic identifies 2 prominent right level II lymph nodes with normal shape but with loss of fatty hilum. The dominant lymph node measures 0.55 × 1.24 cm. There are no other abnormal findings. Current thyroglobulin concentration is less than 0.1 ng/mL (<0.1 μg/L)

with negative thyroglobulin antibodies. The patient is anxious about the ultrasonography findings.

Which of the following is the best next step?

A. Order neck CT
B. Perform ultrasound-guided FNA of the dominant right level 2 lymph node
C. Reassure the patient and repeat ultrasonography in 6 to 12 months

Answer: C) Reassure the patient and repeat ultrasonography in 6 to 12 months

Thyroglobulin is an excellent tumor marker, and the likelihood of metastases skipping to level II without first going to levels VI, IV, and then III, is low. Neck ultrasonography has a high risk of false-positive findings. Thus, the patient can be reassured and ultrasonography can be repeated in 6 to 12 months (Answer C).

Case 2

A 40-year-old woman with diffuse sclerosing variant of papillary thyroid cancer is treated with total thyroidectomy and radioactive iodine. She has recurrent/persistent disease treated with right lateral neck dissection in 1 year later. Five of 17 right level IV and V lymph nodes are positive for metastatic papillary thyroid cancer and 4 of 5 right level II and III lymph nodes are positive. There is a high level II lymph node that is resected, and it does not have metastasis. There is no extranodal extension in any of the lymph nodes.

Neck ultrasonography in clinic identifies 2 prominent right level II lymph nodes with normal shape but with loss of fatty hilum. The dominant lymph node measures 0.55 × 1.24 cm. There are no other abnormal findings. Her thyroglobulin concentration last year was 0.1 ng/mL (0.1 μg/L) with negative thyroglobulin antibodies. Recently, her thyroglobulin concentration was 0.1 ng/mL (0.1 μg/L), and thyroglobulin antibodies were positive at 3 IU/mL (3 kIU/L). The patient is anxious about the ultrasonography findings.

Which of the following is the best next step?

A. Order neck CT

B. Perform ultrasound-guided FNA of the dominant right level 2 lymph node

C. Reassure the patient and repeat ultrasonography in 6 to 12 months

Answer: B) Perform ultrasound-guided FNA of the dominant right level 2 lymph node

Data are mixed on whether the sclerosing variant is a more aggressive variant. This patient had known disease in right level V, IV, III, and II. She is at higher risk for recurrence in right level II. There has been a change, as she now has positive thyroglobulin antibodies, a surrogate marker for disease progression. Thus, the best next step is to perform ultrasound-guided FNA of the dominant right level 2 lymph node (Answer B).

Case 3

A 55-year-old woman underwent total thyroidectomy and central lymph node dissection 10 years ago for a 1.9-cm papillary thyroid cancer. There was no report of positive lymph node metastases. She received treatment with 30 mCi of radioactive iodine.

Current laboratory test results:

TSH = 0.46 mIU/L
Thyroglobulin = <0.1 ng/mL (<0.1 µg/L)
Thyroglobulin antibodies, undetectable

Findings on bedside ultrasonography are reassuring, as no suspicious lymphadenopathy is noted.

Can you stop evaluating with bedside ultrasonography?

A. Yes; following with thyroglobulin, thyroglobulin antibodies, and TSH is adequate

B. No; bedside ultrasonography should be continued yearly until 20 years after diagnosis

C. No; periodic bedside ultrasonography should be continued indefinitely based on thyroid cancer history

Answer: A) Yes; following with thyroglobulin, thyroglobulin antibody, and TSH is adequate

Thyroglobulin is a reliable tumor marker. Some studies suggest that about 75% of recurrences occur in the first 5 years after diagnosis.

Case 3 (continued)

What if...

The patient first underwent total thyroidectomy with central node dissection and radioactive iodine treatment 20 years ago for a 1.9-cm papillary thyroid cancer, but she had recurrence 10 years later and underwent a modified radical neck dissection with 4/25 lymph nodes positive for tall-cell variant of papillary thyroid cancer. There was no extranodal extension. She then had a 1.6-cm prelaryngeal recurrence resected 2 years ago.

Current laboratory test results:

TSH = 0.12 mIU/L
Thyroglobulin = <0.1 ng/mL (<0.1 µg/L)
Thyroglobulin antibodies, stable at 53 IU/mL

Findings on bedside ultrasonography are reassuring, as no suspicious lymphadenopathy is noted.

Can you stop evaluating with bedside ultrasonography?

A. Yes; following with thyroglobulin, thyroglobulin antibodies, and TSH is adequate

B. No; bedside ultrasonography should be continued yearly until 20 years after diagnosis

C. No; periodic bedside ultrasonography should be continued indefinitely based on thyroid cancer history

Answer: C) No; periodic bedside ultrasonography should be continued indefinitely based on thyroid cancer history

She has a history of positive thyroglobulin antibodies, and there are fewer data on when to de-escalate care in the setting of positive thyroglobulin antibodies. In addition, she has had 2 prior recurrences, one occurring 10 years after original diagnosis and one occurring 18 years after original diagnosis. Thus, she has a history of late recurrences. Although the frequency at which bedside ultrasonography should be repeated is unknown, it is likely that she will continue to need bedside ultrasonography in the future (Answer C).

Case 4

A 29-year-old patient was diagnosed with a 2-cm classic variant of papillary thyroid cancer 1 year ago. She is tearful and very worried about recurrence, as well as about future life planning, including pregnancy. Her father recently died of pancreatic cancer.

In addition to continuing to manage her cancer and to reassure when appropriate, which of the following is the best approach to helping her with her cancer-related worry?

A. Let her know that there are online resources available to help cancer survivors

B. Let her know that there are local resources available, such as hospital social workers

C. All of the above

Answer: C) All of the above

Patients can be provided information about online support groups (eg, ThyCa: Thyroid Cancer Survivors' Association, Inc), general information on cancer distress (eg, NCCN patient guidelines on cancer distress), thyroid cancer–specific information on distress and coping (eg, ASCO's Thyroid Cancer: Coping with Treatment and NCI's Thyroid Cancer - Patient Version), as well as access to local resources such as hospital social work and/or psychology (Answer C).

Key Learning Points

- There is not a one-size-fits-all approach to the long-term management of patients with thyroid cancer. The surveillance strategy should be tailored to the patient and the disease.

- In some scenarios, there is an opportunity to de-escalate long-term surveillance.

- Addressing the psychosocial impact of thyroid cancer is part of the long-term management.

Recommended Reading

1. Yang SP, Bach AM, Tuttle RM, Fish SA. Serial neck ultrasound is more likely to identify false-positive abnormalities than clinically significant disease in low-risk papillary thyroid cancer patients. *Endocr Pract.* 2015;21(12):1372-1379. PMID: 26372300

2. Sek KS-Y, Tsang I, Lee XY, et al. Frequent neck US in papillary thyroid cancer likely detects non-actionable findings. *Clin Endocrinol (Oxf).* 2021;94(3):504-512. PMID: 32886805

3. Chou R, Dana T, Brent GA, et al. Serum thyroglobulin measurement following surgery without radioactive iodine for differentiated thyroid cancer: A systematic review. *Thyroid.* 2022;32(6):613-639. PMID: 35412871

4. Applewhite MK, James BC, Kaplan SP, et al. Quality of life in thyroid cancer is similar to that of other cancers with worse survival. *World J Surg.* 2016;40(3):551-561. PMID: 26546191

5. Goldfarb M, Casillas J. Thyroid cancer-specific quality of life and health-related quality of life in young adult thyroid cancer survivors. *Thyroid.* 2016;26(7):923-932. PMID: 27161396

6. Papaleontiou M, Reyes-Gastelum D, Gay BL, et al. Worry in thyroid cancer survivors with a favorable prognosis. *Thyroid.* 2019;29(8):1080-1088. PMID: 31232194

7. American Cancer Society. *Cancer Treatment & Survivorship Facts & Figures 2022-2024.* Atlanta: American Cancer Society; 2022.

Syndromes of Resistance to Thyroid Hormone

Carla Moran, MB PhD. Consultant Endocrinologist, Endocrinology Section, Beacon Hospital Dublin and Department of Endocrinology, St. Vincent's University Hospital, Dublin, Ireland; Email: carla.moran@ucd.ie

Educational Objectives

After reviewing this chapter, learners should be able to:

- Describe the genetic basis and clinical and laboratory findings of the syndromes of resistance to thyroid hormone (RTH).

- Identify patients who should be evaluated for RTH and guide appropriate investigations.

- Summarize the forms of treatment available for RTH α and β.

Significance of the Clinical Problem

The syndromes of RTH are a group of disorders that, via diverse mechanisms, cause relative tissue resistance to the effect of thyroid hormone (TH).

RTH β is the most common form, and it is usually due to heterozygous pathogenic variants in the *THRB* gene, which result in relative TH resistance in organs expressing the β form of the TH receptor. Affected patients have a variable phenotype, but typical clinical features include palpitations; goiter; ear, nose, and throat infections; poor attention; anxiety, low bone mineral density, and increased basal metabolic rate. Some patients develop serious cardiac disease. All patients with RTH β have raised TH levels with nonsuppressed TSH. Most patients require no specific treatment, but, if required, β-adrenergic blockade controls tachycardia. Selected patients with pronounced thyrotoxic features may benefit from treatment with a TH analogue (triiodothyroacetic acid [TRIAC]). Thyroidectomy or radioiodine ablation should be avoided unless absolutely necessary.

RTH α arises due to heterozygous pathogenic variants in the *THRA* gene, which encodes the α form of the TH receptor. Features include childhood developmental delay, growth retardation, dyspraxia, reduced intelligence quotient, low basal metabolic rate, skeletal dysplasia, macrocephaly, dysmorphic facies, and constipation, yet affected patients have normal, or near-normal, TH levels. Levothyroxine therapy improves linear growth, body weight, metabolic rate, constipation, and general well-being.

Defective cellular entry of TH via the MCT8 transporter causes Allan-Herndon-Dudley syndrome. Most affected individuals are male (the condition is inherited in an X-linked recessive manner) and have severely impaired neurological and motor development from childhood. All have raised T_3 with low/low-normal T_4 levels. Recent studies have shown that TRIAC therapy is safe and improves TH biochemistry, body weight, and heart rate.

Inherited deficiency of selenocysteine-containing proteins (including deiodinase enzymes) causes a multisystem disorder with diverse features (growth retardation, muscular dystrophy, male infertility, hearing loss) associated with raised T_4, normal or low T_3, and low selenium levels.

Knowledge of the syndromes of RTH has greatly expanded since the first description of cases more than 50 years ago. We now recognize that reduced sensitivity of TH can occur at multiple levels in the pathway of TH action, with each syndrome having distinct clinical and biochemical features. These conditions can be difficult to recognize and diagnose; RTH β may be mistaken for more common forms of thyrotoxicosis, leading to inappropriate treatment, and RTH α and MCT8 defects are rare and likely underdiagnosed, resulting in missed treatment opportunities.

Practice Gaps

- Many physicians have difficulty differentiating among the potential causes of hyperthyroxinemia with nonsuppressed TSH. Differential diagnoses include assay interference (due to interfering antibodies, medications, or abnormal TH-binding proteins), RTH β, and TSH-secreting pituitary tumors. Diagnosis can be particularly challenging if the patient also has an additional thyroid condition, such as Hashimoto thyroiditis.

- Knowledge of other syndromes of RTH among endocrinologists is limited, leading to underdiagnosis.

- Currently, management of RTH is guided by expert opinion, case series, and limited clinical trials. For each disorder, there is a need for additional research to determine optimal management and treatment strategies.

Discussion
Overview of Thyroid Hormone action

The actions of TH are largely mediated by altering target gene transcription, with several steps being required for normal TH action, including TH entry into cells via specific transporters, conversion of prohormone (T_4) to active hormone (T_3), T_3 binding to nuclear TH receptors, and subsequent changes in TH target gene transcription (*see figure 1*). An understanding of different TH receptor subtypes and their patterns of tissue expression is crucial to understanding the pathogenesis of RTH. Different genes (*THRA*, chromosome 17, *THRB* chromosome 3) encode the TH receptor subtypes, α and β. TH receptor β is most highly expressed in the hypothalamus,

Figure 1. Sites of Resistance to Thyroid Hormone Action

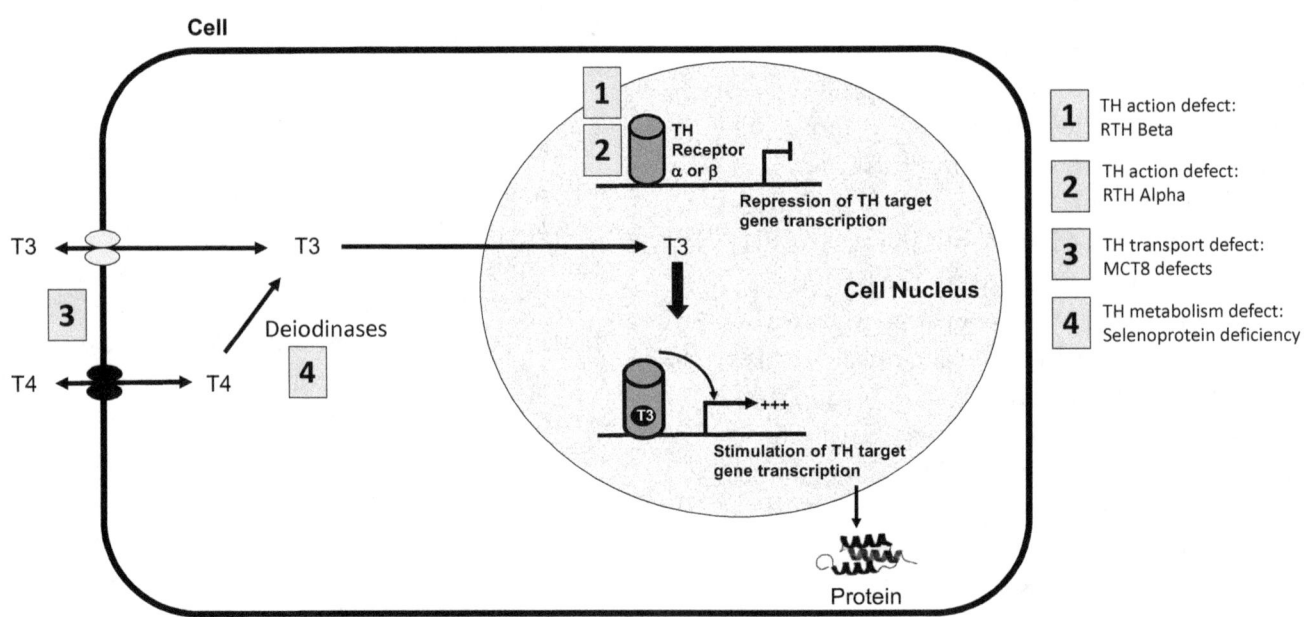

Schematic of the pathway of thyroid hormone action, indicating levels at which resistance occurs in the syndromes of resistance to thyroid hormone. Abbreviation: TH, thyroid hormone.

pituitary, cochlea, retina, liver, and kidney, whereas TH receptor α is the predominant subtype in skeletal muscle, heart, brain, and bone.[1]

Resistance to Thyroid Hormone β

Pathogenesis
RTH β is caused by defective signaling via TH receptor β, resulting in relative resistance to TH action in the hypothalamic-pituitary-thyroid axis and liver, leading to raised circulating T_4 and T_3 with inappropriately nonsuppressed TSH. Elevated, circulating TH, acting on normal receptors in α-expressing tissues, can cause thyrotoxic features.[2]

Clinical Features
Patients with RTH β may be identified through "routine" blood tests and be relatively asymptomatic. Others may come to medical attention with symptoms in childhood and/or adulthood. Childhood features include failure to thrive; difficulty gaining weight; palpitations/tachycardia; goiter; frequent ear, nose, and throat infections; hearing impairment; and inattention/reduced concentration at school or a diagnosis of ADHD (a recognized association). In adults, additional features include dyslipidemia, increased liver fat, arrhythmia, and anxiety. Persistent arrhythmias, cardiomyopathy, and heart failure can occur in severe cases (see figure 2).[3-5]

Investigation
The hallmark of RTH β is the thyroid function test pattern described above, but it is important to exclude other causes, such as TH assay interference. Assay interference may be due to (1) abnormal TH-binding proteins (familial dysalbuminemic hyperthyroxinemia, transthyretin pathogenic variants, TBG deficiency); (2) antiiodothyronine or antiassay reagent antibodies; (3) medication (eg, biotin, chloral hydrate); (4) TH displacement from binding proteins (eg, heparin); or (5) falsely nonsuppressed TSH (eg,

Figure 2. Summary of Features of Resistance to Thyroid Hormone Beta

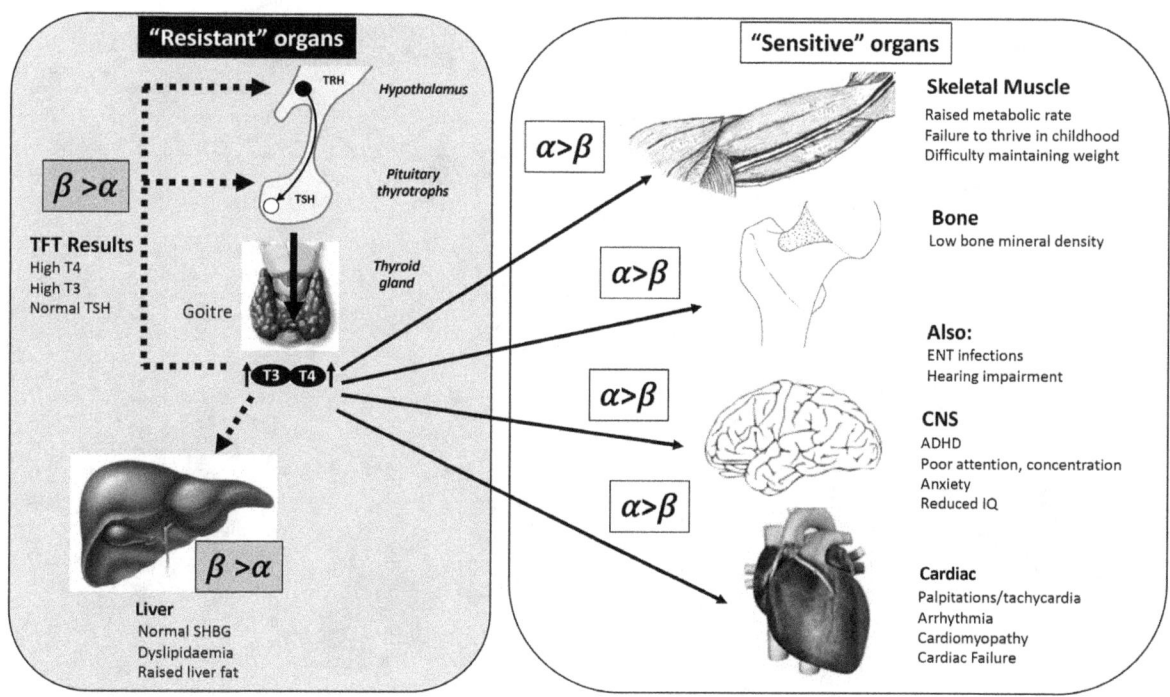

Summary of features of resistance to thyroid hormone β. Abbreviations: ENT, ear, nose, and throat; ADHD, attention-deficit/hyperactivity disorder; IQ, intelligence quotient.

anti-TSH antibodies). Following exclusion of assay interference, diagnoses of RTH β or a TSH-secreting tumor (TSHoma) are considered. A known, pathogenic variant in the *THRB* gene can confirm the diagnosis of RTH β. However, approximately 15% of patients with an RTH β phenotype do not have an identifiable *THRB* pathogenic variant, possibly due to a defect in another gene or (rarely) to somatic mosaicism. Detailed discussion of the differential diagnosis of TSHoma vs RTH β is reviewed in Koulouri at al.[6]

Management

Many patients with RTH β do not require specific treatment. β-Adrenergic blockade is very effective for palpitations and tachycardia. A subset of patients exhibit troublesome "thyrotoxic" symptoms and may benefit from a reduction in TH levels. One difficult aspect of managing such patients is that any systemic treatment (eg, antithyroid drugs) that lowers circulating TH may be beneficial for hormone-sensitive tissues (eg,

heart) but will likely worsen hormone resistance in tissues (eg, liver) expressing the mutant TH receptor β. TRIAC, a TH analogue that selectively acts centrally to inhibit TSH secretion and lower TH levels (but is devoid of thyromimetic activity in peripheral tissues), has been reported to decrease TH levels, heart rate, premature atrial contractions, diarrhea, diaphoresis, goiter size, and hyperactivity.[7-10] In patients with severe RTH β with refractory arrhythmias, cardiomyopathy, or heart failure, the use of antithyroid drugs, alone or in combination with TRIAC, can be considered.[5] Thyroidectomy or radioiodine ablation may be appropriate in life-threatening circumstances. Of note, following such intervention, levothyroxine in a supraphysiological dosage is required to normalize TSH levels and prevent pituitary hyperplasia[11]; hence, caution must be exercised regarding ablative therapies.

Figure 3. Summary of Features of Resistance to Thyroid Hormone Alpha

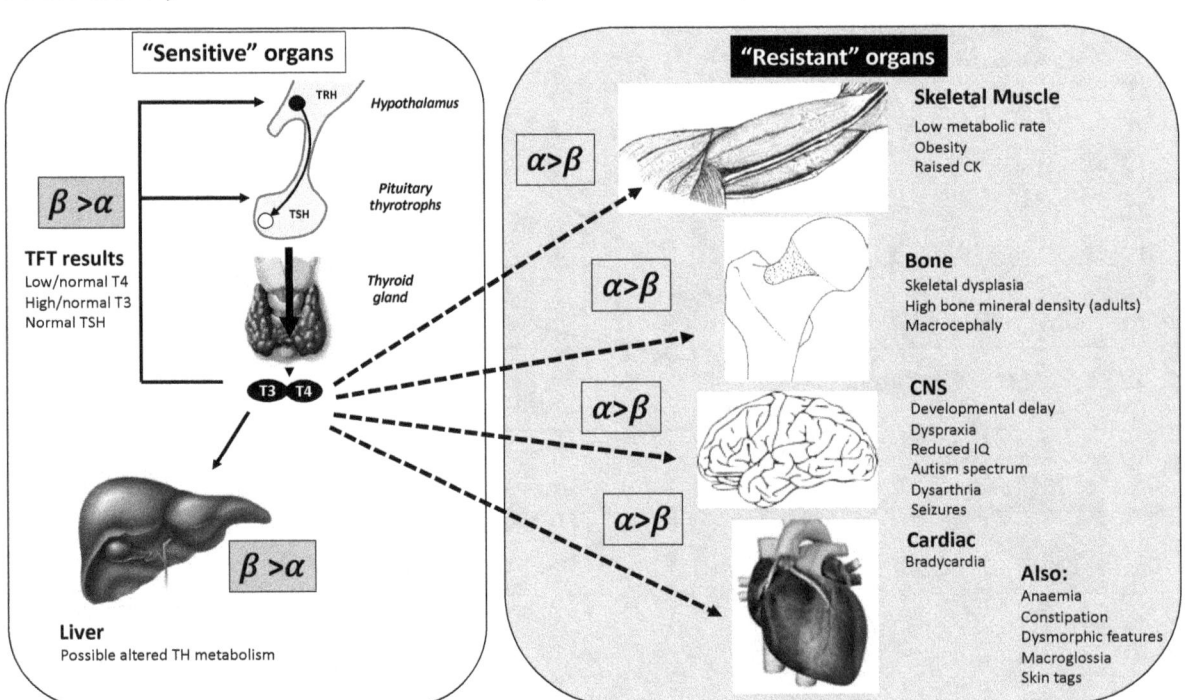

Summary of features of resistance to thyroid hormone α. Abbreviations: TH, thyroid hormone; IQ, intelligence quotient.

Resistance to Thyroid Hormone α

Pathogenesis

RTH α, due to defective signaling via the TH receptor α subtype, is characterized by hormone resistance and a relatively hypothyroid state in TH receptor α–expressing tissues.

Clinical Features

Patients with RTH α exhibit a variable phenotype, often present from birth or early childhood. Features include developmental delay, growth retardation leading to short stature, macrocephaly, skeletal dysplasia, delayed tooth eruption, dyspraxia, dysarthria, ataxic gait, reduced intelligence quotient or autism spectrum disorder, and constipation. Facial features include flattened nasal bridge, elongated philtrum, puffy skin and lips, macroglossia, broad face, hypertelorism, and skin tags (*see figure 3*).

Investigation

Thyroid function test results can be within the reference range, but with a common pattern being borderline-low/low-normal T_4, borderline-high/high-normal T_3 (computing to a raised T_3-to-T_4 ratio), normal TSH, and, in some cases, low reverse T_3. Mild anemia and raised concentrations of creatine kinse and SHBG are common. *THRA* gene sequencing is required for diagnosis.

Management

Levothyroxine therapy in a TSH-suppressive dosage improves growth, increases metabolic rate to limit excessive weight gain, alleviates constipation, increases well-being, and improves emotional affect.[12]

MCT8 Defects

Pathogenesis

Defects in the MCT8 TH transporter, vital for entry of TH into brain, cause profound cerebral hypothyroidism. However, this transporter is not rate-limiting for hormone entry into other tissues (heart, muscle, liver), so the accompanying elevated T_3 levels cause thyrotoxic features in peripheral tissues.

Clinical Features

Most affected patients present in early childhood. Typical features include severe neurodevelopmental delay, hypotonia, reduced lean body mass, feeding difficulties, and tachycardia. Median survival is only 35 years, with mortality often due to pneumonia or sudden death.

Investigation

Thyroid function testing shows raised T_3, low or low-normal T_4, and TSH in the reference range. Sequencing of the *SLC16A2* gene is required for the diagnosis.

Management

Supportive therapies (anticonvulsant medications, nutritional supplementation, anticholinergic agents) can be combined with TRIAC treatment, which is safe and lowers T_3 levels and heart rate, enabling weight gain.[2,13,14]

Defective TH Metabolism

Pathogenesis

Defects in the *SECISBP2* gene (13 cases) or the *TRU-TCA1-1* gene (2 cases), which encode a protein or selenocysteine transfer RNA that controls synthesis of 25 different selenocysteine-containing proteins (including deiodinase enzymes) cause a multisystem disorder with variable phenotypes.

Clinical Features

Affected patients exhibit phenotypes due to selenoprotein deficiencies in specific tissues (eg, muscular dystrophy, male infertility) and also features that reflect loss of antioxidant selenoenzymes (eg, hearing loss, photosensitivity). Growth delay in childhood is common.

Investigation

Altered TH metabolism causes raised T_4, normal or low T_3, raised reverse T_3, and normal or slightly raised TSH, with deficiency of circulating selenoproteins (GPX, SEPP) causing low plasma selenium in all patients. Sequencing of

Table. Summary of Syndromes of Resistance to Thyroid Hormone

	Resistance to thyroid hormone β	Resistance to thyroid hormone α	MCT8 defects	Selenoprotein deficiency
Estimated frequency	1 in 19,000 to 40,000	Unknown; approximately 50 cases described	1 in 70,000 males	Fewer than 20 cases worldwide
Gene(s)	THRB pathogenic variant in approximately 90%	THRA pathogenic variant in all	SLC16A2 pathogenic variant	SECISBP2, TRU-TCA1-1 pathogenic variants
Inheritance pattern	Autosomal dominant Approximately 15% de novo Most are heterozygous	Autosomal dominant At least 20% de novo All heterozygous to date	X -linked (almost exclusively affects males)	Autosomal recessive Homozygous or compound heterozygous
Pathogenesis	Defective signaling through the β form of the TH receptor	Defective signaling through the α form of the TH receptor	Reduced TH transport through the MCT8 TH transporter	Reduced deiodinase activity (deiodinases are selenoproteins)
Clinical features	See figure 2	See figure 3	Psychomotor retardation, hypotonia, seizures, low body weight, tachycardia, reduced life expectancy	Growth retardation, hearing loss, male infertility, muscle weakness, photosensitivity
Laboratory features				
TSH	Normal or ↑	Normal or ↑	Normal	Normal or ↑
T$_4$	↑ to ↑↑↑	Normal or ↓	Normal or ↓	↑ to ↑↑
T$_3$	↑ to ↑↑↑	Normal or ↑	Normal or ↑	Normal or ↓
Reverse T$_3$	↑ to ↑↑↑	Normal or ↓	Normal or ↓	↑
Other	Normal SHBG	Raised creatine kinase, anemia, raised SHBG	Raised SHBG, raised lactate	Low plasma selenium
Diagnosis	THRB sequencing If negative, consider pathogenic variant–negative RTH β	THRA sequencing	SLC16A2 sequencing	SECISBP2, TRU-TCA1-1 sequencing

Abbreviations: TH, thyroid hormone; RTH, resistance to thyroid hormone; ↑, slightly elevated; ↑↑, moderately elevated; ↑↑↑, very elevated.

the SECISBP2 or TRU-TCA1-1 gene is required for diagnosis.

Management
Treatment with liothyronine may improve growth and development. Oral selenium supplementation is ineffective.[2,15]

Clinical Case Vignettes
Case 1

A 61-year-old woman with recently diagnosed Hashimoto thyroiditis is referred by her family practitioner due to persistently abnormal thyroid function test results. Examination reveals a moderate-sized, smooth goiter with no nodules. Her weight is 133.3 lb (60 kg).

Laboratory test results (after being on levothyroxine, 50 mcg once daily for 3 months):

TSH = 35.0 mIU/L (0.4-4.0 mIU/L)
Free T$_4$ = 1.15 ng/dL (0.69-1.55 ng/dL)
(SI: 14.9 pmol/L [9.0-20.0 pmol/L])
TPO antibodies = 1949 mIU/L (<50 mIU/L)

Which of the following is the best next step?

A. Increase the levothyroxine dosage and repeat thyroid function tests in 8 weeks

B. Investigate for assay interference

C. Order *THRA* gene sequencing

D. Order *THRB* gene sequencing

E. Perform pituitary-directed MRI with contrast

Answer: A) Increase the levothyroxine dosage and repeat thyroid function tests in 8 weeks

This patient has an elevated TSH concentration while taking a relatively low dosage of levothyroxine. Her free T_4 is in the mid-normal reference range. Based on her weight, a full replacement dosage would be approximately 100 mcg daily (1.6 mcg × 60 kg = 96 mcg). The best next step is to increase her levothyroxine dosage and repeat thyroid function tests in 6 to 8 weeks (Answer A). Advice on how to take levothyroxine to optimize absorption should also be reiterated.

At this stage, *THRB* gene sequencing (Answer D) and/or investigation for assay interference (Answer B) or TSHoma (Answer E) is not required. Her pattern of thyroid function lab values is not unusual for a patient with primary hypothyroidism on a subtherapeutic dosage of levothyroxine. Although few clinical details are provided, there is nothing mentioned that suggests RTH α, so *THRA* gene sequencing (Answer C) is not required.

Case 1 (continued)

The patient increases her levothyroxine dosage to 100 mcg once daily, and repeated laboratory testing in 2 months shows the following:

TSH = 11.0 mIU/L (0.4-4.0 mIU/L)
Free T_4 = 2.02 ng/dL (0.69-1.55 ng/dL)
  (SI: 26 pmol/L [9-20 pmol/L])
Free T_3 = 4.68 pg/mL (1.95-4.88 pg/mL)
  (SI: 7.2 pmol/L [SI: 3.0-7.5 pmol/L])

Her levothyroxine dosage is further increased to 125 mcg once daily, and repeated laboratory testing in 3 months shows the following:

TSH = 8.0 mIU/L (0.4-4.0 mIU/L)
Free T_4 = 2.19 pg/mL (0.69-1.55 pg/mL)
  (SI: 28.2 pmol/L [9-20 pmol/L])
Free T_3 = 5.4 pg/mL (1.95-4.88 pg/mL)
  (SI: 8.3 pmol/L [3.0-7.5 pmol/L])

The patient reports full adherence to her regimen and is not taking any other medications or supplements. She informs you that her son, who lives abroad, has undergone a thyroidectomy for thyroid disease within the past 6 months.

Which of the following is the best next step?

A. Investigate for assay interference

B. Order *THRB* gene sequencing

C. Perform a malabsorption screen and supervised levothyroxine absorption test

D. Perform a thyrotropin-releasing hormone–stimulation test

E. Perform pituitary-directed MRI with contrast

Answer: A) Investigate for assay interference

It is not unusual for patients on levothyroxine therapy to have a free T_4 level slightly above the reference range, but this patient's pattern of elevated free T_4, elevated free T_3, and nonsuppressed TSH raises a suspicion for resistance within the hypothalamic-pituitary-thyroid axis. First, however, investigation for assay interference (Answer A) (causing either TSH or free T_4 assay interference) must be undertaken prior to proceeding with any other investigations (Answer B).

Intermittent absorption problems can cause a persistently raised TSH on levothyroxine therapy, but here the raised free T_4 and free T_3 indicate that, at least some of the time, thyroxine is being appropriately absorbed. Thus, a malabsorption screen and supervised levothyroxine absorption test (Answer C) are not the best next steps.

A thyrotropin-releasing hormone–stimulation test (Answer D) can be helpful in distinguishing between RTH β and TSHoma, but in a patient with concomitant Hashimoto thyroiditis, the TSH response to thyrotropin-releasing hormone can be exaggerated, so this test is less likely to be discriminatory for this patient.

MRI with contrast (Answer E) should not be performed before excluding assay interference.

Case 1 (continued)

The clinical biochemistry laboratory confirms that assay interference is excluded. Given the family history, *THRB* sequencing identifies a known, pathogenic heterozygous pathogenic variant, M310I. The patient thus has confirmed RTH β. She remains on levothyroxine therapy (125 mcg once daily) and feels well. She has no palpitations, and her pulse rate is 68 beats/min and regular.

Apart from offering screening of family members and monitoring her thyroid function, what additional management should be considered?

A. Formal hearing, intelligence quotient, and attention-deficit/hyperactivity assessments

B. Periodic assessment of bone mineral density and annual thyroid, cardiac, and metabolic risk assessment

C. Propranolol therapy

D. Treatment with TRIAC

E. Nothing, the patient requires no additional treatment and should be discharged

Answer: B) Periodic assessment of bone mineral density and annual thyroid, cardiac, and metabolic risk assessment

While there is no formal guidance regarding the next step, based on clinical experience and the published literature, the best answer is periodic assessment of bone mineral density and annual thyroid, cardiac, and metabolic risk assessment (Answer B).

Propranolol (Answer C) is only required if the patient has tachycardia or palpitations.

TRIAC is only considered for patients with symptoms or signs of excessive effects of TH on TH receptor α–expressing tissues (persistent tachycardia, arrhythmia, cardiac failure, failure to thrive, weight loss, anxiety).

Formal assessments of hearing, intelligence quotient, or attention-deficit/hyperactivity (Answer A) are not required on a routine basis but should be offered if indicated clinically.

Lastly, it is not advisable to discharge this patient (Answer E); her primary care practitioner will most likely not be familiar with RTH β and may not be able to interpret thyroid function test results or advise regarding levothyroxine dosage.

Case 2

A 12-year-old boy is referred to the endocrine clinic for weight gain and suspected central hypothyroidism based on low circulating free T_4 and nonelevated TSH measurements. His mother recalls that his speech and motor development were delayed until 2 years of age but then improved. He attends a mainstream school and has a normal diet. He does not enjoy sports and could not ride a bicycle until 9 years of age. He has no history of seizures.

On physical examination, his height is 50 in (127 cm) (<0.4th percentile) and weight is 110.2 lb (50 kg) (91st percentile). He has no goiter. He has some skin tags around his neck. Findings on neurological examination are normal.

Laboratory test results:

TSH = 3.2 mIU/L (0.4-4.0 mIU/L)
Free T_4 = 0.69 ng/dL (0.69-1.55 ng/dL)
    (SI: 8.9 pmol/L [9-20 pmol/L])
Free T_3 = 5.14 pg/mL (1.95-4.88 pg/mL)
    (SI: 7.9 pmol/L [3.0-7.5 pmol/L])
Creatine kinase = 312 U/L (<250 U/L)
    (SI: 5.21 μkat/L [<4.18 μkat/L])

Which of the following is the most likely diagnosis?

A. Central hypothyroidism

B. *DIO1* (deiodinase type 1) pathogenic variant

C. Iodine deficiency

D. MCT8 defect

E. RTH α

Answer: E) RTH α

This patient has several features that are suggestive of RTH α (Answer E): developmental delay, short stature, increased body weight, skin tags, probable dyspraxia, and a typical biochemical pattern.

The raised free T_3 is not typical of central hypothyroidism (Answer A).

Iodine deficiency (Answer C) is usually associated with a goiter and restrictive diet.

An MCT8 defect (Answer D) is possible, but the neurological features are typically more severe in that condition.

Pathogenic variants in *DIO1* have been recently described; however, these individuals do not have this biochemical pattern.

Key Learning Points

- RTH β should be considered in individuals with raised TH and nonsuppressed TSH, in whom assay interference has been excluded.

- Most individuals with RTH β require no specific treatment; however, I recommend that patients are followed up in the long-term to monitor thyroid function, goiter, bone mineral density, and cardiometabolic status.

- RTH α is characterized by features of untreated congenital or childhood hypothyroidism (developmental delay, short stature, skeletal dysplasia, macrocephaly, dysmorphic facies, constipation, dyspraxia, reduced intelligent quotient) but is associated with normal or near-normal TH concentrations (low-normal/low T_4, high-normal/high T_3).

References

1. Refetoff S, Dumitrescu AM. Syndromes of reduced sensitivity to thyroid hormone: genetic defects in hormone receptors, cell transporters and deiodination. *Best Pract and Res Clin Endocrinol and Metab.* 2007;21(2):277-305. PMID: 17574009

2. Moran C, Schoenmakers N, Visser WEV, Schoenmakers E, Agostini M, Chatterjee K. Genetic disorders of thyroid development, hormone biosynthesis and signalling. *Clin Endocrinol (Oxf).* 2022;97(4):502-514. PMID 35999191

3. Brucker-Davis F, Skarulis MC, Grace MB, et al. Genetic and clinical features of 42 kindreds with resistance to thyroid hormone. *Ann Intern Med.* 1995;123(8):572-583. PMID: 7677297

4. Kahaly GJ, Matthews C, Mohr-Kahaly S, Richards CA, Chatterjee VKK. Cardiac involvement in thyroid hormone resistance. *J Clin Endocrinol Metab.* 2002;87(1):204-212. PMID: 11788648

5. Moran C, Habeb AM, Kahaly GJ, et al. Homozygous resistance to thyroid hormone β: can combined antithyroid drug and triiodothyroacetic acid treatment prevent cardiac failure? *J Endocr Soc.* 2017;1(9):1203-1212. PMID: 29264576

6. Koulouri O, Moran C, Halsall DJ, Chatterjee K, Gurnell M. Pitfalls in the measurement and interpretation of thyroid function tests. *Best Pract Res Clin Endocrinol Metab.* 2013;27(6):745-762. PMID: 24275187

7. Darendelier F, Bas F. Successful therapy with 3,5,'-triiodothyroacetic acid (TRIAC) in pituitary resistance to thyroid hormone. *J Pediatr Endocr Met.* 1997;10(5):535-538. PMID: 9401912

8. Kunitake JM, Hartman N, Henson LC, et al. 3,5,3'-triiodothyroacetic acid therapy for thyroid hormone resistance. *J Clin Endocrinol Metab.* 1989;69(2):461-466. PMID: 2753985

9. Anzai R, Adachi M, Sho N, Muroya K, Asakura Y, Onigata K. Long-term 3,5,3'-triiododothyroacetic acid therapy in a child with hyperthyroidism caused by thyroid hormone resistance: pharmacological study and therapeutic recommendations. *Thyroid.* 2012;22(10):1069-1075. PMID: 22947347

10. Radetti G, Persani L, Molinaro G, et al. Clinical and hormonal outcome after two years of triiodothyroacetic acid treatment in a child with thyroid hormone resistance. *Thyroid.* 1997;7(5):775-778. PMID: 9349583

11. Gurnell M, Rajanayagam O, Barbar I, Jones MK, Chatterjee VK. Reversible pituitary enlargement in the syndrome of resistance to thyroid hormone. *Thyroid.* 1998;8(8):679-682. PMID: 9737363

12. Moran C, Chatterjee VK. Resistance to thyroid hormone due to defective thyroid receptor alpha. *Best Pract Res Clin Endocrinol Metab.* 2015;29(4)647-657. PMID: 26303090

13. Groenweg S, Peeters RP, Moran C, et al. Effectiveness and safety of the tri-iodothyronine analogue Triac in children and adults with MCT8 deficiency: an international single arm, open-label phase 2 trial. *Lancet Diabetes Endocrinol.* 2019;7(9):695-706. PMID: 31377265

14. Groeneweg S, van Geest FS, Abaci A, et al. Disease characteristics of MCT8 deficiency: an international, retrospective, multicentre cohort study. *Lancet Diabetes Endocrinol.* 2020;8(7):594-605. PMID: 32559475

15. Schoenmakers E, Chatterjee K. Human genetic disorders resulting in systemic selenoprotein deficiency. *Int J Mol Sci.* 2021;22(23):12927. PMID: 34884733

Evaluation and Management of Subclinical Hyperthyroidism and Hypothyroidism

Douglas S. Ross, MD. Endocrine Division, Massachusetts General Hospital and Harvard Medical School, Boston, MA; Email: dross@mgh.harvard.edu

Educational Objectives

After reviewing this chapter, learners should be able to:

- Describe the data that support risk stratification for treatment of subclinical hyperthyroidism.

- Explain that documenting adverse clinical effects of subclinical hypothyroidism are insufficient for recommending treatment in the absence of prospective clinical trials, especially in elderly patients.

Significance of the Clinical Problem

Subclinical hyperthyroidism increases the risk of atrial fibrillation and other adverse cardiovascular events, and it reduces bone density and increases fracture risk. These concerns may be minimal in young, healthy patients, but clearly warrant intervention in elderly patients, postmenopausal women who are not receiving antiresorptive treatment for their bones, and patients with underlying cardiovascular disease or osteoporosis. Subclinical hypothyroidism is frequently overtreated due to ubiquitous symptoms attributed to, but not necessarily caused by, subclinical hypothyroidism. Some data suggest that the consequences from the risk of overtreatment in elderly patients may exceed the risk of no treatment. Prospective randomized controlled trials are desperately needed.

Thyroid function tests are frequently ordered for patients with common, nonspecific concerns, such as fatigue, hair loss, palpitations, changes in body weight, and anxiety. Subclinical thyroid disease represents a minimal excess or deficit of thyroid hormone levels, and the term "subclinical" was initially used because patients were asymptomatic when minimal thyroid dysfunction was discovered by screening. Subclinical thyroid disease is common; about 0.7% of the population has subclinical hyperthyroidism, and up to 15% of women older than 65 years have subclinical hypothyroidism.

Clinical investigations have clearly demonstrated potential adverse effects of both subclinical hyperthyroidism and hypothyroidism. However, treatments for subclinical hyperthyroidism—methimazole, radioiodine, or surgery—are not without potential adverse effects. Which patients with subclinical hyperthyroidism should be treated, and the TSH concentration at which should treatment be recommended is based mostly on expert opinion. Few studies have assessed treatment outcomes.

Similarly, symptomatic patients and their physicians have considerable enthusiasm for treating subclinical hypothyroidism. However, some data suggest that the risk of treatment may outweigh the benefits in elderly patients. Well-designed studies are needed to guide recommendations.

Practice Gaps

- Numerous double-blinded studies over several decades have demonstrated that patients with potential hypothyroid symptoms and TSH values less than 10.0 mIU/L do not experience improved symptoms when treated with levothyroxine. Yet most endocrinologists treat these patients.

- Studies demonstrate that the mean and the 97.5th percentile for serum TSH is age-dependent, yet few practices have adopted age-specific reference ranges.

Discussion

Subclinical Hyperthyroidism

Endogenous subclinical hyperthyroidism may be due to autonomy in a nodular or adenomatous goiter, or due to mild Graves disease. One-third of patients with Graves disease progress to overt hyperthyroidism. A study based on a health maintenance organization database found that just over half of the subnormal TSH values (after appropriate exclusions) normalized over short-term follow-up, suggesting that the diagnosis of subclinical hyperthyroidism should be made at least twice before considering treatment.[1] Exogenous subclinical hyperthyroidism is due to overzealous thyroid hormone treatment or intentional suppressive therapy in patients with thyroid cancer.

Subclinical hyperthyroidism is associated with an increase in heart rate, atrial extrasystoles, shortened systolic time intervals, an increase in cardiac muscle mass (which can be prevented by β-adrenergic blockers), both systolic and diastolic dysfunction, and an increased risk of atrial fibrillation.[2] In large epidemiologic studies, it is associated with an increased hazard ratio for total mortality, coronary heart disease mortality, and congestive heart failure.[3]

Subclinical hyperthyroidism is also associated with reduced bone density. Thyroid hormone has a direct resorptive effect on bone, which increases ionized calcium and suppresses PTH, which in turn reduces 1-hydroxylation of 25-hydroxyvitamin D, reducing gut absorption of calcium, and along with calcium losses in the urine, results in a negative calcium balance. During remodeling, the stages are shortened disproportionately, resulting in a deficit of new bone with each remodeling cycle. Also, due to more rapid bone turnover, random trabecular perforations occur more frequently.[4] Postmenopausal women with nodular goiter and subclinical hyperthyroidism have low bone density, and after 18 to 24 months of treatment with antithyroid drugs, their bone density is improved compared with that of untreated control patients.[5] In large epidemiologic studies, subclinical hyperthyroidism is associated with an increased hazard ratio for hip fracture.[6]

Patients with subclinical hyperthyroidism had impaired physical and general health on the SF-36 subscales, but they had improved mental health on the profile of mood states.[7] A prospective 9-year study in adults aged 70 to 79 years demonstrated an increase in incident dementia in patients with a TSH concentration less than 0.1 mIU/L.[8]

While these data demonstrate adverse consequences from untreated subclinical hyperthyroidism, there are few data that guide recommendations for treatment. Cardiovascular disease and arrhythmia are uncommon in younger patients. Reduced bone density can be observed in postmenopausal women ingesting levothyroxine at more than 1.6 mcg/kg body weight, but the threshold for bone loss appears to be closer to 2.0 mcg/kg body weight in premenopausal women.[9]

The task force that wrote the American Thyroid Association (ATA) guidelines for management of hyperthyroidism recommended that patients at high risk who have a TSH concentration less than 0.1 mIU/L be treated: the elderly; postmenopausal women who are not receiving antiresorptive treatment to protect their bones such as estrogen or a bisphosphonate; and patients with known cardiac disease or osteoporosis. The task force also recommended that patients at low risk with a TSH concentration greater than 0.1 mIU/L do not require treatment.

However, the task force could not reach a consensus regarding treatment for patients at low risk with a TSH concentration less than 0.1 mIU/L or patients at high risk with a TSH concentration greater than 0.1 mIU/L, most likely because treatment itself subjects patients to the risks of antithyroid drugs (agranulocytosis and liver failure), radioiodine (thyroid eye disease and radiation concerns), and surgery (recurrent laryngeal nerve damage and hypoparathyroidism). Shared decision-making is important when considering therapy for such patients.

Subclinical Hypothyroidism

Unless patients have had surgery or have received radioiodine, most subclinical hypothyroidism is due to Hashimoto thyroiditis, and it progresses to overt hypothyroidism when TPO antibodies are positive, at about 4% per year. However, in a health maintenance organization database, 62% of patients with elevated TSH had a normal value on repeated measurement, suggesting again that subclinical thyroid disease should be diagnosed at least twice before considering treatment.[1]

In a meta-analysis of 21 studies, treatment of subclinical hypothyroidism did not improve fatigue, quality of life, thyroid-related symptoms, or depressive symptoms. But in epidemiologic studies, a TSH concentration greater than 6.38 to 7.00 mIU/L is associated with an increased hazard ratio for cardiovascular mortality.[10] Subclinical hypothyroidism is associated with increased epicardial adipose tissue, increased carotid intima-media thickness, and reduced flow-mediated endovascular dilatation (the latter is reversible with levothyroxine therapy).[11]

However, arguments for treatment of subclinical hypothyroidism are complicated for 2 reasons. The Leiden 85+ study first reported that mortality was reduced in patients older than 85 years with a slightly elevated TSH.[12] A recent meta-analysis failed to confirm this across several studies,[13] but other data have suggested improved functional mobility, improved cardiovascular fitness and strength, and reduced hip fracture rates in elderly patients with slightly elevated TSH.

In other studies, levothyroxine treatment of subclinical hypothyroidism reduced mortality in younger patients (<65 to 70 years), but it was associated with increased mortality in elderly patients. The current hypothesis is that during periods of unintended overtreatment, elderly persons might experience atrial fibrillation, cognitive impairment, or increased factures. This is supported by a study that found that the hazard ratio for mortality during 7 years of follow-up, divided into 6-month intervals, was higher during periods of low TSH than during periods of high TSH.[14]

Patients exert considerable pressure on health care providers to treat subclinical hypothyroidism because of potential hypothyroid symptoms such as fatigue. Since such treatment is unlikely to result in improved symptoms, this has contributed to patient dissatisfaction with therapies for hypothyroidism.

It is striking that in double-blinded trials, when patients are treated with variable dosages of levothyroxine, they are unable to identify when their TSH is, on average, 1.8 mIU/L vs 9.5 mIU/L.[15] Yet despite the evidence, endocrinologists continue to adjust levothyroxine dosages so that the TSH concentration remains in the lower portion of the normal range.

Low-normal TSH levels may not be optimal for elderly patients. Data suggest that we should adopt age-specific reference ranges for serum TSH.

Clinical Case Vignettes
Case 1

A 32-year-old woman is concerned about fatigue.

Laboratory test results (ordered by her primary care physician):

> TSH = 0.08 mIU/L (0.4-5.0 mIU/L)
> Free T$_4$ = 1.4 ng/dL (0.9-1.8 ng/dL) (SI: 18.0 pmol/L [11.58-23.17 pmol/L])
> Total T$_3$ = 154 ng/dL (60-181 ng/dL) (SI: 2.37 nmol/L [0.92-2.78 nmol/L])
> TRAb, negative

On physical examination, there is some right-sided thyroid fullness. Her BMI is 24 kg/m².

Ultrasonography shows a 16-mm complex thyroid nodule, with a hypoechoic solid portion and no suspicious features. Thyroid scintigraphy with ^{123}I shows an increased concentration of isotope corresponding to the right nodule, with suppression of uptake elsewhere.

The patient is healthy with no other known medical problems. She has no palpitations, insomnia, or anxiety.

Which of the following is the best next step?

A. Advise the patient against pregnancy until her hyperthyroidism has been treated

B. Begin alendronate, 70 mg once weekly

C. Begin atenolol, 25 mg once daily

D. Begin methimazole, 5 mg once daily

E. Discuss treatment options with the patient and decide on follow-up based on her values and preferences

Answer: E) Discuss treatment options with the patient and decide on follow-up based on her values and preferences

Treatment of subclinical hyperthyroidism is controversial, and it should be individualized. Patient values and preferences are important contributors to decision-making when experts themselves cannot agree on the best next step (thus, Answer E is correct). The members of the task force that wrote the ATA guidelines for management of hyperthyroidism were split on whether a patient at low risk requires any treatment for this degree of hyperthyroidism. Surveillance is an option, and it is the option that this patient chose.

If the patient had underlying cardiovascular disease placing her at risk for atrial fibrillation, or if she had a risk factor for osteoporosis later in life, such as recurrent steroid treatment for asthma or a mother with severe osteoporosis, one might encourage her to proceed with treatment now. However, the treatment options all have significant adverse effects: agranulocytosis and liver failure with methimazole (Answer D); development of thyroid eye disease and concern regarding risks from radiation exposure with radioiodine; and recurrent laryngeal nerve damage with surgery. If surveillance is chosen, one could consider a baseline bone density assessment with a 2-year follow-up study to assess whether serial bone loss is greater than expected.

Alendronate (Answer B) would not be appropriate for this premenopausal woman with adequate levels of estradiol, and atenolol (Answer C) is not necessary for a 32-year-old patient in the absence of cardiac symptoms. However, both drugs might be appropriate in a postmenopausal woman who declines treatment directed against her hyperthyroidism.

A TSH value of 0.08 mIU/L is not a contraindication for conception (Answer A). The risk that she might require treatment with propylthiouracil, if she were to become pregnant and her hyperthyroidism progressed, would be included in the discussion of treatment options (Answer E).

If this patient's TSH had been subnormal but greater than 0.1 mIU/L, the ATA Task Force would have recommended surveillance only.

Case 2

A 51-year-old woman sees her primary physician to address fatigue. She is sleeping poorly, she feels her memory is off, and she is having difficulty focusing when working. She has gained 5 lb (2.3 kg) and has noticed some hair loss. Laboratory testing documents a TSH value of 6.48 mIU/L and free T_4 value of 1.2 ng/dL (15.4 pmol/L). She has no known prior medical problems, and her only medication is vitamin D, 1000 IU daily.

Which of the following is the best next step?

A. Begin estradiol, 1 mg, and progesterone, 100 mg daily

B. Begin levothyroxine, 50 mcg daily, and tell the patient she will feel better in 3 to 4 weeks

C. Measure TSH and TPO antibodies again in 4 weeks

D. Measure TPO antibodies and start levothyroxine if elevated

E. Tell the patient she does not currently need treatment

Answer: C) Measure TSH and TPO antibodies again in 4 weeks

A large study based on a health maintenance organization database demonstrated that 62% of elevated TSH values normalized when repeated. This patient's elevated TSH should be verified before considering treatment (Answer C). Numerous double-blinded studies have failed to demonstrate any improvement in potential hypothyroid symptoms with levothyroxine treatment if the pretreatment TSH value is less than 10.0 mIU/L. However, TSH values greater than 7.0 mIU/L are associated with an increase in cardiovascular events in epidemiologic studies. Patients with very high TPO antibodies (normal ranges and the definition of "very high" are assay dependent) have a high likelihood of progressing to overt hypothyroidism within a few years. Thus, many experts use a TSH value of 7.0 mIU/L as their threshold for treatment and may recommend starting treatment in patients with high TPO antibodies at even lower TSH levels to proactively prevent symptoms when overt hypothyroidism becomes manifest. However, high TPO antibody levels (Answer D) may be present for years or decades before the patient develops hypothyroidism.

These evidence-based expert recommendations are largely ignored by practicing endocrinologists, because we all know that if we refuse to treat a patient with potential hypothyroid symptoms and a TSH value above the reference range (Answer E), the patient will find another physician to treat her. Another approach is to suggest a 3-month trial of levothyroxine, but with emphasis on "trial," and inform the patient that you do not anticipate any improvement in her symptoms based on the medical literature. Beginning levothyroxine, 50 mcg daily, and telling her she will feel better in 3 to 4 weeks (Answer B) is inappropriate.

Menopausal symptoms frequently lead to measurement of TSH and a diagnosis of subclinical hypothyroidism. When patients do not respond to levothyroxine therapy, a discussion of menopausal symptoms and the risks and benefits of estrogen replacement should be discussed. A 3-month course of estrogen replacement (Answer A) may be informative for the patient's understanding of the source of her symptoms, but such treatment requires a careful discussion of the risks of postmenopausal estrogen replacement and does not address her elevated TSH concentration.

Case 3

An 89-year-old woman sees her primary care physician to address fatigue. She has noticed some dizziness and lightheadedness. She sleeps poorly, and she has a poor appetite. She falls asleep while watching television in the late afternoon. She has no cardiovascular history and no chest pain, but she occasionally notes palpitations lasting about half a minute. Laboratory testing documents a TSH value of 6.36 mIU/L and a free T_4 value of 1.1 ng/dL (14.2 pmol/L).

She has osteoporosis based on bone density assessment (spine T-score, –2.7; femoral neck T-score, –2.6). She has been on alendronate, 70 mg weekly, for 2 years. She takes vitamin D, 1000 IU daily; calcium, 500 mg twice daily; and a multivitamin. Her BMI is 21 kg/m².

Which of the following is the best next step?

A. Begin levothyroxine, 25 mcg daily

B. Begin levothyroxine, 50 mcg daily

C. Measure TPO antibodies

D. Order a cardiac stress test

E. Repeat TSH measurement in 4 to 8 weeks

Answer: E) Repeat TSH measurement in 4 to 8 weeks

While controversial and the data are inconsistent, several pieces of evidence suggest that elderly patients live longer, have fewer cardiovascular events, and a have reduced fracture rate if mild subclinical hypothyroidism is not treated. In this case, even if the TSH value is similarly elevated on repeated measurement after a 4- to 8- week interval (Answer E), surveillance is likely the better choice until the TSH concentration exceeds 7.0 to 10.0 mIU/L. Uncertainty will remain until prospective randomized controlled trials are published.

The hypothesis is that elderly patients are more susceptible to the adverse effects of thyroid hormone excess, including atrial fibrillation, dementia, and lower bone density with a higher fracture rate. When levothyroxine (Answers A and B) is given to elderly patients, unintentional hormone excess may occur when patients view their levothyroxine as energy pills, or as patients lose weight, perhaps partly due to reduced appetite. With reduced weight and increasing age and frailty, patients may not have their levothyroxine dosage reduced as requirements fall. Subsequent risks of subclinical hyperthyroidism may then exceed the initial risk of subclinical hypothyroidism, leading to increased mortality in some, but not all, studies. The use of age-specific reference ranges for TSH and well-designed treatment trials in elderly patients are critical to addressing this issue. In view of the possible risks of treatment, even if her TPO antibodies were quite elevated (Answer C), or a stress test failed to reveal a concerning arrhythmia or ischemia (Answer D), a TSH value of 6.36 mIU/L is age-appropriate and is likely optimal.

Key Learning Points

- Subclinical hyperthyroidism (TSH <0.1 mIU/L) should be treated in high-risk patients (elderly, postmenopausal women, patients with cardiovascular disease, and patients with osteoporosis). The task force that authored the ATA guidelines for management of hyperthyroidism could not reach a consensus about treatment when the TSH concentration is greater than 0.1 mIU/L.

- Subclinical hyperthyroidism (TSH >0.1 mIU/L) does not need treatment or evaluation in patients who are at low risk. The task force that authored the ATA guidelines could not reach a consensus about treatment when the TSH concentration is less than 0.1 mIU/L.

- Subclinical hypothyroidism (TSH <10.0 mIU/L) is not associated with improved symptoms when treated with levothyroxine.

- Subclinical hypothyroidism (TSH >7.0 mIU/L) is associated with increased cardiovascular events in nonelderly patients. Treatment with levothyroxine appears to be beneficial in younger patients (<65 to 70 years), but treatment may be associated with increased cardiovascular events and fractures in elderly patients. Randomized controlled trials are urgently needed to guide recommendations.

- Age-specific normal reference ranges for TSH should be considered when making therapeutic decisions.

References

1. Meyerovitch J, Rotman-Pikielny P, Sherf M, Battat E, Levy Y, Surks MI. Serum thyrotropin measurements in the community: five-year follow-up in a large network of primary care physicians. *Arch Intern Med* 2007; 167(14):1533-1538. PMID: 17646608

2. Biondi B, Cooper DS. Subclinical hyperthyroidism. *N Engl J Med.* 2018;378(25):2411-2419. PMID: 29924956

3. Collet T-H, Gussekloo J, Bauer DC, et al; Thyroid Studies Collaboration. Subclinical hyperthyroidism and the risk of coronary heart disease and mortality. *Arch Intern Med.* 2012;172(10):799-809. PMID: 22529182

4. Eriksen EF. Normal and pathological remodeling of human trabecular bone: three-dimensional reconstruction of the remodeling sequence in normal and in metabolic bone disease. *Endocr Rev.* 1986;7(4):379-408. PMID: 3536460

5. Mudde AH, Houben AJ, Nieuwenhuijzen Kruseman AC. Bone metabolism during anti-thyroid drug treatment of endogenous subclinical hyperthyroidism. *Clin Endocrinol (Oxf).* 1994;41(4):421-444. PMID: 7955452

6. Blum MR, Bauer DC, Collet T-H, et al. Subclinical thyroid dysfunction and fracture risk: a meta-analysis. *JAMA.* 2015;313(20):2055-2065. PMID: 26010634

7. Samuels MH, Schuff KG, Carlson NE, Carello P, Janowsky JS. Health status, mood, and cognition in experimentally induced subclinical thyrotoxicosis. *J Clin Endocrinol Metab*. 2008;93(5):1730-1736. PMID: 18285414

8. Aubert CE, Bauer DC, da Costa BR, et al; Health ABC Study. The association between subclinical thyroid dysfunction and dementia: the Health, Aging, and Body Composition (Health ABC) Study. *Clin Endocrinol (Oxf)*. 2017;87(5):617-626. PMID: 28850708

9. Garton M, Reid I, Loveridge N, et al. Bone mineral density and metabolism in premenopausal woman taking L-thyroxine replacement therapy. *Clin Endocrinol (Oxf)*. 1994;41(6):747-755. PMID: 7889610

10. Rodondi N, den Elzen WPJ, Bauer DC, et al; Thyroid Studies Collaboration. Subclinical hypothyroidism and the risk of coronary heart disease and mortality. *JAMA*. 2010;304(12):1365-1374. PMID: 20858880

11. Yao K, Zhao T, Zeng L, et al. Non-invasive markers of cardiovascular risk in patients with subclinical hypothyroidism: a systemic review and meta-analysis of 27 case control studies. *Sci Rep*. 2018;8(1):4579. PMID: 29545561

12. Gussekloo J, van Exel E, de Craen AJM, Meinders AE, Frolich M, Westendorp RGJ. Thyroid status, disability and cognitive function, and survival in old age. *JAMA*. 2004;292(21):2591-2599. PMID: 15572717

13. Du Puy RS, Poortvliet RKE, Mooijaart SP, et al. Outcomes of thyroid dysfunction in people aged eighty years and older: an individual patient data meta-analysis of four prospective studies (Towards Understanding Longitudinal International Older People Studies Consortium). *Thyroid*. 2021;31(4):552-562. PMID: 33012278

14. Lillevang-Johansen M, Abrahamsen B, Jorgensen HL, Heiberg Brix T, Hegedus L. Over- and under-treatment of hypothyroidism is associated with excess mortality: a register-based cohort study. *Thyroid*. 2018;28(5):566-574. PMID: 29631518

15. Samuels MH, Kolobova I, Niederhausen M, Janowsky JS. Effects of altering levothyroxine (L-T4) doses on quality of life, mood, and cognition in L-T4 treated subjects. *J Clin Endocrinol Metab*. 2018;103(5):1997-2008. PMID: 29509918

Management of Pediatric Graves Disease

Christiaan F. Mooij, MD, PhD. Department of Pediatric Endocrinology, Emma Children's Hospital, Amsterdam University Medical Centers, University of Amsterdam, The Netherlands; Email: c.mooij@amsterdamumc.nl

A. S. Paul van Trotsenburg, MD, PhD. Department of Pediatric Endocrinology, Emma Children's Hospital, Amsterdam University Medical Centers, University of Amsterdam, The Netherlands; Email: a.s.vantrotsenburg@amsterdamumc.nl

Educational Objectives

After reviewing this chapter, learners should be able to:

- Diagnose Graves disease (GD) and other causes of hyperthyroidism/thyroid hormone excess in children and adolescents.

- Start and supervise medical treatment of pediatric GD.

- Recognize and manage adverse effects of medical treatment of GD.

- Inform young patients and their parents about definitive treatment options for GD.

Significance of the Clinical Problem

Hyperthyroidism caused by GD is a relatively rare condition in children. GD can be diagnosed by documenting a suppressed serum TSH concentration in combination with high or normal free T_4 and free T_3 levels and positive serum TSH-receptor antibodies (TRAb).

Although the treatment options, such as antithyroid drugs (ATD), radioactive iodine (RAI), and thyroid surgery, are similar to those for adults, the advantages and disadvantages of each modality differ in the pediatric population. First-line treatment is medical, consisting of daily oral carbimazole or methimazole with or without temporary β-adrenergic blockade. Longer medical treatment (at least 3 to 5 years) is associated with a higher chance of permanent remission. Total thyroidectomy and RAI are both safe, definitive treatment options for GD. Total thyroidectomy has a low rate of permanent adverse effects, and RAI has several (absolute and relative) contraindications. Children have a significantly lower chance of achieving permanent immunological remission than adults. This requires a different approach.

Practice Gaps

- Children are not small adults, and this has implications for the treatment and prognosis of GD in childhood compared with adulthood.

- Because pediatric GD is a rare condition, treatment should be coordinated by a pediatric endocrinologist.

- Optimal management may be hampered by lack of local resources and experience.

Discussion

Hyperthyroidism and Thyrotoxicosis in Young Patients

Hyperthyroidism is a pathologic condition in which the thyroid gland produces and releases excessive amounts of thyroid hormones (T_4 and T_3). Thyrotoxicosis refers to the clinical picture of excess thyroid hormones. In childhood, overt primary hyperthyroidism is the most common form and is typically caused by underlying thyroid disease that leads to high levels of free T_4 or free T_3, along with fully suppressed TSH (<0.1 mIU/L). Subclinical hyperthyroidism, a milder but rarer form, is characterized by low or suppressed TSH (<0.4 mIU/L) and normal serum free T_4 and free T_3 levels.

In children, GD is the leading cause of hyperthyroidism, typically resulting in severe primary hyperthyroidism.[1] GD is an autoimmune condition that results from the presence of TRAb (also known as thyroid-binding inhibitory immunoglobulin) and leads to an overactive thyroid gland (Graves hyperthyroidism), ocular abnormalities, and localized dermopathy (pretibial myxedema). TRAb act as an agonist, causing excessive thyroid hormone secretion and disrupting pituitary control of the thyroid. These antibodies also promote thyroid gland growth by activating similar, but not identical, signal transduction pathways. In the orbit, TRAb stimulate fibroblasts expressing TSH receptors to produce hyaluronan, which is further enhanced by cross-talk between TSH receptors and IGF-1 receptors. This leads to inflammation behind the eyes, disruption of extraocular muscle fibers, and tissue swelling. TSH-receptor stimulation also causes fibroblasts to differentiate into adipocytes, leading to tissue expansion in the orbit. The underlying cause of GD is not fully understood. However, genetically determined immunological susceptibility appears to interact with environmental factors, such as cigarette smoking, infection, stress, and gut microbiota. Individuals with GD are also more likely to have other autoimmune disorders, such as type 1 diabetes mellitus, celiac disease, and vitiligo, and the condition is more common in individuals with Down syndrome.

Signs and symptoms of hyperthyroidism in children are similar to those in adults, but they may also include accelerated growth and bone maturation, as well as a decline in academic performance. In healthy children, thyroid size increases with age, but in GD, the thyroid gland is frequently symmetrically enlarged, and increased blood flow may result in a thrill or bruit. Thyroid eye disease (Graves orbitopathy), which may cause proptosis and lid retraction, is also common in children with GD, but inflammatory features are typically less severe than in adults. Unfortunately, there is often a delay in the diagnosis of GD in pediatric patients due to suspected behavioral, gastrointestinal, respiratory, or cardiac conditions.

How to Diagnose Hyperthyroidism in Young Patients

For the evaluation of suspected hyperthyroidism in pediatric patients, it is recommended to measure serum levels of free T_4, free T_3, and TSH. As GD is the most common cause of hyperthyroidism, it is important to measure TRAb and, to a lesser extent, TPO antibodies. An elevated free T_3 level is a more sensitive marker of overt hyperthyroidism than free T_4. This biochemical assessment can confirm or rule out the diagnosis of pediatric GD in most cases.

If the clinical presentation suggests GD but TRAb are absent, it is advisable to repeat the antibody measurement after a few weeks. If thyroid autoimmunity is still not confirmed, thyroid ultrasonography, scintigraphy (preferably with ^{99m}Tc-pertechnetate), and additional laboratory investigations may be considered (blood: thyroglobulin antibodies, C-reactive protein, erythrocyte sedimentation rate, α-subunits, thyroglobulin; urine: iodine). (See https://www.ncbi.nlm.nih.gov/pmc/articles/PMC9142815/, *table 2* for the characteristics of GD and other possible causes of hyperthyroidism and thyrotoxicosis in children.) To minimize radiation exposure, thyroid ultrasonography with Doppler blood flow assessment is preferred over scintigraphy. However, scintigraphy is better suited for diagnosing a "hot" autonomous nodule and excluding low iodine uptake thyrotoxicosis.

Treatment of Hyperthyroidism Caused by GD in Young Patients

General Considerations

In view of the harmful consequences of excessive thyroid hormone on multiple organ systems, it is crucial to provide timely treatment for children diagnosed with GD. Occasionally, mild cases of GD may initially manifest as subclinical hyperthyroidism with minimal clinical and biochemical abnormalities, and close monitoring may be necessary to determine the need for treatment. In most cases, medical therapy is first-line treatment. However, if medical therapy is not successful or feasible, definitive treatment options should be considered. The proposed approach to treatment and follow-up is a general one, in which a pediatric endocrinologist should be involved, and may require individualization based on the patient's specific characteristics.[1]

Medical Therapy

Carbimazole, a thionamide, and its active metabolite methimazole, also known as thiamazole, are suitable options for treating hyperthyroidism. Propylthiouracil, however, should not be used in children due to the risk of hepatic failure. Thionamides serve as a preferred substrate for TPO, preventing tyrosine iodination in the thyroglobulin molecule and blocking thyroid hormone synthesis. While there have been suggestions of direct immunomodulatory effects, achieving euthyroidism has a positive impact on autoimmunity.

ATDs can be titrated using thyroid function tests (dose titration) or given in a larger dose to prevent endogenous thyroid hormone production with levothyroxine added later in a replacement dose (block and replace). The appropriate starting dosage of ATD depends on factors such as weight, signs, symptoms, and biochemical severity.

To block thyroid hormone production in most patients, a dose of methimazole 0.5 mg/kg or carbimazole 0.75 mg/kg is recommended; methimazole of 0.6 mg is approximately equivalent to 1.0 mg carbimazole. In patients with mild to moderate disease (eg, free T_4 ≤2.7 ng/dL [≤35 pmol/L] or free T_3 ≤7.8 pg/mL [≤12 pmol/L]), a lower starting dose of 0.15 mg/kg of methimazole or 0.25 mg/kg of carbimazole may be used. Methimazole or carbimazole can be given once daily.

A recent randomized controlled trial found that there is no significant difference in biochemical control between dose titration and block and replace. However, the trial did reveal that block and replace is associated with more adverse events.[2] Therefore, in most situations, dose titration is the preferred treatment.

When there are indications of moderate to severe thyroid hormone excess, it is advisable to administer a β-adrenergic blocker such as propranolol or atenolol, at a dosage appropriate for the patient's age or weight. (In patients with asthma, a cardioselective β-adrenergic blocker should be used). Once the thyroid hormone levels return to normal, the β-adrenergic blocker can be discontinued.

Thyroid status should be evaluated every 4 weeks during the initial 3 months. Subsequently, assessments can be conducted every 2 to 3 months. Hyperthyroidism, akin to ATD, may result in a diminished neutrophil counts and impaired liver function. Therefore, a complete blood cell count and assessment of liver function should be performed before initiating treatment to facilitate proper interpretation of any subsequent investigations.

In the short-term, biochemical euthyroidism can typically be achieved within 4 to 6 weeks of initiating ATD therapy. However, the exact timeline may vary dependent on disease severity, ATD dosage, and patient adherence. While most patients exhibit a normal BMI SD score at the time of diagnosis, in the long-term there is a risk of excessive weight gain after achieving euthyroidism.

Adverse Effects of ATD Treatment

Approximately 15% of pediatric patients diagnosed with GD and treated with ATD, mainly methimazole and carbimazole, experience at least 1 adverse effect or adverse event.[3]

The most common minor adverse effect is a cutaneous reaction, characterized by a pruritic rash and urticaria, with an incidence of around 10%. With carbimazole/methimazole, hepatitis/liver dysfunction is cholestatic and typically resolves upon discontinuation of the ATD, in contrast to the hepatocellular damage associated with propylthiouracil. Major adverse effects, such as agranulocytosis, are rarely reported in pediatric patients with GD. The majority of adverse events occur within the first 3 months of treatment, with a higher incidence rate observed in younger children. It is important to note that severe adverse events may be dose-dependent.

Medical professionals should provide counseling to patients and their families regarding the potential adverse effects of ATD. If agranulocytosis/severe neutropenia is suspected, the patient should discontinue the ATD and undergo a neutrophil count if they exhibit signs or symptoms of infection, such as fever or sore throat. Typically, ATD-associated neutropenia develops within the first month of treatment (median 30 days); however, rare cases have been reported where patients develop neutropenia after several years on treatment. Symptomatic management can be used for some ATD adverse effects, such as rash, knowing that they usually resolve on their own. However, if mucosal blistering is present, which may indicate Stevens-Johnson syndrome, the ATD should be discontinued immediately. An increase in transaminase level (>3 times the upper limit of normal) during treatment should also prompt the cessation of ATD, and liver function tests should be performed in the event of pertinent signs of liver dysfunction. Finally, methimazole or carbimazole should not be readministered to a patient who has experienced a serious complication linked to earlier administration of these drugs.

Criteria for Definitive Treatment

For patients exhibiting adverse effects of ATD, including severe neutropenia or significant liver dysfunction, total thyroidectomy or RAI would be recommended treatment options. Additionally, these therapies may be appropriate in cases where the patient or their parents are unable to report ATD adverse effects due to cognitive impairment, or if the patient has relapsed and does not wish to continue ATD therapy. Finally, longstanding poor adherence to ATD therapy may also warrant consideration of total thyroidectomy or RAI.

Remission and Relapse Rates After ATD treatment

In pediatric patients with GD, the overall remission rate after 2 years of ATD treatment ranges from 20% to 30%. Prolonged treatment duration is associated with an increased remission rate. Specifically, remission rates of 24.1%, 31.0%, and 43.7% have been reported after treatment durations of 1.5 to 2.5, 2.5 to 5, and 5 to 6 years, respectively. In a single study with a treatment duration of 9 years, the remission rate was reported to be 75%.[3]

When to Stop ATD Treatment, Follow-Up After Stopping ATD, and What to Do When There is a Relapse

Treatment duration for pediatric patients with GD should be a minimum of 3 years, and potentially up to 5 years or longer if the patient's characteristics at the initial diagnosis indicate a low probability of remission. ATD can be continued for many years, but it is important to discuss regularly with families the likelihood of long-term remission if ATD is discontinued. Patients who are likely to remit when ATD is stopped usually take a low dosage of ATD and have no detectable TRAb. After 3 years of ATD treatment, TRAb usually decline by a median of 90%, and ATD should not be discontinued if TRAb are elevated. Patients who experience relapse when ATD therapy is discontinued usually do so within 12 months. Therefore, treatment cessation should not typically be done during the period leading up to important educational milestones, such as examinations.

Patients and their families should be educated about the various manifestations of thyrotoxicosis. It is also crucial to emphasize the need for regular thyroid function testing in case of suspected relapse, and in patients who have stopped ATD: every 3 to 4 months in the first year, every 6 months in the second year, and annually thereafter. This testing is not only to monitor the risk of relapse but also the potential development of autoimmune hypothyroidism. After 12 to 24 months, patients can be referred back to their primary care provider with the recommendation to monitor thyroid function annually for at least 10 years, or in the presence of any symptoms or signs of hyperthyroidism.

Some patients who relapse may still remit in the long-term depending on associated features (older age, female sex, race/ethnicity (White), small goiter size, mild biochemical derangement at diagnosis, lower TRAb titer, history of other autoimmune conditions, and duration of ATD treatment). This should be considered when contemplating the role of further ATD.

Definitive Treatment—RAI or Surgery
Definitive treatment is warranted in cases of relapse following ATD treatment, significant or persistent ATD adverse effects, inadequate adherence to treatment, or obstructive symptoms due to a sizable goiter.

RAI Treatment
If RAI is selected as a definitive treatment, it is recommended to aim for thyroid ablation to minimize the risk of relapse and potential malignant transformation of any persistent, viable cells that have been damaged by radiation. There are various methods for calculating appropriate activity, including a fixed approach (with activities ranging from 200 to 800 MBq), limited personalization (15 MBq ^{131}I per gram thyroid tissue; thyroid volume/weight estimated by ultrasonography), or dosimetry aimed at delivering at least 300 Gy to the thyroid gland for functional ablation.

RAI should not be used in certain situations, including during pregnancy (or becoming pregnant within 6 months after RAI), while breastfeeding, in children younger than 5 years (due to higher long-term risk of malignancy), and in patients with active Graves orbitopathy, which may worsen with RAI. There are also relative contraindications, such as age 5 to 10 years old, inactive Graves orbitopathy, and large goiter that may require repeat treatment.

While adverse effects following RAI treatment in pediatric patients with GD are uncommon, some patients experience mild tenderness over the thyroid in the first week after treatment. Observational studies of pediatric patients who received RAI to induce hypothyroidism have reported no cases of malignancy or fertility problems in nearly 4 decades of follow-up. Since the goal of RAI is to completely destroy the thyroid gland, lifelong replacement therapy with levothyroxine is usually necessary. If hyperthyroidism persists after 12 months following RAI treatment, a second course may be considered.[1,4]

Total Thyroidectomy
The primary objective of total thyroidectomy is to eliminate all hyperactive thyroid tissue. This is the most recommended and conclusive treatment option for patients with GD who are younger than 5 years (to 10 years), those who have a (relative) contraindication to RAI treatment, and those with a large or nodular goiter.

The primary benefit of total thyroidectomy is that it immediately resolves hyperthyroidism by removing the source of excess thyroid hormone. However, subsequent hypothyroidism requires lifelong levothyroxine treatment. The mortality rate following thyroidectomy in pediatric patients with GD is extremely low (<0.1%). Nevertheless, there are several postoperative complications that may arise, such as transient hypocalcemia (22.2%) and recurrent laryngeal nerve injury (5.4%). Permanent hypoparathyroidism causing hypocalcemia is observed in 2.5% of cases, while permanent recurrent laryngeal nerve injury occurs in 0.4% of pediatric patients with GD. Although rare, postoperative infection, hemorrhage, and keloid development may occur. High-volume thyroid surgeons are associated with a lower risk of postoperative complications.[1,5]

Prognosis

Discussing the various potential outcomes in managing GD is crucial. The primary treatment objective is to achieve euthyroidism. The most desirable long-term result is permanent functional and immunological remission without medical intervention. Regrettably, some children experience a less favorable outcome, such as persistent thyroid autoimmunity and thyroid stimulation by TRAb, which necessitates prolonged medical therapy or definitive thyroid destructive therapy. Thus, euthyroidism is achieved through long-term ATD treatment or, after definitive treatment, via thyroid hormone replacement. Some children may need thyroid hormone replacement later due to concurrent Hashimoto disease, which progresses to hypothyroidism. Although long-term follow-up studies in adults have revealed that approximately one-quarter of patients in remission develop subclinical or overt Hashimoto hypothyroidism,[6] data in children are insufficient. Another critical long-term outcome is quality of life. In a recent study of young people diagnosed with and treated for GD during childhood, quality of life was found to be lower than that of healthy controls, particularly in the psychosocial domain. Although further research is required in this area, it underscores the importance of additional support for young people with GD, both at school and from a psychological perspective.[7]

Clinical Case Vignettes

Case 1

A 9-year-old girl who had always been healthy is evaluated by a pediatric endocrinologist because of subtle signs of thyrotoxicosis: palpitations and deteriorating school performance. There are no other signs or symptoms.

Laboratory test results (serum) show mild hyperthyroidism:

> TSH = 0.22 mIU/L (0.5-5.0 mIU/L)
> Free T_4 = 2.0 ng/dL (0.9-1.7 ng/dL) (SI: 25.2 pmol/L [12.0-22.0 pmol/L])
> Free T_3 = 3.8 pg/mL (1.8-3.5 pg/mL) (SI: 5.8 pmol/L [2.8-5.3 pmol/L])

Additional diagnostic assessments are performed to elucidate the cause of the hyperthyroidism.

Which of the following diagnostic findings would confirm the diagnosis of GD?

A. Elevated infection parameters (erythrocyte sedimentation rate/C-reactive protein)

B. Negative TPO antibodies

C. Patchy uptake on a ^{99m}Tc scan

D. Positive TRAb

E. Reduced Doppler flow on thyroid ultrasonography

Answer: D) Positive TRAb

The presence of TRAb (Answer D) in patients with hyperthyroidism is indicative of GD.

Case 2

A 14-year-old girl with an unremarkable medical history is evaluated by a pediatric endocrinologist because of severe signs of thyroid hormone excess (palpitations, tremor, heat intolerance, diarrhea, weight loss), a goiter, and signs of Graves orbitopathy.

Biochemical evaluation confirms the diagnosis of GD:

> TSH = <0.01 mIU/L (0.5-5.0 mIU/L)
> Free T_4 = 7.5 ng/dL (0.9-1.7 ng/dL) (SI: 96 pmol/L [12.0-22.0 pmol/L])
> Free T_3 = 10.4 pg/mL (1.8-3.5 pg/mL) (SI: 16.0 pmol/L [2.8-5.3 pmol/L])
> TRAb = 34.1 U/L (0-1.8 U/L)

Methimazole is started (method: dose titration). Because of severe thyrotoxicosis, a β-adrenergic blocker is added.

Two weeks after starting methimazole, she is evaluated for hives and itching all over her body. These signs are interpreted to be probable adverse effects of methimazole.

Which of the following is the best next step in this patient's management?

A. Continue methimazole and start antihistamine treatment

B. Consider definitive treatment (RAI or thyroidectomy)

C. Lower the methimazole dosage

D. Stop methimazole treatment but continue the β-adrenergic blocker

E. Switch from methimazole to propylthiouracil

Answer: A) Continue methimazole and start antihistamine treatment

Cutaneous reactions are among the most common adverse effects of methimazole treatment, and they are generally self-limiting and usually resolve after initiation of antihistamine treatment (Answer A).

Case 2 (continued)

The patient's cutaneous adverse effects of methimazole treatment quickly disappear after antihistamine treatment is started, and the antihistamine is stopped several weeks later. Methimazole normalizes thyroid hormone levels. β-Adrenergic blocker treatment is stopped and the methimazole dosage is adjusted based on the dose-titration principle.

Two years after treatment initiation (regimen, 2.5 mg methimazole daily), biochemical evaluation shows the following results:

TSH = 1.1 mIU/L (0.5-5.0 mIU/L)
Free T$_4$ = 1.4 ng/dL (0.9-1.7 ng/dL) (SI: 17.6 pmol/L [12.0-22.0 pmol/L])
Free T$_3$ = 2.9 pg/mL (1.8-3.5 pg/mL) (SI: 4.5 pmol/L [2.8-5.3 pmol/L])
TRAb = 2.3 U/L (0-1.8 U/L)

Which of the following is the best way to proceed with medical treatment?

A. Continue methimazole treatment for at least 1 more year, but do not stop as long as TRAb are positive

B. Continue methimazole treatment for 1 more year, and then stop treatment

C. Offer definitive treatment because immunological remission is not reached after 2 years of ATD treatment

D. Stop methimazole treatment because she is euthyroid and has been treated with ATD for 2 years

E. Switch to propylthiouracil

Answer: A) Continue methimazole treatment for at least 1 more year, but do not stop as long as TRAb are positive

A minimum treatment duration of 3 years is advised, but treatment should not be stopped as long as TRAb are positive (Answer A).

Case 3

A 15-year-old girl has been treated with methimazole (dose titration) for 3 years because of GD, after which this treatment was stopped. At that time, thyroid function was normal, and TRAb were undetectable. Unfortunately, she presents with recurrent GD after 3 months. Methimazole treatment is restarted, and other treatment strategies are discussed with the patient and her parents: (1) continuation of methimazole treatment because cumulative longer treatment duration is associated with a higher chance of permanent remission; (2) RAI as definitive treatment; (3) total thyroidectomy as definitive treatment. The patient chooses definitive treatment.

Which of the following is an absolute contraindication to RAI treatment?

A. Inactive Graves orbitopathy

B. Large goiter

C. Overt hyperthyroidism at the time of RAI treatment

D. Pregnancy

E. The presence of a thyroid nodule

Answer: D) Pregnancy

Pregnancy (Answer D), breastfeeding, active Graves orbitopathy, and age younger than 5 years are absolute contraindications for RAI treatment in pediatric patients with Graves disease.

References

1. Mooij CF, Cheetham TD, Verburg FA, et al. 2022 European Thyroid Association Guideline for the management of pediatric Graves' disease. *Eur Thyroid J.* 2022;11(1):e210073. PMID: 34981748

2. Wood CL, Morrison N, Cole M, et al. Initial response of young people with thyrotoxicosis to block and replace or dose titration thionamide. *Eur Thyroid J.* 2022;11(1):e210043. PMID: 34981745

3. van Lieshout JM, Mooij CF, van Trotsenburg ASP, Zwaveling-Soonawala N. Methimazole-induced remission rates in pediatric Graves' disease: a systematic review. *Eur J Endocrinol.* 2021;185(2):219-229. PMID: 34061770

4. Lutterman SL, Zwaveling-Soonawala N, Verberne HJ, Verburg FA, van Trotsenburg ASP, Mooij CF. The efficacy and short- and long-term side effects of radioactive iodine treatment in pediatric Graves' disease: a systematic review. *Eur Thyroid J.* 2021;10(5):353-363. PMID: 34540705

5. Zaat AS, Derikx JPM, Zwaveling-Soonawala N, van Trotsenburg ASP, Mooij CF. Thyroidectomy in Pediatric Patients with Graves' Disease: A Systematic Review of Postoperative Morbidity. *Eur Thyroid J.* 2021;10(1):39-51. PMID: 33777818

6. Wiersinga WM. Graves' disease: can it be cured? *Endocrinol Metab.* 2019;34(1):29-38. PMID: 30912336

7. Lane LC, Rankin J, Cheetham T. A survey of the young person's experience of Graves' disease and its management. *Clin Endocrinol (Oxf).* 2021;94(2):330-340. PMID: 33128233

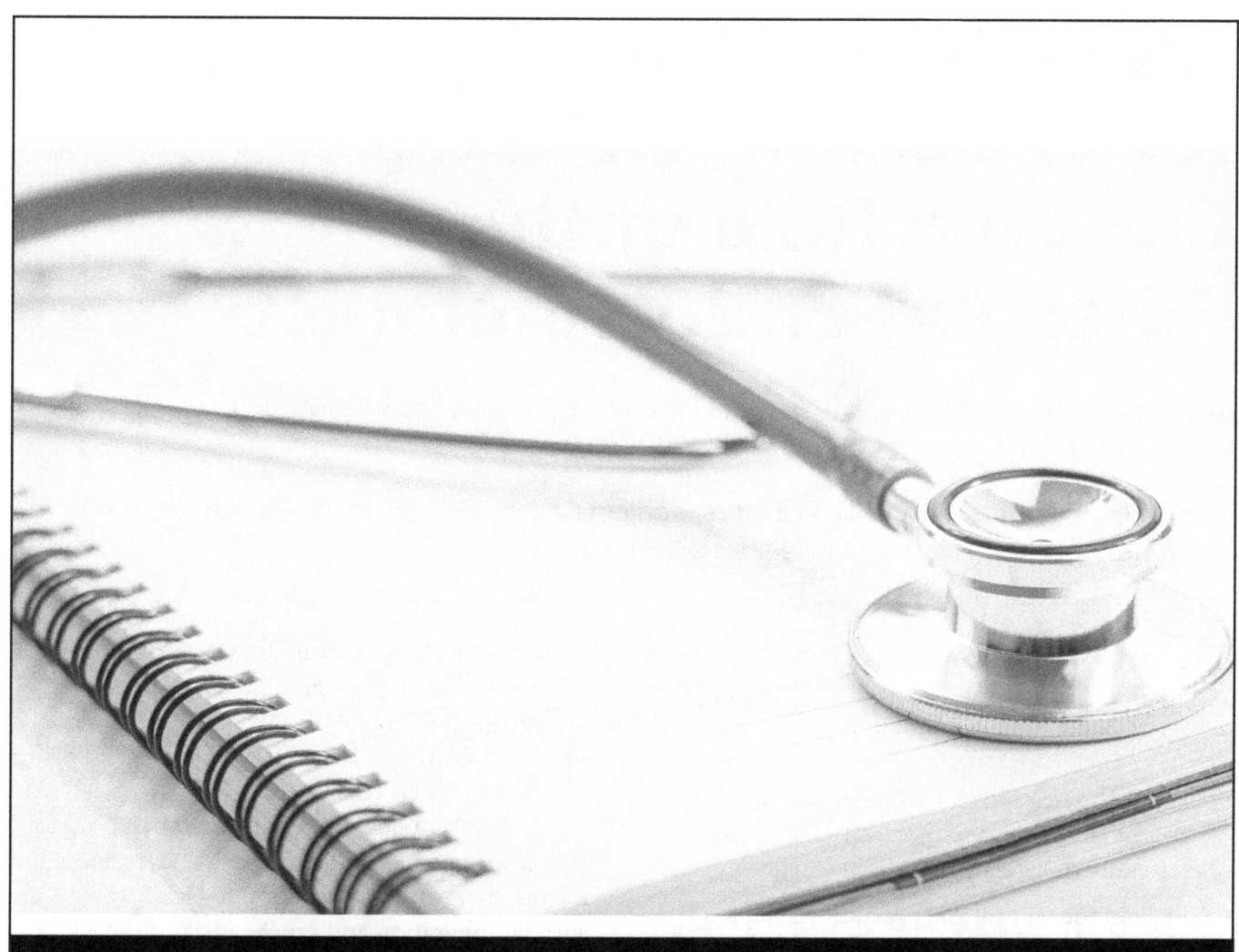

TUMOR BIOLOGY

Radioligand Therapy for Endocrine-Related Cancers: Role of the Referring Endocrinologist

Alan G. Harris, MD, PhD. NYU Langone Grossman School of Medicine, New York, NY; Email: alangharris@gmail.com

Richard A. Feelders, MD, PhD. Erasmus Medical Center, Rotterdam, Netherlands, NYU Langone, New York, NY; Email: r.feelders@erasmusmc.nl

Educational Objectives

After reviewing this chapter, learners should be able to:

- List the indications for which recently approved radioligand therapy (RLT) is used for endocrine-related cancers.

- Explain the clinical and practical challenges faced before, during, and after RLT for endocrine-related cancers.

- Describe the ongoing development of RLT in clinical trials of patients with endocrine-related cancers.

Significance of the Clinical Problem

RLT is an expanding treatment option for patients with specific forms of endocrine-related cancers. The concepts behind targeted radiotherapy in endocrinology are long-established given familiarity with radioiodine treatment of thyroid cancer.[1] More recently, RLT directed against gastroenteropancreatic neuroendocrine cancers (GEP-NETs) with ^{177}Lu-DOTATATE and metastatic castration-resistant prostate cancer with

[177]Lu-vipivotide tetraxetan have been approved. Interest in RLT will remain high as other agents, including ^{177}Lu-EB-FAPI, [212]PbVMT-α-NET, [212]Pb-DOTAMTATE, and [225]Ac-DOTATATE, are in phase 3 clinical trials.

As RLT is a new treatment, major challenges for referring endocrinologists are understanding the optimal patient population for RLT, the correct integration and synchronization of RLT into treatment regimens, and the efficacy and safety expectations to discuss with patients.[2] As awareness regarding RLT increases among patients and prescribers, the challenges with availability of and access to treatment at RLT expert centers are significant. Referral systems for RLT are heterogeneous and generally rely on regional tertiary care centers, which may be distant from patients and their endocrinologists. Focusing on the treatment of GEP-NETs, the use of ^{177}Lu-DOTATATE involves multidisciplinary teams that include endocrinologists, medical and radiation oncologists, nuclear medicine specialists, radiologists, surgeons, pathologists, cardiologists, and others. Coordination of these teams is a crucial part of adequate patient management. Responsibility for communication with patients and their subsequent day-to-day care during and after RLT can fall to the individual endocrinologist. Hence, improved awareness among endocrinologists and other stakeholders regarding the value, strengths, and limitations of RLT for GEP-NETs is needed to optimize referral and patient care.[2]

Peptide receptor radiotherapy (PRRT) is a form of RLT that uses radiolabeled peptides targeting the SSTR2A (somatostatin receptor type 2A), and it can be an effective treatment modality for NETS originating from the gastrointestinal tract and pancreas. The treatment goals can be 3-fold:

(a) To induce sustained tumor control, particularly in patients who show progression while treated with a somatostatin analogue and who often present with widespread metastatic disease.

(b) To control hormonal overproduction by NETs refractory to somatostatin analogue therapy.

(c) To induce tumor shrinkage in patients with localized disease (mainly NETs in the pancreas) to facilitate surgical resection (neoadjuvant treatment).

In many patients, several treatment modalities are possible without the availability of head-to-head comparisons. Thus, it is important to emphasize that treatment decisions should be tailor-made by considering factors such as age, tumor type, tumor grade, hormonal overproduction, mechanical complications, and comorbidities, etc. Each patient should be discussed by a multidisciplinary team including an endocrinologist, oncologist, radiation oncologist, surgeon, nuclear medicine physician, radiologist, gastroenterologist, pathologist, and nurse practitioner.[3,4]

Practice Gaps

- General endocrinologists have a relatively low level of practical experience with RLT. Improved training is needed to integrate RLT guidelines[5] into clinical practice, and better referral pathways should be developed for individual patients to be guided to regional multidisciplinary expert centers.[2]

- There is incomplete information on how to manage RLT as part of a multimodal treatment regimen for GEP-NETs. More experience is needed in the real world regarding the outcomes of RLT for GEP-NETs.

- Management of adverse effects and safety issues specific to RLT and GEP-NETs can fall to the referring endocrinologist. Awareness of these can help to improve patient safety.

Discussion

RLT is a new cancer treatment modality that relies on delivering a therapeutic dose of radiation to cancer cells (eg, GEP-NETs) by targeting receptors that are expressed on the cell surface (eg, somatostatin receptors). The radioligand consists of the ligand (peptide analogue) for the receptor attached to the radioactive particle, which is combined with a chelator and a linker (*figure 1*). In the case of GEP-NET treatment, the RLT consists of the radioactive particle (^{177}Lu) with the chelator DOTA that is attached to a derivative of a somatostatin analogue, octreotate (together called "dotatate"). Lutetium Lu 177 DOTATATE delivers beta radiation, thereby causing its cytotoxic and clinical effects.

Which Patients With GEP-NET Are Eligible for RLT?

Lutetium Lu 177 DOTATATE is indicated for the treatment of somatostatin receptor–positive GEP-NETs, including foregut, midgut, hindgut, and pancreatic NETS in adults. In practical terms, the patient population is limited to those with somatostatin receptor–positive, metastatic (hepatic) GEP-NETs for which curative surgery is not possible and in patients for whom the hepatic tumor burden is moderate and when the disease has progressed on long-acting somatostatin analogues. There are no guidelines assessing metastatic disease burden for eligibility, but GEP-NETs most commonly present with large-volume metastatic

Figure 1. Various component elements necessary for radioligand complex assembly.

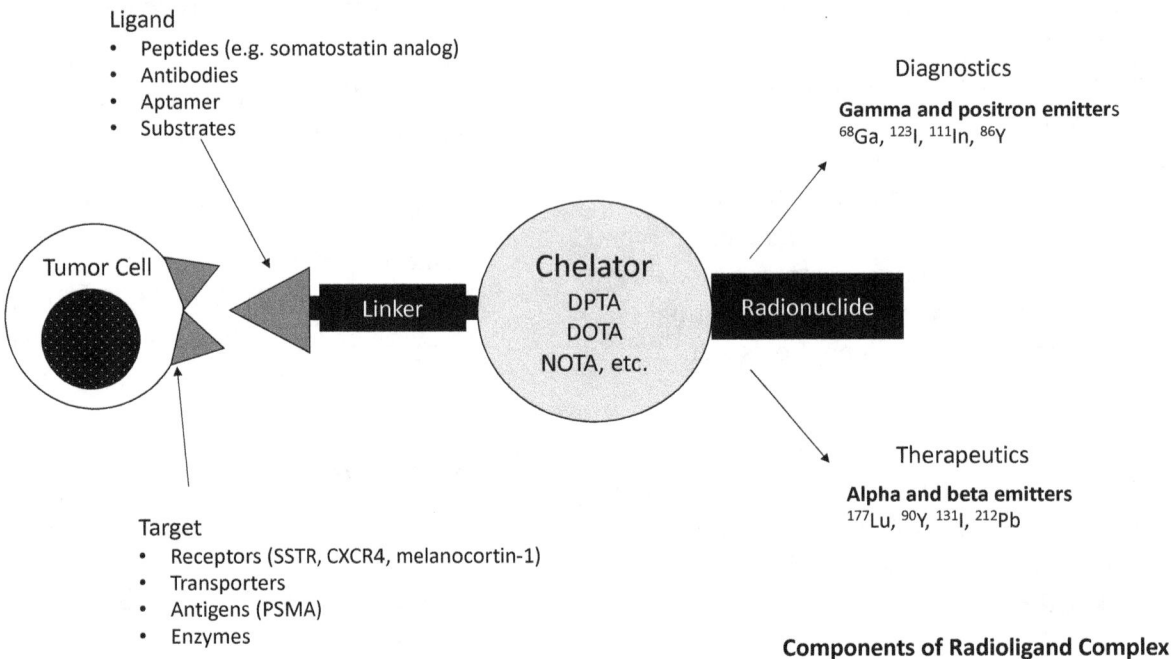

Ligand
- Peptides (e.g. somatostatin analog)
- Antibodies
- Aptamer
- Substrates

Diagnostics

Gamma and positron emitters
^{68}Ga, ^{123}I, ^{111}In, ^{86}Y

Tumor Cell

Chelator
DPTA
DOTA
NOTA, etc.

Linker

Radionuclide

Target
- Receptors (SSTR, CXCR4, melanocortin-1)
- Transporters
- Antigens (PSMA)
- Enzymes

Therapeutics

Alpha and beta emitters
^{177}Lu, ^{90}Y, ^{131}I, ^{212}Pb

Components of Radioligand Complex

---

liver disease that can be controlled with ^{177}Lu-DOTATATE. Other factors to consider before RLT with ^{177}Lu-DOTATATE are the hematological status (absence of grade 2-4 thrombocytopenia), grade 3-4 signs of myelosuppression (anemia, neutropenia), and renal and hepatic toxicity.

When considering RLT, the tumoral expression of somatostatin receptor positivity must be established. Optimally, this involves the endocrinologist referring the patient with GEP-NET for ^{68}Ga-DOTA-SSA (somatostatin analogue) PET. Because of expired pass-through status of ^{68}Ga-DOTATATE, related reimbursement challenges, and flexibility of distribution, ^{64}Cu-DOTATATE is being adopted by PET centers because of its long half-life (12.7 hours). The expression of somatostatin receptor subtype 2A is higher in well-differentiated G1 and G2 GEP-NETs and still partially maintained in G3 tumors. From a prognostic perspective, tumor grade is a determinant of outcome, with lower-grade tumors having improved response to RLT with ^{177}Lu-DOTATATE as compared with high-grade GEP-NETs or neuroendocrine carcinomas.

Safety of RLT for GEP-NETs

When caring for patients with GEP-NETs receiving RLT ^{177}Lu-DOTATATE, the endocrinologist must be vigilant for not only signs related to the underlying disease but also direct effects of RLT on normal organs.[6,7] When relevant adverse events occur, ^{177}Lu-DOTATATE treatment should be withheld until thresholds have been satisfied. Active surveillance for adverse events is required.

Bone Marrow

In the phase 3 study NETTER-1, anemia, thrombocytopenia, and neutropenia of any grade occurred in 81%, 53%, and 26%, respectively, of those receiving ^{177}Lu-DOTATATE. However, grade 3-4 level bone marrow suppression was infrequent, occurring in up to 3%. Onset of thrombocytopenia is gradual and can occur weeks after dosing and may require months to recover.

The following thresholds must be met before permitting treatment with ^{177}Lu-DOTATATE:

Platelet count: >75 × 10⁹/L (grade 0/1 thrombocytopenia)

Neutrophils: >1.0-1.5 × 10⁹/L (grade 0/1/2 neutropenia)

Hemoglobin: >8.0 g/dL (grade 0/1/2 anemia)

In large clinical trials such as NETTER-1 and the Erasmus study,[5] myelodysplastic syndrome occurred in 2.0% to 2.3% of patients who received ¹⁷⁷Lu-DOTATATE. A further 0.5% developed acute leukemia. These events tend to occur late after treatment (years).

Hepatotoxicity

Hyperbilirubinemia greater than 3 times the upper normal limit or a serum albumin concentration less than 30 g/L with an INR above 1.5 while on ¹⁷⁷Lu-DOTATATE treatment is an indication to dose adjust, hold-off, or stop treatment.

In large clinical trials, less than 1% of patients experience significant hepatotoxicity (which may be secondary to hemorrhage of the metastases).

Nephrotoxicity

Lutetium Lu 177 DOTATATE tends to accumulate in the kidney, so kidney function must be monitored. The creatinine clearance threshold is 40 mL min⁻¹ 1.73 m⁻². In large clinical trials, the incidence of significant renal toxicity is less than 1%.

Other rare but important adverse events related to GEP-NETs include acute events such as carcinoid crises due to hormonal and vasoactive amine release caused by cytotoxicity and subacute events such as intestinal ischemia in patients with a high burden of peritoneal and mesenteric metastases. The treating physicians should be well-trained in recognizing and treating these effects (*figure 2*).

Clinical Case Vignettes
Case 1

A 74-year-old woman is referred for treatment of a metastasized pancreatic NET. She initially sought evaluation by her family physician because of weight loss of 33 lb (15 kg) over 12 months. In addition, she has a history of abdominal discomfort that precedes the weight loss and was diagnosed with irritable bowel syndrome. Sometimes she has diarrhea for which she uses loperamide. She reports flushes a couple of times per week with no clear triggering factor. Her medical history includes hypertension, type 2 diabetes mellitus, and glaucoma.

Her primary care physician detected an enlarged liver on physical examination, and subsequent ultrasonography revealed liver lesions suspicious for metastases. Abdominal CT showed a pancreatic tumor with liver metastases. Pathologic examination of a biopsy of one of the lesions demonstrated an NET, grade II (Ki67 index, 6%).

Laboratory test results:

ALT = 82 U/L (<34 U/L) (SI: 1.37 μkat/L [<0.57 μkat/L])

AST = 76 U/L (<31 U/L) (SI: 1.27 μkat/L [<0.52 μkat/L])

Alkaline phosphatase = 190 U/L (<98 U/L)

γ-Glutamyltransferase = 112 U/L (<38 U/L) (SI: 1.87 μkat/L [<0.63 μkat/L])

Figure 2. Dose-modifying toxicity (DMT) algorithm.

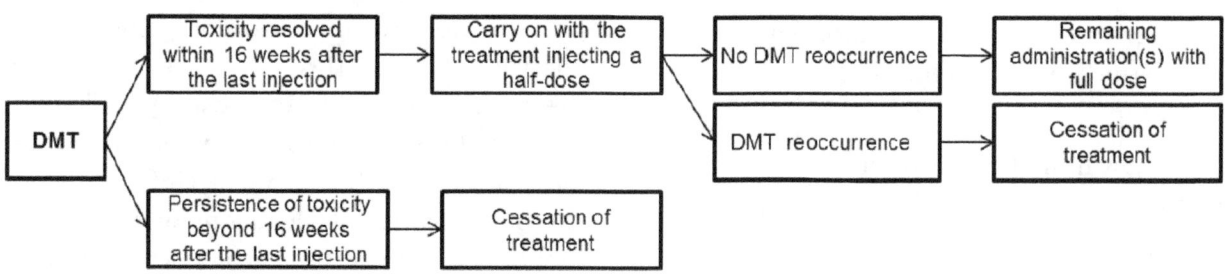

Accessible at: https://www.medicines.org.uk/emc/product/12723/smpc/print.

Bilirubin = 0.58 mg/dL (<0.99 mg/dL) (SI: 10 μmol/L [<17 μmol/L])

Chromogranin A = 308 ng/mL (SI: 308 μg/L)

Neuron specific enolase (NSE) = 11.4 μg/L (<16.3 μg/L)

5-Hydroxyindoleacetic acid (5-HIAA) = 16.6 mg/24 h (<9.6 mg/24 h) (SI: 88 μmol/d [<50 μmol/d])

Additional imaging studies with ^{111}In-pentetreotide scintigraphy (somatostatin receptor imaging) demonstrate a pancreatic NET with liver metastases. There are no lymph node, lung, or bone lesions.

Questions

1. **How often do neuroendocrine pancreas tumors secrete serotonin?**

2. **Which other hormones produced by pancreatic NETs can cause diarrhea?**

3. **Which treatment modality should be started?**

   A. Chemotherapy (capecitabine/temozolomide)

   B. Somatostatin analogue

   C. mTOR inhibitor (everolimus)

   D. PRRT

   E. Tyrosine kinase inhibitor (sunitinib, cabozantinib, lenvatinib)

In the multidisciplinary team discussion, it is decided to start somatostatin analogue therapy (lanreotide, 120 mg every 4 weeks). After 3 lanreotide injections, diarrhea and flushes disappear. After 2.5 years of stable disease with somatostatin analogue treatment, CT and ^{111}In-pentetreotide scintigraphy show progression of the liver lesions (size and number), whereas the primary pancreatic tumor remains stable.

4. **Which treatment modality should be considered?**

   A. Liver-directed therapy (radiofrequency ablation, liver embolization)

   B. PRRT

   C. mTOR inhibitor (everolimus)

   D. Tyrosine kinase inhibitor (sunitinib, cabozantinib, lenvatinib)

   E. Chemotherapy (capecitabine/temozolomide)

The patient is treated with 4 cycles of PRRT with ^{177}Lu-octreotate (cumulative administered activity 29.5 GBq). Post-PRRT imaging shows a decrease in size of both the primary pancreatic tumor and liver metastases on 3 consecutive CT scans, indicating a partial response. After 4 years of stable disease, imaging with ^{68}Ga-DOTATATE PET-CT demonstrates progression of both the primary pancreatic tumor and liver metastases.

5. **Which treatment modality should be considered?**

   A. Retreatment with PRRT

   B. mTOR inhibitor (everolimus)

   C. Tyrosine kinase inhibitor (sunitinib, cabozantinib, lenvatinib)

   D. Chemotherapy (capecitabine/temozolomide)

Based on the continuous avidity on ^{68}Ga-DOTATATE scan and with a progression-free survival benefit of 4 years, the patient is retreated with 2 more cycles of PRRT with ^{177}Lu-octreotate (cumulative administered activity, 244.3 GBq). CT performed 3 months after these 2 cycles shows an unchanged size of the primary pancreatic tumor but an increase in diameter of some of the liver lesions. Subsequent CT 4 months later demonstrates a decrease in tumor size of both the pancreatic tumor and the liver metastases. The initial increase of some liver lesions on the first CT scan after treatment is interpreted as therapy effect ("pseudo-progression"). Currently, the patient has still stable disease 3.5 years after retreatment.

A minority (ie, 8.5%) of pancreatic NETs produce serotonin.[8] Serotonin overproduction is predominantly associated with midgut and lung neuroendocrine tumors. Pancreatic NETs producing gastrin, vasoactive intestinal peptide, and somatostatin are also accompanied by diarrhea.[9] Grade I-II NETs can be stabilized by treatment with "cold" somatostatin analogues.[10,11] The duration of stable disease varies from several months to more than 10 years. Unfortunately, no biomarkers are available that predict treatment response to somatostatin analogues. Somatostatin analogues are generally well-tolerated and can be given lifelong. It is therefore a logical choice to start with a somatostatin analogue as initial treatment of patients with a metastasized grade I-II NET.

All options mentioned in question 4 can be considered to treat progressive disease in this patient. Liver-directed therapy could be an option. Radiofrequency ablation was not possible because of size and number of liver metastases. Liver embolization could be performed, but this can be accompanied by serious adverse effects (eg, pain, tumor necrosis with sepsis), which may be a limiting factor in this older patient. PRRT may have a better efficacy-to-adverse effect ratio compared with that of an mTOR inhibitor (which may also dysregulate the patient's diabetes mellitus), a tyrosine kinase inhibitor, or chemotherapy.

The same arguments can be used for retreatment with PRRT, which can be effective in patients who had benefit from initial PRRT.[12] Considering age and condition of the patient and the initial response to PRRT, it was decided to give 2 additional cycles of PRRT, which resulted in a sustained response.

Case 2

A 54-year-old woman is admitted to the hospital for evaluation of hypoglycemia. In the last 2 months, she has experienced episodes of tremor, sweating, blurred vision, headache, and loss of concentration. These concerns often occur early in the morning and improve with food intake. She has gained 4.4 lb (2 kg). The day before hospital admission, she visited her family physician who documented a point-of-care glucose measurement of 36 mg/dL (2.0 mmol/L).

During a 72-hour fast, hypoglycemia with associated symptoms occurs after 10.5 hours. After blood sampling, glucose is administered intravenously.

Laboratory test results:

Glucose = 21.6 mg/dL (SI: 1.2 mmol/L)
Insulin = 41 μIU/mL (SI: 285.7 pmol/L)
Proinsulin = 379.2 pg/mL (SI: 43 pmol/L)
C-peptide = 3.69 ng/mL (SI: 1.22 nmol/L)

Criteria for endogenous hyperinsulinism are as follows:

- Glucose <39.6 mg/dL (SI: <2.2 mmol/L) with hypoglycemic symptoms
- Insulin >6 μIU/mL (SI: >42 pmol/L)
- Proinsulin >44 pg/mL (SI: >5 pmol/L)
- C-peptide >0.6 ng/mL (SI: >0.2 nmol/L)

A ^{68}Ga-DOTATATE PET-CT shows a somatostatin receptor–avid tumor in the pancreas head with local lymph node and liver metastases. Pathologic examination of a biopsy of one of the liver lesions shows a grade II NET (Ki67 index, 8%) with positive immunohistochemistry staining for insulin.

Questions

1. **How should this patient be treated?**
   A. Frequent meals
   B. Nocturnal tube feeding
   C. Diazoxide
   D. Somatostatin analogue

Treatment is started with frequent meals; diazoxide, 100 mg 3 times daily; and octreotide, 100 mcg 3 times daily subcutaneously.

2. **Why is octreotide started with the short-acting instead of the long-acting formulation?**

Initially, the combination of frequent meals, diazoxide, and octreotide results in normoglycemia for several weeks. Subsequently, however, hypoglycemia recurs for which the diazoxide dosage is increased to 200 mg 3 times daily. This dosage increase is not well-tolerated because the patient develops generalized edema. In addition, nocturnal tube feeding is necessary, but this does not fully prevent hypoglycemia. Follow-up CT 3 months later shows stable disease.

3. Which additional treatment should be considered to induce normoglycemia?

    A. Liver-directed therapy (embolization)

    B. hemotherapy (streptozocin/5-fluorouracil)

    C. PRRT

    D. mTOR inhibitor (everolimus)

    E. Corticosteroids (dexamethasone)

The patient is treated with 4 cycles of PRRT with ^{177}Lu-octreotate (cumulative administered activity, 29.8 GBq). After the first cycle of therapy, glucose levels remain within the normal range and the diazoxide dosage is tapered without recurrent hypoglycemia. Currently, 1 year after PRRT, the patient has stable disease and has not experienced hypoglycemia.

Initial treatment is started with frequent meals, diazoxide, and octreotide to prevent hypoglycemia. In some patients, somatostatin analogues inhibit glucagon secretion more than insulin secretion by the insulinoma, resulting in worsening hypoglycemia.[6] Therefore, if it is decided to start with a somatostatin analogue, a short-acting somatostatin analogue should be selected with careful glucose monitoring. If no worsening occurs in the degree or frequency of hypoglycemia, a long-acting somatostatin analogue can be started.

Considering the severity of hypoglycemia and the adverse events of diazoxide, additional treatment is indicated. In this patient, PRRT was chosen as treatment considering its efficacy in counteracting hypoglycemia in malignant insulinomas[13] (although reported in small series) and its relatively mild adverse effect profile. Of course, other treatment modalities such as liver embolization and chemotherapy can also effectively reduce insulin overproduction.[6] This case is an example of hormonal overproduction by a NET as indication for PRRT in the presence of stable disease.

Case 3

A 64-year-old woman is referred for evaluation and treatment of a pancreatic NET. Over the past 4 months, the patient has had nausea, abdominal discomfort, and weight loss. Physical examination reveals a palpable mass centrally located in the upper abdomen.

Laboratory test results:

> Chromogranin A = 855 ng/mL (27-94 ng/mL)
> (SI: 855 µg/L [27-94 µg/L])
> Neuron specific enolase (NSE) = 156 µg/L
> (<16.3 µg/L)

CT identifies a 14-cm mass originating from the pancreas tail with compression of the stomach. There are collateral vessels in the upper abdomen and obliteration of the lineal vein. Gallium ^{68}Ga-DOTATATE PET-CT shows high uptake in the pancreatic mass. There is a possibly positive lesion in segment 2 of the liver. No lymph node, lung, or bone metastases are observed.

Pancreas biopsy documents a grade II NET (Ki67 index, 19%).

Question

Which treatment modality should be considered?

    A. Surgical resection

    B. Somatostatin analogue

    C. PRRT

    D. mTOR inhibitor (everolimus)

    E. Tyrosine kinase inhibitor

    F. Chemotherapy (capecitabine/temozolomide)

In the multidisciplinary team discussion, PRRT in the neoadjuvant setting was thought to be the best option aiming to reduce tumor size and thereby improve operability and decrease perioperative morbidity.

After treatment with 4 cycles of ^{177}Lu-octreotate (cumulative administered activity, 29.2 GBq), the tumor size decreased to 3.4 cm, and the possible liver lesion was not visible anymore. Subsequently, the patient underwent an uncomplicated surgical resection of the pancreatic NET in combination with a splenectomy. Currently, 4 years after operation, follow-up imaging shows no recurrence or metastases.

The tumor shrinkage after PRRT in this case is exceptional. But several case series have shown that more subtle tumor size reduction induced by neoadjuvant RLT can improve operability of pancreatic NETs.[14]

Case 4

A 62-year-old man is seen for follow-up 4 years after adrenalectomy to remove a pheochromocytoma. The 5.5-cm tumor had a PASS score of 6 out of 20 (PASS score >4 may indicate uncertain biological behavior). Postoperatively, plasma (nor)metanephrine concentrations and blood pressure values normalized. Genetic analysis identified no pathogenic variants predisposing to pheochromocytoma/paraganglioma. At today's clinic visit, the patient reports having paroxysmal palpitations and headache. His blood pressure is 170/110 mm Hg.

Laboratory test results:

> Plasma metanephrine = 297.8 pg/mL (13.8-65.1 pg/mL) (SI: 1.51 nmol/L [0.07-0.33 nmol/L])
> Plasma normetanephrine = 1163.0 pg/mL (42.1-196.0 pg/mL) (SI: 6.35 nmol/L [0.23-1.07 nmol/L])

Imaging with ^{68}Ga-DOTATATE PET-CT shows local recurrence at the left side and multifocal intra-abdominal lesions. An ^{123}I-MIBG scan shows only weak uptake in some of the lesions visible on ^{68}Ga-DOTATATE PET-CT.

Question

Which treatment modality should be considered for this patient?

A. Chemotherapy (cyclophosphamide/vincristine/dacarbazine or temozolomide)

B. ^{131}MIBG therapy

C. PRRT with ^{177}Lu-octreotate

D. Sunitinib

He was treated with 4 cycles of PRRT with ^{177}Lu-octreotate (cumulative administrated activity, 30.3 GBq). Three years after PRRT, the patient has stable disease and normal levels of plasma (nor)metanephrine:

> Metanephrine = 55.2 pg/mL (SI: 0.28 nmol/L)
> Normetanephrine = 144.7 pg/mL (SI: 0.79 nmol/L)

This case demonstrates that PRRT can stabilize tumors and reduce catecholamine production by a malignant pheochromocytoma. For metastasized pheochromocytoma/paraganglioma, only a few therapeutic options are available. The degree of uptake on ^{123}I-MIBG scan and ^{68}Ga-DOTATATE PET-CT can determine the choice of RLT. PRRT can have added value in the treatment of metastasized pheochromocytoma/paraganglioma.[15] Currently, it is not approved by the US FDA, but it is available in clinical trials and as off-label treatment.

References

1. Harris AG, Vinik AI, O Dorisio TM, O Dorisio MS. Radioligand theranostics in the management of neuroendocrine tumors. *Pancreas.* 2020;49(5):599-603. PMID: 32433395

2. Buatti JM, Pryma DA, Kiess AP, et al. A framework for patient-centered pathways of care for radiopharmaceutical therapy: an ASTRO consensus document. *Int J Radiat Oncol Biol Phys.* 2021;109(4):913-922. PMID: 33249143

3. Bodei L, Herrmann K, Schöder H, Scott AM, Lewis JS. Radiotheranostics in oncology: current challenges and emerging opportunities. *Nat Rev Clin Oncol.* 2022;19(8):534-550. PMID: 35725926

4. Hofland J, Brabander T, Verburg FA, Feelders RA, de Herder WW. Peptide receptor radionuclide therapy. *J Clin Endocrinol Metab.* 2022;107(12):3199-3208. PMID: 36198028

5. Hope TA, Bodei L, Chan JA, et al. NANETS/SNMMI consensus statement on patient selection and appropriate use of ^{177}Lu-DOTATATE peptide receptor radionuclide therapy. *J Nucl Med.* 2020;61(2):222-227. PMID: 32015164

6. Brabander T, van der Zwan WA, Teunissen JJM, et al. Long-term efficacy, survival, and safety of [^{177}Lu-DOTA^0,Tyr^3]octreotate in patients with gastroenteropancreatic and bronchial neuroendocrine tumors. *Clin Cancer Res.* 2017;23(16):4617-4624. PMID: 28428192

7. Baum RP, Kulkarni HR, Singh A, et al. Results and adverse events of personalized peptide receptor radionuclide therapy with ^{90}Yttrium and ^{177}Lutetium in 1048 patients with neuroendocrine neoplasms. *Oncotarget.* 2018,9(24):16932-16950. PMID: 29682195

8. Zandee WT, van Adrichem RC, Kamp K, Feelders RA, van Velthuysen MF, de Herder WW. Incidence and prognostic value of serotonin secretion in pancreatic neuroendocrine tumours. *Clin Endocrinol (Oxf)*. 2017;87(2):165-170. PMID: 28464233

9. Hofland J, Kaltsas G, de Herder WW. Advances in the diagnosis and management of well-differentiated neuroendocrine neoplasms. *Endocr Rev*. 2020;41(2):371-403. PMID: 31555796

10. Rinke A, Müller H-H, Schade-Brittinger C, et al; PROMID Study Group. Placebo-controlled, double-blind, prospective, randomized study on the effect of octreotide LAR in the control of tumor growth in patients with metastatic neuroendocrine midgut tumors: a report from the PROMID Study Group. *J Clin Oncol*. 2009;27(28):4656-4663. PMID: 19704057

11. Caplin ME, Pavel M, Ćwikła JB, et al; CLARINET Investigators. Lanreotide in metastatic enteropancreatic neuroendocrine tumors. *N Engl J Med*. 2014;371(3):224-233. PMID: 25014687

12. van der Zwan WA, Brabander T, et al. Salvage peptide receptor radionuclide therapy with [177Lu-DOTA,Tyr3]octreotate in patients with bronchial and gastroenteropancreatic neuroendocrine tumours. *Eur J Nucl Med Mol Imaging*. 2019;46(3):704-717. PMID: 30267116

13. van Schaik E, van Vliet EI, Feelders RA, et al. Improved control of severe hypoglycemia in patients with malignant insulinomas by peptide receptor radionuclide therapy. *J Clin Endocrinol Metab*. 2011;96(11):3381-3389. PMID: 21917872

14. Minczeles NS, van Eijck CHJ, van Gils MJ, et al. Induction therapy with 177Lu-DOTATATE procures long-term survival in locally advanced or oligometastatic pancreatic neuroendocrine neoplasm patients. *Eur J Nucl Med Mol Imaging*. 2022;49(9):3203-3214. PMID: 35230492

15. Zandee WT, Feelders RA, Smit Duijzentkunst DA, et al. Treatment of inoperable or metastatic paragangliomas and pheochromocytomas with peptide receptor radionuclide therapy using 177Lu-DOTATATE. *Eur J Endocrinol*. 2019;181(1):45-53. PMID: 31067510

Managing Medullary Thyroid Carcinoma in Patients With *RET* Pathogenic Variants

Ana Oliveira Hoff, MD. Endocrine Oncology Unit, Department of Endocrinology, Instituto do Cancer do Estado de São Paulo (ICESP), Faculdade de Medicina da Universidade de São Paulo (FMUSP), São Paulo, Brazil; Email: ana.hoff@hc.fm.usp.br

Educational Objectives

As a result of participating in this session, learners should be able to:

- Explain the role of germline and somatic *RET* pathogenic variants in patients with medullary thyroid carcinoma (MTC).

- Describe the presentation and treatment of patients with MTC and multiple endocrine neoplasia (MEN) type 2.

- Identify patients with high-risk MTC that needs systemic treatment.

- Acquire knowledge about RET-targeted therapies, including multikinase inhibitors and the novel highly selective inhibitors.

Significance of the Clinical Problem

The growing knowledge obtained since the discovery of *RET* as the causative gene of hereditary MTC led to profound modification in the management of MEN type 2 and MTC. In addition to facilitating the discovery of new kindreds with MEN type 2, the gene's discovery led to recognition of strong genotype-phenotype correlations that prompted world-recognized recommendations regarding prophylactic thyroidectomy and pheochromocytoma screening. In addition, the identification of somatic *RET*

pathogenic variants in sporadic MTC and the understanding of *RET's* role as a driver gene that encodes a targetable tyrosine kinase receptor led to the development of RET-specific inhibitors with outstanding efficacy and few adverse effects. These drugs are being developed not only for metastatic MTC but for other solid tumors with *RET* fusions, including differentiated thyroid carcinoma and lung cancer. In this session, we will discuss the clinical management of patients with MTC harboring a germline or somatic *RET* pathogenic variant.

Practice Gaps

- Lack of knowledge about genetic drivers in MTC and genetic testing.

- Determining when to start newly approved RET inhibitors and which one to use.

Discussion

MTC is a rare neuroendocrine tumor that arises from the parafollicular cells. These cells produce calcitonin and CEA, which are used as tumor markers. Most cases are sporadic and about 25% are hereditary. When hereditary, MTC is associated with MEN type 2, which is an autosomal dominant syndrome associated not only with MTC but also with pheochromocytoma and primary hyperparathyroidism. The penetrance and aggressiveness of these clinical manifestations correlate with the specific *RET* variant.

The *RET* proto-oncogene is the major driver of MTC. Pathogenic germline variants in the gene are present in more than 99% of patients with hereditary MTC, and somatic variants are present in 50% to 93.8% of patients with sporadic MTC.[1-6] Patients diagnosed with MTC need germline testing; if a *RET* pathogenic variant is found and MEN type 2 is diagnosed, the patient should undergo annual screening for pheochromocytoma and primary hyperparathyroidism, and family members (first-degree relatives) require testing to verify whether they carry the variant. Carriers undergo prophylactic or therapeutic thyroidectomy; the age of prophylactic thyroidectomy is based on aggressiveness of the specific pathogenic variant. The 2015 American Thyroid Association guidelines classified *RET* pathogenic variants into 3 categories: highest risk (M918T), high risk (codon 634 variants and A883F), and moderate risk (all other *RET* pathogenic variants). Prophylactic thyroidectomies are recommended before age 1 year and before age 5 years for highest and high-risk variants, respectively. For moderate-risk variants, thyroidectomy is recommended within the first and second decade of life depending on the known aggressiveness of the specific variant and its behavior within the affected family (earliest age of onset, disease-free survival, and disease-specific mortality).[7]

Patients with hereditary or sporadic MTC who present with clinical evidence of disease need more extensive surgical treatment, as cervical lymph node involvement is common, and surgery is currently the only curative treatment.[8] These patients should undergo careful preoperative evaluation, including serum calcitonin and carcinoembryonic antigen (CEA) measurement, imaging studies, and screening for pheochromocytoma. Despite adequate surgical treatment, up to 65% of patients remain with disease and require long-term follow-up. Of this patient group, approximately 15% to 20% eventually develop progressive metastatic disease

and need systemic treatment.[9] All available treatments were developed based on the acquired knowledge of the important role of the activated RET signaling pathways in tumor development and progression. This session will focus on the importance of the RET-receptor signaling pathway in the development of MTC and in management decisions.

MTC: Clinical Presentation, Initial Treatment, and Follow-up

Except for carriers of *RET* pathogenic variants who, in most cases, undergo surgical treatment without yet developing clinical disease, most patients with MTC present with a thyroid nodule, with or without cervical lymphadenopathy. A smaller proportion of affected patients present with distant metastatic disease. In a recent series from the Mayo Clinic that included 163 patients with MTC diagnosed between 1995 and 2015, mean age at diagnosis was 48.4 ± 18.8 years, 37% had hereditary MTC, 44% presented with a palpable thyroid nodule, 49% presented with cervical lymph node metastases, and 8% presented with distant metastases.[9] These findings are also observed in other cohort series, with lymph node involvement ranging from 38% to 68% and distant metastases present in 6% to 21%.[10-12] Because a significant number of patients present with cervical lymph node involvement, the preoperative workup should include, in addition to measurements of tumor markers, detailed neck ultrasonography, including lateral lymphatic chains. Contrast-enhanced cross-sectional imaging studies are needed to better delineate disease extension, especially when serum calcitonin is greater than 500 pg/mL (>146 pmol/L).[7] Patients should undergo total thyroidectomy with central compartment dissection with or without lateral neck dissections.

Early diagnosis with treatment of disease still confined to the thyroid gland is essential to achieve biochemical cure in MTC. Several studies indicate the prognostic impact of lymph node metastases. One such study evaluated 197 patients with MTC who underwent systematic lymph node dissections in their initial operation. Only 27.4% (54 of 197) were biochemically cured. Cured patients had significantly less extrathyroidal extension and fewer lymph node metastases (median 2 to 4 vs 12 to 16) and were less likely to have AJCC pN1b disease (56% to 76% vs 89.9% to 91.6%) and distant metastases (0 vs 28.4% to 37.1%) than patients who were not cured.[8]

Postoperatively, assessment of therapeutic response is based on serum calcitonin and CEA measurements and neck ultrasonography. Biochemical remission or excellent response is defined by undetectable serum calcitonin, a CEA concentration within the reference range, and normal findings on neck ultrasonography. Biochemical incomplete response includes patients with normal or elevated calcitonin, elevated CEA, and normal findings on neck ultrasonography. Structural incomplete response includes patients with abnormal findings on neck ultrasonography or other imaging study, independent of biomarker levels. After assessing response to surgical treatment, follow-up tests performed, and their frequency, are determined based on extent of residual disease. Serum calcitonin is an excellent tumor marker, as it correlates well with tumor burden and increasing levels reflect disease progression. A serum calcitonin value greater than 150 pg/mL (>43.8 pmol/L) indicates locoregional or distant metastatic disease; therefore, these patients should have follow-up every 6 months with calcitonin and CEA measurement, as well as neck ultrasonography and structural imaging studies.[7] Because common metastatic sites include cervical and mediastinal lymph nodes, lungs, liver, and bones, recommended imaging studies are contrast-enhanced CT of the neck, chest, and abdomen (3-phase) or MRI to assess for liver metastases. For bone metastases, consider ^{68}Ga-DOTATE PET-CT if available; if not available, consider bone scan and/or skeletal MRI.[13,14]

In patients with biochemical incomplete or structural incomplete response, the main goal is to localize disease and determine disease progression so that a decision can be made to continue surveillance, to proceed with local treatments, or to initiate systemic therapy. In addition to imaging studies, serial measurements of tumor markers such as calcitonin and CEA are very helpful. The doubling time of calcitonin and CEA recommended in the 2015 American Thyroid Association guideline identifies patients with disease progression and those at high risk of disease-specific mortality.[15-17] Doubling time can be determined by measuring serum levels of calcitonin and CEA at least 4 points over at least a 2-year period. This calculator can be accessed at the following web address: (https://www.thyroid.org/professionals/calculators/thyroid-cancer-carcinoma/).

Determining when to initiate systemic therapy is still a challenge in clinical practice, as a significant number of patients with metastatic MTC have stable and asymptomatic disease not requiring systemic treatment. Clearly, patients with symptomatic and structural progression of disease are candidates to initiate therapy. Symptoms include diarrhea, flushing, or symptoms related to tumor mass (eg, airway compromise, pleural effusion, skeletal-related events, hypercortisolism from ectopic ACTH secretion, etc). Currently, 4 drugs are approved by the US FDA for treatment of advanced MTC: vandetanib, cabozantinib, selpercatinib, and pralsetinib. Their efficacy and related adverse effects will be summarized.

Genetic Drivers in MTC and Genetic Testing

RET is the most important gene responsible for development and progression of MTC. Germline pathogenic variants in *RET* are present in most patients with hereditary MTC, and somatic pathogenic variants are present in 55% to 85% of patients with sporadic MTC. The most common somatic *RET* variant is M918T, which is present in up to 40% of affected patients and is associated with disease aggressiveness and poor response to therapy. Other somatic *RET* pathogenic variants at residues C611, C618, C620, C630, C634, E768, A883, and S891, as well as small *RET* deletions and/or insertions, have been detected and associated with MTC development.[4,18,19]

RAS is another driver gene (mainly *HRAS* and *KRAS*) in which pathogenic variants can be observed in sporadic tumors. Such variants occur in 20% to 50% of tumors from patients without a *RET* variant.[3] Approximately 20% of sporadic MTC are negative for both *RET* and *RAS* variants, and several studies are underway to try to identify other drivers in MTC.

The identification of pathogenic variants in the *RET* gene, which encodes a tyrosine kinase receptor (RET receptor) that is a targetable kinase, led to a new era of treatment options for patients with advanced MTC. The first kinase inhibitors approved for treatment were less specific and had considerable activity against VEGFR2 and other VEGFR family members in addition to RET, but the new generation of RET inhibitors are significantly more specific. Being more specific means greater efficacy with fewer adverse events, but their use is limited to tumors with a *RET* pathogenic variant.

All index patients with newly diagnosed MTC regardless of disease stage or family history should have genetic counseling and be tested for germline *RET* pathogenic variants. Patients who need to start systemic therapy and do not harbor a germline *RET* pathogenic variant should undergo testing of a tumor sample. Testing may be performed on formalin-fixed, paraffin-embedded tissue, frozen samples, or cytological specimens. Ideally, testing the most recent tumor sample is preferable. Several next-generation sequencing panels are available; multiplexed next-generation sequencing panels are superior to multiple single-gene tests, and testing should be performed in CLIA (Clinical Laboratory Improvement Amendments)-accredited laboratories (or their international equivalent).[20]

Systemic Treatment

Management options for recurrent or residual MTC include close observation for indolent disease, surgical resection of locoregional disease, external-beam radiation therapy/intensity-modulated radiation therapy in selected cases, and local therapies, such as radiofrequency ablation, cryoablation, and embolization. Systemic therapy is indicated for patients with disease progression by Response Evaluation Criteria in Solid Tumors (RECIST) criteria that is not amenable to local treatment and can be considered in patients with stable disease but with uncontrolled symptoms and in patients with unresectable locally advanced disease that is symptomatic or progressing according to RECIST criteria.

Multikinase Inhibitors

Several multikinase inhibitors have been investigated in MTC, including sorafenib, sunitinib, lenvatinib, and pazopanib, but only vandetanib and cabozantinib were investigated in phase 3 trials and approved by several federal regulatory agencies, including the US FDA and European Medicines Agency.

Vandetanib targets RET, VEGFR, and EGF receptors. The ZETA trial included 331 patients with advanced MTC who were randomly assigned 2:1 to receive vandetanib (300 mg daily) or placebo. Inclusion criteria included measurable, unresectable locally advanced or metastatic MTC independent of disease progression. Progression-free survival (PFS) was significantly longer in the vandetanib-treated group than in the placebo group (30.5 vs 19.3 months; hazard ratio, 0.46; 95% CI, 0.31-0.69; $P < .001$). Although no significant difference was observed in overall survival, vandetanib was associated with significant improvements in tumor response rate and reductions in calcitonin and CEA levels.[21] In a post hoc subgroup analysis including patients with disease progression at baseline (n = 184) treated with vandetanib, PFS was significantly better than that observed with placebo (hazard ratio, 0.43; 95% CI, 0.28-0.64; $P < .01$), as well as overall response rate (37% vs 2%; $P < .001$).[22] In the United States, vandetanib access is restricted through a Risk Evaluation and Mitigation Strategy to prevent cardiac toxicity. Grade 3 or higher adverse events occurring in more than 5% of patients treated with vandetanib included diarrhea (11%), hypertension (9%), QTc prolongation (8%), and fatigue (6%).

Cabozantinib targets VEGFR-1 and VEGFR-2, MET, RET and c-KIT receptors. The phase 3 EXAM trial included 330 patients with advanced metastatic MTC that, differently from the ZETA trial, had documented progression. About 40% of these patients had previously received treatment with cytotoxic or other targeted therapies. Patients were randomly assigned (2:1) to cabozantinib (140 mg daily) or placebo. PFS (11.2 vs 4.0 months; hazard ratio = 0.28; 95% CI: 0.19-0.40; $P < .001$) and overall response rate (28 % vs 0%; $P < .001$) were significantly higher in the cabozantinib group than in the placebo group. Further analysis of the data revealed greater efficacy of cabozantinib in patients harboring a *RET* pathogenic variant. When the entire cohort of patients was analyzed for overall survival, no significant difference between the cabozantinib group and placebo group was observed. However, analysis of the subgroup of patients with a *RET* pathogenic variant demonstrated significantly longer overall survival (44.3 vs 18.9 months; hazard ratio, 0.60; 95% CI, 0.38-0.94; $P = 0.03$). PFS was also significantly longer in this patient subgroup (61 vs 17 weeks; hazard ratio, 0.15; 95% CI: 0.08-0.28; $P < .0001$). The adverse effect profile of cabozantinib is similar to that of vandetanib, with the exception of increased rates of palmar plantar erythrodysesthesia, liver function test abnormalities, and decreased rates of QTc prolongation.

No data are available comparing vandetanib with cabozantinib; therefore, the choice of the first regimen is usually individualized according to patient's clinical status, toxicity profile, and drug availability. Cabozantinib has not yet been approved for this indication in several countries.

RET-Specific Inhibitors

In addition to adverse events, both vandetanib and cabozantinib are subject to resistance by *RET* gatekeeper variants (V804M) and/or development of variants in the *RAS* gene (KRAS G12/G13) that result in disease progression. In these cases, the novel highly selective RET inhibitors can be effective therapies. In addition to their potency in inhibiting RET, even with gatekeeper variants, neither drug significantly inhibits VEGF receptors, known to contribute to the adverse events observed with multikinase inhibitors.

In 2020, the US FDA approved both selpercatinib and pralsetinib which are highly selective *RET* kinase inhibitors with very high potency to inhibit different *RET* pathogenic variants, including point mutations and fusions. The LIBRETTO-001 was a phase 1/2 clinical trial investigating safety and efficacy of selpercatinib, 160 mg twice daily, in 143 patients with MTC; 55 patients with *RET* pathogenic variant–positive MTC previously treated with vandetanib, cabozantinib, or both; and 88 patients with *RET* pathogenic variant–positive MTC not previously treated with vandetanib or cabozantinib. The overall response rate was 73% (95% CI, 62%-82%) and the 1-year PFS was 92% (95% CI, 82%-97%) in patients with *RET* pathogenic variant–positive MTC without previous treatment with vandetanib or cabozantinib and 69% (95% CI, 55%-81%), and the 1-year PFS was 82% (95% CI, 69%-90%) in the cohort of patients previously treated. The most common adverse events of grade 3 or higher were hypertension (in 21% of the patients), increased liver enzymes (in 11%), increased AST concentration (in 9%), hyponatremia (in 8%), and diarrhea (in 6%).[23] Only 2% of patients discontinued treatment because of adverse events. In a recent analysis of patient-related outcomes focused on diarrhea and quality of life, there was a significant reduction in reported diarrhea in 43.5% of patients and maintenance or improvement in all health-related quality of life subscales throughout treatment in most patients.[24]

The arrow study, also a phase 1/2, open-label study, included 122 patients with *RET* pathogenic variant–positive MTC (61 patients pretreated with cabozantinib or vandetanib, or both, and 23 treatment-naïve patients) who were treated with pralsetinib, 400 mg orally once daily. The overall response rate was 71% in treatment-naïve patients (95% CI, 48%-89%) and 60% (95% CI, 46%-73%) in pretreated patients. The estimated 1-year PFS after a median follow-up of 15 months was 75% (95% CI, 63%-86%) in pretreated patients and 81% (95% CI, 63%-98%) in treatment-naïve patients. Grade 3 or 4 adverse events included leukopenia, anemia, decreased phosphate, hypocalcemia, hyponatremia, increased liver enzymes, thrombocytopenia, and increased alkaline phosphatase levels.[25]

Both selpercatinib (LIBRETTO-531, NCT04211337) and pralsetinib (AcceleRET-MTC NCT04760288) are being investigated in multicenter, randomized, open-label, phase 3 trials in patients with metastatic and progressive *RET* pathogenic variant–positive MTC without prior kinase inhibitor therapy and compared with cabozantinib or vandetanib as first-line therapies. Both trials will provide important information on how best to sequence these therapies.

Clinical Case Vignettes

Case 1

A 31-year-old man presents for evaluation after his niece was diagnosed with MTC and genetic testing revealed a germline *RET* Cys634Arg pathogenic variant. He has no specific concerns. He undergoes genetic testing, which reveals the presence of the *RET* pathogenic variant. Physical examination findings are unremarkable except for a 2-cm palpable thyroid nodule.

Which of the following is the most appropriate next step?

A. This patient has MTC and needs referral to a head and neck or endocrine surgeon for surgical treatment

B. As he is asymptomatic and this specific *RET* variant is not associated with pheochromocytoma, there is no need to measure urinary catecholamines or plasma metanephrines

C. As he is asymptomatic and treatment can be delayed, proceed first with genetic counseling and a detailed family history to identify other family members who need testing

D. Perform screening for pheochromocytoma; measure serum calcitonin, CEA, and calcium; and perform neck ultrasonography

Answer: D) Perform screening for pheochromocytoma, measure serum calcitonin, CEA, and calcium and perform neck ultrasonography

The *RET* Cys634Arg pathogenic variant is the most common variant associated with MEN type 2A. According to the American Thyroid Association 2015 guideline, it is classified as a high-risk variant associated with MTC in all carriers, with onset in the first decade of life, usually before 5 years of age. In addition, it is associated with pheochromocytoma in 50% of patients and primary hyperparathyroidism in about 20% of patients. Once a germline *RET* variant is detected, all carriers should undergo screening for pheochromocytoma, independent of the specific *RET* variant. In the event that pheochromocytoma is diagnosed, adrenalectomy should be performed before any other surgical procedure. According to the 2015 American Thyroid Association guideline, carriers of a *RET* codon 634 variant should undergo prophylactic thyroidectomy before age 5 years and should start annual screening for pheochromocytoma at age 11 years. Thus, this patient should undergo screening for pheochromocytoma; measurement of serum calcitonin, CEA, and calcium; and neck ultrasonography (Answer D).

Case 1 (continued)

Screening is positive for pheochromocytoma, and right adrenalectomy is performed.

Laboratory test results:

Serum calcitonin = 650 pg/mL (<14.3 pg/mL) (SI: 189.8 pmol/L [<4.2 pmol/L])
CEA = 15 μg/L (<3.0 μg/L)
Serum calcium = 9.2 mg/dL (8.6-10.3 mg/dL) (SI: 2.3 mmol/L [2.2-2.6 mmol/L])

Ultrasonography reveals 2 hypoechoic thyroid nodules: a 2.5-cm nodule in the right lobe and a 0.8-cm nodule in the left lobe in addition to bilateral suspicious lymph nodes. FNA biopsy confirms medullary thyroid carcinoma involving thyroid and bilateral lymph nodes.

Which of the following is the most appropriate management plan?

A. Preoperative serum calcitonin concentration >500 pg/mL (>146 pmol/L) indicates metastatic disease; he should undergo contrast-enhanced CT of the neck, chest, and abdomen, as well as a bone scan; if metastatic disease is identified, he should initiate a multikinase inhibitor or a RET-specific inhibitor because disease is uncurable and surgery is contraindicated

B. Preoperative serum calcitonin concentration >500 pg/mL (>146 pmol/L) indicates metastatic disease; he should undergo contrast-enhanced CT of the neck, chest, and abdomen, as well as a bone scan; if metastatic disease is identified but local disease is resectable, he should undergo total thyroidectomy with central and lateral lymph node dissections

C. As he has a *RET* pathogenic variant and has advanced locoregional disease, the standard of care is neoadjuvant treatment with a RET-specific inhibitor such as selpercatinib

D. As he is older than the recommended age for thyroidectomy, is asymptomatic, and has advanced but indolent locoregional disease, he can be observed and start active surveillance with serum markers and imaging studies

Answer: B) Preoperative serum calcitonin concentration >500 pg/mL (>146 pmol/L) indicates metastatic disease; he should undergo contrast-enhanced CT of the neck, chest, and abdomen, as well as a bone scan; if metastatic disease is identified but local disease is resectable, he should undergo total thyroidectomy with central and lateral lymph node dissections

A preoperative serum calcitonin concentration greater than 500 pg/mL (>146 pmol/L) is suggestive of significant tumor burden and can be associated with distant metastatic disease. It is appropriate, therefore, to proceed with contrast-enhanced imaging studies to evaluate disease extent. In MTC, despite the presence of metastatic disease, appropriate surgical treatment is indicated if disease is resectable. Local control of disease is necessary for longer survival, especially with MTC; a patient can live for several years with stable metastatic disease. Thus, the best next step is contrast-enhanced CT of the neck, chest, and abdomen, as well as a bone scan. If metastatic disease is identified but local disease is resectable, he should undergo total thyroidectomy with central and lateral lymph node dissections (Answer B).

Neoadjuvant treatment with targeted therapy with the goal of tumor reduction to enable surgery is recommended for several solid tumors, including *BRAF*-positive anaplastic and poorly differentiated thyroid cancers. However, neoadjuvant treatment with the highly selective RET inhibitors is still under investigation in MTC. Observation with active monitoring of disease progression (tumor markers and imaging studies) is appropriate after surgical treatment in patients with low tumor burden who are asymptomatic and have indolent metastatic disease.

Case 1 (continued)

After adrenalectomy, the patient undergoes total thyroidectomy with central and lateral lymph node dissections. Staging with imaging studies fails to reveal distant metastatic disease. Pathology reveals multifocal MTC, largest foci of 2.4 cm with 26 metastatic lymph nodes (out of 68) (T2N1bM0 – AJCC 8th stage IVa). Postoperatively, his serum calcitonin concentration is 258 pg/mL (75.3 pmol/L), CEA is within the reference range, and findings on neck ultrasonography are normal, indicating biochemical incomplete response.

Over the next 6 years, he returns for annual follow-up appointments and has no evidence of contralateral pheochromocytoma or structural disease despite a progressive increase in calcitonin concentration. He then goes 5 years with no follow-up until he is diagnosed with primary hyperparathyroidism. He has a total parathyroidectomy with forearm graft.

Laboratory test results:

> Serum calcitonin = 31,825 pg/mL (<14.3 pg/mL)
> (SI: 9292.9 pmol/L [<4.2 pmol/L])
> CEA = 1538 μg/L (<3.0 μg/L)

Imaging studies reveal liver, bone, and lung metastases. He is closely monitored with imaging studies and tumor markers to assess disease progression. Calcitonin and CEA doubling times are longer than 24 months. He undergoes left adrenalectomy for a contralateral pheochromocytoma with resulting adrenal insufficiency. He remains asymptomatic until age 53 years when he starts experiencing diarrhea that is controlled with loperamide.

Which of the following is the most appropriate management plan?

A. Despite having stable metastatic disease and diarrhea controlled by loperamide, he should start systemic treatment with a kinase inhibitor

B. Despite having a *RET* germline pathogenic variant, he should have tumor testing to evaluate for a somatic *RET* pathogenic variant; if a variant is confirmed in the tumor, he is a candidate to be treated with the highly specific RET inhibitors—selpercatinib or pralsetinib

C. As there is no structural evidence of progression, continued surveillance with symptom control is a reasonable therapeutic option

D. Adrenal insufficiency is a contraindication to start multikinase inhibitors, so vandetanib and cabozantinib are not good therapeutic options

Answer: C) As there is no structural evidence of progression, continued surveillance with symptom control is a reasonable therapeutic option

A clear indication to start systemic therapy is progression of structural disease by the RECIST criteria. However, systemic therapy can be considered in patients with symptoms uncontrolled by medical or local treatment and significant tumor burden without progression. At this point, as none of the available drugs are curative and are associated with adverse effects; a patient with stable disease who is asymptomatic or has controlled symptoms can remain under surveillance (Answer C).

If a patient has a germline *RET* pathogenic variant, tumor testing is unnecessary because the tumor cells will also have the *RET* variant. Somatic testing (tumor testing) should be performed in patients who do not have a germline *RET* pathogenic variant.

Case 2

A 38-year-old man presents with an enlarging neck mass. Preoperative workup excludes pheochromocytoma and reveals a 6.6-cm hypoechoic left thyroid nodule with coarse calcifications and left cervical lymphadenopathy. Findings on FNA biopsy are consistent with MTC.

Preoperative laboratory test results:

> Serum calcitonin = 1552 pg/mL (<14.3 pg/mL)
> (SI: 453.2 pmol/L [<4.2 pmol/L])
> CEA = 10 μg/L (<3.0 μg/L)

He has a total thyroidectomy with central and bilateral lymph node dissection. Pathology reveals a 7-cm MTC with vascular invasion and extrathyroidal extension with 26 metastatic lymph nodes removed (out of 96 lymph nodes) and a Ki67 index of 20% (T4N1bM0). Genetic testing does not identify a germline *RET* pathogenic variant.

Postoperatively, his calcitonin concentration is 95 pg/mL (27.7 pmol/L), his CEA concentration is within the reference range, and there are normal findings on imaging studies (neck ultrasonography and CT of the neck, chest, and abdomen), indicating incomplete biochemical response. Follow-up reveals steady rise of serum calcitonin; 1 year later, his serum calcitonin concentration is 437 pg/mL (127.6 pmol/L), CEA concentration is 2.1 ng/mL, and CT of the abdomen reveals subcentimetric hypervascular liver lesions. An

FDG-PET/CT reveals a 2-cm hilar lymph node (SUV 5), small lesions in C7 and T1 (SUV 5.6), and liver lesions with no FDG uptake. A ^{68}Ga-DOTATATE PET-CT is also performed, which shows ^{68}Ga uptake in a 1.1-cm cervical lymph node and a 2-cm hilar lymph node and moderate to high uptake in C7, T1, manubrium, left fifth rib, and liver lesions.

He is treated with 4 doses of ^{177}Lu-DOTATATE peptide receptor radionuclide therapy without significant response.

Which of the following tests is most appropriate now?

A. Next-generation sequencing of formalin-fixed, paraffin-embedded tumor tissue from thyroidectomy

B. A multicancer panel to identify germline pathogenic variants

C. Liquid biopsy with next-generation sequencing

D. RNA-based next-generation sequencing of tumor sample to detect *RET* fusions

Answer: A) Next-generation sequencing of formalin-fixed, paraffin-embedded tumor tissue from thyroidectomy

Systemic treatment is indicated for this patient who has structural progression of disease. Current options include vandetanib, cabozantinib, selpercatinib, and pralsetinib. Selpercatinib and pralsetinib are highly specific to RET and are only indicated in patients with a germline or somatic *RET* pathogenic variant. Vandetanib and cabozantinib are multikinase inhibitors that can be used independent of the *RET* variant status. There is no consensus on the best first-line therapy, but because of higher efficacy and better toxicity profile, selpercatinib or pralsetinib are preferable. However, access to tumor testing and to these specific inhibitors is not universal. When tumor testing is possible, next-generation sequencing of a sample from thyroidectomy can be performed to identify a *RET* somatic pathogenic variant (Answer A).

RET fusions (Answer D) are present in differentiated thyroid cancer and not in MTC.

Liquid biopsy (Answer C) can be performed, but it is less sensitive than next-generation sequencing of the tumor sample.

As patient has had negative *RET* genetic testing, there is no need to perform another germline panel (Answer B), unless there were suspicion of another hereditary syndrome.

Case 2 (continued)

Two somatic *RET* variants are identified: M918T and V804M.

Which of the following is the most appropriate treatment?

A. The presence of V804M indicates resistance to treatment with vandetanib and cabozantinib, so selpercatinib should be started

B. The presence of any *RET* somatic variant is associated with better overall response rate, PFS, and overall survival when treated with cabozantinib and *RET*-specific inhibitors

C. The EXAM trial included patients with progression similar to that of this patient and showed significant improvement in PFS; therefore, cabozantinib is the best option

D. Pralsetinib is resistant to the *RET* V804M variant and should not be used in this patient

Answer: A) The presence of the V804M variant indicates resistance to treatment with vandetanib and cabozantinib, so selpercatinib should be started

The presence of both of *RET* variants indicates that this patient is eligible for treatment with the highly specific RET inhibitors selpercatinib or pralsetinib. The *RET* M918T variant is the most frequent somatic variant. Despite being associated with more aggressive disease, this variant has also been associated with better PFS and overall survival with cabozantinib treatment compared with these metrics in patients without a *RET* variant. Similar findings were observed with vandetanib, although not statistically significant.

The *RET* V804M variant is a gatekeeper mutation that causes resistance to cabozantinib and vandetanib, as it changes conformation of their binding site at the RET receptor. This variant can be observed in patients with MEN type 2 (germline pathogenic variant) or as a somatic variant. In some cases, a resistance variant is associated with disease progression when the patient is treated with vandetanib or cabozantinib. The presence of this specific variant precludes the use of vandetanib or cabozantinib. Thus, selpercatinib should be started (Answer A).

Key Learning Points

- All patients diagnosed with MTC, independent of age and family history, should undergo germline *RET* genetic testing.

- If a germline *RET* pathogenic variant is identified and MEN type 2 is diagnosed, the patient should undergo annual screening for pheochromocytoma and primary hyperparathyroidism, and family members (first-degree relatives) should undergo testing to verify whether they carry the variant.

- Surgery is the only curative treatment. Patients who present with clinically evident disease, independent of *RET* variant status, should have total thyroidectomy and central lymph node dissection. Carriers of a *RET* pathogenic variant without clinically evident disease should undergo prophylactic thyroidectomy.

- Postoperatively, response to surgical treatment is based on serum calcitonin and CEA levels and imaging studies. Frequency of follow-up and determination of which imaging studies to be performed should be based on response to treatment (excellent response, incomplete biochemical response, or structural incomplete response).

- Management options for recurrent or residual MTC include close observation for indolent disease, local therapies in selected patients, and systemic therapy for patients with structural progression of disease.

- Currently approved drugs for metastatic MTC in patients who need systemic therapy include vandetanib, cabozantinib, selpercatinib, and pralsetinib. The decision of which drug to start should include review of comorbidities, performance status, drug availability, and somatic testing availability. If all drugs are available, as well as somatic testing, the decision can be based on the presence or absence of a *RET* pathogenic variant.

References

1. Elisei R, Cosci B, Romei C, et al. Prognostic significance of somatic RET oncogene mutations in sporadic medullary thyroid cancer: a 10-year follow-up study. *J Clin Endocrinol Metab.* 2008;93(3):682-687. PMID: 18073307

2. Romei C, Casella F, Tacito A, et al. New insights in the molecular signature of advanced medullary thyroid cancer: evidence of a bad outcome of cases with double RET mutations. *J Med Genet.* 2016;53(11):729-734. PMID: 27468888

3. Agrawal N, Jiao Y, Sausen M, et al. Exomic sequencing of medullary thyroid cancer reveals dominant and mutually exclusive oncogenic mutations in RET and RAS. *J Clin Endocrinol Metab.* 2013;98(2):E364-E369. PMID: 23264394

4. Heilmann AM, Subbiah V, Wang K, et al. Comprehensive genomic profiling of clinically advanced medullary thyroid carcinoma. *Oncology.* 2016;90(6):339-346. PMID: 27207748

5. Larouche V, Akirov A, Thomas CM, Krzyzanowska MK, Ezzat S. A primer on the genetics of medullary thyroid cancer. *Curr Oncol.* 2019;26(6):389-394. PMID: 31896937

6. Barletta JA, Nosé V, Sadow PM. Genomics and epigenomics of medullary thyroid carcinoma: from sporadic disease to familial manifestations. *Endocr Pathol.* 2021;32(1):35-43. PMID: 33492588

7. Wells SA Jr, Asa SL, Dralle H, et al; American Thyroid Association Guidelines Task Force on Medullary Thyroid Carcionma. Revised American Thyroid Association guidelines for the management of medullary thyroid carcinoma. *Thyroid.* 2015;25(6):567-610. PMID: 25810047

8. Machens A, Lorenz K, Dralle H. Prediction of biochemical cure in patients with medullary thyroid cancer. *Br J Surg.* 2020;107(6):695-704. PMID: 32108330

9. Kotwal A, Erickson D, Geske JR, Hay ID, Castro MR. Predicting outcomes in sporadic and hereditary medullary thyroid carcinoma over two decades. *Thyroid.* 2021;31(4):616-626. PMID: 33108969

10. Mathiesen JS, Kroustrup JP, Vestergaard P, et al. Survival and long-term biochemical cure in medullary thyroid carcinoma in Denmark 1997-2014: a nationwide study. *Thyroid.* 2019;29(3):368-377. PMID: 30618340

11. Twito O, Grozinsky-Glasberg S, Levy S, et al. Clinico-pathologic and dynamic prognostic factors in sporadic and familial medullary thyroid carcinoma: an Israeli multi-center study. *Eur J Endocrinol.* 2019;181(1):13-21. PMID: 31048559

12. Choi JB, Lee SG, Kim MJ, et al. Dynamic risk stratification in medullary thyroid carcinoma: single institution experiences. *Medicine (Baltimore)*. 2018;97(3):e9686. PMID: 29505021

13. Castroneves LA, Coura Filho G, de Freitas RMC, et al. Comparison of 68Ga PET/CT to other imaging studies in medullary thyroid cancer: superiority in detecting bone metastases. *J Clin Endocrinol Metab*. 2018;103(9):3250-3259. PMID: 29846642

14. Haddad RI, Bischoff L, Ball D, et al. Thyroid carcinoma, version 2.2022, NCCN clinical practice guidelines in oncology. *J Natl Compr Canc Netw*. 2022;20(8):925-951. PMID: 35948029

15. Miyauchi A, Onishi T, Morimoto S, et al. Relation of doubling time of plasma calcitonin levels to prognosis and recurrence of medullary thyroid carcinoma. *Ann Surg*. 1984;199(4):461-466. PMID: 6712322

16. Barbet J, Campion L, Kraeber-Bodéré F, Chatal JF, GTE Study Group. Prognostic impact of serum calcitonin and carcinoembryonic antigen doubling-times in patients with medullary thyroid carcinoma. *J Clin Endocrinol Metab*. 2005;90(11):6077-6084. PMID: 16091497

17. Laure Giraudet A, Al Ghulzan A, Aupérin A, et al. Progression of medullary thyroid carcinoma: assessment with calcitonin and carcinoembryonic antigen doubling times. *Eur J Endocrinol*. 2008;158(2):239-246. PMID: 18230832

18. Salvatore D, Santoro M, Schlumberger M. The importance of the RET gene in thyroid cancer and therapeutic implications. *Nat Rev Endocrinol*. 2021;17(5):296-306. PMID: 33603219

19. Ciampi R, Romei C, Ramone T, et al. Genetic landscape of somatic mutations in a large cohort of sporadic medullary thyroid carcinomas studied by next-generation targeted sequencing. *iScience*. 2019;20:324-336. PMID: 31605946

20. Shonka DC Jr, Ho A, Chintakuntlawar AV, et al. American Head and Neck Society Endocrine Surgery Section and International Thyroid Oncology Group consensus statement on mutational testing in thyroid cancer: defining advanced thyroid cancer and its targeted treatment. *Head Neck*. 2022;44(6):1277-1300. PMID: 35274388

21. Wells SA Jr, Robinson BG, Gagel RF, et al. Vandetanib in patients with locally advanced or metastatic medullary thyroid cancer: a randomized, double-blind phase III trial. *J Clin Oncol*. 2012;30(2):134-141. PMID: 22025146

22. Kreissl MC, Bastholt L, Elisei R, et al. Efficacy and safety of vandetanib in progressive and symptomatic medullary thyroid cancer: post hoc analysis from the ZETA Trial. *J Clin Oncol*. 2020;38(24):2773-2781. PMID: 32584630

23. Wirth LJ, Sherman E, Robinson B, et al. Efficacy of selpercatinib in *RET*-altered thyroid cancers. *N Engl J Med*. 2020;383(9):825-835. PMID: 32846061

24. Wirth LJ, Robinson B, Boni V, Tan DSW, McCoach C, Massarelli E, et al. Patient-reported outcomes with selpercatinib treatment among patients with RET-mutant medullary thyroid cancer in the Phase I/II LIBRETTO-001 Trial. *Oncologist*. 2022;27(1):13-21. PMID: 34516023

25. Subbiah V, Hu MI, Wirth LJ, et al. Pralsetinib for patients with advanced or metastatic RET-altered thyroid cancer (ARROW): a multi-cohort, open-label, registrational, phase 1/2 study. *Lancet Diabetes Endocrinol*. 2021;9(8):491-501. PMID: 34118198

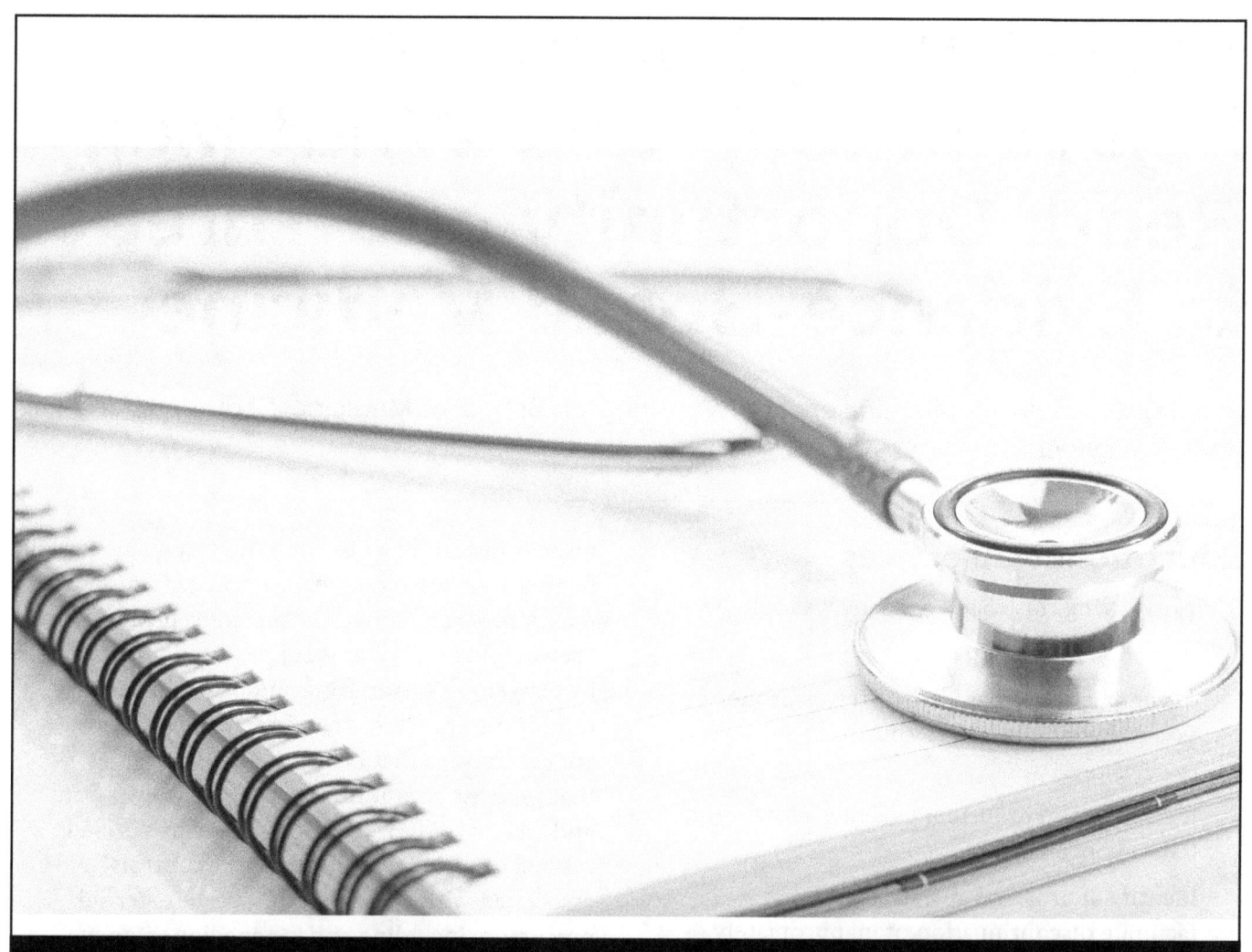

MISCELLANEOUS

"Hormone Optimization," "Rejuvenation," and What Men Read: Opportunity and Threat to Evidence-Based Medicine

Bradley D. Anawalt, MD. University of Washington School of Medicine, Seattle, WA; Email: banawalt@medicine.washington.edu

Educational Objectives

After reviewing this chapter, learners should be able to:

- Recognize clues that identify testosterone assays that might lead to spurious clinical conclusions.

- Identify when to further evaluate a low serum IGF-1 concentration.

- Identify approaches and strategies that facilitate discontinuation of inappropiately prescribed drugs used to "optimize" serum sex steroid hormone and IGF-1 concentrations.

Significance of the Clinical Problem

Over the past 2 decades, there has been a marked increase in the prescription of testosterone to men who are eugonadal or without conclusive evidence of hypogonadism.[1,2] In many countries, clinics that are marketed as "hormone optimizer" or "rejuvenation" clinics have increased in a parallel trend. Testosterone is prescribed liberally to men without risk factors for hypogonadism and who often have normal serum testosterone concentrations.[3] A potpourri of drugs is frequently prescribed: testosterone to increase sexual function, increase vitality, and for favorable changes in muscle and fat; hCG to maintain testicular size and further increase blood testosterone; clomiphene to maintain serum gonadotropin concentrations and spermatogenesis (that is suppressed in normal men by exogenous testoterone and hCG); aromatase inhibitor to prevent a rise in serum estrogen concentrations that occurs with all therapies that increase serum testosterone concentration; and GH or GHRH. (GHRH is often prescribed instead of GH to avoid regulatory controls associated with GH prescription.) Sex steroid precursors including androstenedione ("andro") and dehydroepiandosterone (DHEA) are often recommended by "hormone optimization" clinics, but these prescursors are not typically prescribed or recommended at dosages high enough to increase serum testoterone in men. More modest dosages of DHEA and androstenedione can cause gynecomastia, however. Rarely, nontestosterone androgens (most commonly, nandrolone) are prescribed. Thyroid hormone is sometimes included in hormone optizimation, too, and efforts to raise serum thyroid hormone concentrations within the normal range often result in subclinical or overt thyrotoxicosis. Thyroid hormone will not be discussed further in this Meet the Professor chapter. When administered to normal men without hypogonadism or GH deficiency, all of these drugs have been associated with harm, and none of them have conclusive evidence of benefit.

Practice Gaps

- Widespread prevalence of misleading direct-to-consumer advertising and dissemination of falsehoods and misinformation on the internet and some popular media sources.

- Lack of clinical recognition of the significant variation in the quality and normal ranges of serum testosterone and IGF-1 assays.

- Lack of clinical awareness of the progess toward the standardization and harmonization of serum testosterone assays (led by the Endocrine Society and US Centers for Disease Control and Prevention [CDC]).

- Inappropriate screening for hypogonadism and GH deficiency by some clinicians and unregulated "rejuvenation," "hormone optimization," and "testosterone clinics."

- Failure to recognize that the benefit-to-risk ratio of therapies that raise serum testosterone (or serum gonadotropins and testosterone) shifts from positive in men with androgen deficiency and/or hypogonadotropism and infertility to negative in eugonadal men.

Discussion

Clinical Presentation of Eugonadal Men Who Are Considering "Hormonal Optimization" or "Hormonal Rejuvenation" Therapies

Although endocrinologists always attempt to optimize hormonal therapy for patients with endocrinopathies, I will be referring to "hormone optimization" as defined on a variety of alleged "wellness" internet sites as a health and medical management program "to restore natural hormone levels to their optimal threshold"; note that the optimal threshold is generally not defined. The threshold is often unstated or capriciously set at or near the middle of the normal range. In a study published in December 2022, a secret shopper contacted 7 companies that offered testosterone therapy through online appointments in all 50 states of the United States.[3] The secret shopper followed a script that he had low energy and low libido, and he submitted results from a well-known major commercial laboratory that collaborated with the investigators. The secret shopper had a serum total testosterone concentration of 675 ng/dL (23.43 nmol/L) in a validated testosterone assay (see below under *Management*) with a normal range of 264 to 916 ng/dL (9.2-31.8 nmol/L). Six of the 7 companies offered testosterone therapy to the secret shopper; the single company that did not offer testosterone therapy used the threshold of 450 ng/dL (15.63 nmol/L).

Men of all ages are taking testosterone for "hormone optimization," but middle-aged to older men (35-65 years) might be more likely to request these therapies. Younger men (20-35 years) commonly report that they have the "blood testosterone of an old man." Younger men request "hormone optimization" to increase muscle mass and strength, whereas middle-aged and older men typically are seeking improved mood, energy, vitality, and sexual function. Other common presentations include men who have laboratory results that show very low serum total testosterone (eg, 190 ng/dL [6.60 nmol/L]), but the assay has a low normal range of 160 to 620 ng/dL (5.56-21.53 nmol/L), or men who have a serum total testosterone of 320 ng/dL (11.11 nmol/L) in an assay with a normal range of 335 to 1200 ng/dL (11.63-41.67 nmol/L). A recent survey study of 120 large laboratories in 47 US states demonstrated significant variability in reference ranges.[4] The mean lower limit of normal was only 231 ng/dL (8 nmol/L), and the mean upper limit of normal was 850 ng/dL (29.5 nmol/L) with large standard deviation for both limits. Two important clues for less-useful testosterone assays are automated immunoassays that have lower accuracy and any assay with a reference range that deviates significantly from 264 to 916 ng/dL (9.2-31.8 nmol/L). A caveat is that many laboratories are claiming a normal range of 264 to 916 ng/dL (9.2-31.8 nmol/L) without actually establishing a normal reference range of their assay based on 60 to 100 healthy young men.

The primary information resources for these men are the internet, traditional journalism that is not carefully vetted, and direct-to-consumer advertising. The latest threat to accuracy is artificial intelligence (AI) and GPChat. In February 2023, "What All Men Should Know About Low Testosterone" was AI-generated, purportedly reviewed by human editors and then published in *Men's Journal* by the Arena Group (that also publishes *Sports Illustrated*). There were at least 18 factual errors in this 1-page article (https://futurism.com/neoscope/magazine-mens-journal-errors-ai-health-article). The conclusion read fancifully, "Fortunately, young, healthy men can naturally keep their T levels in check by taking targeted supplements, eating testosterone-boosting meals (including oysters), and monitoring stress levels." The article was taken down, partially edited, and returned to the online site only after the errors were discovered by an investigative journalist.

Management of Low Serum Testosterone ± Low Serum IGF-1 Concentrations

Screening for hypogonadism or GH deficiency is not recommended. However, men who are interested in "hormone optimization" or who have been seen at a "hormone optimization" clinic typically present to endocrinologists with results of serum testosterone concentrations and sometimes serum IGF-1 concentrations. Although most of these men are eugonadal and do not have GH deficiency, a small percentage are hypogonadal and should have a focused history and physical examination for symptoms, risk factors, and signs of androgen deficiency.

The management of men without risk factors for hypogonadism and who request testosterone therapy or "hormone optimization" therapy for improved energy, muscle mass, and/or sexual function is often difficult because they have heightened expectations about the potential benefits of testosterone therapy. However, this is an opportunity to educate these men about healthy lifestyle choices.

The first principle of the management of borderline-low or low serum testosterone concentrations measured at the wrong time or with a total testosterone assay that is suspicious for low quality is to measure serum testosterone with a high-quality assay at least once in a fasting early-morning sample.[4] Because acute illness or a flare of chronic illness may result in suppression of the hypothalamic-pituitary-testicular axis, the morning blood sample must be obtained when the man is at usual baseline health. Many men with a borderline-low or low serum testosterone concentration have a BMI of 30 kg/m^2 or higher, and it is often useful to assess serum SHBG and free testosterone using an accurate method such as calculated free testosterone with one of the validated formulae (eg, the Vermeulen formula) or direct measurement of free testosterone by mass spectrometry after equilibrium dialysis.[4]

Because of this wide variability of total testosterone assay performance and normal range, it is important to use a total testosterone assay (with a normal range of 264-916 ng/dL [9.2-31.8 nmol/L]) that has been validated and harmonized by a trusted, independent, external agency such as the CDC.[5,6] There are several laboratories with CDC-validated and harmonized total testosterone assays in the United States and some in Europe and Asia.[7] These validated and harmonized testosterone assays have the additional advantage of being connected to patient outcomes in 2 of the largest placebo-controlled trials of testosterone therapy in older men: the United States Testosterone Trials and the soon-to-be-published TRAVERSE trial.

The second principle of the management of borderline-low or low-normal serum testosterone concentrations in men with low or very low probability of hypogonadism is education about normal ranges. It is useful to state that the normal range of testosterone has been based on blood samples drawn in the early morning (when testosterone concentrations peak) in normal, healthy young men. A young man who has a low-normal serum testosterone conconcentration has a result that is normal compared with concentrations of other young healthy men. Use of fasting early-morning samples is essential to reduce the variability of the measured testosterone results. It is equally important to confirm low results with at least 1 more sample. For men with a low total testosterone result based on an assay that has not been validated by an external quality control agency and/or has an unusual normal range, I often order measurement of 2 blood testosterone concentrations drawn in the fasting state between 7 and 10 AM.

The third principle of the management of borderline-low or low-normal serum testosterone concentrations is a healthy lifestyle. Many of these men have a high BMI ($\geq$30 kg/m^2). Exercise at least 3 times weekly for 90 minutes is associated with improved sense of well-being, strength, and physical function in men with obesity.[8] Weight loss of 7% to 10% with regular exercise and a hypocaloric diet is associated with a significant increase of average serum testosterone (10%-30% above baseline values) and improved sexual function in men with obesity and low serum testosterone.[9,10] Although broccoli, oysters, and other specific foods have been touted as "testosterone boosters," there is no good evidence or rational mechanism that any specific foods will cause a sustained increase in serum testosterone. Weight loss, not macronutrient proportions, increases serum total testosterone in men with high BMI.

The principles of management of low serum IGF-1 concentrations are similar to those of low serum testosterone concentrations. A number of health conditions, including diabetes mellitus, malnutrition, chronic liver disease, and kidney diseases, may result in a low serum IGF-1 concentration.[11] In addition, serum IGF-1 assays have extremely variable performance and quality.[11] Finally, serum IGF-1 declines with aging, and GH therapy is not indicated for a low serum IGF-1 concentration due to aging.[11] In general, an adult with a slightly low serum IGF-1 or low-normal IGF-1 concentration and no known or suspected cause of GH deficiency needs no further evaluation.

Prevention and Management of Inappropriately Prescribed Testosterone, hCG, Aromatase Inhibitors, Clomiphene, and GH or GHRH

Men who have been initiated on multiple drugs that increase serum testosterone generally have a very high serum testosterone concentration through different mechanisms. Exogenous hCG has LH activity and stimulates Leydig-cell synthesis of testosterone. Aromatase inhibitors block testosterone metabolism resulting in a modest increase in serum testosterone. Aromatase inhibitors and clomiphene, a selective recepter modulator, decrease estradiol-mediated inhibition of gonadotropin secretion and result in serum gonadotropins that are relatively unsuppressed by the high circulating testosterone concentrations from exogenous testosterone and hCG. Dosages of these medications that result in very high serum testosterone concentrations are known to suppress spermatogenesis and fertility and also cause erythrocytosis.[12] There have also been concerns of an association between very supranormal serum testosterone and increased cardiovascular risk, including atherosclerosis, cardiac fibrosis, and cardimyopathy.[12] For men who have been taking the combination of testosterone, hCG, an aromatase inhibitor, and clomiphene, the hCG, aromatase inhibitor, and clomiphene may be stopped immediately. I inform the man that the hCG is more likely to cause gynecomastia (the LH activity increases aromatase activity and estradiol production), the aromatase inhibitor results in increased body fat and decreased bone mass, and clomiphene is associated with venous thromboses including retinal vein thromboses.[13,14] The long-term safety of clomiphene, a hormone with mixed agonist-antagonist estrogen properties for stroke, myocardial infarction, and fracture risk is unknown.[12] Most men are willing to stop these drugs at the first or second visit.

Testosterone therapy might need to be tapered under 2 circumstances: (1) the patient has been taking testosterone and/or hCG for significantly more than 1 year; or (2) the patient is concerned about abrupt withdrawal from all of the medications that increase serum testosterone. For patients who have been taking testosterone alone or testosterone plus hCG for less than 1 year, immediate discontinuation is sensible after informing them of the possibility of hypogonadal symptoms for 1 to 3 months while hypothalamic and pituitary function recover. For patients who have been taking testosterone or testosterone for significantly longer than 1 year, androgen withdrawal with inanition, depression, and symptoms of hypogonadism is more likely. These patients tend to do better with a testosterone taper; they avoid severe withdrawal symptoms, and they like the idea of a slower decrement in serum testosterone.

For those men taking GH and/or androgen precursor as a part of the hormone menu, these may be discontinued immediately, too. Reviewing the lack of evidence of benefit of GH for aging men and the potential accumulating effects that might result in acromegaly is generally persuasive. Because the dosages of androstenedione and DHEA are generally well below the daily dosage of the hundreds of milligrams required to raise serum testosterone in eugonadal men, I generally do not focus on these supplements. Informing the patient that these supplements increase serum estradiol disproportionately more than serum testosterone and thereby increase the risk of gynecomastia is generally enough to persuade them to stop, though.

Clinical Case Vignettes

Case 1

A 32-year-old man requests evaluation for testosterone or clomiphene therapy. He brings in a testosterone result that he states is low according to the American Urology Association (AUA) guidelines. He has no relevant medical history and takes no medications. His BMI is 23.5 kg/m^2 and the rest of his physical examination findings are normal, including no gynecomastia and normal-sized testes.

Laboratory test result (sample drawn fasting at 9 AM while at baseline health):

> Serum total testosterone =
> 290 ng/dL (160-690 ng/dL) (SI: 10.1 nmol/L
> [5.56-24.0 nmol/L])

In addition to reassessment of serum total testosterone with a validated, harmonized assay, which of the following would you tell him?

A. His serum total testosterone is low because the normal range was not determined correctly

B. His serum total testosterone is low because of laboratory error

C. His initial serum testosterone is low, but this result must be confirmed with a validated assay

D. His serum total testosterone is normal, and it is likely higher than reported by this laboratory

E. His serum total testosterone is normal, and it is likely lower than reported by this laboratory

Answer: D) His serum total testosterone is normal, and it is likely higher than reported by this laboratory

A nonharmonized total testosterone assay with a reference range significantly lower than 264 to 916 ng/dL (9.2-31.8 nmol/L) yields spuriously low results. His serum total testosterone is normal, and it is most likely that his serum total testosterone value will be higher using a validated, harmonized assay with a normal range of 264 to 916 ng/dL (9.2-31.8 nmol/L) (Answer D). The testosterone assay used for this man's initial test has a normal range that is low. The lower and upper limits of normal are shifted down. If there is a linear relationship between this assay and a validated, harmonized assay, then the results could be corrected (upwards) based on the slope of the line. Answers A, B, and C are incorrect because his initial serum total testosterone value is normal in this assay. Answers A, B, and C are also wrong because the entire normal range of this assay is shifted downward. Harmonization, if possible, would yield consistently higher results for all measurements. The 2018 AUA guidelines state a threshold of 300 ng/dL (10.42 nmol/L), but that recommendation fails to account for the significant variability of testosterone assays.[15] Furthermore, the threshold is not connected to any clinical outcomes, whereas a CDC-validated assay was used in the Testosterone Trials and TRAVERSE trial.

Case 2

A 65-year-old man with a history of diabetes mellitus seeks a second opinion after going to The Ponce de Leon Clinic. He received a recommendation and prescription for testosterone gel; oral sermorelin (GHRH); and clomiphene, 100 mg daily. He reports no headaches or change in vision. Type 2 diabetes was diagnosed 5 years ago, and he also has hypertension and dyslipidemia. He takes metformin, lisinopril, and atorvastatin. He has no history of head trauma or head irradiation.

Physical examination findings are remarkable for a BMI of 36 kg/m^2 and acanthosis nigricans. He has no significant gynecomastia, and his testes are normal-sized.

He brings his laboratory results from that clinic (sample drawn fasting at 8 AM while at baseline health):

> Serum total testosterone = 245 ng/dL (264- 916 ng/dL) (SI: 8.51 nmol/L [9.2-31.8 nmol/L])
> Serum IGF-1, –1.5 SD for age
> Hemoglobin A$_{1c}$ = 8.2% (66 mmol/mol)
> Estimated glomerular filtration rate = >60 mL/min per 1.73 m^2

In addition to a repeated serum total testosterone measurement plus a calculated free testosterone assessment, which of the following should be recommended?

A. Order a GH-stimulation test with macimorelin

B. Delay GH-stimulation testing until after repeat testosterone results are available

C. No further evaluation for GH deficiency

D. Begin GH therapy

E. Begin taking fenugreek seed extracts and ashwagandha root

Answer: C) No further evaluation for GH deficiency

A low random (screening) serum IGF-1 value does not indicate GH deficiency. Further evaluation for GH deficiency is not indicated (Answer C) because this patient has low probability of GH deficiency due to hypothalamic or pituitary disease. His IGF-1 concentration is not lower than –2 SD for age, and he has type 2 diabetes that may cause a low serum IGF-1.[13] Answers A and B are wrong because there is no reason to do a GH-stimulation test. Although hypogonadism is associated with lower serum IGF-1 concentrations and testosterone therapy increases serum IGF-1 concentrations, there is no reason to do a GH-stimulation test for this patient at any time. Answer D is also wrong because GH therapy is not indicated to attenuate the effects of aging. Fenugreek seed extracts and ashwaganda root (Answer E) are commonly used, but they have not been proven to be safe or effective for increasing serum testosterone concentrations. Although fenugreek seed extracts and ashwagandha root seem to be safe, the studies are short-term.[16] In addition, the studies showing a small increase in serum testosterone are limited by bias, short duration, and metholodological flaws, including lack of reporting the timing of blood sampling for testosterone measurement.[16]

Key Learning Points

- Most men who request "hormone optimization" to improve energy, sense of well-being, and sexual function are eugonadal, but the clinic visit is an opportunity to improve overall health habits.

- For patients who have low probability of hypogonadism, a low pretreatment serum total testosterone concentration measured in an assay that has a normal range that differs significantly from 264 to 916 ng/dL (9.2-31.8 nmol/L) should be reassessed at least once with an accurate testosterone assay.

- In this clinical setting, the most useful testosterone assay is one that has been certified (validated and harmonized) by the US CDC or another agency that has established expertise in assay quality control and harmonization and has a normal range of 264 to 916 ng/dL (9.2-31.8 nmol/L).

- Screening for hypogonadism or GH deficiency is not recommended.

- Most men with a low screening serum IGF-1 value do not have GH deficiency.

- The management of inappropriately prescribed testosterone, hCG, aromatase inhibitor, clomiphene, and GH is anchored on explaining the potential detriments and risks of these drugs and the lack of proven benefits in patient outcomes. hCG, aromatase inhibitors, clomiphene, and GH can and should be stopped immediately.

References

1. Bandari J, Ayyash OM, Emery SL, Wessel CB, Davies BJ. Marketing and testosterone treatment in the USA: a systematic review. *Eur Urol Focus.* 2017;3(4-5):395-340. PMID: 29174614

2. Handelsman DJ. Androgen Physiology, Pharmacology, Use and Misuse. 2020 Oct 5. In: Feingold KR, Anawalt B, Blackman MR, Boyce A, Chrousos G, Corpas E, et al, eds. *Endotext* [Internet]. South Dartmouth (MA): MDText. com, Inc.; 2000-.

3. Dubin JM, Jesse E, Fantus RJ, et al. Guideline-discordant care among direct-to-consumer testosterone therapy platforms. *JAMA Intern Med.* 2022;182(12):1321-1323. PMID: 36369030

4. Le M, Flores D, May D, Gourley E, Nangia AK. Current practices of measuring and reference range reporting of free and total testosterone in the United States. *J Urol.* 2016;195(5):1556-1561. PMID: 25707506

5. Bhasin S, Brito JP, Cunningham GR, et al. Testosterone therapy in men with hypogonadism: an Endocrine Society clinical practice guideline. *J Clin Endocrinol Metab.* 2018;103(5):1715-1744. PMID: 29562364

6. Travison TG, Vesper HW, Orwoll E, et al. Harmonized reference ranges for circulating testosterone levels in men of four cohort studies in the United States and Europe. *J Clin Endocrinol Metab.* 2017;102(4):1161-1167. PMID: 28324103

7. U.S. Department of Health and Human Services, Centers for Disease Control and Prevention. Available at: https://www.cdc.gov/labstandards/hs_certified_participants.html

8. Grossmann M, Matsumoto AM. A perspective on middle-aged and older men with functional hypogonadism: focus on holistic management. *J Clin Endocrinol Metab.* 2017;102(3):1067-1075. PMID: 28359097

9. Esposito K, Giugliano F, Di Palo C, et al. Effect of lifestyle changes on erectile dysfunction in obese men: a randomized controlled trial. *JAMA.* 2004;291(24):2978-2984. PMID: 15213209

10. Maio G, Saraeb S, Marchiori A. Physical activity and PDE5 inhibitors in the treatment of erectile dysfunction: results of a randomized controlled study. *J Sex Med.* 2010;7(6):2201-2208. PMID: 20367777

11. Yuen KCJ, Biller BMK, Radovick S, et al. American Association of Clinical Endocrinologist and American College of Endocrinology guidelines for management of growth hormone deficiency in adults and patients transitioning from pediatric to adult care. *Endocr Pract.* 2019;25(11):1191-1232. PMID: 31760824

12. Pope HG Jr, Wood RI, Rogol A, Nyberg F, Bowers L, Bhasin S. Adverse health consequences of performance-enhancing drugs: an Endocrine Society scientific statement. *Endocr Rev.* 2014;35(3):341-375. PMID: 24423981

13. Anawalt BD. Diagnosis and management of anabolic androgenic steroid use. *J Clin Endocrinol Metab.* 2019;104(7):2490-2500. PMID: 30753550

14. Finkelstein JS, Lee H, Burnett-Bowie SA, et al. Gonadal steroids and body composition, strength, and sexual function in men. *N Engl J Med.* 2013;369(11):1011-1022. PMID: 24024838

15. Mulhall JP, Trost LW, Brannigan RE, et al. Evaluation and management of testosterone deficiency: AUA guideline. *J Urol.* 2018;200(2):423-432. PMID: 29601923

16. Smith SJ, Lopresti AL, Teo SYM, Fairchild TJ. Examining the effects of herbs on testosterone concentrations in men: a systematic review. *Adv Nutr.* 2021;12(3):744-765. PMID: 33150931

Management of Androgen Abuse, Recovery, and Dependence

David J. Handelsman, AO, MBBS, PhD. ANZAC Research Institute, University of Sydney, and Andrology Department, Concord Hospital, NSW 2139, Australia; Email: djh@anzac. edu.au

Educational Objectives

After reviewing this chapter, learners should be able to:

- Recognize and assess androgen abuse and misuse.

- Appreciate importance of perceptive history-taking as key to good management.

- Recognize androgen dependence on the pathophysiological basis of hypothalamic-pituitary-testicular (HPT) axis suppression and gradual recovery (with withdrawal [androgen deficiency]) symptoms) following cessation of exogenous androgen intake.

- Manage androgen dependence and recovery from HPT-axis suppression without contributing to further HPT suppression (which would delay ultimate recovery) while also avoiding new iatrogenic adverse effects.

Significance of the Clinical Problem

Exogenous androgens taken at, or higher than, testosterone replacement dosages, whether prescribed or illicit (nonprescribed), suppress the HPT axis.[1] Following prolonged use of injectable androgens, HPT-axis suppression is long-lasting, with recovery taking months to years since the last injection.[2-5] The major determinant of recovery is time since cessation; thus, resuming androgen intake in any form resets the recovery clock to zero.[2,3] During recovery from HPT-axis suppression, men often experience troublesome but not life-threatening withdrawal symptoms (androgen deficiency) of varying severity and tolerability. Knowing these symptoms are alleviated by resuming androgens, readily available to them from illicit sources, potentially creates a vicious cycle of androgen dependence, fostering resumption of androgen intake. Facilitating the slow, but potentially complete, natural recovery requires breaking this cycle of dependence. This requires supportive management based on establishing trust and respect for expert advice and encouraging persistence with non-use of androgens to allow for recovery. No therapeutics have been proven to accelerate the tempo or extent of natural recovery despite promotion of folkloric treatments (hCG, estrogen blockers), known as "post-cycle therapy" (PCT) by some androgen abusers and their suppliers. Rather, such ad hoc remedies simply prolong androgen abuse by other means, further suppressing the HPT axis and delaying ultimate recovery, as well as introducing risk of additional drug adverse effects. Recent evidence indicates that androgen dependence may also occur following prolonged testosterone administration at standard replacement doses in men without pathologic hypogonadism, most often used as an unapproved elixir of youth to restore energy and/or sexual function to older men experiencing comorbidities of aging.

This form of androgen (testosterone) misuse contributes to the massive increases over recent decades in off-label prescription of testosterone without any new approved indications.[6] Clinical management of androgen abuse and misuse is challenging, requiring the highest clinical skills in supportive management, and the field urgently needs more well-controlled clinical research aiming to identify predictors of HPT-axis recovery in addition to methods to accelerate such recovery.

Androgen abuse, defined as using androgens without valid medical indications or prescription for performance or image enhancement,[1] is a growing clinical and public health problem that is poorly recognized and understudied with few well-designed clinical studies providing sound guidance for management. Alarming cocktails comprising massive doses of multiple androgens simultaneously in pharmacologically irrational combinations are being taken with reckless disregard for harm to self, family, friends, and strangers, and contrary to medical advice, if sought. Androgen abuse lacks the fatal overdose risk of opioid abuse but fosters massive doses with mind-altering, mood-elevating properties. Optimal clinical diagnosis and management based on still-incomplete knowledge requires careful judgment of applied androgen pathophysiology combined with supportive care to promote nonuse during the slow, natural recovery, while avoiding iatrogenic harm from well-intended but misguided, unproven treatments.

Androgen misuse, defined as prescribing testosterone at standard replacement doses for off-label indications that are unproven, ineffective, or harmful,[1] has grown massively over the last 3 decades with a 100-fold increase in global testosterone prescription sales, without a single new approved indication.[6] Over a decade (2000-2011), dramatic increases in testosterone prescribing were evident in Canada (40-fold), in the United States (10-fold, but underestimated in selective private health insurance databases[7]), and in nearly all 41 countries studied.[6] Most testosterone prescription misuse envisages testosterone as an antiaging or sexual tonic, often "justified" by age-related low testosterone (misnamed "hypogonadism"),[8-10] a functional state triggered by concomitant systemic illness and/or comorbidities of aging. The US FDA does not accept "age-related hypogonadism" or its various neologisms (andropause, late-onset or functional hypogonadism) as a valid medical diagnosis or justification for testosterone treatment.[11] This state is best termed nongonadal illness (or sick eugonadal) syndrome,[1] analogous to the nonthyroidal illness (or sick euthyroid) syndrome,[12] which equally does not warrant thyroid hormone treatment.[13]

Androgen dependence is a pivotal issue for both androgen misuse and abuse. It arises in a cycle of withdrawal (androgen deficiency) symptoms after ceasing exogenous androgen intake during prolonged (months) slow recovery from underlying HPT-axis suppression. This creates temptation to resume androgen intake for symptom alleviation, which, together with ready access to illicit or prescription sources of androgens, pose a major challenge to supportive management of recovery.

Recent evidence extends the involvement of androgen dependence to the slow recovery of the HPT axis in men without pathological hypogonadism after prolonged testosterone administration.[2] Men with pathologic hypogonadism have permanent structural or genetic HPT pathology requiring lifelong testosterone replacement for irreversible conditions. In contrast, men without pathologic hypogonadism with mildly reduced blood testosterone still have some ongoing endogenous testosterone production. This remains capable of suppression by exogenous testosterone becoming evident during recovery after ineffective testosterone treatment inevitably ceases. Hence, prescribing testosterone for men without pathologic hypogonadism is likely to create superimposed iatrogenic androgen deficiency symptoms of variable duration and severity when ineffective testosterone treatment ceases, even if they were not originally androgen deficient. This mandates the highest level of caution to first, do no harm (*primum non nocere*).

Practice Gaps

- Failure to recognize androgen abuse.

  - Maintain an index of suspicion with awareness of clinical and laboratory clues.

  - Engage in thorough, perceptive medical history-taking for accurate diagnosis.

  - Be alert to unusually muscular men with obsessive fixation on increasing muscle bulk via weightlifting and/or bodybuilding and diet, gym, or exercise fads.

  - Consider androgen abuse in men presenting with azoospermic infertility after normal puberty and no known testicular pathology.

  - Consider androgen abuse in men seeking prescription of testosterone or adjunctive drugs (hCG, antiestrogens) and/or "health monitoring" for health reassurance while continuing androgen abuse.

- Failure to recognize androgen dependence driving resumption of androgen abuse/misuse due to withdrawal (androgen deficiency) symptoms during slow HPT-axis recovery.

  - Avoid prescribing drugs of abuse on demand by careful evaluation of therapeutic needs.

  - Avoid ineffective health monitoring alone as collusion in perpetuating androgen abuse.

- Failure to recognize the need to provide supportive and encouraging case management giving prognosis for recovery without aggravating underlying HPT-axis suppression and delaying recovery.

  - Provide supportive care comparable to that given in the setting of other addictions.

  - Provide realistic prognosis for recovery based on serial serum LH and FSH measurements.

  - Dismantle myths and unsound advice received driving androgen misuse/abuse.

  - Avoid prescribing androgens in any form, as this resets the recovery clock to zero because the principal determinant of recovery is the time since last androgen dose.

- Failure to appreciate the importance of measuring serum LH and FSH, together with serum testosterone and SHBG, to evaluate HPT-axis suppression and recovery.

Discussion

Diagnosis and Management of Androgen Abuse

Androgens consist of natural potent (testosterone, dihydrotestosterone) or proandrogenic (DHEA, androstenedione) steroids, as well as synthetic steroidal ("anabolic-androgenic steroids") and nonsteroidal ("SARM" [Selective Androgen Receptor Modulator]) androgens. All androgens are both anabolic and androgenic, including the newer nonsteroidal synthetic androgens. Hence the outdated, misleading terms "anabolic-androgenic steroid" and "anabolic steroid" represent oxymorons or redundancies that perpetuate a false distinction between steroidal and nonsteroidal androgens where there is no functional difference.

Androgen abuse typically involves use of massive nontherapeutic doses of multiple androgens in cycles of 2- to 3-month duration with intervening off-treatment periods claimed to reduce adverse effects and/or restore androgen sensitivity.[3,14] In internet and social media chatter, these patterns are referred to as "cycling," "pyramiding," "stacking," "blast and cruise," etc, but lack any rational pharmacologic basis other than rationale for massive dosing. Variations include an annual seasonal cycle to achieve "body-beautiful" image for summer or Mardi Gras, whereas professional bodybuilders may use high doses of androgens continuously for years.

Reasons for use include performance enhancement in sport (doping) or sculpting a hypermuscular or "cut" body image for psychological or occupational reasons. Women constitute only 1% to 2% of androgen abusers, mostly professional bodybuilders or weightlifters introduced to androgen abuse by boyfriends or coaches. The prevalence among females is highly overestimated in epidemiological surveys due to confusing the ambiguous term "steroids" with glucocorticoid use for asthma, allergies, or skin conditions.[15]

Any exogenous androgens at doses at or beyond testosterone replacement therapy suppress the HPT axis, exerting characteristic clinical and laboratory effects. The key to accurate diagnosis is a careful medical history involving an index of suspicion and awareness of diagnostic clues to androgen abuse or misuse. Clinically, androgen abuse should be suspected in highly muscular men who present with unexplained male-factor infertility without known testicular pathology and in those who seek prescriptions for testosterone or related treatments (hCG, antiestrogens), "health monitoring," or combinations of these. Typically, they are preoccupied with muscle building through frequent weightlifting and gym or intense exercise sessions and complain of being unable to further increase muscle size or strength or improve exercise performance or energy with familiar stereotypical symptoms (cyberchondria). The drug history is pivotal. Although a negative history of androgen intake is accurate in men who are not drug-seeking,[16] for drug-seeking men, the drug history is often deceptive and incomplete with denial or nondisclosure, at least initially until trust and respect for medical expertise and integrity are established. Admitted use of over-the-counter diet/nutritional supplements and preoccupation with bodybuilding are suspicious clues to possible nondisclosed illicit androgen intake, often seen as the "next step."

Typically, androgen abusers had a normal puberty and are in good general health (including fertility), but a history of delayed or incomplete puberty may be a clue to undiagnosed congenital hypogonadotropic hypogonadism. A history of isotretinoin prescription (for acne), plastic surgery (for gynecomastia) long after adolescence, or tendon ruptures are salient clues to androgen abuse. Thoughtful exploration of their perceptions and beliefs leading to androgen abuse is important to understand their motivations, which, together with a tailored education to rectify common misunderstandings of androgen pathophysiology, are crucial elements in sustaining no androgen intake to allow for gradual recovery. In addition to a muscular physique, physical examination may reveal relatively small (<15 mL), atrophic (soft consistency) testes, active truncal acne, gynecomastia (or periareolar surgical scars), and tendon ruptures. These findings in young men are telltale clinical clues within an otherwise unremarkable physical examination.

The most direct confirmation of androgen abuse is toxicologic urine drug screen; however, these tests are rarely available in commercial pathology labs. Sophisticated testing (including provision to exclude sample tampering) is restricted to World Anti-Doping Agency (WADA)–accredited antidoping labs and is barred from providing public diagnostic service to avoid athlete gaming. Laboratory tests to diagnose, and manage recovery from, androgen abuse require measuring serum LH, FSH, testosterone, and SHBG serially, together with semen analysis if fertility is an issue. Severe reduction in serum LH and FSH and reduced serum SHBG are characteristic, with undetectable serum LH and FSH virtually pathognomonic of androgen abuse in an otherwise healthy man. Serum testosterone may be elevated if testosterone is being used; otherwise, use of nontestosterone androgens leads to suppressed serum testosterone. However, cross-reactivity with structurally related steroids may distort interpretation of standard testosterone immunoassays, unlike more specific liquid chromatography–tandem mass spectrometry measurements. Among men who abuse androgens, sperm output is usually severely reduced, and they often have azoospermia or near-azoospermia. Hemoglobin may be elevated during androgen abuse, rarely to levels requiring phlebotomy, and is reversed quickly (2 to 3 months) after cessation of androgen intake. Other laboratory tests include lowered HDL cholesterol, thyroxine-binding globulin, and cortisol-binding globulin, which may provide confirmatory diagnostic clues but are not required for diagnosis or management.

Harms from androgen abuse have been well-described and include neuropsychiatric (mood and behavioral disturbance such as reckless, violent, or aggressive behavior), cardiovascular disorders (cardiomyopathy, accelerated atherosclerosis), neuroendocrine manifestations (HPT-axis suppression), erythrocytosis, and hepatotoxicity.[17-19]

During recovery after cessation of all androgen intake, serum LH and FSH provide convenient, cost-effective measures of recovery of the HPT axis. Serial monitoring is particularly useful to encourage persistence with nonuse by showing progress in recovery. Ultimately, all aspects of testicular function recover slowly over 6 to 18+ months, with endocrine function (LH, FSH, testosterone) recovering faster than exocrine function (spermatogenesis, testis volume).[3-5] Androgen-induced lowering of SHBG recovers only partially, possibly reflecting the same mechanism of sustained androgen-induced lowering of serum SHBG observed during male puberty. As a result, late in recovery, mild lowering of serum testosterone proportional to serum SHBG is often observed but does not signify androgen deficiency when serum LH and FSH concentrations (viewed as tissue androgen sensors) return to the reference range.[3] The slower recovery of sperm output and testis size suggests possible cumulative effects of androgen abuse leading to less complete recovery.

Management of androgen abuse requires thoughtful and respectful supportive medical management to encourage maintenance of nonuse (with reminders that any androgen use resets the recovery clock to zero), using evidence of rising serum LH and FSH towards normal as reflecting progressive recovery from HPT-axis suppression. Referral may be required to address additional comorbidities such as underlying

adverse psychological states (anxiety, depression, obsessive-compulsive disorder, body dysmorphia) and other drug abuse (alcohol, marijuana, cocaine, amphetamines, opioids).

Establishing trust and respect for medical expertise is important but challenging, as many androgen abusers regard doctors as unsympathetic, uninformed gatekeepers to prescriptions and health monitoring on demand, and they may be antagonistic to doctors who do not acquiesce to those demands. They are usually influenced by "broscience," an amalgam of internet/social media gossip and amateur pseudoscience, mostly without rational pharmacological basis other than an assumption that more must be better. Success in supporting recovery depends on conveying dispassionate professional judgment firmly rejecting androgen abuse and focusing on positive steps to recovery while avoiding moralistic personal criticism. This requires empathetic understanding of motives coupled with factual education on relevant androgen pathophysiology—displaying sympathy but avoid becoming the hunter captured by the prey (Stockholm syndrome).

Harm minimization for androgen abuse or misuse consists of simply stopping androgen intake to allow for gradual natural recovery. This contrasts with opioid addiction, which risks fatal overdose, blood-borne infection, and criminality, and is mitigated by maintaining opioid addiction under controlled circumstances. By contrast, although androgen withdrawal/recovery involve nonfatal symptoms, continuing androgen abuse by any means risks aggression and violence to others, including family, friends, and even strangers. The gym habitue's maxim "no gain without pain" is equally applicable to overcoming symptoms that signal to the hypothalamus to reinitiate HPT activity. HPT-axis recovery is slow but progressive, depending primarily on the time since last dose.[2,3] Thus, it is crucial to remind those in recovery that resuming androgen intake in any form resets the recovery clock to zero. Similarly, serial measurement of rising serum LH and FSH can provide encouraging prognosis for recovery of testicular function. There is no need for dose tapering of testosterone, as withdrawal does not entail serious adverse effects in contrast to glucocorticoid dependence, where avoiding dangerous adrenal insufficiency (Addisonian crisis) is needed. Both unnecessary tapering or ad hoc PCT continue suppression of the HPT axis and further delay recovery.

Post-Cycle Therapy

Attempts to rectify HPT-axis suppression are advocated in bodybuilding folklore using combinations of testis-stimulating drugs in PCT. These may be used between, or even during, androgen cycles to "restart" the testis. These regimens involve hCG and/or estrogen blockade but without consistency in drugs, dosage, or duration of treatment in regimens lacking fundamental pharmacological rationale. Despite absence of sound clinical trial data, ad hoc use of PCT regimens has been adopted by some doctors; however, anecdotal clinical reports of PCT-style treatments occur when natural recovery is still ongoing. Thus, uncontrolled reports claiming success are equally consistent with natural recovery, casting doubt on the efficacy of these treatments.

Use of hCG is based on the intuitive appeal that compares a functionally suppressed HPT axis to pathologic (congenital or acquired) gonadotropin deficiency. Although hCG treatment increases circulating testosterone while it continues, this prolongs underlying androgen-induced HPT-axis suppression, further delaying ultimate recovery. Furthermore, whereas hCG treatment is effective but slow in pathologic gonadotropin deficiency,[20,21] it usually requires additional FSH administration.[22] On the contrary, in recovery from androgen abuse, androgen-induced suppression of endogenous FSH is exacerbated by hCG administration, thereby counterproductively reducing sperm production further.

Another component of PCT is estrogen blockade using either estrogen-receptor antagonists (clomiphene, tamoxifen, raloxifene, and congeners) that competitively block estrogen receptor action or aromatase inhibitors (anastrozole, letrozole, and congeners) that inhibit estradiol synthesis. Such estrogen blockade inhibits negative androgenic hypothalamic feedback by disrupting testosterone's effects on the brain, which are largely mediated by testosterone's aromatization to estradiol to then act on estrogen receptors. This causes a reflexive rise in LH and FSH and consequently testosterone secretion (only as long as it continues). However, effective estrogen blockade also risks impairing other estrogen-dependent functions, potentially impairing male sexual function, as well as causing imperceptible loss of bone density and structure but risking future fractures.[23] Furthermore, inhibition of male sexual function by estrogen deficiency is overcome by high-dose androgens,[24] providing a perverse incentive to resuming androgen abuse.

Diagnosis and Management of Androgen (Testosterone) Misuse

The most important aspect of managing androgen (testosterone) misuse is prevention. That means not initiating testosterone treatment for men without pathologic hypogonadism, both in leading by example and advocacy to referring doctors. The diagnosis of testosterone misuse depends primarily on identifying the off-label indication for testosterone prescription. Ensuring pathologic hypogonadism has been excluded is important.

A common presentation of testosterone misuse when men are evaluated by Andrology or Endocrinology consultants is a man who was started on testosterone treatment by his own nonspecialist doctor, for obscure or off-label symptomatic complaints. These concerns most often consist of symptoms of low energy and/or sexual dysfunction, reduced gym or exercise performance, or a mixture of these things with a clinical background of obesity (with or without type 2 diabetes) and/or other systemic illnesses. There is usually minimal or no documentation of a cause for low testosterone, nor concomitant measurement of serum LH, FSH, and SHBG required to interpret the testosterone measurement. In these scenarios, after starting testosterone treatment, men might report short-term symptomatic improvement followed by the feeling that, "…the testosterone is no longer working"—a heart-sinking revelation of a placebo reaction to ineffective testosterone treatment. Thoughtful, forward-looking, positive management is required to avoid recriminations about prior mismanagement and for developing an effective pathway for recovery. This includes rectifying undiagnosed or inadequately treated underlying medical conditions associated with the nonspecific symptoms and/or lower testosterone levels. This requires identifying common causes of a nongonadal illness syndrome (obesity ± diabetes, obstructive sleep apnea, depression, liver, kidney or cardiac failure, cardiovascular disease), which should be ameliorated wherever possible, including by implementing appropriate diet/lifestyle/drug/surgery changes for obesity, performing sleep studies, and administering psychological assessment for depression. In addition, appropriate education on relevant androgen pathophysiology, also addressing obsessive fixation on specific testosterone levels, is usually wise.

Full reevaluation of underlying testicular endocrine function with a washout period is not always required if there is evidence of prior normal functioning of the HPT axis. If needed, testosterone intake must cease for an adequate washout period based on the last testosterone product used (4 weeks for transdermal or oral products; 8 weeks for short-acting injectables; 24 weeks for long-acting injectables) before reevaluation of serum testosterone, LH, FSH, and SHBG on 2 or more occasions. The most frequent findings underlying testosterone misuse is the pseudohypogonadism of obesity, with or without type 2 diabetes. In this setting the reduced serum SHBG of obesity is accompanied by proportionate lowering of testosterone but also normal serum LH and FSH as useful tissue androgen sensors.

Clinical Case Vignettes
Case 1

A 35-year-old man is referred by his partner's gynecologist who is investigating infertility due to confirmed azoospermia. He fathered an easily conceived child, now 11 years old, during a 13-year marriage that dissolved 5 years ago. He is in a relationship with a 40-year-old woman, who has 2 biological children aged 17 and 14 years. She had her medicated intrauterine device removed 2.5 years ago and has regular menses without conception. Her serum antimullerian hormone concentration is 0.6 ng/mL (SI: 4.3 pmol/L) (age-specific reference range, 0.12-3.40 ng/mL [SI: 0.9-24.3 pmol/L]). She has an otherwise unremarkable medical history.

The patient completed puberty at similar age to peers and has no significant medical history. He was never a regular cigarette smoker, but he now vapes regularly and is a moderate, social drinker without binging. He has had no headaches or visual disturbance. He has a normal serum prolactin concentration.

He began bodybuilding at age 14 years and started using androgens sourced through his gym as "the next step" over the previous 8 years to make him "…feel and look good." Over the first 3 to 4 years, he used daily injections of testosterone and other injectable androgens (nandrolone) with numerous diet supplements (eg, turkesterone, branched chain amino acids, protein powders, vitamin D, "natural testosterone boosters"). Owing to the COVID-19 pandemic making supplies of illicit androgens unreliable, he stopped injectable androgens abruptly ("cold turkey") but switched intermittently to using various combinations of PCT comprising hCG, clomiphene, and letrozole, maintaining androgen abuse by other means. When first seen, he claimed to have stopped all androgens for several years but complained of reduced sexual function (treated with intermittent use of sildenafil), easy fatigue, and reduced physical performance during weightlifting at regular gym sessions several times per week.

On physical examination, he is highly muscular, heavily tattooed over his trunk and arms, and has a gruff, belligerent manner. He has no acne, gynecomastia, or striae, and testicular volume is 12.5 mL bilaterally (orchidometry) with an atrophic (soft) consistency. His vital signs and visual fields are normal. The rest of his examination findings are unremarkable.

Which of the following is the next most important test(s) to verify a diagnosis of androgen abuse?

A. Hemoglobin and serum SHBG measurement

B. Karyotype and bone density assessment

C. Pituitary MRI

D. Serum LH and FSH measurement

E. Serum lipid panel and liver function tests

F. Serum testosterone measurement

G. Urine drug screen

Answer: D) Serum LH and FSH measurement

In this clinical context, serum LH is a convenient, sensitive, and specific marker of androgen-induced HPT-axis suppression and is also very useful for evaluating progress of recovery. Complete LH and FSH suppression in an otherwise healthy man with prior fertility is virtually pathognomonic of androgen abuse. As LH is pulsatile, the more stable serum FSH can help confirm the diagnosis, unless there is also significant testicular damage (which would be unrelated to androgen abuse) causing a high serum FSH value in its own right. Thus, measuring LH and FSH (Answer D) is the best test to verify this patient's diagnosis.

A urine drug screen (Answer G) is incorrect because sophisticated urine androgen profiling methods used by World Anti-Doping Agency–accredited antidoping labs to identify androgen doping are not available through regular clinical pathology labs whose routine urine drug screens do not usually include abused androgens.

This patient was injecting testosterone, so his serum testosterone concentration (Answer F) could be high or low depending on which androgen and time since the last injection, making it hard to interpret. The measurement also depends on the specificity of the testosterone immunoassay.

Androgen abuse may increase hemoglobin and reduce serum SHBG (Answer A), and although those findings support the diagnosis (and remain useful serially in recovery), they are not specific enough to be diagnostic.

Karyotype and bone density assessment (Answer B) are incorrect because his adult testicular volume and prior fertility exclude Klinefelter syndrome, and androgen abuse has minimal effect on bone density.

He has no symptoms suggestive of a pituitary tumor. He has no visual field defects and a normal serum prolactin concentration. Thus, pituitary MRI (Answer C) is incorrect.

Although androgens may affect serum lipids, those effects are not diagnostic. While hepatotoxicity of oral alkylated androgens may be detected, it is also not diagnostic of androgen abuse per se. Thus, a lipid panel and liver function tests (Answer E) are incorrect.

Case 1 (continued)

Laboratory test results from his first visit:

> Hemoglobin = 16.0 g/dL (13.0-18.0 g/dL)
>   (SI: 160 g/L [130-180 g/L])
> Serum testosterone = 120 ng/dL (286-858 ng/dL)
>   (SI: 4.2 nmol/L [10.0-30.0 nmol/L])
> Serum LH = <0.1 mIU/mL (1.7-8.6 mIU/mL)
>   (SI: <0.1 IU/L [1.7-8.6 IU/L])
> Serum FSH = <0.1 mIU/mL (1.5-12.4 mIU/mL)
>   (SI: <0.1 IU/L [1.5-12.4 IU/L])
> Serum SHBG = 1.18 µg/mL (1.69-8.99 µg/mL)
>   (SI: 10.5 nmol/L [15.0-80.0 nmol/L])
> Serum TSH = 0.5 mIU/L (0.4-3.5 mIU/L)
> Serum prolactin = 18 ng/mL (5-25 ng/mL)
>   (SI: 0.78 nmol/L [0.22-1.09 nmol/L])

At a second visit 2 months later, based on the original completely suppressed serum LH and FSH values, he admits to using "some" androgens to ward off withdrawal symptoms before that visit but states he has not used any since. Today, the following test results show impressive recovery of serum LH and FSH together with proportionate increases in serum SHBG and testosterone.

> Hemoglobin = 16.5 g/dL (SI: 165 g/L)
> Serum testosterone = 229 ng/dL (SI: 7.9 nmol/L)
> Serum LH = 4.3 mIU/mL (SI: 4.3 IU/L)
> Serum FSH = 6.8 mIU/mL (SI: 6.8 IU/L)
> Serum SHBG = 2.90 µg/mL (SI: 25.8 nmol/L)
> Semen analysis = <0.3 million/ejaculate; a few motile sperm (>39 million sperm/ejaculate)

Serum LH is at a level predictive of good hormonal recovery. He is still mildly symptomatic, but supportive discussions encourage him to continue nonuse by reminding him that (1) prognosis for full hormonal recovery is good but slow (up to 18 months), and using any androgens (including PCT) resets the recovery clock back to zero and (2) sperm recovery is slower than hormonal recovery. He agrees to continue to refrain from androgen use and to continue further follow-up.

Four months after the first visit, he states he has not used any androgens; a third set of blood tests confirms similar recovery in serum LH, FSH, SHBG, and testosterone, with a sperm output of 4.5 million (semen volume, 2.5 mL; sperm concentration, 1.5 million sperm/mL). Concerned about his partner's age, he now seeks further advice on fertility options.

Which of the following is the best therapeutic option now?

A. Clomiphene or tamoxifen treatment

B. Clomiphene treatment for his wife

C. hCG treatment

D. Intracytoplasmic sperm injection/in vitro fertilization with ejaculated sperm

E. In vitro fertilization with donor sperm

F. Supportive management, no specific treatment

Answer: D) Intracytoplasmic sperm injection/ in vitro fertilization with ejaculated sperm

In this setting, in vitro fertilization would be the fastest and most reliable way to secure a pregnancy, but it will be limited by the partner's age-related subfertility and cost. As he has some spermatogenesis, although still subnormal, sufficient ejaculated sperm should be available for in vitro fertilization, likely coupled with intracytoplasmic sperm injection (Answer D).

Supportive management (Answer F) would be reasonable if his fertile partner were younger, as his sperm recovery is likely to continue improving, but his partner's age-related fertility is low and declining.

Given the natural history of recovery of HPT axis, including testosterone and sperm production taking up to 18 months, there is no sound evidence that hCG administration (Answer C) is more effective than awaiting natural recovery. Furthermore, hCG treatment suppresses FSH and, in men with any sperm output (like this man), it may reduce sperm production through suppressing serum FSH as well as prolonging HPT-axis suppression and delaying ultimate recovery.

Inhibiting estrogen action either by antiestrogens (clomiphene, tamoxifen) (Answer A) or aromatase inhibitors (letrozole, anastrozole) has no proven effect superior to awaiting natural recovery and may have potential adverse effects on sexual function and bone density.

Clomiphene is not likely to be useful for his wife (Answer B) who has proven fertility (albeit now of advanced gynecological age) and continued regular menstrual periods. Also, the overwhelming likelihood is that the patient's severe oligospermia is the couple's major fertility limitation.

In vitro fertilization with donor sperm (Answer E) is incorrect, as it is not necessary to deny natural paternity when it is achievable either via advanced reproductive technologies (in vitro fertilization with intracytoplasmic sperm injection) or by waiting for sufficient spermatogenesis recovery.

Case 2

A 34-year-old man is referred for management of infertility with azoospermia due to androgen abuse. He is in general good health without financial, domestic, or other stressors. His medical history includes periods of depression treated with sertraline and minor sports injuries. He has had no major injuries, operations, or other forms of reproductive pathology. He is a nonsmoker apart from occasional marijuana use (<1 monthly) and he consumes moderate daily alcohol with weekly binges and uses cocaine rarely.

He was previously married for 10 years with 3 easily conceived children (youngest 7 years old) before divorce 5 years ago. He is in a new 2-year relationship with a 29-year-old woman in good general health. She had no children and stopped oral contraception seeking to become pregnant 6 months previously, but she has not resumed periods and is being evaluated for polycystic ovary syndrome.

The patient's sexual function is adequate for fertility. He does not attend a gym or engage in weightlifting. Testosterone was prescribed by his family doctor 8 years ago for "low T," although his serum testosterone concentration was never low. He used transdermal testosterone gel, 50 mg daily, for 12 months before switching for unclear reasons to injectable testosterone undecanoate, 1000 mg every 12 weeks. The dosing interval was progressively shortened to every 8 weeks, with last injection 2 months prior to his first consultation. He reports that this testosterone treatment was "life-changing" in that he felt calmer and more decisive. He had remained on this treatment for 8 years till first seen but denied using any other prescription or illicit androgens.

On physical examination, he appears healthy, tall, well-muscled, and clinically eugonadal, with no acne, gynecomastia, or hair-pattern changes. Testes are 15 mL bilaterally with firm consistency. He states they are smaller than before he started using androgens.

Laboratory test results:

> Hemoglobin = 15.2 g/dL (13.0-18.0 g/dL)
> (SI: 152 g/L [130-180 g/L])
> Serum testosterone = 369 ng/dL (286-858 ng/dL)
> (SI: 12.9 nmol/L [10.0-30.0 nmol/L])
> Serum LH = <0.1 mIU/mL (1.7-8.6 mIU/mL)
> (SI: <0.1 IU/L [1.7-8.6 IU/L])
> Serum FSH = <0.1 mIU/mL (1.5-12.4 mIU/mL)
> (SI: <0.1 IU/L [1.5-12.4 IU/L])
> Serum SHBG = 3.19 μg/mL (1.69-8.99 μg/mL)
> (SI: 28.4 nmol/L [15.0-80.0 nmol/L])
> Serum ALT = 67 U/L (10-50 U/L) (SI: 1.12 μkat/L
> [0.17-0.84 μkat/L])
> Serum AST = 41 U/L (10-35 U/L) (SI: 0.68 μkat/L
> [0.17-0.58 μkat/L])
> Serum alkaline phosphatase = 116 U/L (30-110 U/L)
> (SI: 1.94 μkat/L [0.50-1.84 μkat/L])

In addition to abstinence from exogenous testosterone, what is the best therapeutic option at this time?

A. Clomiphene or tamoxifen treatment

B. Clomiphene treatment for his wife

C. hCG treatment

D. In vitro fertilization with donor sperm

E. Supportive management, no specific treatment

F. Testicular sperm extraction/intracytoplasmic sperm injection/in vitro fertilization with ejaculated sperm

Answer: E) Supportive management, no specific treatment

The natural history of recovery from androgen use is slow but usually complete if no androgen intake is resumed. Thus, the best recommendation is supportive management and no specific treatment. This patient was also advised to reduce alcohol intake.

Given the natural history of HPT-axis recovery, including testosterone and sperm production taking up to 18 months, there is no sound evidence that hCG administration (Answer C) is more effective than awaiting natural recovery. Furthermore, hCG treatment suppresses FSH and, in men with any sperm output (like this man), it may reduce sperm production through suppressing serum FSH as well as prolonging HPT-axis suppression and delaying ultimate recovery.

Inhibiting estrogen action either by antiestrogens (clomiphene, tamoxifen) (Answer A) or aromatase inhibitors (letrozole, anastrozole) has no proven effect superior to awaiting natural recovery and may have potential adverse effects on sexual function and bone density.

Testicular sperm extraction/intracytoplasmic sperm injection/in vitro fertilization with ejaculated sperm (Answer F) is invasive and costly and may not be necessary.

Clomiphene treatment for his wife (Answer B) would not be effective, as there is no sperm output and, once there is, ovulation induction may not be necessary.

In vitro fertilization with donor sperm (Answer D) is incorrect, as it is not necessary to deny natural paternity when it is achievable either via advanced reproductive technologies (in vitro fertilization with intracytoplasmic sperm injection) or by waiting for sufficient spermatogenesis recovery.

Follow-up laboratory results are shown:

Pregnancy occurred (without in vitro fertilization, ovulation induction, or resumption of testosterone), with estimated conception occurring at 21 months of follow-up.

Case 3

A 56-year-old man is referred for evaluation and management of symptoms of low libido, erectile dysfunction, and low energy (possibly androgen deficiency related to past androgen abuse). About 1 year ago, his local physician declined to continue prior testosterone prescriptions on demand after a diagnosis of prostate cancer.

He had normal puberty and has been married 3 times, with an unplanned pregnancy in the brief first marriage and no children by choice in his 19-year second marriage, or in his 8-year third marriage. He has never smoked cigarettes regularly, drinks alcohol socially, maintains a good diet, takes no medications, and trains regularly in the gym (≥4 times/week). He has no headaches or visual disturbance. He has mild diet-managed type 2 diabetes, a history of depression successfully treated 2 years ago with an antidepressant, and a history of multiple sports-related injuries. He developed screen-detected, biopsy-proven, organ-confined prostate cancer (Gleeson 6, 8% cells), which, after 12 months of monitoring with PSA measurement, was

Date	Serum testosterone	Serum LH	Serum FSH	Serum SHBG	Semen analysis
First visit	369 ng/dL (SI: 12.9 nmol/L)	<0.1 mIU/mL (SI: <0.1 IU/L)	<0.1 mIU/mL (SI: <0.1 IU/L)	3.19 µg/mL (SI: 28.4 nmol/L)	0
+ 1 month	200 ng/dL (SI: 7.0 nmol/L)	<0.1 mIU/mL (SI: <0.1 IU/L)	<0.1 mIU/mL (SI: <0.1 IU/L)	2.39 µg/mL (SI: 21.3 nmol/L)	0
+ 3 months	251 ng/dL (SI: 8.8 nmol/L)	1.4 mIU/mL (SI: 1.4 IU/L)	3.2 mIU/mL (SI: 3.2 IU/L)	3.37 µg/mL (SI: 30.0 nmol/L)	0.2 million/ejac
+ 7 months	180 ng/dL (SI: 6.3 nmol/L)	4.3 mIU/mL (SI: 4.3 IU/L)	7.9 mIU/mL (SI: 7.9 IU/L)	3.00 µg/mL (SI: 26.7 nmol/L)	0.2 million/ejac
+ 9 months	223 ng/dL (SI: 7.8 nmol/L)	3.2 mIU/mL (SI: 3.2 IU/L)	7.7 mIU/mL (SI: 7.7 IU/L)	2.70 µg/mL (SI: 24.0 nmol/L)	25.3 million/ejac
+ 18 months	277 ng/dL (SI: 9.7 nmol/L)	3.6 mIU/mL (SI: 3.6 IU/L)	6.4 mIU/mL (SI: 6.4 IU/L)	2.27 µg/mL (SI: 20.2 nmol/L)	152 million/ejac

Reference ranges: serum testosterone, 286-858 ng/dL (SI: 10-30 nmol/L); serum LH, 1.7-8.6 mIU/mL (SI: 1.7-8.6 IU/L); serum FSH, 1.5-12.4 mIU/mL (SI: 1.5-12.4 IU/L); SHBG, 1.69-8.99 µg/mL (SI: 15.0–80.0 nmol/L); semen analysis, >39 million/ejac.

treated by definitive ionizing irradiation, completed 3 months prior to his first visit.

He was a competitive bodybuilder and boxer for 8 years in Zimbabwe until age 26 years. In the 1980s and 1990s, he took multiple intermittent cycles of high-dosage injectables (testosterone, nandrolone), oral androgens (metandienone), and diet supplements. After retiring as a bodybuilder, he used injectable testosterone intermittently ever since, obtained on prescription from many doctors ostensibly to maintain his sexual function. He states that phosphodiesterase 5 inhibitors cause headaches. His testosterone intake ceased abruptly between for 5 years in his early 30s when he was living in a country where testosterone was not available to him. He noticed consistent loss of sexual function but remained otherwise well. In 2005, he migrated to Australia where he was prescribed testosterone by an antiaging doctor (later deregistered for supplying drugs of abuse) for about 14 years, until his diagnosis of prostate cancer.

On physical examination, he is tall and muscular with a BMI of 31.2 kg/m². His blood pressure is 118/76 mm Hg. He has no acne or gynecomastia, and testes are 10 mL bilaterally (orchidometry) with atrophic (soft) consistency. He has normal leg reflexes and arterial pulses and normal visual fields. The rest of his physical examination findings are unremarkable.

Laboratory test results:

> Hemoglobin = 14.1 g/dL (13.0-18.0 g/dL)
>   (SI: 141 g/L [130-180 g/L])
> Serum testosterone = 63 ng/dL (286-858 ng/dL)
>   (SI: 2.2 nmol/L [10.0-30.0 nmol/L])
> Serum LH = 6.0 mIU/mL (1.7-8.6 mIU/mL)
>   (SI: 6.0 IU/L [1.7-8.6 IU/L])
> Serum FSH = 8.3 mIU/mL (1.5-12.4 mIU/mL)
>   (SI: 8.3 IU/L [1.5-12.4 IU/L])
> Serum SHBG = 2.92 µg/mL (1.69-8.99 µg/mL)
>   (SI: 26.0 nmol/L [15.0-80.0 nmol/L])
> Serum PSA = 1.66 ng/mL (0.3-3.5 ng/mL)
>   (SI: 1.66 µg/L [0.3-3.5 µg/L])
> Serum prolactin = 15 ng/mL (5-25 ng/mL)
>   (SI: 0.65 nmol/L [0.22-1.09 nmol/L])

Which additional diagnostic test is required to complete the evaluation?

A. Bone density assessment

B. Iron studies (serum ferritin and transferrin saturation)

C. Karyotype analysis

D. Olfactory function test

E. Pituitary MRI

Answer: A) Bone density assessment

Bone density is a valuable, convenient integrated measure of androgen exposure. This patient's DXA showed normal Z-scores of 0.8 and 0.9 (spine and hip), indicating adequate long-term androgen exposure.

Karyotype analysis (Answer C) is incorrect because his testicular size and prior fertility exclude Klinefelter syndrome.

He has no clinical signs or symptoms of a pituitary tumor, a normal serum prolactin concentration, and nonsuppressed LH and FSH concentrations. Thus, pituitary MRI (Answer E) is incorrect.

He completed normal puberty, developed adult-sized testes, and is fertile, thus excluding Kallmann syndrome (anosmic congenital hypogonadotropic hypogonadism). An olfactory function test (Answer D) is not necessary.

His background and clinical features do not suggest hemochromatosis, so iron studies (Answer B) are not indicated.

Case 3 (continued)

Which of the following is the main cause of his currently low serum testosterone concentration?

A. HPT-axis suppression from androgen abuse

B. Testicular scatter irradiation

C. Klinefelter syndrome

D. Kallmann syndrome

Answer: B) Testicular scatter irradiation

Follow-up laboratory test results are shown:

Analyte	First visit	+6 months	+12 months	+30 months
Hemoglobin	14.1 g/dL (SI: 141 g/L)	...	...	14.1 g/dL (SI: 141 g/L)
Serum testosterone	63 ng/dL (SI: nmol/L)	51 ng/dL (SI: nmol/L)	74 ng/dL (SI: nmol/L)	163 ng/dL (SI: nmol/L)
Serum LH	6.0 mIU/mL (SI: 6.0 IU/L)	7.3 mIU/mL (SI: 7.3 IU/L)	4.9 mIU/mL (SI: 4.9 IU/L)	1.6 mIU/mL (SI: 1.6 IU/L)
Serum FSH	8.3 mIU/mL (SI: 8.3 IU/L)	10.9 mIU/mL (SI: 10.9 IU/L)	10.3 mIU/mL (SI: 10.3 IU/L)	3.2 mIU/mL (SI: 3.2 IU/L)
Serum SHBG	2.92 µg/mL (SI: 26.0 nmol/L)	3.37 µg/mL (SI: 30.0 nmol/L)	2.51 µg/mL (SI: 22.3 nmol/L)	2.39 µg/mL (SI: 21.3 nmol/L)
Serum PSA	1.66 ng/mL (SI: 1.66 µg/L)	3.67 ng/mL (SI: 3.67 µg/L)	2.57 ng/mL (SI: 2.57 µg/L)	0.93 ng/mL (SI: 0.93 µg/L)

Recent pelvic irradiation (Answer B) has sufficient scatter to impair testicular function.

He has nonsuppressed serum LH and FSH, so HPT-axis suppression from androgen abuse (Answer A) is incorrect.

He completed normal puberty, has adult-sized (but atrophic) testes, and has proven fertility, so Klinefelter syndrome (Answer C) and Kallmann syndrome (Answer D) are unlikely diagnoses.

Despite primary hypogonadism and his wish for testosterone for symptom alleviation, it was agreed to wait until his serum PSA concentration plateaued following prostate irradiation. Low-dosage testosterone gel (50 mg daily) was started 18 months after first consultation. The patient thought this made a "big difference" with increased energy for exercise and improved concentration despite persistently low serum testosterone. However, sexual function remained poor despite a brief testosterone dosage increase to 100 mg daily.

Key Learning Points

- A careful medical history with an index of suspicion for diagnostic clinical and laboratory clues is pivotal in recognizing and managing androgen abuse and misuse.

- Be aware of androgen dependence during prolonged HPT-axis recovery.

- Always measure serum LH and FSH together with serum testosterone and SHBG to evaluate androgen abuse, misuse, and deficiency.

- Undetectable serum LH and FSH in an otherwise healthy postpubertal man is virtually pathognomonic of androgen abuse.

- Serial measurement of serum LH and FSH is a simple, valuable, and cost-effective guide to the stages of recovery. Rising levels are indicative of recovery.

- Recovery of testicular function is gradual over 6 to 18 months with endocrine function (steroidogenesis) restored faster than exocrine function (spermatogenesis), but residual and possibly cumulative effects of androgen abuse on testis volume and serum SHBG are characteristic.

References

1. Handelsman DJ. Androgen misuse and abuse. *Endocr Rev.* 2021;42(4):457-501. PMID: 33484556

2. Handelsman DJ, Desai R, Conway AJ, et al. Recovery of male reproductive endocrine function after ceasing prolonged testosterone undecanoate injections. *Eur J Endocrinol.* 2022;186(3):307-318. PMID: 35000898

3. Shankara-Narayana N, Yu C, Savkovic S, et al. Rate and Extent of Recovery from Reproductive and Cardiac Dysfunction Due to Androgen Abuse in Men. *J Clin Endocrinol Metab.* 2020;105(6):1827-1839. PMID: 32030409

4. Rasmussen JJ, Selmer C, Ostergren PB, et al. Former abusers of anabolic androgenic steroids exhibit decreased testosterone levels and hypogonadal symptoms years after cessation: a case-control study. *PLoS One.* 2016;11(8):e0161208. PMID: 27532478

5. Kanayama G, Hudson JI, DeLuca J, et al. Prolonged hypogonadism in males following withdrawal from anabolic-androgenic steroids: an under-recognized problem. *Addiction.* 2015;110(5):823-831. PMID: 25598171

6. Handelsman DJ. Global trends in testosterone prescribing, 2000-2011: expanding the spectrum of prescription drug misuse. *Med J Aust.* 2013;199(8):548-551. PMID: 24138381

7. Baillargeon J, Kuo Y-F, Westra JR, Urban RJ, Goodwin JS. Testosterone prescribing in the United States, 2002-2016. *JAMA.* 2018;320(2):200-202. PMID: 29998328

8. Jasuja GK, Bhasin S, Rose AJ, et al. Provider and site-level determinants of testosterone prescribing in the Veterans Healthcare System. *J Clin Endocrinol Metab.* 2017;102(9):3226-3233. PMID: 28911150

9. Jasuja GK, Bhasin S, Reisman JI, et al. Who gets testosterone? Patient characteristics associated with testosterone prescribing in the Veteran Affairs System: a Cross-Sectional Study. *J Gen Intern Med* 2017;32(3):304-311. PMID: 27995426

10. Handelsman DJ. Pharmacoepidemiology of testosterone: curbing off-label prescribing. *Pharmacoepidemiol Drug Saf.* 2017;26(10):1248-1255. PMID: 28833745

11. Nguyen CP, Hirsch MS, Moeny D, Kaul S, Mohamoud M, Joffe HV. Testosterone and "age-related hypogonadism"--FDA Concerns. *N Engl J Med.* 2015;373(8):689-691. PMID: 26287846

12. Pappa TA, Vagenakis AG, Alevizaki M. The nonthyroidal illness syndrome in the non-critically ill patient. *Eur J Clin Invest.* 2011;41(2):212-220. PMID: 20964678

13. Lee S, Farwell AP. Euthyroid sick syndrome. *Compr Physiol.* 2016;6(2):1071-1080. PMID: 27065175

14. Smit DL, Buijs MM, de Hon O, den Heijer M, de Ronde W. Disruption and recovery of testicular function during and after androgen abuse: the HAARLEM study. *Hum Reprod.* 2021;36(4):880-890. PMID: 33550376

15. Kanayama G, Boynes M, Hudson JI, Field AE, Pope HG Jr. Anabolic steroid abuse among teenage girls: an illusory problem? *Drug Alcohol Depend.* 2007;88(2-3):156-162. PMID: 17127018

16. Shankara-Narayana N, Brooker L, Goebel C, Speers N, Handelsman DJ. Reliability of drug history and hormonal profiling for verification of androgen abuse. figshare. Dataset2022. https://doi.org/10.6084/m9.figshare.18130667.v1. Accessed March 2022.

17. Nieschlag E, Vorona E. Doping with anabolic androgenic steroids (AAS): adverse effects on non-reproductive organs and functions. *Rev Endocr Metab Disord.* 2015;16(3):199-211. PMID: 26373946

18. Nieschlag E, Vorona E. Mechanisms in endocrinology: medical consequences of doping with anabolic androgenic steroids: effects on reproductive functions. *Eur J Endocrinol.* 2015;173(2):R47-R58. PMID: 25805894

19. Pope HG Jr, Wood RI, Rogol A, Nyberg F, Bowers L, Bhasin S. Adverse health consequences of performance-enhancing drugs: an Endocrine Society scientific statement. *Endocr Rev.* 2014;35(3):341-375. PMID: 24423981

20. Liu PY, Baker HWG, Jayadev V, Zacharin M, Conway AJ, Handelsman DJ. Induction of spermatogenesis and fertility during gonadotropin treatment of gonadotropin-deficient infertile men: predictors of fertility outcome. *J Clin Endocrinol Metab.* 2009;94(3):801-808. PMID: 19066302

21. Rastrelli G, Corona G, Mannucci E, Maggi M. Factors affecting spermatogenesis upon gonadotropin-replacement therapy: a meta-analytic study. *Andrology.* 2014;2(6):794-808. PMID: 25271205

22. Matsumoto AM, Karpas AE, Bremner WJ. Chronic human chorionic-gonadotropin administration in normal men: evidence that follicle-stimulating hormone is necessary for the maintenance of quantitatively normal spermatogenesis in man. *J Clin Endocr Metab.* 1986;62(6):1184-1192. PMID: 3084535

23. Finkelstein JS, Lee H, Burnett-Bowie SA, et al. Gonadal steroids and body composition, strength, and sexual function in men. *N Engl J Med.* 2013;369(11):1011-1022. PMID: 24024838

24. Sartorius GA, Ly LP, Handelsman DJ. Male sexual function can be maintained without aromatization: randomized placebo-controlled trial of dihydrotestosterone (DHT) in healthy, older men for 24 months. *J Sex Med.* 2014;11(10):2562-2570. PMID: 24751323

www.ingramcontent.com/pod-product-compliance
Lightning Source LLC
Chambersburg PA
CBHW080410190526
45161CB00003B/190